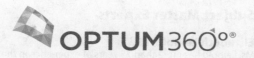

EXPERT

HCPCS Level II

A resourceful compilation of HCPCS codes
Supports HIPAA compliance

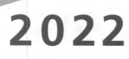

2022   optum360coding.com

Publisher's Notice

The Optum360 *2022 HCPCS Level II* is designed to be an accurate and authoritative source of information about this government coding system. Every effort has been made to verify the accuracy of the listings, and all information is believed reliable at the time of publication. Absolute accuracy cannot be guaranteed, however. This publication is made available with the understanding that the publisher is not engaged in rendering legal or other services that require a professional license.

Our Commitment to Accuracy

Optum360 is committed to producing accurate and reliable materials. To report corrections, please email accuracy@optum.com. You can also reach customer service by calling 1.800.464.3649, option 1.

To view Optum360 updates/correction notices, please visit http://www.optum360coding.com/ProductUpdates/

Acknowledgments

Gregory A. Kemp, MA, *Product Manager*

Stacy Perry, *Manager, Desktop Publishing*

Elizabeth Leibold, RHIT, *Subject Matter Expert*

Jacqueline Petersen, RHIA, CHDA, CPC, *Subject Matter Expert*

Tracy Betzler, *Senior Desktop Publishing Specialist*

Hope M. Dunn, *Senior Desktop Publishing Specialist*

Katie Russell, *Desktop Publishing Specialist*

Lynn Speirs, *Editor*

Subject Matter Experts

Elizabeth Leibold, RHIT

Ms. Leibold has more than 25 years of experience in the health care profession. She has served in a variety of roles, ranging from patient registration to billing and collections, and has an extensive background in both physician and hospital outpatient coding and compliance. She has worked for large health care systems and health information management services companies, and has wide-ranging experience in facility and professional component coding, along with CPT expertise in interventional procedures, infusion services, emergency department, observation, and ambulatory surgery coding. Her areas of expertise include chart-to-claim coding audits and providing staff education to both tenured and new coding staff. She is an active member of the American Health Information Management Association (AHIMA).

Jacqueline Petersen, RHIA, CHDA, CPC

Ms. Petersen is a Clinical/Technical editor with Optum360. She has served as Senior Clinical Product Research Analyst with Optum360 developing business requirements for edits to support correct coding and reimbursement for claims processing applications. Her experience includes development of data-driven and system rules for both professional and facility claims and in-depth analysis of claims data inclusive of ICD-10-CM, CPT, HCPCS, and modifiers. Her background also includes consulting work for Optum, serving as a SME, providing coding and reimbursement education to internal and external clients. Ms. Petersen is a member of the American Academy of Professional Coders (AAPC), and the American Health Information Management Association (AHIMA).

Welcome to over 25 years of coding expertise.

Every medical organization knows that medical documentation and coding accuracy are vital to the revenue cycle. As a leading health services business, Optum360® has proudly created industry-leading coding, billing and reimbursement solutions for more than 25 years. Serving the broad health market, including physicians, health care organizations, payers and government, we help health systems reduce costs and achieve timely and accurate revenue.

You'll find ICD-10-CM/PCS, CPT®, HCPCS, DRG, specialty and reference content across our full suite of medical coding, billing and reimbursement products. And to ensure you have expert insight and the right information at your fingertips, our subject matter experts have incorporated proprietary features into these resources. These include supplementary edits and notations, coding tips and tools, and appendixes — making each product comprehensive and easy to use. Think of it as coding resources built by coders, for coders like you.

Your coding, billing and reimbursement product team,

Ryan Nichole Greg LaJuana
Ken
Jacqui Denise Leanne
Marianne Elizabeth Nann
Anita Debbie Karen

Put Optum360 medical coding, billing and reimbursement content at your fingertips today. Choose what works for you.

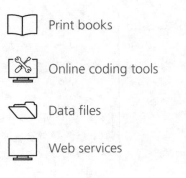

- Print books
- Online coding tools
- Data files
- Web services

Visit us at **optum360coding.com** to browse our products, or call us at **1-800-464-3649, option 1,** for more information.

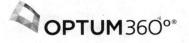

OPTUM360°®

CPT is a registered trademark of the American Medical Association.

At our core, we're about coding.

Essential medical code sets are just that — essential to your revenue cycle. In our ICD-10-CM/PCS, CPT®, HCPCS and DRG coding tools, we apply our collective coding expertise to present these code set resources in a way that is comprehensive, plus easy to use and apply. Print books are budget-friendly and easily referenced, created with intuitive features and formats, such as visual alerts, color-coding and symbols to identify important coding notes and instructions — plus, great coding tips.

Find the same content, tips and features of our code books in a variety of formats. Choose from print products, online coding tools, data files or web services.

Your coding, billing and reimbursement product team,

Ryan   Nichole   Greg   LaJuana
        Ken   Denise
Jacqui   Marianne   Leanne
        Anita   Debbie   Elizabeth   Nann
                         Karen

Put Optum360 medical coding, billing and reimbursement content at your fingertips today. Choose what works for you.

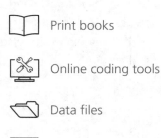

Print books

Online coding tools

Data files

Web services

Visit us at **optum360coding.com** to browse our products, or call us at **1-800-464-3649, option 1,** for more information.

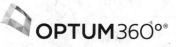

Contents

Introduction

About HCPCS Codes

HCPCS Level II codes, except for the dental code series, are developed and maintained by a joint editorial panel consisting of the Centers for Medicare and Medicaid Services (CMS), the Blue Cross Blue Shield Association, and the Health Insurance Association of America. HCPCS Level II codes may be used throughout the United States in all Medicare regions. They consist of one alpha character (A through V) followed by four digits. Optum360 does not change the code descriptions other than correcting typographical errors. For 2022, there are some codes that appear to be duplicates. CMS has indicated that each of the codes is used to report a specific condition or service. At press time, CMS had not provided further clarification regarding these codes. Additional information may be found on the CMS website, https://www.cms.gov/Medicare/Coding/HCPCSReleaseCodeSets/index.html.

Any supplier or manufacturer can submit a request for coding modification to the HCPCS Level II National codes. A document explaining the HCPCS modification process, as well as a detailed format for submitting a recommendation for a modification to HCPCS Level II codes, is available on the HCPCS website at https://www.cms.gov/Medicare/Coding/MedHCPCSGenInfo/HCPCS_Coding_Questions. Besides the information requested in this format, a requestor should also submit any additional descriptive material, including the manufacturer's product literature and information that is believed would be helpful in furthering CMS's understanding of the medical features of the item for which a coding modification is being recommended. The HCPCS coding review process is an ongoing, continuous process.

The dental (D) codes are not included in the official 2022 HCPCS Level II code set. The American Dental Association (ADA) holds the copyright on those codes and instructed CMS to remove them. As a result, Optum360 has removed them from this product; however, Optum360 has additional resources available for customers requiring the dental codes. Please visit www.optum360coding.com or call 1.800.464.3649.

Note: The expanded Medically Unlikely Edit (MUE) tables containing HCPCS/CPT codes, MUE values, MUE adjudication indicators, and MUE rationale are no longer published in this book. They will be available on the Optum360 website for users of the *HCPCS Level II Expert* at www.optum360coding.com/2022HCPCSMUE.

> Password: o360mue22

The table containing the Medicare national average payment (NAP) for services, supplies (DME, orthotics, prosthetics, etc.), drugs, biologicals, and nonphysician procedures using HCPCS Level II codes are available at www.optum360coding.com/2022MedAvgPay.

> Password: o360map22

How to Use HCPCS Level II

Coders should keep in mind that the insurance companies and government do not base payment solely on what was done for the patient. They need to know why the services were performed. In addition to using the HCPCS coding system for procedures and supplies, coders must also use the ICD-10-CM coding system to denote the diagnosis. This book will not discuss ICD-10-CM codes, which can be found in a current ICD-10-CM code book for diagnosis codes. To locate a HCPCS Level II code, follow these steps:

1. Identify the services or procedures that the patient received.

   Example:

   Patient administered PSA exam.

2. Look up the appropriate term in the index.

   Example:

   Screening
       prostate specific antigen test (PSA)

   Coding Tip: Coders who are unable to find the procedure or service in the index can look in the table of contents for the type of procedure or device to narrow the code choices. Also, coders should remember to check the unlisted procedure guidelines for additional choices.

3. Assign a tentative code.

   Example:

   Code G0103

   Coding Tip: To the right of the terminology, there may be a single code or multiple codes, a cross-reference, or an indication that the code has been deleted. Tentatively assign all codes listed.

4. Locate the code or codes in the appropriate section. When multiple codes are listed in the index, be sure to read the narrative of all codes listed to find the appropriate code based on the service performed.

   Example:

   G0103   **Prostate cancer screening; prostate specific antigen test (PSA)**

5. Check for color bars, symbols, notes, and references.

   G0103   **Prostate cancer screening; prostate specific antigen test (PSA)**   ♂ A

6. Review the appendixes for the reference definitions and other guidelines for coverage issues that apply.

7. Determine whether any modifiers should be appended.

8. Assign the code.

   Example:

   The code assigned is G0103.

Coding Standards

Levels of Use

Coders may find that the same procedure is coded at two or even three levels. Which code is correct? There are certain rules to follow if this should occur.

When both a CPT and a HCPCS Level II code have virtually identical narratives for a procedure or service, the CPT code should be used. If, however, the narratives are not identical (e.g., the CPT code narrative is generic, whereas the HCPCS Level II code is specific), the Level II code should be used.

Be sure to check for a national code when a CPT code description contains an instruction to include additional information, such as describing a specific medication. For example, when billing Medicare or Medicaid for supplies, avoid using CPT code 99070 Supplies and materials (except spectacles), provided by the physician over and above those usually included with the office visit or other services rendered (list drugs, trays, supplies, or materials provided). There are many HCPCS Level II codes that specify supplies in more detail.

Special Reports

Submit a special report with the claim when a new, unusual, or variable procedure is provided or a modifier is used. Include the following information:

- A copy of the appropriate report (e.g., operative, x-ray), explaining the nature, extent, and need for the procedure
- Documentation of the medical necessity of the procedure

- Documentation of the time and effort necessary to perform the procedure

How To Use Optum360 HCPCS Level II Books

Organization of Optum360 HCPCS Level II Expert

The Optum360 2022 *HCPCS Level II* contains mandated changes and new codes for use as of January 1, 2022. Deleted codes have also been indicated and cross-referenced to active codes when possible. New codes have been added to the appropriate sections, eliminating the time-consuming step of looking in two places for a code. However, keep in mind that the information in this book is a reproduction of the 2022 HCPCS; additional information on coverage issues may have been provided to Medicare contractors after publication. All contractors periodically update their systems and records throughout the year. If this book does not agree with your contractor, it is either because of a mid-year update or correction, or a specific local or regional coverage policy.

HCPCS Code Index

Because HCPCS is organized by code number rather than by service or supply name, the index enables the coder to locate any code without looking through individual ranges of codes. Just look up the medical or surgical supply, service, orthotic, or prosthetic in question to find the appropriate codes. This index also refers to many of the brand names by which these items are known.

Appendixes

Appendix 1: Table of Drugs and Biologicals

The brand names of drugs and biologicals listed are examples only and may not include all products available for that type. The table lists HCPCS codes from any available section including A codes, C codes, J codes, S codes, and Q codes under brand and generic names with amount, route of administration, and code numbers. While every effort is made to make the table comprehensive, it is not all-inclusive.

Appendix 2: Modifiers

This appendix identifies current modifiers. A modifier is a two-position alpha or numeric code that is appended to a CPT or HCPCS code to clarify the services being reported. Modifiers provide a means by which a service can be altered without changing the procedure code. They add more information, such as anatomical site, to the code. In addition, they help eliminate the appearance of duplicate billing and unbundling. Modifiers are used to increase the accuracy in reimbursement and coding consistency, ease editing, and capture payment data.

Appendix 3: Abbreviations and Acronyms

This appendix contains a list of abbreviations and acronyms found throughout the HCPCS code set that may be helpful. It is not an all-inclusive list.

Appendix 4: Medicare Internet-only Manuals (IOMs)

Previously, this appendix contained a verbatim printout of the Medicare Internet-only Manual references pertaining to specific codes. This appendix now contains a link to the IOMs on the Centers for Medicare and Medicaid Services website. The IOM references to applicable to specific codes can still be found at the code level.

Appendix 5: New, Revised, and Deleted Codes

This appendix is a complete list of all new, revised, and deleted HCPCS codes for the current year. New and revised codes are listed along with their current code descriptors. Deleted codes are provided as a list of codes.

Appendix 6: Place of Service and Type of Service

This appendix contains lists of place-of-service codes that should be used on professional claims and type-of-service codes used by the Medicare Common Working File.

Appendix 7: Crosswalk of Deleted Codes

This appendix is a cross-reference from a deleted code to an active code when one is available. The deleted code cross-reference will also appear under the deleted code description in the tabular section of the book.

Appendix 8: Glossary

This appendix contains general terms and definitions that could be helpful for coding and reimbursement.

Appendix 9: Quality Payment Program (QPP)

Previously, this appendix contained lists of the numerators and denominators applicable to the Medicare PQRS. However, with the implementations of the Quality Payment Program mandated by passage of the Medicare Access and Chip Reauthorization Act (MACRA) of 2015, the PQRS system will be obsolete. This appendix now contains information pertinent to that legislation as well as a brief overview of the proposed changes for the following year as available by date of this publication.

Color-coded Coverage Instructions

The Optum360 *HCPCS Level II* book provides colored symbols for each coverage and reimbursement instruction. A legend to these symbols is provided on the bottom of each two-page spread.

Green Color Bar—Special Coverage Instructions

A green bar for "special coverage instructions" over a code means that special coverage instructions apply to that code. These special instructions are also typically given in the form of Medicare Internet Only Manuals (IOM) reference numbers.

| A4336 | Incontinence supply, urethral insert, any type, each |

Yellow Color Bar—Carrier Discretion

Issues that are left to "carrier discretion" are covered with a yellow bar. Contact the carrier for specific coverage information on those codes.

| A9581 | Injection, gadoxetate disodium, 1 ml |

Pink Color Bar—Not Covered by or Invalid for Medicare

Codes that are not covered by or are invalid for Medicare are covered by a pink bar. The pertinent Medicare Internet-only Manuals (IOMs) reference numbers are also given explaining why a particular code is not covered. These numbers refer to the appendixes, where the Medicare references are listed.

| A4264 | Permanent implantable contraceptive intratubal occlusion device(s) and delivery system |

Code Icons

Codes in the Optum360 *HCPCS Level II* follow the AMA CPT book conventions to indicate new, revised, and deleted codes.

A black circle (●) precedes a new code.

| ● S0013 | Esketamine, nasal spray, 1 mg |

A black triangle (▲) precedes a code with revised terminology or rules.

| ▲ Q4176 | Neopatch or Therion, per sq cm |

A circle (○) precedes a recycled/reinstated code.

| ○ G0044 | Patients with moderate or severe mitral stenosis |

Codes deleted from the current active codes appear with a strike-out.

| A4397 | ~~Irrigation supply; sleeve, each~~ |

☑ Quantity Alert

Many codes in HCPCS report quantities that may not coincide with quantities available in the marketplace. For instance, a HCPCS code for an ostomy pouch with skin barrier reports each pouch, but the product is generally sold in a package of 10; "10" must be indicated in the quantity box on the CMS claim form to ensure proper reimbursement. This symbol indicates that care should be taken to verify quantities in this code. These quantity alerts do not represent Medicare Unlikely Edits (MUEs) and should not be used for MUEs.

☑ J0120	Injection, tetracycline, up to 250 mg

♀ Female Only

This icon identifies procedures that some payers may consider female only.

A4261	Cervical cap for contraceptive use	♀

♂ Male Only

This icon identifies procedures that some payers may consider male only.

A4326	Male external catheter with integral collection chamber, anytype, each	♂

Ⓐ Age Edit

This icon denotes codes intended for use with a specific age group, such as neonate, newborn, pediatric, and adult. Carefully review the code description to ensure that the code reported most appropriately reflects the patient's age.

Q2037	Influenza virus vaccine, split virus, when administered to individuals 3 years of age and older, for intramuscular use (FLUVIRIN)	Ⓐ

Ⓜ Maternity

This icon identifies procedures that by definition should only be used for maternity patients generally between 12 and 55 years of age.

H1001	Prenatal care, at-risk enhanced service; antepartum management	Ⓜ

A2–Z3 ASC Payment Indicators

Codes designated as being paid by ASC groupings that were effective at the time of printing are denoted by the group number.

G0105	Colorectal cancer screening; colonoscopy on individual at high risk	A2

♿ DMEPOS

Use this icon to identify when to consult the CMS durable medical equipment, prosthetics, orthotics, and supplies (DMEPOS) for payment of this durable medical item. For modifiers NU, RR, and UE: These modifiers are for use when DME equipment is either new, used, or rented. The RR modifiers must also be used in conjunction with rental modifiers KH, KI, or KJ.

E0988	Manual wheelchair accessory, lever-activated, wheel drive, pair	♿

⊘ Skilled Nursing Facility (SNF)

Use this icon to identify certain items and services excluded from SNF consolidated billing. These items may be billed directly to the Medicare contractor by the provider or supplier of the service or item.

A4653	Peritoneal dialysis catheter anchoring device, belt, each	⊘

Drugs commonly reported with a code are listed underneath by brand or generic name.

C9254	Injection, lacosamide, 1 mg
	Use this code for VIMPAT.

CMS does not use consistent terminology when a code for a specific procedure is not listed. The code description may include any of the following terms: unlisted, not otherwise classified (NOC), unspecified, unclassified, other, and miscellaneous. If unsure there is no code for the service or supply provided or used, provide adequate documentation to the payer. Check with the payer for more information.

A0999	Unlisted ambulance service

CMS: This notation appears when instruction pertaining to a code appears in a CMS Internet-only Manual (IOM). Previously, appendix 4 contained a verbatim printout of the Medicare Internet-only Manual references pertaining to specific codes. This appendix now contains a link to the IOMs on the Centers for Medicare and Medicaid Services website. The IOM references applicable to specific codes can still be found at the code level.

A4618	Breathing circuits
	CMS: 100-04, 20, 100.2

AHA: American Hospital Association *Coding Clinic® for HCPCS* citations help in finding expanded information about specific codes and their usage.

A4290	Sacral nerve stimulation test lead, each
	AHA: 1Q, '02, 9

A-Y OPPS Status Indicators

Status indicators identify how individual HCPCS Level II codes are paid or not paid under the OPPS. The same status indicator is assigned to all the codes within an ambulatory payment classification (APC). Consult the payer or resource to learn which CPT codes fall within various APCs. Status indicators for HCPCS and their definitions follow:

A   Services furnished to a hospital outpatient that are paid under a fee schedule or payment system other than OPPS, for example:

- Ambulance Services
- Clinical Diagnostic Laboratory Services
- Non-Implantable Prosthetic and Orthotic Devices
- Physical, Occupational, and Speech Therapy
- Diagnostic Mammography
- Screening Mammography

B   Codes that are not recognized by OPPS when submitted on an outpatient hospital Part B bill type (12x and 13x)

C   Inpatient Procedures

E   Items, Codes, and Services:

- Not covered by any Medicare outpatient benefit category
- Statutorily excluded by Medicare
- Not reasonable and necessary

F   Corneal Tissue Acquisition; Certain CRNA Services and Hepatitis B Vaccines

G   Pass-Through Drugs and Biologicals

H   Pass-Through Device Categories

JI   Hospital Part B services paid through a comprehensive APC

K   Nonpass-Through Drugs and Nonimplantable Biologicals, Including Therapeutic Radiopharmaceuticals

L   Influenza Vaccine; Pneumococcal Pneumonia Vaccine

M   Items and Services Not Billable to the MAC

N   Items and Services Packaged into APC Rates

P   Partial Hospitalization

Q1   STVX-Packaged Codes

Q2   T-Packaged Codes

Q3   Codes That May Be Paid Through a Composite APC

NI   Conditionally Packaged Laboratory Tests

R   Blood and Blood Products

S   Significant Procedure, Not Discounted when Multiple

T   Significant Procedure, Multiple Procedure Reduction Applies

U   Brachytherapy Sources

V   Clinic or Emergency Department Visit

Y   Nonimplantable Durable Medical Equipment

A	**L8440**	Prosthetic shrinker, below knee, each
B	**Q4005**	Cast supplies, long arm cast, adult (11 years +), plaster
C	**G0341**	Percutaneous islet cell transplant, includes portal vein catheterization and infusion
E	**A0021**	Ambulance service, outside state per mile, transport (Medicaid only)
F	**V2785**	Processing, preserving and transporting corneal tissue
G	**C9460**	Injection, cangrelor, 1 mg
H	**C2613**	Lung biopsy plug with delivery system
K	**J1750**	Injection, iron dextran, 50 mg
L	**Q2036**	Influenza virus vaccine, split virus, when administered to individuals 3 years of age and older, for intramuscular use (FLULAVAL)
M	**G0333**	Pharmacy dispensing fee for inhalation drug(s); initial 30-day supply as a beneficiary
N	**A4220**	Refill kit for implantable infusion pump
P	**G0129**	Occupational therapy services requiring the skills of a qualified occupational therapist, furnished as a component of a partial hospitalization treatment program, per session (45 minutes or more)
Q3	**C8935**	Magnetic resonance angiography without contrast, upper extremity
R	**P9010**	Blood (whole), for transfusion, per unit
S	**G0117**	Glaucoma screening for high risk patients furnished by an optometrist or ophthalmologist
T	**C9727**	Insertion of implants into the soft palate; minimum of 3 implants
U	**A9527**	Iodine I-125, sodium iodide solution, therapeutic, per millicurie
V	**G0101**	Cervical or vaginal cancer screening; pelvic and clinical breast examination
Y	**A5500**	For diabetics only, fitting (including follow-up), custom preparation and supply of off-the-shelf depth-inlay shoe manufactured to accommodate multidensity insert(s), per shoe

A2 –Z3 ASC Payment Indicators

This icon identifies the ASC status payment indicators. They indicate how the ASC payment rate was derived and/or how the procedure, item, or service is treated under the ASC payment system. For more information about these indicators and how they affect billing, consult Optum360's *Revenue Cycle Pro*.

A2 Surgical procedure on ASC list in CY 2007 or later; payment based on OPPS relative payment weight

C5 Inpatient procedure

F4 Corneal tissue acquisition, hepatitis B vaccine; paid at reasonable cost

G2 Non-office-based surgical procedure added in CY 2008 or later; payment based on OPPS relative payment weight

H2 Brachytherapy source paid separately when provided integral to a surgical procedure on ASC list; payment based on OPPS rate

J7 OPPS pass-through device paid separately when provided integral to a surgical procedure on ASC list; payment based on OPPS rate

J8 Device-intensive procedure paid at adjusted rate

K2 Drugs and biologicals paid separately when provided integral to a surgical procedure on ASC list; payment based on OPPS rate

K7 Unclassified drugs and biologicals; payment contractor-priced

L1 Influenza vaccine; pneumococcal vaccine; packaged item/service; no separate payment made

L6 New Technology Intraocular Lens (NTIOL); special payment

N1 Packaged service/item; no separate payment made

P2 Office-based surgical procedure added to ASC list in CY 2008 or later with MPFS nonfacility PE RVUs; payment based on OPPS relative payment weight

P3 Office-based surgical procedure added to ASC list in CY 2008 or later with MPFS nonfacility PE RVUs; payment based on MPFS nonfacility PE RVUs

R2 Office-based surgical procedure added to ASC list in CY 2008 or later without MPFS nonfacility PE RVUs; payment based on OPPS relative payment weight

Z2 Radiology service paid separately when provided integral to a surgical procedure on ASC list; payment based on OPPS relative payment weight

Z3 Radiology service paid separately when provided integral to a surgical procedure on ASC list; payment based on MPFS nonfacility PE RVUs

F4 V2785 Processing, preserving and transporting corneal tissue

H2 A9527 Iodine I-125, sodium iodide solution, therapeutic per millicurie

J7 C1841 Retinal prosthesis, includes all internal and external components

K2 C9132 Prothrombin complex concentrate (human), Kcentra, per IU of Factor IX activity

K7 C9399 Unclassified drugs or biologicals

L1 Q2037 Influenza virus vaccine, split virus, when administered to individuals 3 years of age and older, for intramuscular use (FLUVIRIN)

N1 C9353 Microporous collagen implantable slit tube (NeuraWrap Nerve Protector), per cm length

Z3 G0130 Single energy x-ray absorptiometry (SEXA) bone density study, one or more sites; appendicular skeleton (peripheral) (e.g., radius, wrist, heel)

Z2 C8911 Magnetic resonance angiography without contrast followed by with contrast, chest (excluding myocardium)

Infusion — *continued*
Sipuleucel-T autologous CD54+, Q2043
supplies, A4222, A4223
syringe cartridge, non-insulin pump, K0552
therapy, home, S9347, S9351, S9497-S9504
Inhalation drugs
acetylcysteine, J7608
albuterol, J7609, J7610, J7611
Alupent, J7668-J7669
atropine, J7635-J7636
Atrovent, J7644
Azmacort, J7684
beclomethasone, J7622
betamethasone, J7624
bitolterol mesylate, J7628-J7629
Brcanyl, J7680-J7681
Brethine, J7680-J7681
budesonide, J7626-J7627, J7633-J7634
colistimethate sodium, S0142
cromolyn sodium, J7631
dexamethasone, J7637-J7638
dornase alpha, J7639
flunisolide, J7641
formoterol, J7606, J7640
Gastrocrom, J7631
glycopyrrolate, J7642-J7643
iloprost, Q4074
Intal, J7631
ipratropium bromide, J7644-J7645
isoetharine HCl, J7647-J7650
isoproterenol HCl, J7657-J7660
levalbuterol, J7607, J7614, J7615
metaproterenol sulfate, J7667-J7670
methacholine chloride, J7674
Mucomyst, J7608
Mucosil, J7608
Nasalcrom, J7631
NOC, J7699
pentamidine isethionate, J7676
Pulmicort Respules, J7627
terbutaline sulfate, J7680-J7681
Tobi, J7682
tobramycin, J7682, J7685
Tornalate, J7628-J7629
triamcinolone, J7683-J7684
Initial
ECG, Medicare, G0403-G0405
physical exam, Medicare, G0402
Injectable
bulking agent
urinary tract, L8603-L8606
vocal cord, L8607
Injection — *see also* Table of Drugs
adjustment, bariatric band, S2083
bulking agent
urinary tract, L8603-L8606
vocal cord, L8607
contrast material, during MRI, A9576-A9579, Q9953
dermal filler for LDS, G0429
sacroiliac joint, G0259-G0260
subretinal, C9770
supplies for self-administered, A4211, A4224-A4225
InnovaMatrix AC, A2001
Inpatient telehealth pharmacologic management, G0459
Insert
convex, for ostomy, A5093
diabetic, for shoe, A5512-A5514
foot insert/plate, L3031
implant
prosthetic socket, gasket or seal, L7700
soft palate, C9727
Insertion
cardioverter-defibrillator system, G0448
central venous access device
inside-out technique, C9780
intrauterine system, S4981
tray, A4310-A4316
Instillation fecal microbiota, G0455
Integra
Bilayer Matrix Wound Dressing, Q4104
Dermal Regeneration Template, Q4105

Integra — *continued*
Flowable, Q4114
Matrix, Q4108
Meshed Bilayer Wound Matrix, C9363
MOZAIK Osteoconductive Scaffold Putty, C9359
MOZAIK Osteoconductive Scaffold Strip, C9362
InteguPLY, Q4126
Interbody cage
anterior/lateral, personalized, C1831
Interface
cough stimulating device, A7020
oral with suction pump, A7047
Interfyl, Q4171
Intermittent
limb compression device, E0676
peritoneal dialysis system, E1592
positive pressure breathing (IPPB) machine, E0500
Interphalangeal joint, prosthetic implant, L8658
Interrogation, remote evaluation
cardiovascular, G2066
Interscapular thoracic prosthesis
endoskeletal, L6570
upper limb, L6350-L6370
Interspinous process distraction device, C1821
Intervention
alcohol and/or drug, H0050
leak of endoluminal contents, G9305-G9306
Intrafallopian transfer
complete cycle, gamete, S4013
complete cycle, zygote, S4014
donor egg cycle, S4023
incomplete cycle, S4017
Intraocular lenses, C1780, C1840, Q1004-Q1005, S0596, V2630-V2632
new technology
category 4, Q1004
category 5, Q1005
presbyopia correcting function, V2788
refractive correcting, S0596
telescopic, C1840
Intraoperative
near-infrared fluorescence
lymphatic mapping, C9756
major extrahepatic bile ducts, C9776
Intratubal occlusion device, A4264
Intrauterine device
copper contraceptive, J7300
etonogestrel, J7307
levonorgestrel-releasing, J7296-J7298, S4981
other, S4989
Progestacert, S4989
Introducer sheath
guiding, C1766, C1892, C1893
other than guiding, C1894, C2629
Inversion device, A9285
Investigational device exemption (IDE) study
interatrial shunt, transcatheter, C9760
Iodine 125, A9527, A9532, C2638-C2639
Iodine I-131
albumin, A9524
iobenguane sulfate, A9508
sodium iodide, A9517
Iodine swabs/wipes, A4247
IPD
system, E1592
IPPB machine, E0500
delivery device, A9274, E0784, S5560-S5561, S5565-S5571
home infusion administration, S9353
intermediate acting, S5552
long acting, S5553
NPH, J1815, S5552
outpatient IV treatment, G9147
rapid onset, S5550-S5551
Ipratropium bromide
administered through DME, J7644-J7645
Iris Preventix pressure relief/reduction mattress, E0184
Iris prosthesis, C1839
Iris therapeutic overlays, E0199

IRM ankle-foot orthotic, L1950
Iron
sucrose, J1756
Irrigation supplies, A4320, A4322, A4355, A4398-A4400, A4436-A4437
Surfit
irrigation sleeve, A4436-A4437
night drainage container set, A5102
Visi-flow irrigator, A4398, A4399
Irrigation/evacuation system, bowel
control unit, E0350
disposable supplies for, E0352
Islet cell transplant
laparoscopy, G0342
laparotomy, G0343
percutaneous, G0341
Isocal, enteral nutrition, B4150
HCN, B4152
Isoetharine
inhalation solution
concentrated, J7647
unit dose, J7649-J7650
Isolates, B4150, B4152
Isoproterenol HCl
administered through DME, J7657-J7660
Isosulfan blue, Q9968
Isotein, enteral nutrition, B4153
IV, G0459
administration set, non-PVC, S1016
infusion, OPPS, C8957
pole, E0776, K0105
solution
10% LMD, J7100
5% dextrose/normal saline, J7042
D-5-W, J7070
dextran, J7100, J7110
Gentran, J7100, J7110
normal saline, A4217, J7030-J7040, J7050
Rheomacrodex, J7100
Ringer's lactate, J7120
tubing extension set, S1015

J

Jace tribrace, L1832
Jacket
scoliosis, L1300, L1310
J-cell battery, replacement for blood glucose monitor, A4234
Jejunostomy tube, B4087-B4088
Joint device, C1776
transcutaneous electrical stimulation, E0762

K

Kaltostat, alginate dressing, A6196-A6199
Kartop Patient Lift, toilet or bathroom (*see also* Lift), E0625
Keramatrix, Kerasorb, Q4165
Keratectomy photorefractive, S0810
Keratoprosthesis, C1818
Kerecis Omega3, Q4158
Keroxx, Q4202
Keto-Diastix, box of 100 glucose/ketone urine test strips, A4250
Key-Pred
-25,-50, J2650
Kidney
ESRD supply, A4651-A4913
system, E1510
wearable artificial, E1632
Kingsley gloves, above hands, L6890
Kits
asthma, S8097
enteral feeding supply (syringe) (pump) (gravity), B4034-B4036
fistula cannulation (set), A4730
parenteral nutrition, B4220-B4224
surgical dressing (tray), A4550
tracheostomy, A4625
Knee
Adjustabrace 3, L2999
disarticulation, prosthesis, K1022, L5150-L5160, L5312
extension/flexion device, E1812

Knee — *continued*
immobilizer, L1830
joint, miniature, L5826
Knee-O-Prene Hinged Wraparound Knee Support, L1810
locks, L2405-L2425
Masterbrace 3, L2999
Masterhinge Adjustabrace 3, L2999
orthotic (KO), E1810, L1810, L1820, L1830-L1860, L1851-L1852
Knee Support, L2000-L2038, L2126-L2136
Knee-O-Prene Hinged Knee Sleeve, L1810
Knee-O-Prene Hinged Wraparound Knee Support, L1810
KnitRite
prosthetic
sheath, L8400-L8415
sock, L8420-L8435
stump sock, L8470-L8485
K-Y Lubricating Jelly, A4332, A4402
Kyphosis pad, L1020, L1025

L

Labor care (not resulting in delivery), S4005
Laboratory tests
chemistry, P2028-P2038
miscellaneous, Q0111-Q0115
Lacrimal duct implant
permanent, A4263
temporary, A4262
Laminotomy, C9757
Lancet, A4258, A4259
Laparoscopy, surgical
esophagomyotomy, S2079
Laryngectomy
tube, A7520-A7522
Larynx, artificial, L8500
Laser
application, S8948
assisted uvulopalatoplasty (LAUP), S2080
in situ keratomileusis, S0800
myringotomy, S2225
Laser skin piercing device, for blood collection, E0620
replacement lens, A4257
LAUP, S2080
Lead
adaptor
neurostimulator, C1883
pacing, C1883
cardioverter, defibrillator, C1777, C1895, C1896
environmental, home evaluation, T1029
neurostimulator, C1778
neurostimulator/test kit, C1897
pacemaker, C1779, C1898, C1899
ventricular, C1900
Leg
bag, A4358, A5112
extensions for walker, E0158
Nextep Contour Lower Leg Walker, L2999
Nextep Low Silhouette Lower Leg Walkers, L2999
rest, elevating, K0195
rest, wheelchair, E0990
strap, A5113, A5114, K0038, K0039
Legg Perthes orthotic, A4565, L1700-L1755
Lens
aniseikonic, V2118, V2318
contact, V2500-V2599
deluxe feature, V2702
eye, S0504-S0508, S0580-S0590, S0596, V2100-V2615, V2700-V2799
intraocular, C1780, C1840, V2630-V2632
low vision, V2600-V2615
mirror coating, V2761
occupational multifocal, V2786
polarization, V2762
polycarbonate, V2784
progressive, V2781
skin piercing device, replacement, A4257
telescopic, C1840
tint, V2744
addition, V2745
Lenticular lens
bifocal, V2221

Index

Needle — Ostomy

Ostomy — *continued*
pouch, A4416-A4420, A4423-A4434
drainable, A4412-A4413, S5056-A5057
pediatric, A5061-A5062
skin barrier, A4411, A4414-A4415
extended wear, A4407-A4410
paste, A4405-A4406
wipes or swabs, A5120
vent, A4366
Otto Bock prosthesis
battery charger, six volt, L7362
battery, six volt, L7360
hook adapter, L6628
lamination collar, L6629
pincher tool, L6810
wrist, L6629
Outpatient hospital clinic visit, G0463
Overlay, mattress, E0371-E0373
Ovulation induction, S4042
Owens & Minor
cervical collar, L0140
cervical helmet, L0120
Oximeter, E0445
probe, A4606
Oxi-Uni-Pak, E0430
Oxygen
accessory, E1352
ambulance, A0422
battery
charger, E1357
pack, E1356
chamber, hyperbaric, topical, A4575
concentrator, E1390, E1391
portable, rental, E1392
gaseous, K0738, S8120
liquid, S8121
mask, A4620
medication supplies, A4611-A4627
portable, E0433, E0443-E0444, E0447, K0738
power adapter, E1358
rack/stand, E1355
regulator, E1353
respiratory equipment/supplies, A4611-A4627, E0424-E0480
Oxi-Uni-Pak, E0430
supplies and equipment, E0425-E0444, E0433, E0455, E1353-E1406
tent, E0455
tubing, A4616
water vapor enriching system, E1405, E1406
wheeled cart, E1354

P

Pacemaker
dual chamber
non-rate responsive, C2619
rate responsive, C1785
lead, C1779, C1898, C1899
monitor, E0610, E0615
other than single or dual chamber, C2621
single chamber
non-rate responsive, C2620
rate responsive, C1786
Pacer manual wheelchair, K0003
Packing strips, A6407
Pad
abdominal, L1270
adhesive, A6203-A6205, A6212-A6214, A6219-A6221, A6237-A6239, A6245-A6247, A6254-A6256
alginate, A6196-A6199
alternating pressure, E0181
arm, K0019
Asis, L1250
condylar, L2810
crutch, A4635
fluid circulating, cold, with pump, E0218
gel pressure, E0185, E0196
gluteal, L2650
gradient pressure pads, S8421-S8429
heating, E0210, E0215, E0217, E0249
heel, L3480, L3485
kyphosis, L1020, L1025

Pad — *continued*
lumbar, L1030, L1040, L1240
nonadhesive (dressing), A6209-A6211, A6216-A6218, A6222-A6224, A6228-A6230, A6234-A6236, A6242-A6244
orthotic device interface, E1820
pressure, E0181-E0182
replacement, infrared heat system, A4639
rib gusset, L1280
sheepskin, E0188, E0189
shoe, L3430-L3485
stabilizer, L3170
sternal, L1050
thoracic, L1060, L1260
triceps, L6100
trochanteric, L1290
truss, L8320, L8330
water circulating, heat, unit, E0249
water circulating, heat, with pump, E0217
water pressure, E0198
Pail, for use with commode chair, E0167
Pain, G9250-G9251
PalinGen Flow or ProMatrX (fluid), Q4174
PalinGen or PalinGen XPlus Membrane, Q4173
Palladium, C2640-C2641
Pan, for use with commode chair, E0167
Pancreas, S1034-S1037
artificial device system, S1034
replacement external receiver, S1037
replacement external transmitter, S1036
replacement invasive disposable subcutaneous sensor, S1035
Pantoprazole sodium, C9113, S0164
Papanicolaou (Pap) screening smear, P3000, P3001, Q0091
Paraffin, A4265
bath unit, E0235
Paramedic intercept, S0207-S0208
Paranasal sinus ultrasound, S9024
Parenteral nutrition
administration kit, B4224
home infusion therapy, S9364-S9368
pump, B9004, B9006
solution, B4164-B5200
supplies, not otherwise classified, B9999
supply kit, B4220, B4222
Parenting class, S9444
infant safety, S9447
Parking fee, nonemergency transport, A0170
Partial hospitalization, S0201
PASRR, T2010-T2011
Passive motion
continuous exercise device, E0936
Paste, conductive, A4558
conductive, A4558
coupling for ultrasound, A4559
Pathogen(s)
reduced, platelets, P9073
test for platelets, P9100
Pathology and laboratory tests
molecular pathology, G0452
surgical
prostate, G0416
Pathology screening tests, P3000-P3001, Q0091
Patient lift, E0625, E0637, E0639, E0640
Patten Bottom, Legg Perthes orthotic, L1755
Pavlik harness, hip orthotic, L1650
Payment, home health bundled care improvement initiative, G9187
Peak flow meter, S8110
portable, S8096
Pediatric hip abduction splint
Orthomedics, L1640
Orthomerica, L1640
Pediculosis treatment, A9180
PEFR, peak expiratory flow rate meter, A4614
Pelvic and breast exam, G0101
Pelvic belt/harness/boot, E0944
Penicillin G
potassium, J2540
procaine, aqueous, J2510
Penlet II lancet device, A4258
Penlet lancet device, A4258
Percussor, E0480

Percutaneous
access system, A4301
arteriovenous fistula creation
using radiofrequency energy, G2171
using thermal resistance energy, G2170
image-guided lumbar decompression (PILD), G0276
transluminal coronary atherectomy, C9602-C9603
transluminal revascularization, C9604-C9608
Perflexane lipid microspheres, Q9955
Perflutren lipid microsphere, Q9957
Peripheral
catheter infusion, C1751
Perlstein, ankle-foot orthotic, L1920
Permacol, C9364
Peroneal strap, L0980
Peroxide, A4244
Personal care item, S5199
Personal care services, T1019-T1020
Personalized
anterior/lateral interbody cage, C1831
Pessary, A4561-A4562
PET imaging
any site, NOS, G0235
breast, G0252
whole body, G0219
Pharmacy
compounding and dispensing, S9430
dispensing fee
inhalation drugs
per 30 days, Q0513
per 90 days, Q0514
supply fee
initial immunosuppressive drugs, Q0510
oral anticancer antiemetic or immunosuppressive drug, Q0511-Q0512
Pharmaplast disposable insulin syringes, per syringe, A4206
Phelps, ankle-foot orthotic, L1920
Pheresis, platelets, P9034-P9037, P9053
pathogen reduced, P9073
Philadelphia tracheotomy cervical collar, L0172
Philly One-piece Extrication collar, L0150
pHisoHex solution, A4246
Photocoagulation, G0186
Phototherapy
home visit service (Bili-Lite), S9098
keratectomy (PKT), S0812
light (bilirubin), E0202
Physical exam
for college, S0622
related to surgical procedure, S0260
Physical therapy, S8990
shoulder stretch device, E1841
Physical therapy/therapist
home health setting, G0151, S9131
performed by assistant, G2168
Physician management
home care
episodic, S0272
hospice monthly, S0271
standard monthly, S0270
Physician quality reporting system (PQRS)
See Quality payment program (QPP)
Physician review
home INR testing, G0250
Physician supervision, G0181-G0182
Pillow
abduction, E1399
decubitus care, E0190
nasal, A7029
positioning, E0190
Pinworm examination, Q0113
Placement
applicator, breast, C9726
interstitial device radiotherapy, other than prostate, C9728
occlusive, G0269
Plan of care, T2024

Planning
cancer treatment, S0353-S0354
Plasma
autologous platelet rich plasma, G0460, G0465
cryoprecipitate reduced, P9044
pathogen reduced, P9025
frozen, P9058-P9060
multiple donor, pooled, frozen, P9023, P9070-P9071
protein fraction, P9043, P9048
single donor, fresh frozen, P9017
Plastazote, L3002, L3252, L3253, L3265, L5654-L5658
Plaster
bandages
Orthoflex Elastic Plaster Bandages, A4580
Specialist Plaster Bandages, A4580
Genmould Creamy Plaster, A4580
Specialist J-Splint Plaster Roll Immobilizer, A4580
Specialist Plaster Roll Immobilizer, A4580
Specialist Plaster Splints, A4580
Platelets, P9019-P9020, P9031-P9037, P9052-P9053, P9055
apheresis/pheresis, P9052, P9055
concentrate, each unit, P9019
pathogen(s)
reduced, platelets, P9073
test, P9100
pheresis, P9034-P9037, P9053
pathogen reduced, P9073
rich plasma, each unit, P9020
Platform attachment
forearm crutch, E0153
walker, E0154
Platform, for home blood glucose monitor, A4255
Plumbing, for home ESRD equipment, A4870
Plurivest, Q4153
Pneumatic nebulizer
administration set
small volume
disposable, A7004
filtered, A7006
non-disposable, A7005
non-filtered, A7003
Polaris, E0601
Polaris Lt, E0601
Polycose, enteral nutrition
liquid, B4155
powder, B4155
PolyCyte, Q4241
Poor blood, each unit, P9016
Port
indwelling, C1788
Portable
equipment transfer, R0070-R0076
hemodialyzer system, E1635
home suction pump, K0743
nebulizer, E0570
oxygen contents
gaseous, E0443
liquid, E0444, E0447
oxygen system
gaseous, E0430-E0431
liquid, E0433-E0435
x-ray equipment, Q0092
Portagen Powder, enteral nutrition, B4150
Posey restraints, E0700
Positive airway pressure device supply, A7046
Postcoital examination, Q0115
Postdischarge services
LVRS surgery, G0305
Postural drainage board, E0606
Potassium
hydroxide (KOH) preparation, Q0112
Pouch
Active Life convex one-piece urostomy, A4421
closed, A4387, A5052
drainable, A4388-A4389, A5056-A5057, A5061
fecal collection, A4330
Little Ones Sur-fit mini, A5054

Technology based services
FQHC or RHC, G0071
Telehealth
brief communication, technology based, G2251-G2252
consultation
emergency department, G0425-G0427
inpatient, G0406-G0408, G0425-G0427
critical care, G0508-G0509
facility fee, Q3014
inpatient pharmacologic management, G0459
transmission, T1014
Telemonitoring
patient in home, includes equipment, S9110
Television
amplifier, V5270
caption decoder, V5271
TenderCloud electric air pump, E0182
TenderFlo II, E0187
TenderGel II, E0196
Tenderlet lancet device, A4258
TenoGlide Tendon Protector Sheet, C9356
TENS, A4595, E0720-E0749
Neuro-Pulse, E0720
Tensix, Q4146
Tent, oxygen, E0455
Terminal devices, L6703-L6715, L6721-L6722
Terumo disposable insulin syringes, up to 1 cc, per syringe, A4206
Test materials, home monitoring, G0249
Testing
comparative genomic hybridization, S3870
Coronavirus (2019-nCoV) diagnostic panel, U0001-U0002
with High throughput technologies, U0003-U0004
developmental, G0451
drug, G0480-G0483, G0659
genetic, S3800, S3840-S3842, S3844-S3846, S3849-S3850, S3852-S3853, S3861
Warfarin responsiveness, genetic technique, G9143
Thalassemia, genetic test
alpha, S3845
hemoglobin E beta, S3846
Thallous chloride TI 201, A9505
TheraGenesis, A2008
Therapeutic
agent, A4321
procedures, respiratory, G0239
Therapeutic radiopharmaceutical
sodium iodide I-131, A9530
Therapy
activity, G0176, H2032
beta-blocker, G9188-G9192
convulsive, G2000
infusion, Q0081
lymphedema, S8950
nutrition, reassessment, G0270-G0271
respiratory, G0237-G0239
transcatheter microinfusion, C9759
TheraSkin, Q4121
Therion, Q4176
Thermalator T-12-M, E0239
Thermometer
oral, A4931
rectal, A4932
Thickener, food, B4100
Thinning solvent, NuHope, 2 oz bottle, A4455
Thomas
heel wedge, foot orthotic, L3465, L3470
Thoracic-lumbar-sacral orthotic (TLSO)
flexible with trunk support, L0450-L0457
sagittal control, L0466-L0467
sagittal-coronal control, L0468-L0469, L0490-L0492
scoliosis, L1200-L1290
triplanar control, L0458-L0464, L0470-L0488
Threshold
current perception, G0255
Thumb-O-Prene Splint, L3999

Thymol turbidity, blood, P2033
Thyrotropin
alpha, J3240
Tibia
Specialist Tibial Pre-formed Fracture Brace, L2116
Toad finger splint, A4570
Ticarcillin disodium and clavulanate potassium, S0040
Tip (cane, crutch, walker) replacement, A4637
Tire, wheelchair, E2214, E2220
Tissue
connective
human, C1762
non-human, C1763
localization and excision device, C1819
marker, A4648
Tissue marker, A4648
TLSO, L0450-L0492, L1200-L1290
Tobramycin
inhalation solution, J7682, J7685
sulfate, J3260
unit dose, J7682
Toe
holder, E0952
Specialist Toe Insert for Specialist Closed-Back Cast Boot and Specialist Health/Post Operative Shoe, A9270
Toilet accessories, E0167-E0175, E0243, E0244, E0625
raised toilet seat, E0244
Combo-Seat Universal, E0244
Moore, E0244
Sure-Safe, E0244
seat lift, E0172
transfer bench, E0247, E0248
Toll, non-emergency transport, A0170
Tomosynthesis, diagnostic, G0279
Topical hyperbaric oxygen chamber, A4575
Topographic brain mapping, S8040
Toronto, Legg Perthes orthotic, L1700
Total hip resurfacing, S2118
Total Universal Buck's Boot, E0870
Tourniquet, for dialysis, A4929
TPN, home infusion therapy, S9364-S9368
Tracer blood glucose
meter, E0607
strips, box of 50, A4253
Tracer II Diabetes Care System, E0607
Tracer Wheelchairs, E1240, E1250, E1260, E1270, E1280, E1285, E1290, E1295
Tracheal suction catheter, A4624
Tracheoesophageal prosthesis supplies, L8511-L8514
Tracheostoma
adhesive disc, A7506
filter, A7504
filter holder, A7503, A7507, A7509
housing, A7505, A7508
replacement diaphragm, faceplate, A7502
valve, A7501
Tracheostomy
care kit, A4629
filter, A4481
mask, A7525
speaking valve, L8501
supplies, A4623-A4626, A4628, A4629, A7523-A7526, S8189
tube, A7520-A7522
Traction equipment, E0840-E0948
cervical equipment
not requiring frame, E0855
stand or frame, E0849
device
cervical, E0856
extremity, E0870, E0880
Total Universal Buck's Boot, E0870
head harness/halter, cervical, E0942
occipital-pull head halter, E0942
overdoor, cervical, E0860
Exo-Static, E0860
pelvic, E0890, E0900
Secure-All universal, belt, E0890
Training
child development, T1027
diabetes, G0108, G0109

Training — *continued*
home care, S5108-S5116
INR monitoring device, G0248
medication, H0034
skills, H2014
Tramacal, enteral nutrition, B4154
TranCyte, Q4182
Transbronchial ablation, C9751
Transcatheter
microinfusion therapy, C9759
NYHA IDE study
interatrial shunt implantation, C9760
Transcutaneous electrical nerve stimulator (TENS), E0720-E0749
distal nerve, K1023
trigeminal nerve, K1015-K1016
Transducer protector, dialysis, E1575
Transesophageal doppler, G9157
Transfer (shoe orthoses), L3600-L3640
Transfer board or device, E0705
Transfer system, E1036
Transfusion, blood products, at home, S9538
Transmitter
interstitial glucose monitor, A9277
Transmitting coil/cable, L8629
Transparent film (for dressing), A6257-A6259
Transplant
autologous chondrocyte, J7330
bone marrow, allogeneic, S2150
islet cell, G0341-G0343
islet cell tissue, allogeneic, S2102
lobar lung, S2060
multivisceral organs, S2054
pancreas/kidney, S2065
renal, documentation, G9231
small intestine and liver allografts, S2053
stem cell, S2142
Transport chair, E1037-E1038
heavy weight, E1039
Transportation
ambulance, A0021-A0999
corneal tissue, V2785
EKG (portable), R0076
extra attendant, A0424
handicapped, A0130
nonemergency, A0080-A0210, T2001-T2005, T2049
mileage, S0215
parking fees, A0170
service, including ambulance, A0021-A0999
taxi, nonemergency, A0100
toll, nonemergency, A0170
volunteer, nonemergency, A0080, A0090
waiting time, T2007
x-ray (portable), R0070, R0075
TranZgraft, Q4126
Trapeze bar, E0910-E0912, E0940
Trauma response team, G0390
Traum-aid, enteral nutrition, B4154
Travasorb, enteral nutrition, B4150
Hepatic, B4154
HN, B4153
MCT, B4154
Renal, B4154
Travel allowance, P9603-P9604
Traveler manual wheelchair, K0001
Tray
insertion, A4310-A4316, A4354
irrigation, A4320
surgical (*see also* kits), A4550
wheelchair, E0950
Treatment
fracture
pelvic bone, G0412-G0415
nursing facility acute care, G9679-G9684
outpatient IV insulin, G9147
Treatment planning and care coordination
cancer, S0353-S0354
comprehensive, advanced illness, S0311
Trifocal, glass or plastic, V2300-V2399
Trim nails, G0127
Truform prosthetic shrinker, L8440-L8465
TruSkin, Q4167
Truss, L8300-L8330
Tub
transfer bench, E0247-E0248

Tube/Tubing
anchoring device, A5200
blood, A4750, A4755
chest
drain valve, A7040
drainage container, A7041
CPAP device, A7037
gastrostomy/jejunostomy, B4087-B4088
irrigation, A4355
microcapillary, calibrated, A4651
sealant, A4652
nasogastric, B4081, B4082
oxygen, A4616
serum clotting time, A4771
stomach, B4083
suction pump, each, A7002
tire, E2212-E2213, E2215
tracheostomy or laryngotomy plug, A7527
urinary drainage, A4331
with integrated heating element, A4604
Tumor
destruction
embolization, S2095
infiltrating lymphocyte therapy, S2107
Turtle Neck safety collars, E0942

U

Ulcers
electromagnetic therapy, G0329
Ultra Blood Glucose
monitor, E0607
test strips, box of 50, A4253
UltraCare vest-style body holder, E0700
Ultrafast computed tomography, S8092
Ultrafine disposable insulin syringes, per syringe, A4206
Ultralightweight wheelchair, K0005
Ultrasound
ablation, C9734
uterine, C9734
aerosol generator, E0574
guidance
multifetal pregnancy reduction, S8055
radiation therapy field placement, G6001
paranasal sinus, S9024
therapeutic intervention, C9734
Ultraviolet light-therapy
bulb, A4633
cabinet, E0691-E0694
system panel, E0691-E0693
Underpads, disposable, A4554
Unilet lancet device, A4258
Unipuncture control system, dialysis, E1580
Unistik lancet device, A4258
Universal
remover for adhesives, A4455
socket insert
above knee, L5694
below knee, L5690
telescoping versarail bed rail, E0310
Up-Draft Neb-U-Mist, E0580
Upper extremity addition, locking elbow, L6693
Upper extremity fracture orthotic, L3980-L3999
Upper limb prosthesis, L6000-L7499
Ureteroscopy
for ureteral calculi, S2070
Urethral clamp/compression device, A4360
Urethral insert, A4336
Urgent care, S9088
global fee, S9083
Urinal, E0325, E0326
Urinary
catheter, A4338-A4346, A4351-A4353
catheter irrigation, A4321
collection and retention (supplies), A4310-A4358
incontinence repair device, C1771, C2631
incontinence supplies, A4310-A4421, A4423-A4434, A5051-A5093, A5102-A5114, A5120-A5200
leg bag, A5105, A5112
tract implant, collagen, L8603

Index

Urine — Wound

Wound — *continued*
  therapy
    negative pressure
      supplies, A6550
Wound matrix, A2001-A2010, Q4100-Q4255
WoundEx, Q4163
WoundEx Flow, Q4162
WoundFix, WoundFix Plus, WoundFix Xplus, Q4217
Wrap
  abdominal aneurysm, M0301

Wrap — *continued*
  cold/heat, A9273
  compression, A6545
Wrist
  brace, cock-up, L3908
  disarticulation prosthesis, L6050, L6055
  hand/finger orthotic (WHFO), E1805, E1825, L3806-L3808
  Specialist Pre-Formed Ulnar Fracture Brace, L3982

X

Xcaliber power wheelchair, K0014
XCellerate, Q4234
XCelliStem, A2004
XCM Biologic Tissue Matrix, Q4142
Xenon Xe-133, A9558
X-ray
  equipment
    portable, Q0092, R0070, R0075
XWRAP, Q4204

Y

Y set tubing for peritoneal dialysis, A4719
Yttrium 90
  ibritumomab tiuxeton, A9543
  microsphere
    brachytherapy, C2616
    procedure, S2095

Z

ZIFT, S4014

Transportation Services Including Ambulance A0021-A0999

This code range includes ground and air ambulance, nonemergency transportation (taxi, bus, automobile, wheelchair van), and ancillary transportation-related fees.

HCPCS Level II codes for ambulance services must be reported with modifiers that indicate pick-up origins and destinations. The modifier describing the arrangement (QM, QN) is listed first. The modifiers describing the origin and destination are listed second. Origin and destination modifiers are created by combining two alpha characters from the following list. Each alpha character, with the exception of X, represents either an origin or a destination. Each pair of alpha characters creates one modifier. The first position represents the origin and the second the destination. The modifiers most commonly used are:

D	Diagnostic or therapeutic site other than "P" or "H" when these are used as origin codes
E	Residential, domiciliary, custodial facility (other than 1819 facility)
G	Hospital-based ESRD facility
H	Hospital
I	Site of transfer (e.g., airport or helicopter pad) between modes of ambulance transport
J	Free standing ESRD facility
N	Skilled nursing facility (SNF)
P	Physician's office
R	Residence
S	Scene of accident or acute event
X	Intermediate stop at physician's office on way to hospital (destination code only)

Note: Modifier X can only be used as a destination code in the second position of a modifier. See S0215. For Medicaid, see T codes and T modifiers.

Ambulance Transport and Supplies

A0021 Ambulance service, outside state per mile, transport (Medicaid only) E
CMS: 100-04,15,20.4

A0080 Nonemergency transportation, per mile - vehicle provided by volunteer (individual or organization), with no vested interest E
CMS: 100-04,15,20.4

A0090 Nonemergency transportation, per mile - vehicle provided by individual (family member, self, neighbor) with vested interest E
CMS: 100-04,15,20.4

A0100 Nonemergency transportation; taxi E
CMS: 100-04,15,20.4

A0110 Nonemergency transportation and bus, intra- or interstate carrier E
CMS: 100-04,15,20.4

A0120 Nonemergency transportation: mini-bus, mountain area transports, or other transportation systems E
CMS: 100-04,15,20.4

A0130 Nonemergency transportation: wheelchair van E
CMS: 100-04,15,20.4

A0140 Nonemergency transportation and air travel (private or commercial) intra- or interstate E
CMS: 100-04,15,20.4

A0160 Nonemergency transportation: per mile - caseworker or social worker E
CMS: 100-04,15,20.4

A0170 Transportation ancillary: parking fees, tolls, other E
CMS: 100-04,15,20.4

A0180 Nonemergency transportation: ancillary: lodging-recipient E
CMS: 100-04,15,20.4

A0190 Nonemergency transportation: ancillary: meals, recipient E
CMS: 100-04,15,20.4

A0200 Nonemergency transportation: ancillary: lodging, escort E
CMS: 100-04,15,20.4

A0210 Nonemergency transportation: ancillary: meals, escort E
CMS: 100-04,15,20.4

A0225 Ambulance service, neonatal transport, base rate, emergency transport, one way E
CMS: 100-02,10,10.1.2; 100-02,10,10.2.1; 100-02,10,30.1; 100-02,10,30.1.1; 100-04,15,20.4

A0380 BLS mileage (per mile) E ☑
See code(s): A0425
CMS: 100-02,10,10.1.2; 100-02,10,10.2.1; 100-02,10,10.3.3; 100-02,10,30.1; 100-02,10,30.1.1; 100-04,15,20.4; 100-04,15,30.2

A0382 BLS routine disposable supplies E
CMS: 100-02,10,10.1.2; 100-02,10,10.2.1; 100-02,10,30.1; 100-02,10,30.1.1; 100-04,15,20.4

A0384 BLS specialized service disposable supplies; defibrillation (used by ALS ambulances and BLS ambulances in jurisdictions where defibrillation is permitted in BLS ambulances) E
CMS: 100-02,10,10.1.2; 100-02,10,10.2.1; 100-02,10,30.1; 100-02,10,30.1.1; 100-04,15,20.4

A0390 ALS mileage (per mile) E ☑
See code(s): A0425
CMS: 100-02,10,10.1.2; 100-02,10,10.2.1; 100-02,10,10.3.3; 100-02,10,30.1; 100-02,10,30.1.1; 100-04,15,20.4; 100-04,15,30.2

A0392 ALS specialized service disposable supplies; defibrillation (to be used only in jurisdictions where defibrillation cannot be performed in BLS ambulances) E
CMS: 100-02,10,10.1.2; 100-02,10,10.2.1; 100-02,10,30.1; 100-02,10,30.1.1; 100-04,15,20.4

A0394 ALS specialized service disposable supplies; IV drug therapy E
CMS: 100-02,10,10.1.2; 100-02,10,10.2.1; 100-02,10,30.1; 100-02,10,30.1.1; 100-04,15,20.4

A0396 ALS specialized service disposable supplies; esophageal intubation E
CMS: 100-02,10,10.1.2; 100-02,10,10.2.1; 100-02,10,30.1; 100-02,10,30.1.1; 100-04,15,20.4

A0398 ALS routine disposable supplies E
CMS: 100-02,10,10.1.2; 100-02,10,10.2.1; 100-02,10,30.1; 100-02,10,30.1.1; 100-04,15,20.4

Waiting Time

Units	Time
1	1/2 to 1 hr.
2	1 to 1-1/2 hrs.
3	1-1/2 to 2 hrs.
4	2 to 2-1/2 hrs.
5	2-1/2 to 3 hrs.
6	3 to 3-1/2 hrs.
7	3-1/2 to 4 hrs.
8	4 to 4-1/2 hrs.
9	4-1/2 to 5 hrs.
10	5 to 5-1/2 hrs.

A0420 Ambulance waiting time (ALS or BLS), one-half (1/2) hour increments E
CMS: 100-02,10,10.1.2; 100-02,10,10.2.1; 100-02,10,30.1; 100-02,10,30.1.1; 100-04,15,20.4

Special Coverage Instructions   Noncovered by Medicare   Carrier Discretion   ☑ Quantity Alert   ● New Code   ○ Recycled/Reinstated   ▲ Revised Code

Medical and Surgical Supplies

A0422 — A2009

Other Ambulance Services

A0422 **Ambulance (ALS or BLS) oxygen and oxygen supplies, life sustaining situation** E
CMS: 100-02,10,10.1.2; 100-02,10,10.2.1; 100-02,10,30.1; 100-02,10,30.1.1; 100-04,15,20.4

A0424 **Extra ambulance attendant, ground (ALS or BLS) or air (fixed or rotary winged); (requires medical review)** E
Pertinent documentation to evaluate medical appropriateness should be included when this code is reported.
CMS: 100-02,10,10.1.2; 100-02,10,10.2.1; 100-02,10,30.1; 100-02,10,30.1.1; 100-04,15,20.4; 100-04,15,30.2.1

A0425 **Ground mileage, per statute mile** A ☑
CMS: 100-02,10,10.1.2; 100-02,10,10.2.1; 100-02,10,10.2.2; 100-02,10,10.3.3; 100-02,10,20; 100-02,10,30.1; 100-02,10,30.1.1; 100-02,10.20; 100-04,15,10.3; 100-04,15,20.1.4; 100-04,15,20.4; 100-04,15,20.6; 100-04,15,30; 100-04,15,30.1.2; 100-04,15,30.2.1; 100-04,15,40
AHA: 4Q, '12, 1

A0426 **Ambulance service, advanced life support, nonemergency transport, level 1 (ALS 1)** A
CMS: 100-02,10,10.1.2; 100-02,10,10.2.1; 100-02,10,10.2.2; 100-02,10,10.3.3; 100-02,10,20; 100-02,10,30.1; 100-02,10,30.1.1; 100-02,10.20; 100-04,15,10.3; 100-04,15,20.1.4; 100-04,15,20.4; 100-04,15,30; 100-04,15,30.1.2; 100-04,15,30.2; 100-04,15,30.2.1; 100-04,15,40
AHA: 4Q, '12, 1

A0427 **Ambulance service, advanced life support, emergency transport, level 1 (ALS 1 - emergency)** A
CMS: 100-02,10,10.1.2; 100-02,10,10.2.1; 100-02,10,10.2.2; 100-02,10,10.3.3; 100-02,10,20; 100-02,10,30.1; 100-02,10,30.1.1; 100-02,10.20; 100-04,15,10.3; 100-04,15,20.1.4; 100-04,15,20.4; 100-04,15,30; 100-04,15,30.1.2; 100-04,15,30.2; 100-04,15,30.2.1; 100-04,15,40
AHA: 4Q, '12, 1

A0428 **Ambulance service, basic life support, nonemergency transport, (BLS)** A
CMS: 100-02,10,10.1.2; 100-02,10,10.2.1; 100-02,10,10.2.2; 100-02,10,10.3.3; 100-02,10,20; 100-02,10,30.1; 100-02,10,30.1.1; 100-02,10.20; 100-04,15,10.3; 100-04,15,20.1.4; 100-04,15,20.4; 100-04,15,20.6; 100-04,15,30; 100-04,15,30.1.2; 100-04,15,30.2; 100-04,15,30.2.1; 100-04,15,40
AHA: 4Q, '12, 1

A0429 **Ambulance service, basic life support, emergency transport (BLS, emergency)** A
CMS: 100-02,10,10.1.2; 100-02,10,10.2.1; 100-02,10,10.2.2; 100-02,10,10.3.3; 100-02,10,20; 100-02,10,30.1; 100-02,10,30.1.1; 100-02,10.20; 100-04,15,10.3; 100-04,15,20.1.4; 100-04,15,20.4; 100-04,15,30; 100-04,15,30.1.2; 100-04,15,30.2; 100-04,15,30.2.1; 100-04,15,40
AHA: 4Q, '12, 1

A0430 **Ambulance service, conventional air services, transport, one way (fixed wing)** A
CMS: 100-02,10,10.1.2; 100-02,10,10.2.1; 100-02,10,10.2.2; 100-02,10,10.3.3; 100-02,10,20; 100-02,10,30.1; 100-02,10,30.1.1; 100-02,10.20; 100-04,15,10.3; 100-04,15,20.1.4; 100-04,15,20.3; 100-04,15,20.4; 100-04,15,30; 100-04,15,30.1.2; 100-04,15,30.2; 100-04,15,30.2.1; 100-04,15,40
AHA: 4Q, '12, 1

A0431 **Ambulance service, conventional air services, transport, one way (rotary wing)** A
CMS: 100-02,10,10.1.2; 100-02,10,10.2.1; 100-02,10,10.2.2; 100-02,10,10.3.3; 100-02,10,20; 100-02,10,30.1; 100-02,10,30.1.1; 100-02,10.20; 100-04,15,10.3; 100-04,15,20.1.4; 100-04,15,20.3; 100-04,15,20.4; 100-04,15,30; 100-04,15,30.1.2; 100-04,15,30.2; 100-04,15,30.2.1; 100-04,15,40
AHA: 4Q, '12, 1

A0432 **Paramedic intercept (PI), rural area, transport furnished by a volunteer ambulance company which is prohibited by state law from billing third-party payers** A
CMS: 100-02,10,10.1.2; 100-02,10,10.2.1; 100-02,10,10.2.2; 100-02,10,10.3.3; 100-02,10,20; 100-02,10,30.1; 100-02,10,30.1.1; 100-02,10.20; 100-04,15,10.3; 100-04,15,20.1.4; 100-04,15,20.4; 100-04,15,30; 100-04,15,30.1.2; 100-04,15,30.2; 100-04,15,30.2.1; 100-04,15,40
AHA: 4Q, '12, 1

A0433 **Advanced life support, level 2 (ALS 2)** A
CMS: 100-02,10,10.1.2; 100-02,10,10.2.1; 100-02,10,10.2.2; 100-02,10,10.3.3; 100-02,10,20; 100-02,10,30.1; 100-02,10,30.1.1; 100-02,10.20; 100-04,15,10.3; 100-04,15,20.1.4; 100-04,15,20.4; 100-04,15,30; 100-04,15,30.1.2; 100-04,15,30.2; 100-04,15,30.2.1; 100-04,15,40
AHA: 4Q, '12, 1

A0434 **Specialty care transport (SCT)** A
CMS: 100-02,10,10.1.2; 100-02,10,10.2.1; 100-02,10,10.2.2; 100-02,10,10.3.3; 100-02,10,20; 100-02,10,30.1; 100-02,10,30.1.1; 100-02,10.20; 100-04,15,10.3; 100-04,15,20.1.4; 100-04,15,20.4; 100-04,15,30; 100-04,15,30.1.2; 100-04,15,30.2; 100-04,15,30.2.1; 100-04,15,40
AHA: 4Q, '12, 1

A0435 **Fixed wing air mileage, per statute mile** A
CMS: 100-02,10,10.1.2; 100-02,10,10.2.1; 100-02,10,10.2.2; 100-02,10,10.3.3; 100-02,10,20; 100-02,10,30.1; 100-02,10,30.1.1; 100-02,10.20; 100-04,15,10.3; 100-04,15,20.1.4; 100-04,15,20.3; 100-04,15,20.4; 100-04,15,30; 100-04,15,30.1.2; 100-04,15,30.2; 100-04,15,30.2.1; 100-04,15,40
AHA: 4Q, '12, 1

A0436 **Rotary wing air mileage, per statute mile** A
CMS: 100-02,10,10.1.2; 100-02,10,10.2.1; 100-02,10,10.2.2; 100-02,10,10.3.3; 100-02,10,20; 100-02,10,30.1; 100-02,10,30.1.1; 100-02,10.20; 100-04,15,10.3; 100-04,15,20.1.4; 100-04,15,20.3; 100-04,15,20.4; 100-04,15,30; 100-04,15,30.1.2; 100-04,15,30.2; 100-04,15,30.2.1; 100-04,15,40
AHA: 4Q, '12, 1

A0888 **Noncovered ambulance mileage, per mile (e.g., for miles traveled beyond closest appropriate facility)** E
CMS: 100-02,10,10.1.2; 100-02,10,10.2.1; 100-02,10,20; 100-02,10,30.1; 100-02,10,30.1.1; 100-04,15,20.4; 100-04,15,30.1.2; 100-04,15,30.2.4

A0998 **Ambulance response and treatment, no transport** E
CMS: 100-02,10,10.1.2; 100-02,10,10.2.1; 100-02,10,30.1; 100-02,10,30.1.1; 100-04,15,20.4

A0999 **Unlisted ambulance service** A
CMS: 100-02,10,10.1; 100-02,10,10.1.2; 100-02,10,10.2.1; 100-02,10,20; 100-02,10,30.1; 100-02,10,30.1.1; 100-04,15,20.4

Medical and Surgical Supplies A2001-A9999

This section covers a wide variety of medical, surgical, and some durable medical equipment (DME) related supplies and accessories. DME-related supplies, accessories, maintenance, and repair required to ensure the proper functioning of this equipment is generally covered by Medicare under the prosthetic devices provision.

Skin Substitutes

● **A2001** **InnovaMatrix AC, per sq cm**

● **A2002** **Mirragen Advanced Wound Matrix, per sq cm**

● **A2003** **bio-ConneKt Wound Matrix, per sq cm**

● **A2004** **XCelliStem, per sq cm**

● **A2005** **Microlyte Matrix, per sq cm**

● **A2006** **NovoSorb SynPath dermal matrix, per sq cm**

● **A2007** **Restrata, per sq cm**

● **A2008** **TheraGenesis, per sq cm**

● **A2009** **Symphony, per sq cm**

Special Coverage Instructions   Noncovered by Medicare   Carrier Discretion   ☑ Quantity Alert ● New Code   ○ Recycled/Reinstated   ▲ Revised Code

2 — A Codes   A Age Edit   M Maternity Edit   ♀ Female Only   ♂ Male Only   A-Y OPPS Status Indicators   © 2021 Optum360, LLC

● **A2010**   Apis, per sq cm

Injection Supplies

A4206   Syringe with needle, sterile, 1 cc or less, each   N ☑

A4207   Syringe with needle, sterile 2 cc, each   N ☑

A4208   Syringe with needle, sterile 3 cc, each   N ☑

A4209   Syringe with needle, sterile 5 cc or greater, each   N ☑

A4210   Needle-free injection device, each   E ☑
Sometimes covered by commercial payers with preauthorization and physician letter stating need (e.g., for insulin injection in young children).

A4211   Supplies for self-administered injections   N
When a drug that is usually injected by the patient (e.g., insulin or calcitonin) is injected by the physician, it is excluded from Medicare coverage unless administered in an emergency situation (e.g., diabetic coma).

A4212   Noncoring needle or stylet with or without catheter   N

A4213   Syringe, sterile, 20 cc or greater, each   N ☑

A4215   Needle, sterile, any size, each   N

A4216   Sterile water, saline and/or dextrose, diluent/flush, 10 ml   N ☑ ⅋

A4217   Sterile water/saline, 500 ml   N ☑ ⅋ (AU)
CMS: 100-04,20,30.9

A4218   Sterile saline or water, metered dose dispenser, 10 ml   N ☑

A4220   Refill kit for implantable infusion pump   N

A4221   Supplies for maintenance of noninsulin drug infusion catheter, per week (list drugs separately)   N ⅋

A4222   Infusion supplies for external drug infusion pump, per cassette or bag (list drugs separately)   N ⅋

A4223   Infusion supplies not used with external infusion pump, per cassette or bag (list drugs separately)   N ☑

A4224   Supplies for maintenance of insulin infusion catheter, per week   N ⅋

A4225   Supplies for external insulin infusion pump, syringe type cartridge, sterile, each   N ⅋

A4226   Supplies for maintenance of insulin infusion pump with dosage rate adjustment using therapeutic continuous glucose sensing, per week

A4230   Infusion set for external insulin pump, nonneedle cannula type   N ☑
Covered by some commercial payers as ongoing supply to preauthorized pump.

A4231   Infusion set for external insulin pump, needle type   N ☑
Covered by some commercial payers as ongoing supply to preauthorized pump.

A4232   Syringe with needle for external insulin pump, sterile, 3 cc   E ☑
Covered by some commercial payers as ongoing supply to preauthorized pump.

Batteries

A4233   Replacement battery, alkaline (other than J cell), for use with medically necessary home blood glucose monitor owned by patient, each   E ☑ ⅋ (NU)

A4234   Replacement battery, alkaline, J cell, for use with medically necessary home blood glucose monitor owned by patient, each   E ☑ ⅋ (NU)

A4235   Replacement battery, lithium, for use with medically necessary home blood glucose monitor owned by patient, each   E ☑ ⅋ (NU)

A4236   Replacement battery, silver oxide, for use with medically necessary home blood glucose monitor owned by patient, each   E ☑ ⅋ (NU)

Other Supplies

A4244   Alcohol or peroxide, per pint   N ☑

A4245   Alcohol wipes, per box   N ☑

A4246   Betadine or pHisoHex solution, per pint   N ☑

A4247   Betadine or iodine swabs/wipes, per box   N ☑

A4248   Chlorhexidine containing antiseptic, 1 ml   N ☑

A4250   Urine test or reagent strips or tablets (100 tablets or strips)   E ☑
CMS: 100-02,15,110

Dipstick urinalysis: The strip is dipped and color-coded squares are read at timed intervals (e.g., pH immediately; ketones at 15 seconds, etc.). Results are compared against a reference chart

A4252   Blood ketone test or reagent strip, each   E ☑

A4253   Blood glucose test or reagent strips for home blood glucose monitor, per 50 strips   N ☑ ⅋ (NU)
Medicare covers glucose strips for diabetic patients using home glucose monitoring devices prescribed by their physicians.

A4255   Platforms for home blood glucose monitor, 50 per box   N ☑ ⅋
Some Medicare contractors cover monitor platforms for diabetic patients using home glucose monitoring devices prescribed by their physicians. Some commercial payers also provide this coverage to noninsulin dependent diabetics.

A4256   Normal, low, and high calibrator solution/chips   N ⅋
Some Medicare contractors cover calibration solutions or chips for diabetic patients using home glucose monitoring devices prescribed by their physicians. Some commercial payers also provide this coverage to noninsulin dependent diabetics.

A4257   Replacement lens shield cartridge for use with laser skin piercing device, each   E ☑ ⅋
AHA: 1Q, '02, 5

A4258   Spring-powered device for lancet, each   N ☑ ⅋
Some Medicare contractors cover lancing devices for diabetic patients using home glucose monitoring devices prescribed by their physicians. Medicare jurisdiction: DME regional contractor. Some commercial payers also provide this coverage to noninsulin dependent diabetics.

A4259   Lancets, per box of 100   N ☑ ⅋
Medicare covers lancets for diabetic patients using home glucose monitoring devices prescribed by their physicians. Medicare jurisdiction: DME regional contractor. Some commercial payers also provide this coverage to noninsulin dependent diabetics.

Special Coverage Instructions   Noncovered by Medicare   Carrier Discretion   ☑ Quantity Alert   ● New Code   ○ Recycled/Reinstated   ▲ Revised Code

© 2021 Optum360, LLC   A2-Z3 ASC Pmt   CMS: IOM   AHA: Coding Clinic   ⅋ DMEPOS Paid   ⊘ SNF Excluded   A Codes — 3

Medical and Surgical Supplies

A4261 — A4314

Code	Description	
A4261	Cervical cap for contraceptive use	M ♀ E
A4262	Temporary, absorbable lacrimal duct implant, each	N ☑
	Always report concurrent to the implant procedure.	
A4263	Permanent, long-term, nondissolvable lacrimal duct implant, each	N ☑
	Always report concurrent to the implant procedure.	
A4264	Permanent implantable contraceptive intratubal occlusion device(s) and delivery system	M ♀ E ☑
A4265	Paraffin, per pound	N ☑ ♿
A4266	Diaphragm for contraceptive use	M ♀ E
A4267	Contraceptive supply, condom, male, each	♂ E ☑
A4268	Contraceptive supply, condom, female, each	M ♀ E ☑
A4269	Contraceptive supply, spermicide (e.g., foam, gel), each	M ♀ E ☑
A4270	Disposable endoscope sheath, each	N ☑
A4280	Adhesive skin support attachment for use with external breast prosthesis, each	N ☑ ♿

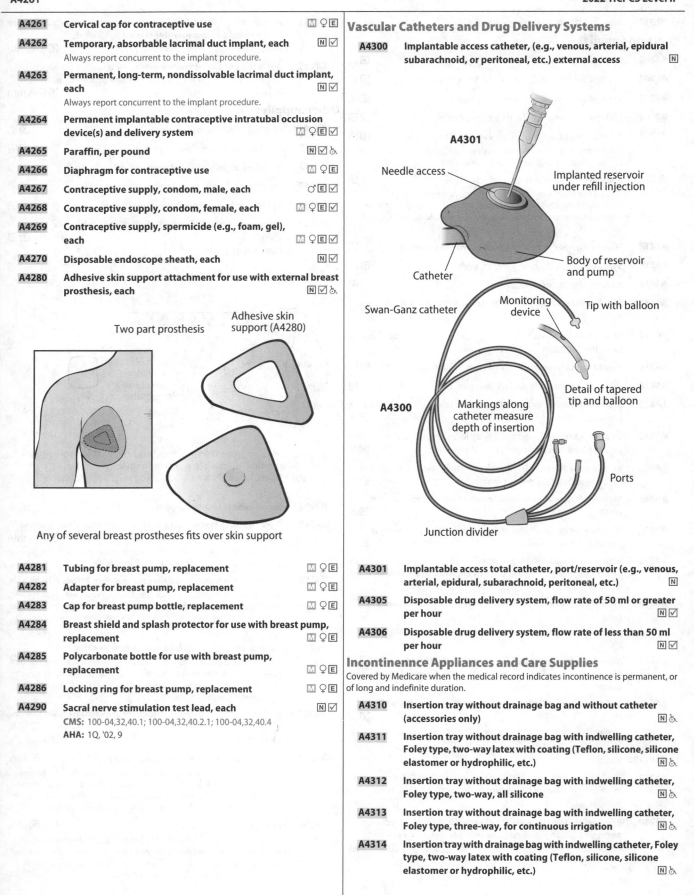

Two part prosthesis

Adhesive skin support (A4280)

Any of several breast prostheses fits over skin support

Code	Description	
A4281	Tubing for breast pump, replacement	M ♀ E
A4282	Adapter for breast pump, replacement	M ♀ E
A4283	Cap for breast pump bottle, replacement	M ♀ E
A4284	Breast shield and splash protector for use with breast pump, replacement	M ♀ E
A4285	Polycarbonate bottle for use with breast pump, replacement	M ♀ E
A4286	Locking ring for breast pump, replacement	M ♀ E
A4290	Sacral nerve stimulation test lead, each	N ☑
	CMS: 100-04,32,40.1; 100-04,32,40.2.1; 100-04,32,40.4	
	AHA: 1Q, '02, 9	

Vascular Catheters and Drug Delivery Systems

Code	Description	
A4300	Implantable access catheter, (e.g., venous, arterial, epidural subarachnoid, or peritoneal, etc.) external access	N

A4301

Needle access — Implanted reservoir under refill injection

Catheter — Body of reservoir and pump

Swan-Ganz catheter — Monitoring device — Tip with balloon

Detail of tapered tip and balloon

A4300 — Markings along catheter measure depth of insertion

Ports

Junction divider

Code	Description	
A4301	Implantable access total catheter, port/reservoir (e.g., venous, arterial, epidural, subarachnoid, peritoneal, etc.)	N
A4305	Disposable drug delivery system, flow rate of 50 ml or greater per hour	N ☑
A4306	Disposable drug delivery system, flow rate of less than 50 ml per hour	N ☑

Incontinennce Appliances and Care Supplies

Covered by Medicare when the medical record indicates incontinence is permanent, or of long and indefinite duration.

Code	Description	
A4310	Insertion tray without drainage bag and without catheter (accessories only)	N ♿
A4311	Insertion tray without drainage bag with indwelling catheter, Foley type, two-way latex with coating (Teflon, silicone, silicone elastomer or hydrophilic, etc.)	N ♿
A4312	Insertion tray without drainage bag with indwelling catheter, Foley type, two-way, all silicone	N ♿
A4313	Insertion tray without drainage bag with indwelling catheter, Foley type, three-way, for continuous irrigation	N ♿
A4314	Insertion tray with drainage bag with indwelling catheter, Foley type, two-way latex with coating (Teflon, silicone, silicone elastomer or hydrophilic, etc.)	N ♿

Special Coverage Instructions   Noncovered by Medicare   Carrier Discretion   ☑ Quantity Alert   ● New Code   ○ Recycled/Reinstated   ▲ Revised Code

A4315	Insertion tray with drainage bag with indwelling catheter, Foley type, two-way, all silicone N &
A4316	Insertion tray with drainage bag with indwelling catheter, Foley type, three-way, for continuous irrigation N &
A4320	Irrigation tray with bulb or piston syringe, any purpose N &
A4321	Therapeutic agent for urinary catheter irrigation N &
A4322	Irrigation syringe, bulb or piston, each N ☑ &
A4326	Male external catheter with integral collection chamber, any type, each ♂ N ☑ &
A4327	Female external urinary collection device; meatal cup, each ♀ N ☑ &
A4328	Female external urinary collection device; pouch, each A ♀ N ☑ &
A4330	Perianal fecal collection pouch with adhesive, each N ☑ &
A4331	Extension drainage tubing, any type, any length, with connector/adaptor, for use with urinary leg bag or urostomy pouch, each N ☑ &
A4332	Lubricant, individual sterile packet, each N ☑ &
A4333	Urinary catheter anchoring device, adhesive skin attachment, each N ☑ &
A4334	Urinary catheter anchoring device, leg strap, each N ☑ &
A4335	Incontinence supply; miscellaneous N
A4336	Incontinence supply, urethral insert, any type, each N ☑ &
A4337	Incontinence supply, rectal insert, any type, each N
A4338	Indwelling catheter; Foley type, two-way latex with coating (Teflon, silicone, silicone elastomer, or hydrophilic, etc.), each N ☑ &
A4340	Indwelling catheter; specialty type, (e.g., Coude, mushroom, wing, etc.), each N ☑ &
A4344	Indwelling catheter, Foley type, two-way, all silicone, each N ☑ &
A4346	Indwelling catheter; Foley type, three-way for continuous irrigation, each N ☑ &
A4349	Male external catheter, with or without adhesive, disposable, each ♂ N ☑ &
A4351	Intermittent urinary catheter; straight tip, with or without coating (Teflon, silicone, silicone elastomer, or hydrophilic, etc.), each N &
A4352	Intermittent urinary catheter; Coude (curved) tip, with or without coating (Teflon, silicone, silicone elastomeric, or hydrophilic, etc.), each N ☑ &
A4353	Intermittent urinary catheter, with insertion supplies N &
A4354	Insertion tray with drainage bag but without catheter N &
A4355	Irrigation tubing set for continuous bladder irrigation through a three-way indwelling Foley catheter, each N ☑ &
A4356	External urethral clamp or compression device (not to be used for catheter clamp), each N ☑ &
A4357	Bedside drainage bag, day or night, with or without antireflux device, with or without tube, each N ☑ &
A4358	Urinary drainage bag, leg or abdomen, vinyl, with or without tube, with straps, each N ☑ &
A4360	Disposable external urethral clamp or compression device, with pad and/or pouch, each N ☑ &

Ostomy Supplies

A4361	Ostomy faceplate, each N ☑ &
A4362	Skin barrier; solid, 4 x 4 or equivalent; each N ☑ &
A4363	Ostomy clamp, any type, replacement only, each E &
A4364	Adhesive, liquid or equal, any type, per oz N ☑ &
A4366	Ostomy vent, any type, each N ☑ &
A4367	Ostomy belt, each N ☑ &
A4368	Ostomy filter, any type, each N ☑ &
A4369	Ostomy skin barrier, liquid (spray, brush, etc.), per oz N ☑ &
A4371	Ostomy skin barrier, powder, per oz N ☑ &
A4372	Ostomy skin barrier, solid 4 x 4 or equivalent, standard wear, with built-in convexity, each N ☑ &
A4373	Ostomy skin barrier, with flange (solid, flexible or accordion), with built-in convexity, any size, each N ☑ &

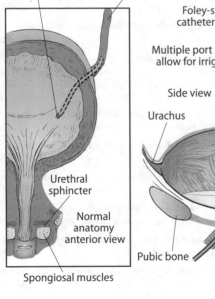

Ureteral orifice
Left ureter
Urethral sphincter
Normal anatomy anterior view
Spongiosal muscles

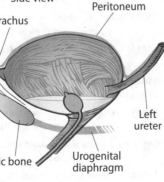

Foley-style indwelling catheter (A4344–A4346)

Multiple port indwelling catheters allow for irrigation and drainage

Side view
Urachus
Peritoneum
Left ureter
Pubic bone
Urogenital diaphragm

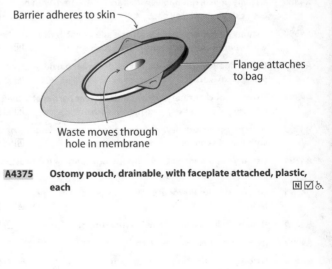

Faceplate flange and skin barrier combination (A4373)

Barrier adheres to skin
Flange attaches to bag
Waste moves through hole in membrane

A4375	Ostomy pouch, drainable, with faceplate attached, plastic, each N ☑ &

Medical and Surgical Supplies

A4376 — A4427

A4376 Ostomy pouch, drainable, with faceplate attached, rubber, each　N ☑ &

Colostomy pouch with faceplate and drain (A4376)

A4377 Ostomy pouch, drainable, for use on faceplate, plastic, each　N ☑ &

A4378 Ostomy pouch, drainable, for use on faceplate, rubber, each　N ☑ &

A4379 Ostomy pouch, urinary, with faceplate attached, plastic, each　N ☑ &

A4380 Ostomy pouch, urinary, with faceplate attached, rubber, each　N ☑ &

A4381 Ostomy pouch, urinary, for use on faceplate, plastic, each　N ☑ &

A4382 Ostomy pouch, urinary, for use on faceplate, heavy plastic, each　N ☑ &

A4383 Ostomy pouch, urinary, for use on faceplate, rubber, each　N ☑ &

A4384 Ostomy faceplate equivalent, silicone ring, each　N ☑ &

A4385 Ostomy skin barrier, solid 4 x 4 or equivalent, extended wear, without built-in convexity, each　N ☑ &

A4387 Ostomy pouch, closed, with barrier attached, with built-in convexity (one piece), each　N ☑ &

A4388 Ostomy pouch, drainable, with extended wear barrier attached, (one piece), each　N ☑ &

A4389 Ostomy pouch, drainable, with barrier attached, with built-in convexity (one piece), each　N ☑ &

A4390 Ostomy pouch, drainable, with extended wear barrier attached, with built-in convexity (one piece), each　N ☑ &

A4391 Ostomy pouch, urinary, with extended wear barrier attached (one piece), each　N ☑ &

A4392 Ostomy pouch, urinary, with standard wear barrier attached, with built-in convexity (one piece), each　N ☑ &

A4393 Ostomy pouch, urinary, with extended wear barrier attached, with built-in convexity (one piece), each　N ☑ &

A4394 Ostomy deodorant, with or without lubricant, for use in ostomy pouch, per fl oz　N ☑ &

A4395 Ostomy deodorant for use in ostomy pouch, solid, per tablet　N ☑ &

A4396 Ostomy belt with peristomal hernia support　N &

A4397 ~~Irrigation supply; sleeve, each~~

A4398 Ostomy irrigation supply; bag, each　N ☑ &

A4399 Ostomy irrigation supply; cone/catheter, with or without brush　N &

A4400 Ostomy irrigation set　N &

A4402 Lubricant, per oz　N ☑ &

A4404 Ostomy ring, each　N ☑ &

A4405 Ostomy skin barrier, nonpectin-based, paste, per oz　N ☑ &

A4406 Ostomy skin barrier, pectin-based, paste, per oz　N ☑ &

A4407 Ostomy skin barrier, with flange (solid, flexible, or accordion), extended wear, with built-in convexity, 4 x 4 in or smaller, each　N ☑ &

A4408 Ostomy skin barrier, with flange (solid, flexible or accordion), extended wear, with built-in convexity, larger than 4 x 4 in, each　N ☑ &

A4409 Ostomy skin barrier, with flange (solid, flexible or accordion), extended wear, without built-in convexity, 4 x 4 in or smaller, each　N ☑ &

A4410 Ostomy skin barrier, with flange (solid, flexible or accordion), extended wear, without built-in convexity, larger than 4 x 4 in, each　N ☑ &

A4411 Ostomy skin barrier, solid 4 x 4 or equivalent, extended wear, with built-in convexity, each　N ☑ &

A4412 Ostomy pouch, drainable, high output, for use on a barrier with flange (two-piece system), without filter, each　N ☑ &

A4413 Ostomy pouch, drainable, high output, for use on a barrier with flange (two-piece system), with filter, each　N ☑ &

A4414 Ostomy skin barrier, with flange (solid, flexible or accordion), without built-in convexity, 4 x 4 in or smaller, each　N ☑ &

A4415 Ostomy skin barrier, with flange (solid, flexible or accordion), without built-in convexity, larger than 4 x 4 in, each　N ☑ &

A4416 Ostomy pouch, closed, with barrier attached, with filter (one piece), each　N ☑ &

A4417 Ostomy pouch, closed, with barrier attached, with built-in convexity, with filter (one piece), each　N ☑ &

A4418 Ostomy pouch, closed; without barrier attached, with filter (one piece), each　N ☑ &

A4419 Ostomy pouch, closed; for use on barrier with nonlocking flange, with filter (two piece), each　N ☑ &

A4420 Ostomy pouch, closed; for use on barrier with locking flange (two piece), each　N ☑ &

A4421 Ostomy supply; miscellaneous　N

Determine if an alternative HCPCS Level II or a CPT code better describes the service being reported. This code should be used only if a more specific code is unavailable.

A4422 Ostomy absorbent material (sheet/pad/crystal packet) for use in ostomy pouch to thicken liquid stomal output, each　N ☑ &

A4423 Ostomy pouch, closed; for use on barrier with locking flange, with filter (two piece), each　N ☑ &

A4424 Ostomy pouch, drainable, with barrier attached, with filter (one piece), each　N ☑ &

A4425 Ostomy pouch, drainable; for use on barrier with nonlocking flange, with filter (two-piece system), each　N ☑ &

A4426 Ostomy pouch, drainable; for use on barrier with locking flange (two-piece system), each　N ☑ &

A4427 Ostomy pouch, drainable; for use on barrier with locking flange, with filter (two-piece system), each　N ☑ &

Special Coverage Instructions　　Noncovered by Medicare　　Carrier Discretion　　☑ Quantity Alert　● New Code　○ Recycled/Reinstated　▲ Revised Code

6 — A Codes　　　Ⓐ Age Edit　　Ⓜ Maternity Edit　　♀ Female Only　　♂ Male Only　　Ⓐ-Ⓨ OPPS Status Indicators　　© 2021 Optum360, LLC

A4428	Ostomy pouch, urinary, with extended wear barrier attached, with faucet-type tap with valve (one piece), each	N ✎ &
A4429	Ostomy pouch, urinary, with barrier attached, with built-in convexity, with faucet-type tap with valve (one piece), each	N ☑ &
A4430	Ostomy pouch, urinary, with extended wear barrier attached, with built-in convexity, with faucet-type tap with valve (one piece), each	N ☑ &
A4431	Ostomy pouch, urinary; with barrier attached, with faucet-type tap with valve (one piece), each	N ☑ &
A4432	Ostomy pouch, urinary; for use on barrier with nonlocking flange, with faucet-type tap with valve (two piece), each	N ☑ &
A4433	Ostomy pouch, urinary; for use on barrier with locking flange (two piece), each	N ☑ &
A4434	Ostomy pouch, urinary; for use on barrier with locking flange, with faucet-type tap with valve (two piece), each	N ☑ &
A4435	Ostomy pouch, drainable, high output, with extended wear barrier (one-piece system), with or without filter, each	N &
● A4436	Irrigation supply; sleeve, reusable, per month	
● A4437	Irrigation supply; sleeve, disposable, per month	

Miscellaneous Supplies

A4450	Tape, nonwaterproof, per 18 sq in	N ☑ & (AU, AV, AW)
	See also code A4452.	
	CMS: 100-04,20,30.9	
A4452	Tape, waterproof, per 18 sq in	N ☑ & (AU, AV, AW)
	See also code A4450.	
	CMS: 100-04,20,30.9	
○ A4453	Rectal catheter for use with the manual pump-operated enema system, replacement only	
A4455	Adhesive remover or solvent (for tape, cement or other adhesive), per oz	N ☑ &
A4456	Adhesive remover, wipes, any type, each	N ☑ &
A4458	Enema bag with tubing, reusable	N
A4459	Manual pump-operated enema system, includes balloon, catheter and all accessories, reusable, any type	N
A4461	Surgical dressing holder, nonreusable, each	N ☑ &
A4463	Surgical dressing holder, reusable, each	N ☑ &
A4465	Nonelastic binder for extremity	N
A4467	Belt, strap, sleeve, garment, or covering, any type	E
A4470	Gravlee jet washer	N
A4480	VABRA aspirator	♀ N
	CMS: 100-03,230.6; 100-03,240.4	
A4481	Tracheostoma filter, any type, any size, each	N ☑ &
A4483	Moisture exchanger, disposable, for use with invasive mechanical ventilation	N &
A4490	Surgical stockings above knee length, each	E ☑
	CMS: 100-02,15,110	
A4495	Surgical stockings thigh length, each	E ☑
	CMS: 100-02,15,110	
A4500	Surgical stockings below knee length, each	E ☑
	CMS: 100-02,15,110	
A4510	Surgical stockings full-length, each	E ☑
	CMS: 100-02,15,110	

A4520	Incontinence garment, any type, (e.g., brief, diaper), each	E ☑
A4550	Surgical trays	B
A4553	Nondisposable underpads, all sizes	E
A4554	Disposable underpads, all sizes	E ☑
A4555	Electrode/transducer for use with electrical stimulation device used for cancer treatment, replacement only	E
A4556	Electrodes (e.g., apnea monitor), per pair	N ☑ &
	If service is not separately payable, or incident to a physician's service, bill through the local carrier. If other, bill the DME MAC.	
	Some payers only cover apnea monitors for newborn or pediatric use. Review specific carrier policy for apnea monitors and supplies.	
A4557	Lead wires (e.g., apnea monitor), per pair	N ☑ &
	If service is not separately payable, or incident to a physician's service, bill through the local carrier. If other, bill the DME MAC.	
	Some payers only cover apnea monitors for newborn or pediatric use. Review specific carrier policy for apnea monitors and supplies.	
A4558	Conductive gel or paste, for use with electrical device (e.g., TENS, NMES), per oz	N ☑ &
A4559	Coupling gel or paste, for use with ultrasound device, per oz	N ☑ &
A4561	Pessary, rubber, any type	♀ N &
A4562	Pessary, nonrubber, any type	♀ N &
	Medicare jurisdiction: DME regional contractor.	
A4563	Rectal control system for vaginal insertion, for long term use, includes pump and all supplies and accessories, any type each	
A4565	Slings	N &
A4566	Shoulder sling or vest design, abduction restrainer, with or without swathe control, prefabricated, includes fitting and adjustment	E
A4570	Splint	E
	Dressings applied by a physician are included as part of the professional service.	
A4575	Topical hyperbaric oxygen chamber, disposable	A
A4580	Cast supplies (e.g., plaster)	E
	See Q4001-Q4048.	
A4590	Special casting material (e.g., fiberglass)	E
	See Q4001-Q4048.	
A4595	Electrical stimulator supplies, 2 lead, per month, (e.g., TENS, NMES)	N &
	CMS: 100-03,10.2	
A4600	Sleeve for intermittent limb compression device, replacement only, each	E ☑
A4601	Lithium-ion battery, rechargeable, for nonprosthetic use, replacement	E
A4602	Replacement battery for external infusion pump owned by patient, lithium, 1.5 volt, each	N & (NU)
A4604	Tubing with integrated heating element for use with positive airway pressure device	N & (NU)
	CMS: 100-04,36,50.14	
A4605	Tracheal suction catheter, closed system, each	N ☑ & (NU)
A4606	Oxygen probe for use with oximeter device, replacement	N
A4608	Transtracheal oxygen catheter, each	N ☑ &

Supplies for Oxygen and Related Respiratory Equipment

| A4611 | Battery, heavy-duty; replacement for patient-owned ventilator | E |

Special Coverage Instructions   Noncovered by Medicare   Carrier Discretion   ☑ Quantity Alert   ● New Code   ○ Recycled/Reinstated   ▲ Revised Code

© 2021 Optum360, LLC   A2-Z3 ASC Pmt   CMS: IOM   AHA: Coding Clinic   & DMEPOS Paid   ⊘ SNF Excluded   A Codes — 7

Medical and Surgical Supplies

A4612 — A4721

A4612	**Battery cables; replacement for patient-owned ventilator**	E
A4613	**Battery charger; replacement for patient-owned ventilator**	E ☑
A4614	**Peak expiratory flow rate meter, hand held**	N 🦽
A4615	**Cannula, nasal**	N 🦽
	CMS: 100-04,20,100.2	
A4616	**Tubing (oxygen), per foot**	N ☑ 🦽
	CMS: 100-04,20,100.2	
A4617	**Mouthpiece**	N 🦽
	CMS: 100-04,20,100.2	
A4618	**Breathing circuits**	N 🦽 (NU, RR, UE)
	CMS: 100-04,20,100.2	
A4619	**Face tent**	N 🦽 (NU)
	CMS: 100-04,20,100.2	
A4620	**Variable concentration mask**	N 🦽
	CMS: 100-04,20,100.2	
A4623	**Tracheostomy, inner cannula**	N 🦽
A4624	**Tracheal suction catheter, any type other than closed system, each**	N ☑ 🦽 (NU)
A4625	**Tracheostomy care kit for new tracheostomy**	N 🦽
A4626	**Tracheostomy cleaning brush, each**	N ☑ 🦽
A4627	**Spacer, bag or reservoir, with or without mask, for use with metered dose inhaler**	E
	CMS: 100-02,15,110	
A4628	**Oropharyngeal suction catheter, each**	N ☑ 🦽 (NU)
A4629	**Tracheostomy care kit for established tracheostomy**	N 🦽

Replacement Supplies for DME

A4630	**Replacement batteries, medically necessary, transcutaneous electrical stimulator, owned by patient**	E ☑ 🦽 (NU)
A4633	**Replacement bulb/lamp for ultraviolet light therapy system, each**	E ☑ 🦽 (NU)
A4634	**Replacement bulb for therapeutic light box, tabletop model**	N
A4635	**Underarm pad, crutch, replacement, each**	E ☑ 🦽 (NU, UE)
A4636	**Replacement, handgrip, cane, crutch, or walker, each**	E ☑ 🦽 (NU, RR, UE)
	CMS: 100-04,36,50.15	
A4637	**Replacement, tip, cane, crutch, walker, each**	E ☑ 🦽 (NU, UE)
	CMS: 100-04,36,50.15	
A4638	**Replacement battery for patient-owned ear pulse generator, each**	E ☑ 🦽 (NU, RR, UE)
A4639	**Replacement pad for infrared heating pad system, each**	E ☑ 🦽 (RR)
A4640	**Replacement pad for use with medically necessary alternating pressure pad owned by patient**	E 🦽 (NU, RR, UE)

Radiopharmaceuticals

A4641	**Radiopharmaceutical, diagnostic, not otherwise classified**	N ☑
	CMS: 100-04,13,60.3; 100-04,13,60.3.2	
	AHA: 4Q, '05, 1-6; 3Q, '04, 1-10	
A4642	**Indium In-111 satumomab pendetide, diagnostic, per study dose, up to 6 mCi**	N ☑
	Use this code for Oncoscint.	
	AHA: 4Q, '05, 1-6; 3Q, '04, 1-10; 2Q, '02, 8-9	

Miscellaneous Supplies

A4648	**Tissue marker, implantable, any type, each**	N ☑
	AHA: 3Q, '13, 9	
A4649	**Surgical supply; miscellaneous**	N
	Determine if an alternative HCPCS Level II or a CPT code better describes the service being reported. This code should be used only if a more specific code is unavailable.	
A4650	**Implantable radiation dosimeter, each**	N ☑ ⊘
A4651	**Calibrated microcapillary tube, each**	N ☑ ⊘
	AHA: 1Q, '02, 5	
A4652	**Microcapillary tube sealant**	N ⊘
	AHA: 1Q, '02, 5	

Dialysis Supplies

A4653	**Peritoneal dialysis catheter anchoring device, belt, each**	N ☑ ⊘
A4657	**Syringe, with or without needle, each**	N ☑ ⊘
	CMS: 100-04,8,60.2.1; 100-04,8,60.4.4; 100-04,8,60.4.6.3	
	AHA: 1Q, '02, 5	
A4660	**Sphygmomanometer/blood pressure apparatus with cuff and stethoscope**	N ⊘
A4663	**Blood pressure cuff only**	N ⊘
A4670	**Automatic blood pressure monitor**	E
A4671	**Disposable cycler set used with cycler dialysis machine, each**	B ☑ ⊘
A4672	**Drainage extension line, sterile, for dialysis, each**	B ☑ ⊘
A4673	**Extension line with easy lock connectors, used with dialysis**	B ⊘
A4674	**Chemicals/antiseptics solution used to clean/sterilize dialysis equipment, per 8 oz**	B ☑ ⊘
A4680	**Activated carbon filter for hemodialysis, each**	N ☑ ⊘
A4690	**Dialyzer (artificial kidneys), all types, all sizes, for hemodialysis, each**	N ⊘
A4706	**Bicarbonate concentrate, solution, for hemodialysis, per gallon**	N ☑ ⊘
	AHA: 1Q, '02, 5	
A4707	**Bicarbonate concentrate, powder, for hemodialysis, per packet**	N ☑ ⊘
	AHA: 1Q, '02, 5	
A4708	**Acetate concentrate solution, for hemodialysis, per gallon**	N ☑ ⊘
	AHA: 1Q, '02, 5	
A4709	**Acid concentrate, solution, for hemodialysis, per gallon**	N ☑ ⊘
	AHA: 1Q, '02, 5	
A4714	**Treated water (deionized, distilled, or reverse osmosis) for peritoneal dialysis, per gallon**	N ☑ ⊘
A4719	**"Y set" tubing for peritoneal dialysis**	N ⊘
	AHA: 1Q, '02, 5	
A4720	**Dialysate solution, any concentration of dextrose, fluid volume greater than 249 cc, but less than or equal to 999 cc, for peritoneal dialysis**	N ☑ ⊘
	AHA: 1Q, '02, 5	
A4721	**Dialysate solution, any concentration of dextrose, fluid volume greater than 999 cc but less than or equal to 1999 cc, for peritoneal dialysis**	N ☑ ⊘
	AHA: 1Q, '02, 5	

■ Special Coverage Instructions   ■ Noncovered by Medicare   ■ Carrier Discretion   ☑ Quantity Alert   ● New Code   ○ Recycled/Reinstated   ▲ Revised Code

8 — A Codes   Ⓐ Age Edit   Ⓜ Maternity Edit   ♀ Female Only   ♂ Male Only   Ⓐ-Ⓨ OPPS Status Indicators   © 2021 Optum360, LLC

Code	Description	Symbols
A4722	Dialysate solution, any concentration of dextrose, fluid volume greater than 1999 cc but less than or equal to 2999 cc, for peritoneal dialysis	N ☑ ⊘
	AHA: 1Q, '02, 5	
A4723	Dialysate solution, any concentration of dextrose, fluid volume greater than 2999 cc but less than or equal to 3999 cc, for peritoneal dialysis	N ☑ ⊘
	AHA: 1Q, '02, 5	
A4724	Dialysate solution, any concentration of dextrose, fluid volume greater than 3999 cc but less than or equal to 4999 cc, for peritoneal dialysis	N ☑ ⊘
	AHA: 1Q, '02, 5	
A4725	Dialysate solution, any concentration of dextrose, fluid volume greater than 4999 cc but less than or equal to 5999 cc, for peritoneal dialysis	N ☑ ⊘
	AHA: 1Q, '02, 5	
A4726	Dialysate solution, any concentration of dextrose, fluid volume greater than 5999 cc, for peritoneal dialysis	N ☑ ⊘
	AHA: 1Q, '02, 5	
A4728	Dialysate solution, nondextrose containing, 500 ml	B ☑ ⊘
A4730	Fistula cannulation set for hemodialysis, each	N ☑ ⊘
A4736	Topical anesthetic, for dialysis, per g	N ☑ ⊘
	AHA: 1Q, '02, 5	
A4737	Injectable anesthetic, for dialysis, per 10 ml	N ☑ ⊘
	AHA: 1Q, '02, 5	
A4740	Shunt accessory, for hemodialysis, any type, each	N ⊘
A4750	Blood tubing, arterial or venous, for hemodialysis, each	N ☑
A4755	Blood tubing, arterial and venous combined, for hemodialysis, each	N ☑
A4760	Dialysate solution test kit, for peritoneal dialysis, any type, each	N ☑ ⊘
A4765	Dialysate concentrate, powder, additive for peritoneal dialysis, per packet	N ☑ ⊘
A4766	Dialysate concentrate, solution, additive for peritoneal dialysis, per 10 ml	N ☑ ⊘
	AHA: 1Q, '02, 5	
A4770	Blood collection tube, vacuum, for dialysis, per 50	N ☑ ⊘
A4771	Serum clotting time tube, for dialysis, per 50	N ☑ ⊘
A4772	Blood glucose test strips, for dialysis, per 50	N ☑ ⊘
A4773	Occult blood test strips, for dialysis, per 50	N ☑ ⊘
A4774	Ammonia test strips, for dialysis, per 50	N ☑ ⊘
A4802	Protamine sulfate, for hemodialysis, per 50 mg	N ☑ ⊘
	AHA: 1Q, '02, 5	
A4860	Disposable catheter tips for peritoneal dialysis, per 10	N ☑ ⊘
A4870	Plumbing and/or electrical work for home hemodialysis equipment	N ⊘
A4890	Contracts, repair and maintenance, for hemodialysis equipment	N
A4911	Drain bag/bottle, for dialysis, each	N ☑ ⊘
	AHA: 1Q, '02, 5	
A4913	Miscellaneous dialysis supplies, not otherwise specified	N ⊘
	Pertinent documentation to evaluate medical appropriateness should be included when this code is reported. Determine if an alternative HCPCS Level II or a CPT code better describes the service being reported. This code should be used only if a more specific code is unavailable. CMS: 100-04,8,20; 100-04,8,60.2.1	

Code	Description	Symbols
A4918	Venous pressure clamp, for hemodialysis, each	N ☑ ⊘
A4927	Gloves, nonsterile, per 100	N ☑ ⊘
A4928	Surgical mask, per 20	N ☑ ⊘
	AHA: 1Q, '02, 5	
A4929	Tourniquet for dialysis, each	N ☑ ⊘
	AHA: 1Q, '02, 5	
A4930	Gloves, sterile, per pair	N ☑ ⊘
A4931	Oral thermometer, reusable, any type, each	N ☑ ⊘
A4932	Rectal thermometer, reusable, any type, each	N ☑

Ostomy Pouches and Supplies

A5051	Ostomy pouch, closed; with barrier attached (one piece), each	N ☑ ও
A5052	Ostomy pouch, closed; without barrier attached (one piece), each	N ☑ ও
A5053	Ostomy pouch, closed; for use on faceplate, each	N ☑ ও
A5054	Ostomy pouch, closed; for use on barrier with flange (two piece), each	N ☑ ও
A5055	Stoma cap	N ও
A5056	Ostomy pouch, drainable, with extended wear barrier attached, with filter, (one piece), each	N ☑ ও
A5057	Ostomy pouch, drainable, with extended wear barrier attached, with built in convexity, with filter, (one piece), each	N ☑ ও
A5061	Ostomy pouch, drainable; with barrier attached, (one piece), each	N ☑ ও
A5062	Ostomy pouch, drainable; without barrier attached (one piece), each	N ☑ ও
A5063	Ostomy pouch, drainable; for use on barrier with flange (two-piece system), each	N ☑ ও
A5071	Ostomy pouch, urinary; with barrier attached (one piece), each	N ☑ ও
A5072	Ostomy pouch, urinary; without barrier attached (one piece), each	N ☑ ও
A5073	Ostomy pouch, urinary; for use on barrier with flange (two piece), each	N ☑ ও
A5081	Stoma plug or seal, any type	N ও
A5082	Continent device; catheter for continent stoma	N ও
A5083	Continent device, stoma absorptive cover for continent stoma	N ও
A5093	Ostomy accessory; convex insert	N ও

Incontinence Supplies

Code	Description	Symbols
A5102	Bedside drainage bottle with or without tubing, rigid or expandable, each	N ☑ ও
A5105	Urinary suspensory with leg bag, with or without tube, each	N ☑ ও
A5112	Urinary drainage bag, leg or abdomen, latex, with or without tube, with straps, each	N ☑ ও
A5113	Leg strap; latex, replacement only, per set	E ☑ ও
A5114	Leg strap; foam or fabric, replacement only, per set	E ☑ ও
A5120	Skin barrier, wipes or swabs, each	N ☑ ও (AU, AV)
A5121	Skin barrier; solid, 6 x 6 or equivalent, each	N ☑ ও
A5122	Skin barrier; solid, 8 x 8 or equivalent, each	N ☑ ও
A5126	Adhesive or nonadhesive; disk or foam pad	N ও

Special Coverage Instructions   Noncovered by Medicare   Carrier Discretion   ☑ Quantity Alert   ● New Code   ○ Recycled/Reinstated   ▲ Revised Code

© 2021 Optum360, LLC   A2–Z3 ASC Pmt   CMS: IOM   AHA: Coding Clinic   ও DMEPOS Paid   ⊘ SNF Excluded   A Codes — 9

A5131   Appliance cleaner, incontinence and ostomy appliances, per 16 oz   N ☑ &

A5200   Percutaneous catheter/tube anchoring device, adhesive skin attachment   N &

Diabetic Shoes, Fitting, and Modifications

According to Medicare, documentation from the prescribing physician must certify the diabetic patient has one of the following conditions: peripheral neuropathy with evidence of callus formation; history of preulcerative calluses; history of ulceration; foot deformity; previous amputation; or poor circulation. The footwear must be fitted and furnished by a podiatrist, pedorthist, orthotist, or prosthetist.

A5500   For diabetics only, fitting (including follow-up), custom preparation and supply of off-the-shelf depth-inlay shoe manufactured to accommodate multidensity insert(s), per shoe   Y ☑ &
CMS: 100-02,15,140

A5501   For diabetics only, fitting (including follow-up), custom preparation and supply of shoe molded from cast(s) of patient's foot (custom molded shoe), per shoe   Y ☑ &
CMS: 100-02,15,140

A5503   For diabetics only, modification (including fitting) of off-the-shelf depth-inlay shoe or custom molded shoe with roller or rigid rocker bottom, per shoe   Y ☑ &
CMS: 100-02,15,140

A5504   For diabetics only, modification (including fitting) of off-the-shelf depth-inlay shoe or custom molded shoe with wedge(s), per shoe   Y ☑ &
CMS: 100-02,15,140

A5505   For diabetics only, modification (including fitting) of off-the-shelf depth-inlay shoe or custom molded shoe with metatarsal bar, per shoe   Y ☑ &
CMS: 100-02,15,140

A5506   For diabetics only, modification (including fitting) of off-the-shelf depth-inlay shoe or custom molded shoe with off-set heel(s), per shoe   Y ☑ &
CMS: 100-02,15,140

A5507   For diabetics only, not otherwise specified modification (including fitting) of off-the-shelf depth-inlay shoe or custom molded shoe, per shoe   Y ☑ &
CMS: 100-02,15,140

A5508   For diabetics only, deluxe feature of off-the-shelf depth-inlay shoe or custom molded shoe, per shoe   Y ☑
CMS: 100-02,15,140

A5510   For diabetics only, direct formed, compression molded to patient's foot without external heat source, multiple-density insert(s) prefabricated, per shoe   N ☑
CMS: 100-02,15,140
AHA: 1Q, '02, 5

A5512   For diabetics only, multiple density insert, direct formed, molded to foot after external heat source of 230 degrees Fahrenheit or higher, total contact with patient's foot, including arch, base layer minimum of 1/4 inch material of Shore A 35 durometer or 3/16 inch material of Shore A 40 durometer (or higher), prefabricated, each   Y ☑ &

A5513   For diabetics only, multiple density insert, custom molded from model of patient's foot, total contact with patient's foot, including arch, base layer minimum of 3/16 inch material of Shore A 35 durometer (or higher), includes arch filler and other shaping material, custom fabricated, each   Y ☑ &

A5514   For diabetics only, multiple density insert, made by direct carving with CAM technology from a rectified CAD model created from a digitized scan of the patient, total contact with patient's foot, including arch, base layer minimum of 3/16 inch material of Shore A 35 durometer (or higher), includes arch filler and other shaping material, custom fabricated, each

Dressings

A6000   Noncontact wound-warming wound cover for use with the noncontact wound-warming device and warming card   E
AHA: 1Q, '02, 5

A6010   Collagen based wound filler, dry form, sterile, per g of collagen   N ☑ &
AHA: 1Q, '02, 5

A6011   Collagen based wound filler, gel/paste, per g of collagen   N ☑ &

A6021   Collagen dressing, sterile, size 16 sq in or less, each   N ☑ &

A6022   Collagen dressing, sterile, size more than 16 sq in but less than or equal to 48 sq in, each   N ☑ &

A6023   Collagen dressing, sterile, size more than 48 sq in, each   N ☑ &

A6024   Collagen dressing wound filler, sterile, per 6 in   N ☑ &

A6025   Gel sheet for dermal or epidermal application, (e.g., silicone, hydrogel, other), each   N ☑

A6154   Wound pouch, each   N ☑ &

A6196   Alginate or other fiber gelling dressing, wound cover, sterile, pad size 16 sq in or less, each dressing   N ☑ &

A6197   Alginate or other fiber gelling dressing, wound cover, sterile, pad size more than 16 sq in but less than or equal to 48 sq in, each dressing   N ☑ &

A6198   Alginate or other fiber gelling dressing, wound cover, sterile, pad size more than 48 sq in, each dressing   N ☑

A6199   Alginate or other fiber gelling dressing, wound filler, sterile, per 6 in   N ☑ &

A6203   Composite dressing, sterile, pad size 16 sq in or less, with any size adhesive border, each dressing   N ☑ &

A6204   Composite dressing, sterile, pad size more than 16 sq in, but less than or equal to 48 sq in, with any size adhesive border, each dressing   N ☑ &

A6205   Composite dressing, sterile, pad size more than 48 sq in, with any size adhesive border, each dressing   N ☑

A6206   Contact layer, sterile, 16 sq in or less, each dressing   N ☑

A6207   Contact layer, sterile, more than 16 sq in but less than or equal to 48 sq in, each dressing   N ☑ &

A6208   Contact layer, sterile, more than 48 sq in, each dressing   N ☑

A6209   Foam dressing, wound cover, sterile, pad size 16 sq in or less, without adhesive border, each dressing   N ☑ &

A6210   Foam dressing, wound cover, sterile, pad size more than 16 sq in but less than or equal to 48 sq in, without adhesive border, each dressing   N ☑ &

A6211   Foam dressing, wound cover, sterile, pad size more than 48 sq in, without adhesive border, each dressing   N ☑ &

A6212   Foam dressing, wound cover, sterile, pad size 16 sq in or less, with any size adhesive border, each dressing   N ☑ &

A6213   Foam dressing, wound cover, sterile, pad size more than 16 sq in but less than or equal to 48 sq in, with any size adhesive border, each dressing   N ☑

Special Coverage Instructions   Noncovered by Medicare   Carrier Discretion   ☑ Quantity Alert   ● New Code   ○ Recycled/Reinstated   ▲ Revised Code

10 — A Codes   Ⓐ Age Edit   Ⓜ Maternity Edit   ♀ Female Only   ♂ Male Only   Ⓐ-Ⓨ OPPS Status Indicators   © 2021 Optum360, LLC

A6214 Foam dressing, wound cover, sterile, pad size more than 48 sq in, with any size adhesive border, each dressing N ☑ &

A6215 Foam dressing, wound filler, sterile, per g N ☑

A6216 Gauze, nonimpregnated, nonsterile, pad size 16 sq in or less, without adhesive border, each dressing N ☑ &

A6217 Gauze, nonimpregnated, nonsterile, pad size more than 16 sq in but less than or equal to 48 sq in, without adhesive border, each dressing N ☑ &

A6218 Gauze, nonimpregnated, nonsterile, pad size more than 48 sq in, without adhesive border, each dressing N ☑

A6219 Gauze, nonimpregnated, sterile, pad size 16 sq in or less, with any size adhesive border, each dressing N ☑ &

A6220 Gauze, nonimpregnated, sterile, pad size more than 16 sq in but less than or equal to 48 sq in, with any size adhesive border, each dressing N ☑ &

A6221 Gauze, nonimpregnated, sterile, pad size more than 48 sq in, with any size adhesive border, each dressing N ☑

A6222 Gauze, impregnated with other than water, normal saline, or hydrogel, sterile, pad size 16 sq in or less, without adhesive border, each dressing N ☑ &

A6223 Gauze, impregnated with other than water, normal saline, or hydrogel, sterile, pad size more than 16 sq in but less than or equal to 48 sq in, without adhesive border, each dressing N ☑ &

A6224 Gauze, impregnated with other than water, normal saline, or hydrogel, sterile, pad size more than 48 sq in, without adhesive border, each dressing N ☑ &

A6228 Gauze, impregnated, water or normal saline, sterile, pad size 16 sq in or less, without adhesive border, each dressing N ☑

A6229 Gauze, impregnated, water or normal saline, sterile, pad size more than 16 sq in but less than or equal to 48 sq in, without adhesive border, each dressing N ☑ &

A6230 Gauze, impregnated, water or normal saline, sterile, pad size more than 48 sq in, without adhesive border, each dressing N ☑

A6231 Gauze, impregnated, hydrogel, for direct wound contact, sterile, pad size 16 sq in or less, each dressing N ☑ &

A6232 Gauze, impregnated, hydrogel, for direct wound contact, sterile, pad size greater than 16 sq in but less than or equal to 48 sq in, each dressing N ☑ &

A6233 Gauze, impregnated, hydrogel, for direct wound contact, sterile, pad size more than 48 sq in, each dressing N ☑ &

A6234 Hydrocolloid dressing, wound cover, sterile, pad size 16 sq in or less, without adhesive border, each dressing N ☑ &

A6235 Hydrocolloid dressing, wound cover, sterile, pad size more than 16 sq in but less than or equal to 48 sq in, without adhesive border, each dressing N ☑ &

A6236 Hydrocolloid dressing, wound cover, sterile, pad size more than 48 sq in, without adhesive border, each dressing N ☑ &

A6237 Hydrocolloid dressing, wound cover, sterile, pad size 16 sq in or less, with any size adhesive border, each dressing N ☑ &

A6238 Hydrocolloid dressing, wound cover, sterile, pad size more than 16 sq in but less than or equal to 48 sq in, with any size adhesive border, each dressing N ☑ &

A6239 Hydrocolloid dressing, wound cover, sterile, pad size more than 48 sq in, with any size adhesive border, each dressing N ☑

A6240 Hydrocolloid dressing, wound filler, paste, sterile, per oz N ☑ &

A6241 Hydrocolloid dressing, wound filler, dry form, sterile, per g N ☑ &

A6242 Hydrogel dressing, wound cover, sterile, pad size 16 sq in or less, without adhesive border, each dressing N ☑ &

A6243 Hydrogel dressing, wound cover, sterile, pad size more than 16 sq in but less than or equal to 48 sq in, without adhesive border, each dressing N ☑ &

A6244 Hydrogel dressing, wound cover, sterile, pad size more than 48 sq in, without adhesive border, each dressing N ☑ &

A6245 Hydrogel dressing, wound cover, sterile, pad size 16 sq in or less, with any size adhesive border, each dressing N ☑ &

A6246 Hydrogel dressing, wound cover, sterile, pad size more than 16 sq in but less than or equal to 48 sq in, with any size adhesive border, each dressing N ☑ &

A6247 Hydrogel dressing, wound cover, sterile, pad size more than 48 sq in, with any size adhesive border, each dressing N ☑ &

A6248 Hydrogel dressing, wound filler, gel, per fl oz N ☑ &

A6250 Skin sealants, protectants, moisturizers, ointments, any type, any size N

Surgical dressings applied by a physician are included as part of the professional service. Surgical dressings obtained by the patient to perform homecare as prescribed by the physician are covered.

A6251 Specialty absorptive dressing, wound cover, sterile, pad size 16 sq in or less, without adhesive border, each dressing N ☑ &

A6252 Specialty absorptive dressing, wound cover, sterile, pad size more than 16 sq in but less than or equal to 48 sq in, without adhesive border, each dressing N ☑ &

A6253 Specialty absorptive dressing, wound cover, sterile, pad size more than 48 sq in, without adhesive border, each dressing N ☑ &

A6254 Specialty absorptive dressing, wound cover, sterile, pad size 16 sq in or less, with any size adhesive border, each dressing N ☑ &

A6255 Specialty absorptive dressing, wound cover, sterile, pad size more than 16 sq in but less than or equal to 48 sq in, with any size adhesive border, each dressing N ☑ &

A6256 Specialty absorptive dressing, wound cover, sterile, pad size more than 48 sq in, with any size adhesive border, each dressing N ☑

A6257 Transparent film, sterile, 16 sq in or less, each dressing N ☑ &

Surgical dressings applied by a physician are included as part of the professional service. Surgical dressings obtained by the patient to perform homecare as prescribed by the physician are covered. Use this code for Polyskin, Tegaderm, and Tegaderm HP.

A6258 Transparent film, sterile, more than 16 sq in but less than or equal to 48 sq in, each dressing N ☑ &

Surgical dressings applied by a physician are included as part of the professional service. Surgical dressings obtained by the patient to perform homecare as prescribed by the physician are covered.

A6259 Transparent film, sterile, more than 48 sq in, each dressing N ☑ &

Surgical dressings applied by a physician are included as part of the professional service. Surgical dressings obtained by the patient to perform homecare as prescribed by the physician are covered.

A6260 Wound cleansers, any type, any size N

Surgical dressings applied by a physician are included as part of the professional service. Surgical dressings obtained by the patient to perform homecare as prescribed by the physician are covered.

Special Coverage Instructions   Noncovered by Medicare   Carrier Discretion   ☑ Quantity Alert   ● New Code   ○ Recycled/Reinstated   ▲ Revised Code

© 2021 Optum360, LLC   A2–Z3 ASC Pmt   CMS: IOM   AHA: Coding Clinic   & DMEPOS Paid   ⊘ SNF Excluded   A Codes — 11

Medical and Surgical Supplies

A6261 — A6536

A6261 Wound filler, gel/paste, per fl oz, not otherwise specified Ⓝ ☑
Surgical dressings applied by a physician are included as part of the professional service. Surgical dressings obtained by the patient to perform homecare as prescribed by the physician are covered.

A6262 Wound filler, dry form, per g, not otherwise specified Ⓝ ☑

A6266 Gauze, impregnated, other than water, normal saline, or zinc paste, sterile, any width, per linear yd Ⓝ ☑ ♿
Surgical dressings applied by a physician are included as part of the professional service. Surgical dressings obtained by the patient to perform homecare as prescribed by the physician are covered.

A6402 Gauze, nonimpregnated, sterile, pad size 16 sq in or less, without adhesive border, each dressing Ⓝ ☑ ♿
Surgical dressings applied by a physician are included as part of the professional service. Surgical dressings obtained by the patient to perform homecare as prescribed by the physician are covered.

A6403 Gauze, nonimpregnated, sterile, pad size more than 16 sq in but less than or equal to 48 sq in, without adhesive border, each dressing Ⓝ ☑ ♿
Surgical dressings applied by a physician are included as part of the professional service. Surgical dressings obtained by the patient to perform homecare as prescribed by the physician are covered.

A6404 Gauze, nonimpregnated, sterile, pad size more than 48 sq in, without adhesive border, each dressing Ⓝ ☑

A6407 Packing strips, nonimpregnated, sterile, up to 2 in in width, per linear yd Ⓝ ☑ ♿

A6410 Eye pad, sterile, each Ⓝ ☑ ♿

A6411 Eye pad, nonsterile, each Ⓝ ☑ ♿

A6412 Eye patch, occlusive, each Ⓝ ☑

A6413 Adhesive bandage, first aid type, any size, each Ⓔ ☑

A6441 Padding bandage, nonelastic, nonwoven/nonknitted, width greater than or equal to 3 in and less than 5 in, per yd Ⓝ ☑ ♿

A6442 Conforming bandage, nonelastic, knitted/woven, nonsterile, width less than 3 in, per yd Ⓝ ☑ ♿

A6443 Conforming bandage, nonelastic, knitted/woven, nonsterile, width greater than or equal to 3 in and less than 5 in, per yd Ⓝ ☑ ♿

A6444 Conforming bandage, nonelastic, knitted/woven, nonsterile, width greater than or equal to 5 in, per yd Ⓝ ☑ ♿

A6445 Conforming bandage, nonelastic, knitted/woven, sterile, width less than 3 in, per yd Ⓝ ☑ ♿

A6446 Conforming bandage, nonelastic, knitted/woven, sterile, width greater than or equal to 3 in and less than 5 in, per yd Ⓝ ☑ ♿

A6447 Conforming bandage, nonelastic, knitted/woven, sterile, width greater than or equal to 5 in, per yd Ⓝ ☑ ♿

A6448 Light compression bandage, elastic, knitted/woven, width less than 3 in, per yd Ⓝ ☑ ♿

A6449 Light compression bandage, elastic, knitted/woven, width greater than or equal to 3 in and less than 5 in, per yd Ⓝ ☑ ♿

A6450 Light compression bandage, elastic, knitted/woven, width greater than or equal to 5 in, per yd Ⓝ ☑ ♿

A6451 Moderate compression bandage, elastic, knitted/woven, load resistance of 1.25 to 1.34 ft lbs at 50% maximum stretch, width greater than or equal to 3 in and less than 5 in, per yd Ⓝ ☑ ♿

A6452 High compression bandage, elastic, knitted/woven, load resistance greater than or equal to 1.35 ft lbs at 50% maximum stretch, width greater than or equal to 3 in and less than 5 in, per yd Ⓝ ☑ ♿

A6453 Self-adherent bandage, elastic, nonknitted/nonwoven, width less than 3 in, per yd Ⓝ ☑ ♿

A6454 Self-adherent bandage, elastic, nonknitted/nonwoven, width greater than or equal to 3 in and less than 5 in, per yd Ⓝ ☑ ♿

A6455 Self-adherent bandage, elastic, nonknitted/nonwoven, width greater than or equal to 5 in, per yd Ⓝ ☑ ♿

A6456 Zinc paste impregnated bandage, nonelastic, knitted/woven, width greater than or equal to 3 in and less than 5 in, per yd Ⓝ ☑ ♿

A6457 Tubular dressing with or without elastic, any width, per linear yd Ⓝ ♿

A6460 Synthetic resorbable wound dressing, sterile, pad size 16 sq in or less, without adhesive border, each dressing

A6461 Synthetic resorbable wound dressing, sterile, pad size more than 16 sq in but less than or equal to 48 sq in, without adhesive border, each dressing

Compression Garments

A6501 Compression burn garment, bodysuit (head to foot), custom fabricated Ⓝ ♿

A6502 Compression burn garment, chin strap, custom fabricated Ⓝ ♿

A6503 Compression burn garment, facial hood, custom fabricated Ⓝ ♿

A6504 Compression burn garment, glove to wrist, custom fabricated Ⓝ ♿

A6505 Compression burn garment, glove to elbow, custom fabricated Ⓝ ♿

A6506 Compression burn garment, glove to axilla, custom fabricated Ⓝ ♿

A6507 Compression burn garment, foot to knee length, custom fabricated Ⓝ ♿

A6508 Compression burn garment, foot to thigh length, custom fabricated Ⓝ ♿

A6509 Compression burn garment, upper trunk to waist including arm openings (vest), custom fabricated Ⓝ ♿

A6510 Compression burn garment, trunk, including arms down to leg openings (leotard), custom fabricated Ⓝ ♿

A6511 Compression burn garment, lower trunk including leg openings (panty), custom fabricated Ⓝ ♿

A6512 Compression burn garment, not otherwise classified Ⓝ

A6513 Compression burn mask, face and/or neck, plastic or equal, custom fabricated Ⓑ ♿

A6530 Gradient compression stocking, below knee, 18-30 mm Hg, each Ⓔ ☑

A6531 Gradient compression stocking, below knee, 30-40 mm Hg, each Ⓝ ☑ ♿ (AW)

A6532 Gradient compression stocking, below knee, 40-50 mm Hg, each Ⓝ ☑ ♿ (AW)

A6533 Gradient compression stocking, thigh length, 18-30 mm Hg, each Ⓔ ☑

A6534 Gradient compression stocking, thigh length, 30-40 mm Hg, each Ⓔ ☑

A6535 Gradient compression stocking, thigh length, 40-50 mm Hg, each Ⓔ ☑

A6536 Gradient compression stocking, full-length/chap style, 18-30 mm Hg, each Ⓔ ☑

Special Coverage Instructions   Noncovered by Medicare   Carrier Discretion   ☑ Quantity Alert   ● New Code   ○ Recycled/Reinstated   ▲ Revised Code

A6537 Gradient compression stocking, full-length/chap style, 30-40 mm Hg, each   E ☑

A6538 Gradient compression stocking, full-length/chap style, 40-50 mm Hg, each   E ☑

A6539 Gradient compression stocking, waist length, 18-30 mm Hg, each   E ☑

A6540 Gradient compression stocking, waist length, 30-40 mm Hg, each   E ☑

A6541 Gradient compression stocking, waist length, 40-50 mm Hg, each   E ☑

A6544 Gradient compression stocking, garter belt   E

A6545 Gradient compression wrap, nonelastic, below knee, 30-50 mm Hg, each   N ☑ & (AW)

A6549 Gradient compression stocking/sleeve, not otherwise specified   E

A6550 Wound care set, for negative pressure wound therapy electrical pump, includes all supplies and accessories   N ☑ &
CMS: 100-02,7,40.1.2.8

Respiratory Supplies

A7000 Canister, disposable, used with suction pump, each   Y ☑ & (NU)

A7001 Canister, nondisposable, used with suction pump, each   Y ☑ & (NU)

A7002 Tubing, used with suction pump, each   Y ☑ & (NU)

A7003 Administration set, with small volume nonfiltered pneumatic nebulizer, disposable   Y & (NU)

A7004 Small volume nonfiltered pneumatic nebulizer, disposable   Y & (NU)

A7005 Administration set, with small volume nonfiltered pneumatic nebulizer, nondisposable   Y & (NU)

A7006 Administration set, with small volume filtered pneumatic nebulizer   Y & (NU)

A7007 Large volume nebulizer, disposable, unfilled, used with aerosol compressor   Y & (NU)

A7008 Large volume nebulizer, disposable, prefilled, used with aerosol compressor   Y & (NU)

A7009 Reservoir bottle, nondisposable, used with large volume ultrasonic nebulizer   Y & (NU)

A7010 Corrugated tubing, disposable, used with large volume nebulizer, 100 ft   Y ☑ & (NU)

A7012 Water collection device, used with large volume nebulizer   Y & (NU)

A7013 Filter, disposable, used with aerosol compressor or ultrasonic generator   Y & (NU)

A7014 Filter, nondisposable, used with aerosol compressor or ultrasonic generator   Y & (NU)

A7015 Aerosol mask, used with DME nebulizer   Y & (NU)

A7016 Dome and mouthpiece, used with small volume ultrasonic nebulizer   Y & (NU)

A7017 Nebulizer, durable, glass or autoclavable plastic, bottle type, not used with oxygen   Y & (NU, RR, UE)

A7018 Water, distilled, used with large volume nebulizer, 1000 ml   Y ☑ &

A7020 Interface for cough stimulating device, includes all components, replacement only   Y & (NU)

A7025 High frequency chest wall oscillation system vest, replacement for use with patient-owned equipment, each   N ☑ & (RR)

A7026 High frequency chest wall oscillation system hose, replacement for use with patient-owned equipment, each   Y ☑ & (NU)

A7027 Combination oral/nasal mask, used with continuous positive airway pressure device, each   Y ☑ & (NU)

A7028 Oral cushion for combination oral/nasal mask, replacement only, each   Y ☑ & (NU)

A7029 Nasal pillows for combination oral/nasal mask, replacement only, pair   Y ☑ & (NU)

A7030 Full face mask used with positive airway pressure device, each   Y ☑ & (NU)
CMS: 100-04,36,50.14

A7031 Face mask interface, replacement for full face mask, each   Y ☑ & (NU)
CMS: 100-04,36,50.14

A7032 Cushion for use on nasal mask interface, replacement only, each   Y ☑ & (NU)
CMS: 100-03,240.4; 100-04,36,50.14

A7033 Pillow for use on nasal cannula type interface, replacement only, pair   Y ☑ & (NU)
CMS: 100-03,240.4; 100-04,36,50.14

A7034 Nasal interface (mask or cannula type) used with positive airway pressure device, with or without head strap   Y & (NU)
CMS: 100-03,240.4; 100-04,36,50.14

A7035 Headgear used with positive airway pressure device   Y & (NU)
CMS: 100-03,240.4; 100-04,36,50.14

A7036 Chinstrap used with positive airway pressure device   Y & (NU)
CMS: 100-03,240.4; 100-04,36,50.14

A7037 Tubing used with positive airway pressure device   Y & (NU)
CMS: 100-03,240.4; 100-04,36,50.14

A7038 Filter, disposable, used with positive airway pressure device   Y & (NU)
CMS: 100-04,36,50.14

A7039 Filter, nondisposable, used with positive airway pressure device   Y & (NU)
CMS: 100-04,36,50.14

A7040 One way chest drain valve   N &

A7041 Water seal drainage container and tubing for use with implanted chest tube   N &

A7044 Oral interface used with positive airway pressure device, each   Y ☑ & (NU)
CMS: 100-03,240.4; 100-04,36,50.14

A7045 Exhalation port with or without swivel used with accessories for positive airway devices, replacement only   Y & (NU, RR, UE)
CMS: 100-03,240.4; 100-04,36,50.14

A7046 Water chamber for humidifier, used with positive airway pressure device, replacement, each   Y ☑ & (NU)
CMS: 100-04,36,50.14

A7047 Oral interface used with respiratory suction pump, each   N ☑ & (NU)

A7048 Vacuum drainage collection unit and tubing kit, including all supplies needed for collection unit change, for use with implanted catheter, each   N &

Tracheostomy Supplies

A7501 Tracheostoma valve, including diaphragm, each   N ☑ &

Special Coverage Instructions   Noncovered by Medicare   Carrier Discretion   ☑ Quantity Alert   ● New Code   ○ Recycled/Reinstated   ▲ Revised Code

A7502	Replacement diaphragm/faceplate for tracheostoma valve, each — N ☑ ᗒ
A7503	Filter holder or filter cap, reusable, for use in a tracheostoma heat and moisture exchange system, each — N ☑ ᗒ
A7504	Filter for use in a tracheostoma heat and moisture exchange system, each — N ☑ ᗒ
A7505	Housing, reusable without adhesive, for use in a heat and moisture exchange system and/or with a tracheostoma valve, each — N ☑ ᗒ
A7506	Adhesive disc for use in a heat and moisture exchange system and/or with tracheostoma valve, any type each — N ☑ ᗒ
A7507	Filter holder and integrated filter without adhesive, for use in a tracheostoma heat and moisture exchange system, each — N ☑ ᗒ
A7508	Housing and integrated adhesive, for use in a tracheostoma heat and moisture exchange system and/or with a tracheostoma valve, each — N ☑ ᗒ
A7509	Filter holder and integrated filter housing, and adhesive, for use as a tracheostoma heat and moisture exchange system, each — N ☑ ᗒ
A7520	Tracheostomy/laryngectomy tube, noncuffed, polyvinyl chloride (PVC), silicone or equal, each — N ☑ ᗒ
A7521	Tracheostomy/laryngectomy tube, cuffed, polyvinyl chloride (PVC), silicone or equal, each — N ☑ ᗒ
A7522	Tracheostomy/laryngectomy tube, stainless steel or equal (sterilizable and reusable), each — N ☑ ᗒ
A7523	Tracheostomy shower protector, each — N ☑
A7524	Tracheostoma stent/stud/button, each — N ☑ ᗒ
A7525	Tracheostomy mask, each — N ☑ ᗒ
A7526	Tracheostomy tube collar/holder, each — N ☑ ᗒ
A7527	Tracheostomy/laryngectomy tube plug/stop, each — N ☑ ᗒ

Protective Helmet

A8000	Helmet, protective, soft, prefabricated, includes all components and accessories — Y ᗒ (NU, RR, UE)
A8001	Helmet, protective, hard, prefabricated, includes all components and accessories — Y ᗒ (NU, RR, UE)
A8002	Helmet, protective, soft, custom fabricated, includes all components and accessories — Y ᗒ (NU, RR, UE)
A8003	Helmet, protective, hard, custom fabricated, includes all components and accessories — Y ᗒ (NU, RR, UE)
A8004	Soft interface for helmet, replacement only — Y ᗒ (NU, RR, UE)

Other Supplies and Devices

A9150	Nonprescription drugs — B
A9152	Single vitamin/mineral/trace element, oral, per dose, not otherwise specified — E ☑
A9153	Multiple vitamins, with or without minerals and trace elements, oral, per dose, not otherwise specified — E ☑
A9155	Artificial saliva, 30 ml — B ☑
A9180	Pediculosis (lice infestation) treatment, topical, for administration by patient/caretaker — E
A9270	Noncovered item or service — E CMS: 100-04,11,100.1; 100-04,20,30.9; 100-04,23,20.9.1.1 AHA: 1Q, '14, 7; 3Q, '04, 1-10
A9272	Wound suction, disposable, includes dressing, all accessories and components, any type, each — E ☑

A9273	Cold or hot fluid bottle, ice cap or collar, heat and/or cold wrap, any type — E
A9274	External ambulatory insulin delivery system, disposable, each, includes all supplies and accessories — E ☑
A9275	Home glucose disposable monitor, includes test strips — E
A9276	Sensor; invasive (e.g., subcutaneous), disposable, for use with interstitial continuous glucose monitoring system, 1 unit = 1 day supply — E ☑
A9277	Transmitter; external, for use with interstitial continuous glucose monitoring system — E
A9278	Receiver (monitor); external, for use with interstitial continuous glucose monitoring system — E
A9279	Monitoring feature/device, stand-alone or integrated, any type, includes all accessories, components and electronics, not otherwise classified — E
A9280	Alert or alarm device, not otherwise classified — E
A9281	Reaching/grabbing device, any type, any length, each — E ☑
A9282	Wig, any type, each — E ☑
A9283	Foot pressure off loading/supportive device, any type, each — E ☑
A9284	Spirometer, nonelectronic, includes all accessories — N
A9285	Inversion/eversion correction device — A
A9286	Hygienic item or device, disposable or nondisposable, any type, each — E
A9300	Exercise equipment — E

Radiopharmaceuticals

A9500	Technetium Tc-99m sestamibi, diagnostic, per study dose — N M ☑ ◯ Use this code for Cardiolite. AHA: 2Q, '06, 5; 4Q, '05, 1-6; 3Q, '04, 1-10
A9501	Technetium Tc-99m teboroxime, diagnostic, per study dose — N M ☑ ◯
A9502	Technetium Tc-99m tetrofosmin, diagnostic, per study dose — N M ☑ ◯ Use this code for Myoview. AHA: 2Q, '06, 5; 4Q, '05, 1-6; 3Q, '04, 1-10
A9503	Technetium Tc-99m medronate, diagnostic, per study dose, up to 30 mCi — N M ☑ ◯ Use this code for CIS-MDP, Draximage MDP-10, Draximage MDP-25, MDP-Bracco, Technetium Tc-99m MPI-MDP. AHA: 4Q, '05, 1-6; 3Q, '04, 1-10; 2Q, '02, 8-9
A9504	Technetium Tc-99m apcitide, diagnostic, per study dose, up to 20 mCi — N M ☑ ◯ Use this code for Acutect. AHA: 4Q, '05, 1-6; 3Q, '04, 1-10; 2Q, '02, 8-9; 4Q, '01, 5
A9505	Thallium Tl-201 thallous chloride, diagnostic, per mCi — N M ☑ ◯ Use this code for MIBG, Thallous Chloride USP. AHA: 4Q, '05, 1-6; 3Q, '04, 1-10; 2Q, '02, 8-9
A9507	Indium In-111 capromab pendetide, diagnostic, per study dose, up to 10 millicuries — N M ☑ ◯ Use this code for Prostascint. AHA: 4Q, '05, 1-6; 3Q, '04, 1-10
A9508	Iodine I-131 iobenguane sulfate, diagnostic, per 0.5 mCi — N M ☑ ◯ Use this code for MIBG. AHA: 4Q, '05, 1-6; 3Q, '04, 1-10; 2Q, '02, 8-9

Special Coverage Instructions   Noncovered by Medicare   Carrier Discretion   ☑ Quantity Alert   ● New Code   ◯ Recycled/Reinstated   ▲ Revised Code

A9509 Iodine I-123 sodium iodide, diagnostic, per mCi N N1 ☑

A9510 Technetium Tc-99m disofenin, diagnostic, per study dose, up to 15 mCi N N1 ☑
Use this code for Hepatolite.
AHA: 4Q, '05, 1-6; 3Q, '04, 1-10

A9512 Technetium Tc-99m pertechnetate, diagnostic, per mCi N N1 ☑
Use this code for Technelite, Ultra-Technelow.
AHA: 4Q, '05, 1-6; 3Q, '04, 1-10

A9513 Lutetium Lu 177, dotatate, therapeutic, 1 mCi
Use this code for Lutathera.

A9515 Choline C-11, diagnostic, per study dose up to 20 mCi G N1 ☑

A9516 Iodine I-123 sodium iodide, diagnostic, per 100 mcCi, up to 999 mcCi N N1 ⊘
AHA: 4Q, '05, 1-6; 3Q, '04, 1-10

A9517 Iodine I-131 sodium iodide capsule(s), therapeutic, per mCi K ☑ ⊘
AHA: 3Q, '08, 6; 4Q, '05, 1-6; 3Q, '04, 1-10

A9520 Technetium Tc-99m, tilmanocept, diagnostic, up to 0.5 mCi N N1 ☑

A9521 Technetium Tc-99m exametazime, diagnostic, per study dose, up to 25 mCi N N1 ☑ ⊘
Use this code for Ceretec.
AHA: 4Q, '05, 1-6; 3Q, '04, 1-10

A9524 Iodine I-131 iodinated serum albumin, diagnostic, per 5 mcCi N N1 ☑ ⊘
AHA: 4Q, '05, 1-6; 3Q, '04, 1-10

A9526 Nitrogen N-13 ammonia, diagnostic, per study dose, up to 40 mCi N N1 ☑ ⊘
CMS: 100-04,13,60.3; 100-04,13,60.3.2
AHA: 4Q, '05, 1-6; 3Q, '04, 1-10

A9527 Iodine I-125, sodium iodide solution, therapeutic, per mCi U H2 ☑ ⊘
AHA: 3Q, '16, 11

A9528 Iodine I-131 sodium iodide capsule(s), diagnostic, per mCi N N1 ☑ ⊘
AHA: 4Q, '05, 1-6; 3Q, '04, 1-10

A9529 Iodine I-131 sodium iodide solution, diagnostic, per mCi N N1 ☑ ⊘
AHA: 4Q, '05, 1-6; 3Q, '04, 1-10

A9530 Iodine I-131 sodium iodide solution, therapeutic, per mCi K ☑ ⊘
AHA: 4Q, '05, 1-6; 3Q, '04, 1-10

A9531 Iodine I-131 sodium iodide, diagnostic, per mcCi (up to 100 mcCi) N N1 ☑ ⊘
AHA: 4Q, '05, 1-6; 3Q, '04, 1-10

A9532 Iodine I-125 serum albumin, diagnostic, per 5 mcCi N N1 ☑ ⊘
AHA: 4Q, '05, 1-6; 3Q, '04, 1-10

A9536 Technetium Tc-99m depreotide, diagnostic, per study dose, up to 35 mCi N N1 ⊘
AHA: 4Q, '05, 1-6

A9537 Technetium Tc-99m mebrofenin, diagnostic, per study dose, up to 15 mCi N N1 ☑ ⊘
AHA: 4Q, '05, 1-6

A9538 Technetium Tc-99m pyrophosphate, diagnostic, per study dose, up to 25 mCi N N1 ☑ ⊘
Use this code for CIS-PYRO, Phosphostec, Technescan Pyp Kit.
AHA: 4Q, '05, 1-6

A9539 Technetium Tc-99m pentetate, diagnostic, per study dose, up to 25 mCi N N1 ☑
Use this code for AN-DTPA, DTPA, MPI-DTPA Kit-Chelate, MPI Indium DTPA IN-111, Pentate Calcium Trisodium, Pentate Zinc Trisodium.
AHA: 4Q, '05, 1-6

A9540 Technetium Tc-99m macroaggregated albumin, diagnostic, per study dose, up to 10 mCi N N1 ☑ ⊘
AHA: 4Q, '05, 1-6

A9541 Technetium Tc-99m sulfur colloid, diagnostic, per study dose, up to 20 mCi N N1 ☑ ⊘
AHA: 4Q, '05, 1-6

A9542 Indium In-111 ibritumomab tiuxetan, diagnostic, per study dose, up to 5 mCi N N1 ☑ ⊘
Use this code for Zevalin.
AHA: 4Q, '05, 1-6

A9543 Yttrium Y-90 ibritumomab tiuxetan, therapeutic, per treatment dose, up to 40 mCi K ☑ ⊘
AHA: 4Q, '05, 1-6

A9546 Cobalt Co-57/58, cyanocobalamin, diagnostic, per study dose, up to 1 mcCi N N1 ☑ ⊘
AHA: 4Q, '05, 1-6

A9547 Indium In-111 oxyquinoline, diagnostic, per 0.5 mCi N N1 ☑ ⊘
AHA: 4Q, '05, 1-6

A9548 Indium In-111 pentetate, diagnostic, per 0.5 mCi N N1 ☑ ⊘
AHA: 4Q, '05, 1-6

A9550 Technetium Tc-99m sodium glucepate, diagnostic, per study dose, up to 25 mCi N N1 ☑ ⊘
AHA: 4Q, '05, 1-6

A9551 Technetium Tc-99m succimer, diagnostic, per study dose, up to 10 mCi N N1 ☑ ⊘
Use this code for MPI-DMSA Kidney Reagent.
AHA: 4Q, '05, 1-6

A9552 Fluorodeoxyglucose F-18 FDG, diagnostic, per study dose, up to 45 mCi N N1 ☑ ⊘
CMS: 100-03,220.6.13; 100-03,220.6.17; 100-04,13,60.15; 100-04,13,60.16; 100-04,13,60.3.2
AHA: 3Q, '08, 7, 8; 4Q, '05, 1-6

A9553 Chromium Cr-51 sodium chromate, diagnostic, per study dose, up to 250 mcCi N N1 ☑ ⊘
Use this code for Chromitope Sodium.
AHA: 4Q, '05, 1-6

A9554 Iodine I-125 sodium iothalamate, diagnostic, per study dose, up to 10 mcCi N N1 ☑ ⊘
Use this code for Glofil-125.
AHA: 4Q, '05, 1-6

A9555 Rubidium Rb-82, diagnostic, per study dose, up to 60 mCi N N1 ☑ ⊘
Use this code for Cardiogen 82.
CMS: 100-03,220.6.1; 100-04,13,60.3.2
AHA: 4Q, '05, 1-6

A9556 Gallium Ga-67 citrate, diagnostic, per mCi N N1 ☑ ⊘
AHA: 4Q, '05, 1-6

A9557 Technetium Tc-99m bicisate, diagnostic, per study dose, up to 25 mCi N N1 ☑ ⊘
Use this code for Neurolite.
AHA: 4Q, '05, 1-6

A9558 Xenon Xe-133 gas, diagnostic, per 10 mCi N N1 ☑ ⊘
AHA: 4Q, '05, 1-6

A9559 Cobalt Co-57 cyanocobalamin, oral, diagnostic, per study dose, up to 1 mcCi N M ☑ ⊘
AHA: 4Q, '05, 1-6

A9560 Technetium Tc-99m labeled red blood cells, diagnostic, per study dose, up to 30 mCi N M ☑ ⊘
AHA: 3Q, '08, 7, 8; 4Q, '05, 1-6

A9561 Technetium Tc-99m oxidronate, diagnostic, per study dose, up to 30 mCi N M ☑ ⊘
Use this code for TechneScan.
AHA: 4Q, '05, 1-6

A9562 Technetium Tc-99m mertiatide, diagnostic, per study dose, up to 15 mCi N M ☑ ⊘
Use this code for TechneScan MAG-3.
AHA: 4Q, '05, 1-6

A9563 Sodium phosphate P-32, therapeutic, per mCi K ☑ ⊘
AHA: 4Q, '05, 1-6

A9564 Chromic phosphate P-32 suspension, therapeutic, per mCi E ☑ ⊘
Use this code for Phosphocol (P32).
AHA: 4Q, '05, 1-6

A9566 Technetium Tc-99m fanolesomab, diagnostic, per study dose, up to 25 mCi N M ☑ ⊘
AHA: 4Q, '05, 1-6

A9567 Technetium Tc-99m pentetate, diagnostic, aerosol, per study dose, up to 75 mCi N M ☑ ⊘
Use this code for AN-DTPA, DTPA, MPI-DTPA Kit-Chelate, MPI Indium DTPA IN-111, Pentate Calcium Trisodium, Pentate Zinc Trisodium.
AHA: 4Q, '05, 1-6

A9568 Technetium Tc-99m arcitumomab, diagnostic, per study dose, up to 45 mCi N M ☑ ⊘
Use this code for CEA Scan.

A9569 Technetium Tc-99m exametazime labeled autologous white blood cells, diagnostic, per study dose N M ☑ ⊘
AHA: 1Q, '08, 6

A9570 Indium In-111 labeled autologous white blood cells, diagnostic, per study dose N M ☑ ⊘

A9571 Indium In-111 labeled autologous platelets, diagnostic, per study dose N M ☑ ⊘

A9572 Indium In-111 pentetreotide, diagnostic, per study dose, up to 6 mCi N M ☑ ⊘
Use this code for Ostreoscan.

A9575 Injection, gadoterate meglumine, 0.1 ml N M ☑
Use this code for Dotarem.
AHA: 1Q, '14, 6

A9576 Injection, gadoteridol, (ProHance multipack), per ml N M ☑

A9577 Injection, gadobenate dimeglumine (MultiHance), per ml N M ☑
AHA: 1Q, '08, 6

A9578 Injection, gadobenate dimeglumine (MultiHance multipack), per ml N M ☑

A9579 Injection, gadolinium-based magnetic resonance contrast agent, not otherwise specified (NOS), per ml N M ☑
Use this code for Omniscan, Magnevist.
CMS: 100-03,1,220.2
AHA: 1Q, '08, 6

A9580 Sodium fluoride F-18, diagnostic, per study dose, up to 30 mCi N M ☑ ⊘
CMS: 100-03,220.6.19; 100-04,13,60.18; 100-04,13,60.3.2

A9581 Injection, gadoxetate disodium, 1 ml N M ☑
Use this code for Eovist.

A9582 Iodine I-123 iobenguane, diagnostic, per study dose, up to 15 mCi N M ☑

A9583 Injection, gadofosveset trisodium, 1 ml N M ☑
Use this code for Ablavar, Vasovist.

A9584 Iodine I-123 ioflupane, diagnostic, per study dose, up to 5 mCi N M ☑
Use this code for DaTscan.

A9585 Injection, gadobutrol, 0.1 ml N M ☑
Use this code for Gadavist.

A9586 Florbetapir F18, diagnostic, per study dose, up to 10 mCi N M ☑
Use this code for Amyvid.
CMS: 100-04,17, 80.12
AHA: 3Q, '14, 7; 1Q, '14, 6

A9587 Gallium Ga-68, dotatate, diagnostic, 0.1 mCi G M ☑
Use this code for Netspot.
CMS: 100-04,13,60.3.2
AHA: 1Q, '17, 9-10

A9588 Fluciclovine F-18, diagnostic, 1 mCi G M ☑
Use this code for Axumin.
CMS: 100-04,13,60.3.2
AHA: 1Q, '17, 9-10

A9589 Instillation, hexaminolevulinate HCl, 100 mg
Use this code for Cysview.
CMS: 100-04,13,60.3.2

A9590 Iodine I-131, iobenguane, 1 mCi K2
Use this code for Azedra.
CMS: 100-04,13,60.3.2

A9591 Fluoroestradiol f 18, diagnostic, 1 mCi K2
Use this code for Cerianna.
CMS: 100-04,13,60.3.2

● **A9592** Copper Cu-64, dotatate, diagnostic, 1 mCi K2
Use this code for Detectnet.
CMS: 100-04,13,60.3.2

● **A9593** Gallium Ga-68 PSMA-11, diagnostic, (UCSF), 1 mCi K2
CMS: 100-04,13,60.3.2

● **A9594** Gallium Ga-68 PSMA-11, diagnostic, (UCLA), 1 mCi K2
CMS: 100-04,13,60.3.2

● **A9595** Piflufolastat f-18, diagnostic, 1 mCi K2
Use this code for Pylarify.
CMS: 100-04,13,60.3.2

A9597 Positron emission tomography radiopharmaceutical, diagnostic, for tumor identification, not otherwise classified N M ☑
CMS: 100-04,13,60.3.2
AHA: 1Q, '17, 9-10; 1Q, '17, 8

A9598 Positron emission tomography radiopharmaceutical, diagnostic, for nontumor identification, not otherwise classified N M ☑
CMS: 100-04,13,60.3.2
AHA: 1Q, '17, 9-10; 1Q, '17, 8

A9600 Strontium Sr-89 chloride, therapeutic, per mCi K ☑ ⊘
Use this code for Metastron.
AHA: 4Q, '05, 1-6; 3Q, '04, 1-10; 2Q, '02, 8-9

A9604 Samarium Sm-153 lexidronam, therapeutic, per treatment dose, up to 150 mCi K ☑
Use this code for Quadramet.

A9606 Radium RA-223 dichloride, therapeutic, per UCI K ☑
Use this code for Xofigo.

Special Coverage Instructions   Noncovered by Medicare   Carrier Discretion   ☑ Quantity Alert ● New Code ○ Recycled/Reinstated ▲ Revised Code

16 — A Codes   A Age Edit   M Maternity Edit   ♀ Female Only   ♂ Male Only   A-Y OPPS Status Indicators   © 2021 Optum360, LLC

A9698	Nonradioactive contrast imaging material, not otherwise classified, per study	N NI ☑ ⊘
	AHA: 1Q, '17, 8; 4Q, '05, 1-6	
A9699	Radiopharmaceutical, therapeutic, not otherwise classified	N ☑ ⊘
	AHA: 4Q, '05, 1-6; 3Q, '04, 1-10	
A9700	Supply of injectable contrast material for use in echocardiography, per study	N NI
	AHA: 1Q, '17, 8; 2Q, '03, 7; 4Q, '01, 5	

Miscellaneous

A9900	Miscellaneous DME supply, accessory, and/or service component of another HCPCS code	Y
A9901	DME delivery, set up, and/or dispensing service component of another HCPCS code	A
A9999	Miscellaneous DME supply or accessory, not otherwise specified	Y

Enteral and Parenteral Therapy (side tab)

B4034 — B4159 (side tab)

Enteral and Parenteral Therapy B4034-B9999
This section includes codes for supplies, formulae, nutritional solutions, and infusion pumps.

Enteral Formulae and Enteral Medical Supplies

B4034 Enteral feeding supply kit; syringe fed, per day, includes but not limited to feeding/flushing syringe, administration set tubing, dressings, tape ☑Y ☑
CMS: 100-03,180.2; 100-04,20,160.2

B4035 Enteral feeding supply kit; pump fed, per day, includes but not limited to feeding/flushing syringe, administration set tubing, dressings, tape ☑Y ☑
CMS: 100-03,180.2; 100-04,20,160.2

B4036 Enteral feeding supply kit; gravity fed, per day, includes but not limited to feeding/flushing syringe, administration set tubing, dressings, tape ☑Y ☑
CMS: 100-03,180.2; 100-04,20,160.2

B4081 Nasogastric tubing with stylet ☑Y
CMS: 100-03,180.2; 100-04,20,160.2

Many types of stylets are used. Some may be fitted with lights or optics. Others are used as guides

B4082 Nasogastric tubing without stylet ☑Y
CMS: 100-03,180.2; 100-04,20,160.2

B4083 Stomach tube - Levine type ☑Y
CMS: 100-03,180.2; 100-04,20,160.2

B4087 Gastrostomy/jejunostomy tube, standard, any material, any type, each Ⓐ ☑
CMS: 100-03,180.2

B4088 Gastrostomy/jejunostomy tube, low-profile, any material, any type, each Ⓐ ☑
CMS: 100-03,180.2

B4100 Food thickener, administered orally, per oz Ⓔ ☑
CMS: 100-03,180.2

B4102 Enteral formula, for adults, used to replace fluids and electrolytes (e.g., clear liquids), 500 ml = 1 unit ☑Y ☑
CMS: 100-03,180.2

B4103 Enteral formula, for pediatrics, used to replace fluids and electrolytes (e.g., clear liquids), 500 ml = 1 unit ☑Y ☑
CMS: 100-03,180.2

B4104 Additive for enteral formula (e.g., fiber) Ⓔ
CMS: 100-03,180.2

B4105 In-line cartridge containing digestive enzyme(s) for enteral feeding, each
CMS: 100-03,180.2

B4149 Enteral formula, manufactured blenderized natural foods with intact nutrients, includes proteins, fats, carbohydrates, vitamins and minerals, may include fiber, administered through an enteral feeding tube, 100 calories = 1 unit ☑Y ☑
CMS: 100-03,180.2

B4150 Enteral formula, nutritionally complete with intact nutrients, includes proteins, fats, carbohydrates, vitamins and minerals, may include fiber, administered through an enteral feeding tube, 100 calories = 1 unit ☑Y ☑
Use this code for Enrich, Ensure, Ensure HN, Ensure Powder, Isocal, Lonalac Powder, Meritene, Meritene Powder, Osmolite, Osmolite HN, Portagen Powder, Sustacal, Renu, Sustagen Powder, Travasorb.
CMS: 100-03,180.2; 100-04,20,160.2

B4152 Enteral formula, nutritionally complete, calorically dense (equal to or greater than 1.5 kcal/ml) with intact nutrients, includes proteins, fats, carbohydrates, vitamins and minerals, may include fiber, administered through an enteral feeding tube, 100 calories = 1 unit ☑Y ☑
Use this code for Magnacal, Isocal HCN, Sustacal HC, Ensure Plus, Ensure Plus HN.
CMS: 100-03,180.2; 100-04,20,160.2

B4153 Enteral formula, nutritionally complete, hydrolyzed proteins (amino acids and peptide chain), includes fats, carbohydrates, vitamins and minerals, may include fiber, administered through an enteral feeding tube, 100 calories = 1 unit ☑Y ☑
Use this code for Criticare HN, Vivonex t.e.n. (Total Enteral Nutrition), Vivonex HN, Vital (Vital HN), Travasorb HN, Isotein HN, Precision HN, Precision Isotonic.
CMS: 100-03,180.2; 100-04,20,160.2

B4154 Enteral formula, nutritionally complete, for special metabolic needs, excludes inherited disease of metabolism, includes altered composition of proteins, fats, carbohydrates, vitamins and/or minerals, may include fiber, administered through an enteral feeding tube, 100 calories = 1 unit ☑Y ☑
Use this code for Hepatic-aid, Travasorb Hepatic, Travasorb MCT, Travasorb Renal, Traum-aid, Tramacal, Aminaid.
CMS: 100-03,180.2; 100-04,20,160.2

B4155 Enteral formula, nutritionally incomplete/modular nutrients, includes specific nutrients, carbohydrates (e.g., glucose polymers), proteins/amino acids (e.g., glutamine, arginine), fat (e.g., medium chain triglycerides) or combination, administered through an enteral feeding tube, 100 calories = 1 unit ☑Y ☑
Use this code for Propac, Gerval Protein, Promix, Casec, Moducal, Controlyte, Polycose Liquid or Powder, Sumacal, Microlipids, MCT Oil, Nutri-source.
CMS: 100-03,180.2; 100-04,20,160.2

B4157 Enteral formula, nutritionally complete, for special metabolic needs for inherited disease of metabolism, includes proteins, fats, carbohydrates, vitamins and minerals, may include fiber, administered through an enteral feeding tube, 100 calories = 1 unit ☑Y ☑
CMS: 100-03,180.2

B4158 Enteral formula, for pediatrics, nutritionally complete with intact nutrients, includes proteins, fats, carbohydrates, vitamins and minerals, may include fiber and/or iron, administered through an enteral feeding tube, 100 calories = 1 unit ☑Y ☑
CMS: 100-03,180.2

B4159 Enteral formula, for pediatrics, nutritionally complete soy based with intact nutrients, includes proteins, fats, carbohydrates, vitamins and minerals, may include fiber and/or iron, administered through an enteral feeding tube, 100 calories = 1 unit ☑Y ☑
CMS: 100-03,180.2

☑ Special Coverage Instructions Noncovered by Medicare Carrier Discretion ☑ Quantity Alert ● New Code ○ Recycled/Reinstated ▲ Revised Code
Ⓐ Age Edit Ⓜ Maternity Edit ♀ Female Only ♂ Male Only Ⓐ-Ⓨ OPPS Status Indicators © 2021 Optum360, LLC

B4160   Enteral formula, for pediatrics, nutritionally complete calorically dense (equal to or greater than 0.7 kcal/ml) with intact nutrients, includes proteins, fats, carbohydrates, vitamins and minerals, may include fiber, administered through an enteral feeding tube, 100 calories = 1 unit ☒ ☑
CMS: 100-03,180.2

B4161   Enteral formula, for pediatrics, hydrolyzed/amino acids and peptide chain proteins, includes fats, carbohydrates, vitamins and minerals, may include fiber, administered through an enteral feeding tube, 100 calories = 1 unit ☒ ☑
CMS: 100-03,180.2

B4162   Enteral formula, for pediatrics, special metabolic needs for inherited disease of metabolism, includes proteins, fats, carbohydrates, vitamins and minerals, may include fiber, administered through an enteral feeding tube, 100 calories = 1 unit ☒ ☑
CMS: 100-03,180.2

Parenteral Nutrition Solutions and Supplies

B4164   Parenteral nutrition solution: carbohydrates (dextrose), 50% or less (500 ml = 1 unit), home mix ☒ ☑
CMS: 100-03,180.2; 100-04,20,160.2

B4168   Parenteral nutrition solution; amino acid, 3.5%, (500 ml = 1 unit) - home mix ☒ ☑
CMS: 100-03,180.2; 100-04,20,160.2

B4172   Parenteral nutrition solution; amino acid, 5.5% through 7%, (500 ml = 1 unit) - home mix ☒ ☑
CMS: 100-03,180.2; 100-04,20,160.2

B4176   Parenteral nutrition solution; amino acid, 7% through 8.5%, (500 ml = 1 unit) - home mix ☒ ☑
CMS: 100-03,180.2; 100-04,20,160.2

B4178   Parenteral nutrition solution: amino acid, greater than 8.5% (500 ml = 1 unit) - home mix ☒ ☑
CMS: 100-03,180.2; 100-04,20,160.2

B4180   Parenteral nutrition solution: carbohydrates (dextrose), greater than 50% (500 ml = 1 unit), home mix ☒ ☑
CMS: 100-03,180.2; 100-04,20,160.2

B4185   Parenteral nutrition solution, not otherwise specified, 10 g lipids ☒ ☑
CMS: 100-03,180.2

B4187   Omegaven, 10 g lipids
CMS: 100-03,180.2

B4189   Parenteral nutrition solution: compounded amino acid and carbohydrates with electrolytes, trace elements, and vitamins, including preparation, any strength, 10 to 51 g of protein, premix ☒ ☑
CMS: 100-03,180.2; 100-04,20,160.2

B4193   Parenteral nutrition solution: compounded amino acid and carbohydrates with electrolytes, trace elements, and vitamins, including preparation, any strength, 52 to 73 g of protein, premix ☒ ☑
CMS: 100-03,180.2; 100-04,20,160.2

B4197   Parenteral nutrition solution; compounded amino acid and carbohydrates with electrolytes, trace elements and vitamins, including preparation, any strength, 74 to 100 g of protein - premix ☒ ☑
CMS: 100-03,180.2; 100-04,20,160.2

B4199   Parenteral nutrition solution; compounded amino acid and carbohydrates with electrolytes, trace elements and vitamins, including preparation, any strength, over 100 g of protein - premix ☒ ☑
CMS: 100-03,180.2; 100-04,20,160.2

B4216   Parenteral nutrition; additives (vitamins, trace elements, Heparin, electrolytes), home mix, per day ☒
CMS: 100-03,180.2; 100-04,20,160.2

B4220   Parenteral nutrition supply kit; premix, per day ☒
CMS: 100-03,180.2; 100-04,20,160.2

B4222   Parenteral nutrition supply kit; home mix, per day ☒
CMS: 100-03,180.2; 100-04,20,160.2

B4224   Parenteral nutrition administration kit, per day ☒
CMS: 100-03,180.2; 100-04,20,160.2

B5000   Parenteral nutrition solution: compounded amino acid and carbohydrates with electrolytes, trace elements, and vitamins, including preparation, any strength, renal - Amirosyn RF, NephrAmine, RenAmine - premix ☒
Use this code for Amirosyn-RF, NephrAmine, RenAmin.
CMS: 100-03,180.2; 100-04,20,160.2

B5100   Parenteral nutrition solution compounded amino acid and carbohydrates with electrolytes, trace elements, and vitamins, including preparation, any strength, hepatic-HepatAmine-premix ☒
Use this code for FreAmine HBC, HepatAmine.
CMS: 100-03,180.2; 100-04,20,160.2

B5200   Parenteral nutrition solution compounded amino acid and carbohydrates with electrolytes, trace elements, and vitamins, including preparation, any strength, stress-branch chain amino acids-FreAmine-HBC-premix ☒
CMS: 100-03,180.2; 100-04,20,160.2

Enteral and Parenteral Pumps

B9002   Enteral nutrition infusion pump, any type ☒
CMS: 100-03,180.2; 100-04,20,160.2

B9004   Parenteral nutrition infusion pump, portable ☒
CMS: 100-03,180.2; 100-04,20,160.2

B9006   Parenteral nutrition infusion pump, stationary ☒
CMS: 100-03,180.2; 100-04,20,160.2

B9998   NOC for enteral supplies ☒
CMS: 100-03,180.2

B9999   NOC for parenteral supplies ☒
Determine if an alternative HCPCS Level II or a CPT code better describes the service being reported. This code should be used only if a more specific code is unavailable.
CMS: 100-03,180.2

Special Coverage Instructions   Noncovered by Medicare   Carrier Discretion   ☑ Quantity Alert   ● New Code   ○ Recycled/Reinstated   ▲ Revised Code

© 2021 Optum360, LLC   A2–Z3 ASC Pmt   CMS: IOM   AHA: Coding Clinic   ⅄ DMEPOS Paid   ⊘ SNF Excluded   B Codes — 19

Outpatient PPS C1052-C9899

This section reports drug, biological, and device codes that must be used by OPPS hospitals. Non-OPPS hospitals, Critical Access Hospitals (CAHs), Indian Health Service Hospitals (HIS), hospitals located in American Samoa, Guam, Saipan, or the Virgin Islands, and Maryland waiver hospitals may report these codes at their discretion. The codes can only be reported for facility (technical) services.

The C series of HCPCS may include device categories, new technology procedures, and drugs, biologicals and radiopharmaceuticals that do not have other HCPCS codes assigned. Some of these items and services are eligible for transitional pass-through payments for OPPS hospitals, have separate APC payments, or are items that are packaged. Hospitals are encouraged to report all appropriate C codes regardless of payment status.

C1052 Hemostatic agent, gastrointestinal, topical J7

C1062 Intravertebral body fracture augmentation with implant (e.g., metal, polymer) J7

C1713 Anchor/screw for opposing bone-to-bone or soft tissue-to-bone (implantable) N N1
AHA: 3Q, '16, 15-19; 3Q, '16, 10-15; 3Q, '15, 2; 2Q, '10, 3; 3Q, '02, 4-5; 1Q, '01, 6

C1714 Catheter, transluminal atherectomy, directional N N1
AHA: 3Q, '16, 10-15; 4Q, '04, 4-5; 4Q, '03, 8; 3Q, '02, 4-5; 1Q, '01, 6

C1715 Brachytherapy needle N N1 ⊘
AHA: 3Q, '16, 10-15; 3Q, '02, 4-5; 1Q, '01, 6

C1716 Brachytherapy source, nonstranded, gold-198, per source U H2 ☑ ⊘
AHA: 3Q, '16, 11; 3Q, '16, 10-15; 2Q, '07, 11; 4Q, '04, 8; 2Q, '04, 10; 3Q, '02, 4-5; 1Q, '01, 6

C1717 Brachytherapy source, nonstranded, high dose rate iridium-192, per source U H2 ☑ ⊘
AHA: 3Q, '16, 11; 3Q, '16, 10-15; 2Q, '07, 11; 4Q, '04, 8; 2Q, '04, 10; 3Q, '02, 4-5; 1Q, '01, 6

C1719 Brachytherapy source, nonstranded, nonhigh dose rate iridium-192, per source U H2 ☑ ⊘
AHA: 3Q, '16, 11; 3Q, '16, 10-15; 2Q, '07, 11; 4Q, '04, 8; 2Q, '04, 10; 3Q, '02, 4-5; 1Q, '01, 6

C1721 Cardioverter-defibrillator, dual chamber (implantable) N N1
CMS: 100-04,14,40.8
AHA: 3Q, '16, 10-15; 4Q, '04, 4-5; 3Q, '02, 4-5; 1Q, '01, 6

C1722 Cardioverter-defibrillator, single chamber (implantable) N N1
CMS: 100-04,14,40.8
AHA: 3Q, '16, 10-15; 2Q, '06, 11; 4Q, '04, 4-5; 3Q, '02, 4-5; 1Q, '01, 6

C1724 Catheter, transluminal atherectomy, rotational N N1
AHA: 3Q, '16, 9; 3Q, '16, 10-15; 4Q, '04, 4-5; 4Q, '03, 8; 3Q, '02, 4-5; 1Q, '01, 6

C1725 Catheter, transluminal angioplasty, nonlaser (may include guidance, infusion/perfusion capability) N N1
To appropriately report drug-coated transluminal angioplasty catheters, use HCPCS code C2623.
AHA: 3Q, '16, 15-19; 3Q, '16, 10-15; 4Q, '04, 4-5; 4Q, '03, 8; 3Q, '02, 4-5; 1Q, '01, 6

C1726 Catheter, balloon dilatation, nonvascular N N1
AHA: 3Q, '16, 15-19; 3Q, '16, 10-15; 3Q, '02, 4-5; 1Q, '01, 6

C1727 Catheter, balloon tissue dissector, nonvascular (insertable) N N1
AHA: 3Q, '16, 15-19; 3Q, '16, 10-15; 3Q, '02, 4-5; 1Q, '01, 6

C1728 Catheter, brachytherapy seed administration N N1 ⊘
AHA: 3Q, '16, 10-15; 3Q, '02, 4-5; 1Q, '01, 6

C1729 Catheter, drainage N N1
AHA: 3Q, '16, 15-19; 3Q, '16, 10-15; 3Q, '02, 4-5; 1Q, '01, 6

C1730 Catheter, electrophysiology, diagnostic, other than 3D mapping (19 or fewer electrodes) N N1
AHA: 3Q, '16, 15-19; 3Q, '16, 10-15; 4Q, '04, 4-5; 3Q, '02, 4-5; 3Q, '01, 4-5; 1Q, '01, 6

C1731 Catheter, electrophysiology, diagnostic, other than 3D mapping (20 or more electrodes) N N1
AHA: 3Q, '16, 15-19; 3Q, '16, 10-15; 4Q, '04, 4-5; 3Q, '02, 4-5; 1Q, '01, 6

C1732 Catheter, electrophysiology, diagnostic/ablation, 3D or vector mapping N N1
AHA: 3Q, '16, 15-19; 3Q, '16, 10-15; 4Q, '04, 4-5; 3Q, '02, 4-5; 3Q, '01, 4-5; 1Q, '01, 6

C1733 Catheter, electrophysiology, diagnostic/ablation, other than 3D or vector mapping, other than cool-tip N N1
AHA: 3Q, '16, 15-19; 3Q, '16, 10-15; 4Q, '04, 4-5; 3Q, '02, 4-5; 3Q, '01, 4-5; 1Q, '01, 6

C1734 Orthopedic/device/drug matrix for opposing bone-to-bone or soft tissue-to bone (implantable) J7

C1748 Endoscope, single-use (i.e. disposable), upper GI, imaging/illumination device (insertable) J7

C1749 Endoscope, retrograde imaging/illumination colonoscope device (implantable) N N1
AHA: 3Q, '16, 10-15

C1750 Catheter, hemodialysis/peritoneal, long-term N N1
AHA: 3Q, '16, 10-15; 4Q, '15, 6; 4Q, '12, 9; 4Q, '03, 8; 3Q, '02, 4-5; 1Q, '01, 6

C1751 Catheter, infusion, inserted peripherally, centrally or midline (other than hemodialysis) N N1
AHA: 3Q, '16, 10-15; 3Q, '14, 5; 4Q, '04, 4-5; 4Q, '03, 8; 3Q, '02, 4-5; 3Q, '01, 4-5; 1Q, '01, 6

C1752 Catheter, hemodialysis/peritoneal, short-term N N1
AHA: 3Q, '16, 10-15; 4Q, '03, 8; 3Q, '02, 4-5; 1Q, '01, 6

C1753 Catheter, intravascular ultrasound N N1
AHA: 3Q, '16, 10-15; 4Q, '03, 8; 3Q, '02, 4-5; 1Q, '01, 6

C1754 Catheter, intradiscal N N1
AHA: 3Q, '16, 10-15; 4Q, '03, 8; 3Q, '02, 4-5; 1Q, '01, 6

C1755 Catheter, intraspinal N N1
AHA: 3Q, '16, 10-15; 4Q, '03, 8; 3Q, '02, 4-5; 1Q, '01, 6

C1756 Catheter, pacing, transesophageal N N1
AHA: 4Q, '03, 8; 3Q, '02, 4-5; 1Q, '01, 6

C1757 Catheter, thrombectomy/embolectomy N N1
AHA: 3Q, '16, 10-15; 4Q, '03, 8; 3Q, '02, 4-5; 1Q, '01, 6

C1758 Catheter, ureteral N N1
AHA: 3Q, '16, 10-15; 4Q, '03, 8; 3Q, '02, 4-5; 1Q, '01, 6

C1759 Catheter, intracardiac echocardiography N N1
AHA: 3Q, '16, 10-15; 4Q, '03, 8; 3Q, '02, 4-5; 3Q, '01, 4-5; 1Q, '01, 6

C1760 Closure device, vascular (implantable/insertable) N N1
AHA: 3Q, '16, 15-19; 3Q, '16, 10-15; 4Q, '03, 8; 3Q, '02, 4-5; 1Q, '01, 6

● **C1761** Catheter, transluminal intravascular lithotripsy, coronary J7

C1762 Connective tissue, human (includes fascia lata) N N1
AHA: 3Q, '16, 9; 3Q, '16, 15-19; 3Q, '16, 10-15; 3Q, '15, 2; 4Q, '03, 8; 3Q, '03, 11; 3Q, '02, 4-5; 1Q, '01, 6

C1763 Connective tissue, nonhuman (includes synthetic) N N1
AHA: 3Q, '16, 9; 3Q, '16, 15-19; 3Q, '16, 10-15; 4Q, '10, 1; 2Q, '10, 3; 4Q, '03, 8; 3Q, '03, 11; 3Q, '02, 4-5; 1Q, '01, 6

C1764 Event recorder, cardiac (implantable) N N1
CMS: 100-04,14,40.8
AHA: 3Q, '16, 10-15; 2Q, '15, 8; 4Q, '03, 8; 3Q, '02, 4-5; 1Q, '01, 6

Special Coverage Instructions   Noncovered by Medicare   Carrier Discretion   ☑ Quantity Alert   ● New Code   ○ Recycled/Reinstated   ▲ Revised Code

© 2021 Optum360, LLC   A2-Z3 ASC Pmt   CMS: IOM   AHA: Coding Clinic   DMEPOS Paid   ⊘ SNF Excluded   C Codes — 21

C1765   **Adhesion barrier**   N N1
AHA: 3Q, '16, 15-19; 3Q, '16, 10-15

C1766   **Introducer/sheath, guiding, intracardiac electrophysiological, steerable, other than peel-away**   N N1
AHA: 3Q, '16, 10-15; 4Q, '04, 4-5; 3Q, '02, 4-5; 3Q, '01, 4-5

C1767   **Generator, neurostimulator (implantable), nonrechargeable**   N N1
CMS: 100-04,14,40.8; 100-04,32,40.1; 100-04,32,40.2.1; 100-04,32,40.2.4; 100-04,32,40.4
AHA: 3Q, '16, 10-15; 4Q, '06, 4; 4Q, '04, 4-5; 4Q, '03, 8; 3Q, '02, 4-5; 1Q, '02, 9; 1Q, '01, 6

C1768   **Graft, vascular**   N N1
AHA: 3Q, '16, 10-15; 4Q, '03, 8; 3Q, '02, 4-5; 1Q, '01, 6

C1769   **Guide wire**   N N1
AHA: 3Q, '16, 10-15; 3Q, '16; 3Q, '14, 5; 2Q, '07, 6; 4Q, '03, 8; 3Q, '02, 4-5; 3Q, '01, 4-5; 1Q, '01, 6

C1770   **Imaging coil, magnetic resonance (insertable)**   N N1
AHA: 3Q, '16, 10-15; 4Q, '03, 8; 3Q, '02, 4-5; 1Q, '01, 6

C1771   **Repair device, urinary, incontinence, with sling graft**   N N1
CMS: 100-04,14,40.8
AHA: 3Q, '16, 15-19; 3Q, '16, 10-15; 4Q, '03, 8; 3Q, '02, 4-5; 3Q, '01, 4-5; 1Q, '01, 6

C1772   **Infusion pump, programmable (implantable)**   N N1
CMS: 100-04,14,40.8
AHA: 3Q, '16, 10-15; 4Q, '04, 4-5; 3Q, '02, 4-5; 1Q, '01, 6

C1773   **Retrieval device, insertable (used to retrieve fractured medical devices)**   N N1
AHA: 3Q, '16, 15-19; 3Q, '16, 10-15; 4Q, '03, 8; 3Q, '02, 4-5; 1Q, '01, 6

C1776   **Joint device (implantable)**   N N1
CMS: 100-04,14,40.8
AHA: 3Q, '16, 3; 3Q, '16, 15-19; 3Q, '16, 10-15; 3Q, '10, 6; 4Q, '08, 6, 8; 3Q, '02, 4-5; 3Q, '01, 4-5; 1Q, '01, 6

C1777   **Lead, cardioverter-defibrillator, endocardial single coil (implantable)**   N N1
AHA: 3Q, '16, 10-15; 2Q, '06, 11; 4Q, '04, 4-5; 3Q, '02, 4-5; 1Q, '01, 6

C1778   **Lead, neurostimulator (implantable)**   N N1
CMS: 100-04,14,40.8; 100-04,32,40.1; 100-04,32,40.2.1; 100-04,32,40.2.4; 100-04,32,40.4
AHA: 3Q, '16, 10-15; 4Q, '11, 10; 3Q, '02, 4-5; 1Q, '02, 9; 1Q, '01, 6

C1779   **Lead, pacemaker, transvenous VDD single pass**   N N1
CMS: 100-04,14,40.8
AHA: 3Q, '16, 15-19; 3Q, '16, 10-15; 4Q, '04, 4-5; 3Q, '02, 4-5; 1Q, '01, 6

C1780   **Lens, intraocular (new technology)**   N N1
AHA: 3Q, '16, 15-19; 3Q, '16, 10-15; 3Q, '02, 4-5; 1Q, '01, 6

C1781   **Mesh (implantable)**   N N1
Use this code for OrthADAPT Bioimplant.
AHA: 3Q, '16, 15-19; 3Q, '16, 10-15; 2Q, '12, 3; 2Q, '10, 3; 2Q, '10, 2, 3; 3Q, '02, 4-5; 1Q, '01, 6

C1782   **Morcellator**   N N1
AHA: 3Q, '16, 15-19; 3Q, '16, 10-15; 3Q, '02, 4-5; 1Q, '01, 6

C1783   **Ocular implant, aqueous drainage assist device**   N N1
AHA: 1Q, '17, 5; 3Q, '16, 10-15

C1784   **Ocular device, intraoperative, detached retina**   N N1
AHA: 3Q, '16, 15-19; 3Q, '16, 10-15; 3Q, '02, 4-5; 1Q, '01, 6

C1785   **Pacemaker, dual chamber, rate-responsive (implantable)**   N N1
CMS: 100-04,14,40.8; 100-04,21,320.4.7; 100-04,32,320.4.1; 100-04,32,320.4.2; 100-04,32,320.4.4; 100-04,32,320.4.6; 100-04,32,320.4.7
AHA: 3Q, '16, 10-15; 4Q, '03, 8; 3Q, '02, 4-5; 1Q, '01, 6

C1786   **Pacemaker, single chamber, rate-responsive (implantable)**   N N1
CMS: 100-04,14,40.8; 100-04,21,320.4.7; 100-04,32,320.4.1; 100-04,32,320.4.2; 100-04,32,320.4.4; 100-04,32,320.4.6; 100-04,32,320.4.7
AHA: 3Q, '16, 10-15; 4Q, '04, 4-5; 4Q, '03, 8; 3Q, '02, 4-5; 1Q, '01, 6

C1787   **Patient programmer, neurostimulator**   N N1
AHA: 3Q, '16, 15-19; 3Q, '16, 10-15; 4Q, '03, 8; 3Q, '02, 4-5; 1Q, '01, 6

C1788   **Port, indwelling (implantable)**   N N1
AHA: 3Q, '16, 10-15; 3Q, '14, 5; 4Q, '04, 4-5; 4Q, '03, 8; 3Q, '02, 4-5; 3Q, '01, 4-5; 1Q, '01, 6

C1789   **Prosthesis, breast (implantable)**   N N1
AHA: 3Q, '16, 10-15; 4Q, '03, 8; 3Q, '02, 4-5; 1Q, '01, 6

C1813   **Prosthesis, penile, inflatable**   N N1
CMS: 100-04,14,40.8
AHA: 3Q, '16, 10-15; 4Q, '03, 8; 3Q, '02, 4-5; 1Q, '01, 6

C1814   **Retinal tamponade device, silicone oil**   N N1
AHA: 3Q, '16, 15-19; 3Q, '16, 10-15; 2Q, '06, 12

C1815   **Prosthesis, urinary sphincter (implantable)**   N N1
CMS: 100-04,14,40.8
AHA: 3Q, '16, 10-15; 4Q, '03, 8; 3Q, '02, 4-5; 1Q, '01, 6

C1816   **Receiver and/or transmitter, neurostimulator (implantable)**   N N1
AHA: 3Q, '16, 10-15; 4Q, '03, 8; 3Q, '02, 4-5; 1Q, '01, 6

C1817   **Septal defect implant system, intracardiac**   N N1
AHA: 3Q, '16, 15-19; 3Q, '16, 10-15; 4Q, '03, 8; 3Q, '02, 4-5; 1Q, '01, 6

C1818   **Integrated keratoprosthesis**   N N1
AHA: 3Q, '16, 15-19; 3Q, '16, 10-15; 4Q, '03, 4-5

C1819   **Surgical tissue localization and excision device (implantable)**   N N1
AHA: 3Q, '16, 10-15; 1Q, '04, 10

C1820   **Generator, neurostimulator (implantable), with rechargeable battery and charging system**   N N1
Use to report neurostimulator generators that are not high frequency.
CMS: 100-04,14,40.8; 100-04,32,40.2.1; 100-04,32,40.2.4; 100-04,32,40.4; 100-04,4,10.12
AHA: 3Q, '16, 10-15; 2Q, '16, 7; 1Q, '16, 9

C1821   **Interspinous process distraction device (implantable)**   N N1
AHA: 3Q, '16, 10-15; 2Q, '09, 1

C1822   **Generator, neurostimulator (implantable), high frequency, with rechargeable battery and charging system**   N N1
Use to report neurostimulator generators that are high frequency.
AHA: 3Q, '16, 10-15; 2Q, '16, 7; 1Q, '16, 9

C1823   **Generator, neurostimulator (implantable), nonrechargeable, with transvenous sensing and stimulation leads**   J7
CMS: 100-04,4,260.1; 100-04,4,260.1.1

C1824   **Generator, cardiac contractility modulation (implantable)**   J7

C1825   **Generator, neurostimulator (implantable), nonrechargeable with carotid sinus baroreceptor stimulation lead(s)**   J7

C1830   **Powered bone marrow biopsy needle**   N N1
AHA: 3Q, '16, 10-15; 4Q, '11, 10

● **C1831**   **Personalized, anterior and lateral interbody cage (implantable)**   J7

● **C1832**   **Autograft suspension, including cell processing and application, and all system components**

● **C1833**   **Monitor, cardiac, including intracardiac lead and all system components (implantable)**

C1839   **Iris prosthesis**   J7

Special Coverage Instructions   Noncovered by Medicare   Carrier Discretion   ☑ Quantity Alert   ● New Code   ○ Recycled/Reinstated   ▲ Revised Code

   A Age Edit   M Maternity Edit   ♀ Female Only   ♂ Male Only   A-Y OPPS Status Indicators   © 2021 Optum360, LLC

C1840 Lens, intraocular (telescopic) N N1
AHA: 3Q, '16, 10-15; 3Q, '12, 10; 4Q, '11, 10

C1841 Retinal prosthesis, includes all internal and external components N J7
AHA: 1Q, '17, 6; 3Q, '16, 10-15

C1842 Retinal prosthesis, includes all internal and external components; add-on to C1841 E J7
In the ASC setting, C1842 must be reported with C1841 and CPT code 0100T.
AHA: 1Q, '17, 6

C1849 Skin substitute, synthetic, resorbable, per sq cm N1

C1874 Stent, coated/covered, with delivery system N N1
AHA: 3Q, '16, 15-19; 3Q, '16, 10-15; 4Q, '04, 4-5; 3Q, '04, 11-13; 4Q, '03, 8; 3Q, '02, 7; 3Q, '02, 4-5; 3Q, '01, 4-5; 1Q, '01, 6

C1875 Stent, coated/covered, without delivery system N N1
AHA: 3Q, '16, 15-19; 3Q, '16, 10-15; 4Q, '04, 4-5; 4Q, '03, 8; 3Q, '02, 7; 3Q, '02, 4-5; 1Q, '01, 6

C1876 Stent, noncoated/noncovered, with delivery system N N1
AHA: 3Q, '16, 15-19; 3Q, '16, 10-15; 4Q, '04, 4-5; 4Q, '03, 8; 3Q, '02, 7; 3Q, '02, 4-5; 3Q, '01, 4-5; 1Q, '01, 6

C1877 Stent, noncoated/noncovered, without delivery system N N1
AHA: 3Q, '16, 10-15; 4Q, '04, 4-5; 4Q, '03, 8; 3Q, '02, 7; 3Q, '02, 4-5; 3Q, '01, 4-5; 1Q, '01, 6

C1878 Material for vocal cord medialization, synthetic (implantable) N N1
AHA: 3Q, '16, 15-19; 3Q, '16, 10-15; 3Q, '02, 4-5; 1Q, '01, 6

C1880 Vena cava filter N N1
AHA: 3Q, '16, 10-15; 4Q, '03, 8; 3Q, '02, 4-5; 1Q, '01, 6

C1881 Dialysis access system (implantable) N N1
CMS: 100-04,14,40.8
AHA: 3Q, '16, 10-15; 4Q, '03, 8; 3Q, '02, 4-5; 1Q, '01, 6

C1882 Cardioverter-defibrillator, other than single or dual chamber (implantable) N N1
CMS: 100-04,14,40.8
AHA: 3Q, '16, 15-19; 3Q, '16, 10-15; 2Q, '12, 9; 2Q, '06, 11; 4Q, '04, 4-5; 3Q, '02, 4-5; 1Q, '01, 6

C1883 Adaptor/extension, pacing lead or neurostimulator lead (implantable) N N1
CMS: 100-04,32,40.1; 100-04,32,40.2.1; 100-04,32,40.2.4; 100-04,32,40.4
AHA: 3Q, '16, 15-19; 3Q, '16, 10-15; 3Q, '02, 4-5; 1Q, '02, 9; 1Q, '01, 6

C1884 Embolization protective system N N1
AHA: 3Q, '16, 15-19; 3Q, '16, 10-15; 3Q, '14, 5

C1885 Catheter, transluminal angioplasty, laser N N1
AHA: 3Q, '16, 15-19; 3Q, '16, 10-15; 1Q, '16, 5; 4Q, '04, 4-5; 4Q, '03, 8; 3Q, '02, 4-5; 1Q, '01, 6

C1886 Catheter, extravascular tissue ablation, any modality (insertable) N N1
AHA: 3Q, '16, 10-15

C1887 Catheter, guiding (may include infusion/perfusion capability) N N1
AHA: 3Q, '16, 15-19; 3Q, '16, 10-15; 4Q, '04, 4-5; 3Q, '02, 4-5; 3Q, '01, 4-5; 1Q, '01, 6

C1888 Catheter, ablation, noncardiac, endovascular (implantable) N N1
AHA: 3Q, '16, 15-19; 3Q, '16, 10-15

C1889 Implantable/insertable device, not otherwise classified N N1

C1890 No implantable/insertable device used with device-intensive procedures J7
CMS: 100-04,4,260.1; 100-04,4,260.1.1

C1891 Infusion pump, nonprogrammable, permanent (implantable) N N1
CMS: 100-04,14,40.8
AHA: 3Q, '16, 10-15; 4Q, '04, 4-5; 4Q, '03, 8; 3Q, '02, 4-5; 1Q, '01, 6

C1892 Introducer/sheath, guiding, intracardiac electrophysiological, fixed-curve, peel-away N N1
AHA: 3Q, '16, 15-19; 3Q, '16, 10-15; 4Q, '04, 4-5; 3Q, '02, 4-5; 1Q, '01, 6

C1893 Introducer/sheath, guiding, intracardiac electrophysiological, fixed-curve, other than peel-away N N1
AHA: 3Q, '16, 10-15; 4Q, '04, 4-5; 3Q, '02, 4-5; 1Q, '01, 6

C1894 Introducer/sheath, other than guiding, other than intracardiac electrophysiological, nonlaser N N1
AHA: 3Q, '16, 9; 3Q, '16, 10-15; 3Q, '02, 4-5; 1Q, '01, 6

C1895 Lead, cardioverter-defibrillator, endocardial dual coil (implantable) N N1
AHA: 3Q, '16, 10-15; 2Q, '06, 11; 4Q, '04, 4-5; 3Q, '02, 4-5; 1Q, '01, 6

C1896 Lead, cardioverter-defibrillator, other than endocardial single or dual coil (implantable) N N1
AHA: 3Q, '16, 10-15; 2Q, '06, 11; 4Q, '04, 4-5; 3Q, '02, 4-5; 1Q, '01, 6

C1897 Lead, neurostimulator test kit (implantable) N N1
CMS: 100-04,14,40.8; 100-04,32,40.1; 100-04,32,40.2.1; 100-04,32,40.2.4; 100-04,32,40.4
AHA: 3Q, '16, 10-15; 3Q, '02, 4-5; 1Q, '02, 9; 1Q, '01, 6

C1898 Lead, pacemaker, other than transvenous VDD single pass N N1
CMS: 100-04,14,40.8
AHA: 3Q, '16, 10-15; 3Q, '02, 8; 3Q, '02, 4-5; 3Q, '01, 4-5; 1Q, '01, 6

C1899 Lead, pacemaker/cardioverter-defibrillator combination (implantable) N N1
AHA: 3Q, '16, 10-15; 4Q, '04, 4-5; 3Q, '02, 4-5; 1Q, '01, 6

C1900 Lead, left ventricular coronary venous system N N1
CMS: 100-04,14,40.8
AHA: 3Q, '16, 15-19; 3Q, '16, 10-15; 4Q, '04, 4-5

C1982 Catheter, pressure generating, one-way valve, intermittently occlusive J7

C2596 Probe, image guided, robotic, waterjet ablation J7

C2613 Lung biopsy plug with delivery system N N1
AHA: 3Q, '16, 10-15; 3Q, '15, 7

C2614 Probe, percutaneous lumbar discectomy N N1
AHA: 3Q, '16, 10-15

C2615 Sealant, pulmonary, liquid N N1
AHA: 3Q, '16, 15-19; 3Q, '16, 10-15; 4Q, '03, 8; 3Q, '02, 4-5; 1Q, '01, 6

C2616 Brachytherapy source, nonstranded, yttrium-90, per source U H2 ☑ ⊘
AHA: 3Q, '16, 11; 3Q, '16, 10-15; 2Q, '07, 11; 4Q, '04, 8; 2Q, '04, 10; 3Q, '03, 11; 3Q, '02, 4-5

C2617 Stent, noncoronary, temporary, without delivery system N N1
AHA: 3Q, '16, 15-19; 3Q, '16, 10-15; 3Q, '16; 4Q, '04, 4-5; 4Q, '03, 8; 3Q, '02, 4-5; 1Q, '01, 6

C2618 Probe/needle, cryoablation N N1
AHA: 3Q, '16, 10-15; 4Q, '04, 4-5; 4Q, '03, 8; 3Q, '02, 4-5; 1Q, '01, 6

C2619 Pacemaker, dual chamber, nonrate-responsive (implantable) N N1
CMS: 100-04,14,40.8; 100-04,21,320.4.7; 100-04,32,320.4.1; 100-04,32,320.4.2; 100-04,32,320.4.4; 100-04,32,320.4.6; 100-04,32,320.4.7
AHA: 3Q, '16, 10-15; 3Q, '02, 4-5; 3Q, '01, 4-5; 1Q, '01, 6

Special Coverage Instructions   Noncovered by Medicare   Carrier Discretion   ☑ Quantity Alert   ● New Code   ○ Recycled/Reinstated   ▲ Revised Code

© 2021 Optum360, LLC   A2-Z4 ASC Pmt   CMS: IOM   AHA: Coding Clinic   ⅃ DMEPOS Paid   ⊘ SNF Excluded   C Codes — 23

C2620 Pacemaker, single chamber, nonrate-responsive (implantable) N N1
CMS: 100-04,14,40.8; 100-04,21,320.4.7; 100-04,32,320.4.1; 100-04,32,320.4.2; 100-04,32,320.4.4; 100-04,32,320.4.6; 100-04,32,320.4.7
AHA: 3Q, '16, 10-15; 4Q, '04, 4-5; 4Q, '03, 8; 3Q, '02, 4-5; 1Q, '01, 6

C2621 Pacemaker, other than single or dual chamber (implantable) N N1
CMS: 100-04,14,40.8
AHA: 3Q, '16, 15-19; 3Q, '16, 10-15; 4Q, '03, 8; 3Q, '02, 8; 3Q, '02, 4-5; 1Q, '01, 6

C2622 Prosthesis, penile, noninflatable N N1
CMS: 100-04,14,40.8
AHA: 3Q, '16, 10-15; 4Q, '03, 8; 3Q, '02, 4-5; 1Q, '01, 6

C2623 Catheter, transluminal angioplasty, drug-coated, nonlaser N N1
AHA: 3Q, '16, 10-15

C2624 Implantable wireless pulmonary artery pressure sensor with delivery catheter, including all system components N N1
AHA: 3Q, '16, 10-15; 3Q, '15, 1-2

C2625 Stent, noncoronary, temporary, with delivery system N N1
AHA: 3Q, '16, 15-19; 3Q, '16, 10-15; 2Q, '15, 9; 4Q, '04, 4-5; 4Q, '03, 8; 3Q, '02, 4-5; 1Q, '01, 6

C2626 Infusion pump, nonprogrammable, temporary (implantable) N N1
CMS: 100-04,14,40.8
AHA: 3Q, '16, 15-19; 3Q, '16, 10-15; 4Q, '04, 4-5; 3Q, '02, 4-5; 1Q, '01, 6

C2627 Catheter, suprapubic/cystoscopic N N1
AHA: 3Q, '16, 15-19; 3Q, '16, 10-15; 4Q, '03, 8; 3Q, '02, 4-5; 1Q, '01, 6

C2628 Catheter, occlusion N N1
AHA: 3Q, '16, 10-15; 4Q, '04, 4-5; 4Q, '03, 8; 3Q, '02, 4-5; 1Q, '01, 6

C2629 Introducer/sheath, other than guiding, other than intracardiac electrophysiological, laser N N1
AHA: 3Q, '16, 10-15; 3Q, '02, 4-5; 1Q, '01, 6

C2630 Catheter, electrophysiology, diagnostic/ablation, other than 3D or vector mapping, cool-tip N N1
AHA: 3Q, '16, 15-19; 3Q, '16, 10-15; 3Q, '02, 4-5; 1Q, '01, 6

C2631 Repair device, urinary, incontinence, without sling graft N N1
CMS: 100-04,14,40.8
AHA: 3Q, '16, 15-19; 3Q, '16, 10-15; 4Q, '03, 8; 3Q, '02, 4-5; 1Q, '01, 6

C2634 Brachytherapy source, nonstranded, high activity, iodine-125, greater than 1.01 mCi (NIST), per source U H2
AHA: 3Q, '16, 11; 2Q, '07, 11; 2Q, '05, 8; 4Q, '04, 8

C2635 Brachytherapy source, nonstranded, high activity, palladium-103, greater than 2.2 mCi (NIST), per source U H2
AHA: 3Q, '16, 11; 2Q, '07, 11; 2Q, '05, 8; 4Q, '04, 8

C2636 Brachytherapy linear source, nonstranded, palladium-103, per 1 mm U H2
AHA: 3Q, '16, 11; 2Q, '07, 11; 4Q, '04, 8

C2637 Brachytherapy source, nonstranded, ytterbium-169, per source B
AHA: 3Q, '16, 11; 2Q, '07, 11; 3Q, '05, 7

C2638 Brachytherapy source, stranded, iodine-125, per source U H2
AHA: 3Q, '16, 11

C2639 Brachytherapy source, nonstranded, iodine-125, per source U H2
AHA: 3Q, '16, 11

C2640 Brachytherapy source, stranded, palladium-103, per source U H2
AHA: 3Q, '16, 11

C2641 Brachytherapy source, nonstranded, palladium-103, per source U H2
AHA: 3Q, '16, 11

C2642 Brachytherapy source, stranded, cesium-131, per source U H2
AHA: 3Q, '16, 11

C2643 Brachytherapy source, nonstranded, cesium-131, per source U H2
AHA: 3Q, '16, 11

C2644 Brachytherapy source, cesium-131 chloride solution, per mCi U
AHA: 3Q, '16, 11

C2645 Brachytherapy planar source, palladium-103, per sq mm U H2
AHA: 3Q, '16, 11

C2698 Brachytherapy source, stranded, not otherwise specified, per source U H2
AHA: 3Q, '16, 11

C2699 Brachytherapy source, nonstranded, not otherwise specified, per source U H2
AHA: 3Q, '16, 11

C5271 Application of low cost skin substitute graft to trunk, arms, legs, total wound surface area up to 100 sq cm; first 25 sq cm or less wound surface area T G2

C5272 Application of low cost skin substitute graft to trunk, arms, legs, total wound surface area up to 100 sq cm; each additional 25 sq cm wound surface area, or part thereof (list separately in addition to code for primary procedure) N N1

C5273 Application of low cost skin substitute graft to trunk, arms, legs, total wound surface area greater than or equal to 100 sq cm; first 100 sq cm wound surface area, or 1% of body area of infants and children T G2

C5274 Application of low cost skin substitute graft to trunk, arms, legs, total wound surface area greater than or equal to 100 sq cm; each additional 100 sq cm wound surface area, or part thereof, or each additional 1% of body area of infants and children, or part thereof (list separately in addition to code for primary procedure) N N1

C5275 Application of low cost skin substitute graft to face, scalp, eyelids, mouth, neck, ears, orbits, genitalia, hands, feet, and/or multiple digits, total wound surface area up to 100 sq cm; first 25 sq cm or less wound surface area T G2

C5276 Application of low cost skin substitute graft to face, scalp, eyelids, mouth, neck, ears, orbits, genitalia, hands, feet, and/or multiple digits, total wound surface area up to 100 sq cm; each additional 25 sq cm wound surface area, or part thereof (list separately in addition to code for primary procedure) N N1

C5277 Application of low cost skin substitute graft to face, scalp, eyelids, mouth, neck, ears, orbits, genitalia, hands, feet, and/or multiple digits, total wound surface area greater than or equal to 100 sq cm; first 100 sq cm wound surface area, or 1% of body area of infants and children T G2

C5278 Application of low cost skin substitute graft to face, scalp, eyelids, mouth, neck, ears, orbits, genitalia, hands, feet, and/or multiple digits, total wound surface area greater than or equal to 100 sq cm; each additional 100 sq cm wound surface area, or part thereof, or each additional 1% of body area of infants and children, or part thereof (list separately in addition to code for primary procedure) N N1

Special Coverage Instructions   Noncovered by Medicare   Carrier Discretion   ☑ Quantity Alert   ● New Code   ○ Recycled/Reinstated   ▲ Revised Code

24 — C Codes   A Age Edit   M Maternity Edit   ♀ Female Only   ♂ Male Only   A-Y OPPS Status Indicators   © 2021 Optum360, LLC

C8900 Magnetic resonance angiography with contrast, abdomen 〔Q3〕〔Z2〕⊘
CMS: 100-04,13,40.1.1; 100-04,13,40.1.2

C8901 Magnetic resonance angiography without contrast, abdomen 〔Q3〕〔Z2〕⊘
CMS: 100-04,13,40.1.1; 100-04,13,40.1.2

C8902 Magnetic resonance angiography without contrast followed by with contrast, abdomen 〔Q3〕〔Z2〕⊘
CMS: 100-04,13,40.1.1; 100-04,13,40.1.2

C8903 Magnetic resonance imaging with contrast, breast; unilateral 〔Q3〕〔Z2〕⊘

C8905 Magnetic resonance imaging without contrast followed by with contrast, breast; unilateral 〔Q3〕〔Z2〕⊘

C8906 Magnetic resonance imaging with contrast, breast; bilateral 〔Q3〕〔Z2〕⊘

C8908 Magnetic resonance imaging without contrast followed by with contrast, breast; bilateral 〔Q3〕〔Z2〕⊘

C8909 Magnetic resonance angiography with contrast, chest (excluding myocardium) 〔Q3〕〔Z2〕⊘
CMS: 100-04,13,40.1.1; 100-04,13,40.1.2

C8910 Magnetic resonance angiography without contrast, chest (excluding myocardium) 〔Q3〕〔Z2〕⊘
CMS: 100-04,13,40.1.1; 100-04,13,40.1.2

C8911 Magnetic resonance angiography without contrast followed by with contrast, chest (excluding myocardium) 〔Q3〕〔Z2〕⊘
CMS: 100-04,13,40.1.1; 100-04,13,40.1.2

C8912 Magnetic resonance angiography with contrast, lower extremity 〔Q3〕〔Z2〕⊘
CMS: 100-04,13,40.1.1; 100-04,13,40.1.2

C8913 Magnetic resonance angiography without contrast, lower extremity 〔Q3〕〔Z2〕⊘
CMS: 100-04,13,40.1.1; 100-04,13,40.1.2

C8914 Magnetic resonance angiography without contrast followed by with contrast, lower extremity 〔Q3〕〔Z2〕⊘
CMS: 100-04,13,40.1.1; 100-04,13,40.1.2

C8918 Magnetic resonance angiography with contrast, pelvis 〔Q3〕〔Z2〕⊘
CMS: 100-04,13,40.1.1; 100-04,13,40.1.2
AHA: 4Q, '03, 4-5

C8919 Magnetic resonance angiography without contrast, pelvis 〔Q3〕〔Z2〕⊘
CMS: 100-04,13,40.1.1; 100-04,13,40.1.2
AHA: 4Q, '03, 4-5

C8920 Magnetic resonance angiography without contrast followed by with contrast, pelvis 〔Q3〕〔Z2〕⊘
CMS: 100-04,13,40.1.1; 100-04,13,40.1.2
AHA: 4Q, '03, 4-5

C8921 Transthoracic echocardiography (TTE) with contrast, or without contrast followed by with contrast, for congenital cardiac anomalies; complete 〔S〕
CMS: 100-04,4,200.7.2
AHA: 3Q, '12, 8; 2Q, '08, 9

C8922 Transthoracic echocardiography (TTE) with contrast, or without contrast followed by with contrast, for congenital cardiac anomalies; follow-up or limited study 〔S〕
AHA: 2Q, '08, 9

C8923 Transthoracic echocardiography (TTE) with contrast, or without contrast followed by with contrast, real-time with image documentation (2D), includes M-mode recording, when performed, complete, without spectral or color doppler echocardiography 〔S〕
AHA: 2Q, '08, 9

C8924 Transthoracic echocardiography (TTE) with contrast, or without contrast followed by with contrast, real-time with image documentation (2D), includes M-mode recording when performed, follow-up or limited study 〔S〕
AHA: 2Q, '08, 9

C8925 Transesophageal echocardiography (TEE) with contrast, or without contrast followed by with contrast, real time with image documentation (2D) (with or without M-mode recording); including probe placement, image acquisition, interpretation and report 〔S〕
AHA: 2Q, '08, 9

C8926 Transesophageal echocardiography (TEE) with contrast, or without contrast followed by with contrast, for congenital cardiac anomalies; including probe placement, image acquisition, interpretation and report 〔S〕
AHA: 2Q, '08, 9

C8927 Transesophageal echocardiography (TEE) with contrast, or without contrast followed by with contrast, for monitoring purposes, including probe placement, real time (2D) image acquisition and interpretation leading to ongoing (continuous) assessment of (dynamically changing) cardiac pumping function and to therapeutic measures on an immediate time basis 〔S〕
AHA: 2Q, '08, 9

C8928 Transthoracic echocardiography (TTE) with contrast, or without contrast followed by with contrast, real-time with image documentation (2D), includes M-mode recording, when performed, during rest and cardiovascular stress test using treadmill, bicycle exercise and/or pharmacologically induced stress, with interpretation and report 〔S〕
AHA: 2Q, '08, 9

C8929 Transthoracic echocardiography (TTE) with contrast, or without contrast followed by with contrast, real-time with image documentation (2D), includes M-mode recording, when performed, complete, with spectral doppler echocardiography, and with color flow doppler echocardiography 〔S〕

C8930 Transthoracic echocardiography (TTE) with contrast, or without contrast followed by with contrast, real-time with image documentation (2D), includes M-mode recording, when performed, during rest and cardiovascular stress test using treadmill, bicycle exercise and/or pharmacologically induced stress, with interpretation and report; including performance of continuous electrocardiographic monitoring, with physician supervision 〔S〕
AHA: 3Q, '12, 8

C8931 Magnetic resonance angiography with contrast, spinal canal and contents 〔Q3〕〔Z2〕

C8932 Magnetic resonance angiography without contrast, spinal canal and contents 〔Q3〕〔Z2〕

C8933 Magnetic resonance angiography without contrast followed by with contrast, spinal canal and contents 〔Q3〕〔Z2〕

C8934 Magnetic resonance angiography with contrast, upper extremity 〔Q3〕〔Z2〕

C8935 Magnetic resonance angiography without contrast, upper extremity 〔Q3〕〔Z2〕

C8936 Magnetic resonance angiography without contrast followed by with contrast, upper extremity 〔Q3〕〔Z2〕

Special Coverage Instructions   Noncovered by Medicare   Carrier Discretion   ☑ Quantity Alert   ● New Code   ○ Recycled/Reinstated   ▲ Revised Code

© 2021 Optum360, LLC   〔A2–Z3〕 ASC Pmt   CMS: IOM   AHA: Coding Clinic   ✧ DMEPOS Paid   ⊘ SNF Excluded   C Codes — 25

C8937 Computer-aided detection, including computer algorithm analysis of breast MRI image data for lesion detection/characterization, pharmacokinetic analysis, with further physician review for interpretation (list separately in addition to code for primary procedure)

C8957 Intravenous infusion for therapy/diagnosis; initiation of prolonged infusion (more than 8 hours), requiring use of portable or implantable pump ⓈS
CMS: 100-04,4,230.2
AHA: 3Q, '08, 7, 8; 4Q, '05, 15

C9046 Cocaine HCl nasal solution for topical administration, 1 mg K2
Use this code for Goprelto.

C9047 Injection, caplacizumab-yhdp, 1 mg K2
Use this code for Cablivi.

C9065 Injection, romidepsin, non-lyophilized (e.g. liquid), 1 mg
To report, see ~J9314, J9318

C9067 Gallium Ga-68, Dotatoc, diagnostic, 0.01 mCi K2

C9068 Copper Cu-64, dotatate, diagnostic, 1 mCi
To report, see ~A9592

C9069 Injection, belantamab mafodotin-blmf, 0.5 mg
To report, see ~J9037

C9070 Injection, tafasitamab-cxix, 2 mg
To report, see ~J9349

C9071 Injection, viltolarsen, 10 mg
To report, see ~J1427

C9072 Injection, immune globulin (Asceniv), 500 mg
To report, see ~J1554

C9073 Brexucabtagene autoleucel, up to 200 million autologous anti-CD19 CAR positive viable T cells, including leukapheresis and dose preparation procedures, per therapeutic dose
To report, see ~Q2053

C9074 Injection, lumasiran, 0.5 mg
To report, see ~J0224

C9075 Injection, casimersen, 10 mg
To report, see ~J1426

C9076 Lisocabtagene maraleucel, up to 110 million autologous anti-CD19 CAR-positive viable T cells, including leukapheresis and dose preparation procedures, per therapeutic dose
To report, see ~Q2054

C9077 Injection, cabotegravir and rilpivirine, 2 mg/3 mg
To report, see ~J0741

C9078 Injection, trilaciclib, 1 mg
To report, see ~J1448

C9079 Injection, evinacumab-dgnb, 5 mg
To report, see ~J1305

C9080 Injection, melphalan flufenamide HCl, 1 mg
To report, see ~J9247

C9081 Idecabtagene vicleucel, up to 460 million autologous anti-BCMA CAR-positive viable T cells, including leukapheresis and dose preparation procedures, per therapeutic dose
To report, see ~Q2055

C9082 Injection, dostarlimab-gxly, 100 mg
To report, see ~J9272

C9083 Injection, amivantamab-vmjw, 10 mg
To report, see ~J9061

● **C9084** Injection, loncastuximab tesirine-lpyl, 0.1 mg K2
Use this code for Zynlonta.

● **C9085** Injection, avalglucosidase alfa-ngpt, 4 mg
Use this code for Nexviazyme.

● **C9086** Injection, anifrolumab-fnia, 1 mg
Use this code for Saphnelo.

● **C9087** Injection, cyclophosphamide, (AuroMedics), 10 mg

● **C9088** Instillation, bupivacaine and meloxicam, 1 mg/0.03 mg
Use this code for Zynrelef.

● **C9089** Bupivacaine, collagen-matrix implant, 1 mg
Use this code for Xaracoll.

C9113 Injection, pantoprazole sodium, per vial N M1 ☑
Use this code for Protonix.
AHA: 1Q, '02, 5

C9122 Mometasone furoate sinus implant, 10 mcg (Sinuva)
To report, see ~J7402

C9132 Prothrombin complex concentrate (human), Kcentra, per IU of Factor IX activity
To report, see ~J7168

C9248 Injection, clevidipine butyrate, 1 mg N K2 ☑
Use this code for Cleviprex.

C9250 Human plasma fibrin sealant, vapor-heated, solvent-detergent (Artiss), 2 ml K K2 ☑

C9254 Injection, lacosamide, 1 mg N M1 ☑
Use this code for VIMPAT.

C9257 Injection, bevacizumab, 0.25 mg K K2 ☑
Use this code for Avastin.
CMS: 100-03,110.17
AHA: 3Q, '13, 9

C9285 Lidocaine 70 mg/tetracaine 70 mg, per patch N M1 ☑
Use this code for SYNERA.
AHA: 3Q, '11, 9

C9290 Injection, bupivacaine liposome, 1 mg N K2 ☑
Use this code for EXPAREL.
AHA: 2Q, '12, 7

C9293 Injection, glucarpidase, 10 units K ☑
Use this code for Voraxaze.

Special Coverage Instructions   Noncovered by Medicare   Carrier Discretion   ☑ Quantity Alert ● New Code   ○ Recycled/Reinstated   ▲ Revised Code

26 — C Codes   Ⓐ Age Edit   Ⓜ Maternity Edit   ♀ Female Only   ♂ Male Only   Ⓐ-Ⓨ OPPS Status Indicators   © 2021 Optum360, LLC

C9352 Microporous collagen implantable tube (NeuraGen Nerve Guide), per cm length N N1 ☑
AHA: 1Q, '08, 6

Damaged nerve

Healthy nerve

Artificial nerve conduit

A synthetic "bridge" is affixed to each end of a severed nerve with sutures. This procedure is performed using an operating microscope

C9353 Microporous collagen implantable slit tube (NeuraWrap Nerve Protector), per cm length N N1 ☑
AHA: 1Q, '08, 6

C9354 Acellular pericardial tissue matrix of nonhuman origin (Veritas), per sq cm N N1 ☑
AHA: 1Q, '08, 6

C9355 Collagen nerve cuff (NeuroMatrix), per 0.5 cm length N N1 ☑
AHA: 1Q, '08, 6

C9356 Tendon, porous matrix of cross-linked collagen and glycosaminoglycan matrix (TenoGlide Tendon Protector Sheet), per sq cm N N1 ☑
AHA: 3Q, '08, 6

C9358 Dermal substitute, native, nondenatured collagen, fetal bovine origin (SurgiMend Collagen Matrix), per 0.5 sq cm N N1 ☑
AHA: 2Q, '12, 7; 3Q, '08, 6

C9359 Porous purified collagen matrix bone void filler (Integra Mozaik Osteoconductive Scaffold Putty, Integra OS Osteoconductive Scaffold Putty), per 0.5 cc N N1 ☑
AHA: 3Q, '15, 2

C9360 Dermal substitute, native, nondenatured collagen, neonatal bovine origin (SurgiMend Collagen Matrix), per 0.5 sq cm N N1 ☑
AHA: 2Q, '12, 7

C9361 Collagen matrix nerve wrap (NeuroMend Collagen Nerve Wrap), per 0.5 cm length N N1 ☑

C9362 Porous purified collagen matrix bone void filler (Integra Mozaik Osteoconductive Scaffold Strip), per 0.5 cc N N1 ☑
AHA: 2Q, '10, 8

C9363 Skin substitute (Integra Meshed Bilayer Wound Matrix), per sq cm N N1 ☑
CMS: 100-04,4,260.1; 100-04,4,260.1.1
AHA: 2Q, '12, 7; 2Q, '10, 8

C9364 Porcine implant, Permacol, per sq cm N N1 ☑

C9399 Unclassified drugs or biologicals A K7
CMS: 100-02,15,50.5; 100-04,17,90.3; 100-04,32,400; 100-04,32,400.1; 100-04,32,400.2; 100-04,32,400.2.1; 100-04,32,400.2.2; 100-04,32,400.2.3; 100-04,32,400.2.4; 100-04,32,400.3; 100-04,32,400.4; 100-04,32,400.5; 100-04,4,260.1; 100-04,4,260.1.1
AHA: 1Q, '17, 8; 1Q, '17, 1-3; 4Q, '16, 10; 4Q, '14, 5; 2Q, '14, 8; 2Q, '13, 5; 1Q, '13, 9; 1Q, '08, 6; 4Q, '05, 7, 9; 4Q, '04, 3

C9460 Injection, cangrelor, 1 mg G K2 ☑
Use this code for Kengreal.
AHA: 1Q, '16, 6-8

C9462 Injection, delafloxacin, 1 mg G K2
Use this code for Baxdela.

C9482 Injection, sotalol HCl, 1 mg G K2 ☑
AHA: 4Q, '16, 9

C9488 Injection, conivaptan HCl, 1 mg G K2 ☑
Use this code for Vaprisol.

C9600 Percutaneous transcatheter placement of drug eluting intracoronary stent(s), with coronary angioplasty when performed; single major coronary artery or branch J J8

C9601 Percutaneous transcatheter placement of drug-eluting intracoronary stent(s), with coronary angioplasty when performed; each additional branch of a major coronary artery (list separately in addition to code for primary procedure) N N1

C9602 Percutaneous transluminal coronary atherectomy, with drug eluting intracoronary stent, with coronary angioplasty when performed; single major coronary artery or branch J J8

C9603 Percutaneous transluminal coronary atherectomy, with drug-eluting intracoronary stent, with coronary angioplasty when performed; each additional branch of a major coronary artery (list separately in addition to code for primary procedure) N N1

C9604 Percutaneous transluminal revascularization of or through coronary artery bypass graft (internal mammary, free arterial, venous), any combination of drug-eluting intracoronary stent, atherectomy and angioplasty, including distal protection when performed; single vessel J J8

C9605 Percutaneous transluminal revascularization of or through coronary artery bypass graft (internal mammary, free arterial, venous), any combination of drug-eluting intracoronary stent, atherectomy and angioplasty, including distal protection when performed; each additional branch subtended by the bypass graft (list separately in addition to code for primary procedure) N N1

C9606 Percutaneous transluminal revascularization of acute total/subtotal occlusion during acute myocardial infarction, coronary artery or coronary artery bypass graft, any combination of drug-eluting intracoronary stent, atherectomy and angioplasty, including aspiration thrombectomy when performed, single vessel J
CMS: 100-04,4,260.1; 100-04,4,260.1.1

C9607 Percutaneous transluminal revascularization of chronic total occlusion, coronary artery, coronary artery branch, or coronary artery bypass graft, any combination of drug-eluting intracoronary stent, atherectomy and angioplasty; single vessel J J8

Special Coverage Instructions   Noncovered by Medicare   Carrier Discretion   ☑ Quantity Alert ● New Code ○ Recycled/Reinstated ▲ Revised Code

© 2021 Optum360, LLC   A2-Z3 ASC Pmt   CMS: IOM   AHA: Coding Clinic   ᗒ DMEPOS Paid   ⊘ SNF Excluded   C Codes — 27

Outpatient PPS

C9608 — C9773

C9608 Percutaneous transluminal revascularization of chronic total occlusion, coronary artery, coronary artery branch, or coronary artery bypass graft, any combination of drug-eluting intracoronary stent, atherectomy and angioplasty; each additional coronary artery, coronary artery branch, or bypass graft (list separately in addition to code for primary procedure) ⓃN1

C9725 Placement of endorectal intracavitary applicator for high intensity brachytherapy Ⓣ G2 ⊘
AHA: 3Q, '05, 7

C9726 Placement and removal (if performed) of applicator into breast for intraoperative radiation therapy, add-on to primary breast procedure ⓃN1
AHA: 2Q, '07, 10

C9727 Insertion of implants into the soft palate; minimum of three implants Ⓣ G2 ☑

C9728 Placement of interstitial device(s) for radiation therapy/surgery guidance (e.g., fiducial markers, dosimeter), for other than the following sites (any approach): abdomen, pelvis, prostate, retroperitoneum, thorax, single or multiple Ⓢ J8

C9733 Nonophthalmic fluorescent vascular angiography Q2

C9734 Focused ultrasound ablation/therapeutic intervention, other than uterine leiomyomata, with magnetic resonance (MR) guidance J
AHA: 3Q, '13, 9; 2Q, '13, 9

C9738 Adjunctive blue light cystoscopy with fluorescent imaging agent (list separately in addition to code for primary procedure) ⓃN1

C9739 Cystourethroscopy, with insertion of transprostatic implant; one to three implants ♂ J J8
AHA: 2Q, '14, 8

C9740 Cystourethroscopy, with insertion of transprostatic implant; four or more implants ♂ J J8
AHA: 2Q, '14, 8

C9751 Bronchoscopy, rigid or flexible, transbronchial ablation of lesion(s) by microwave energy, including fluoroscopic guidance, when performed, with computed tomography acquisition(s) and 3D rendering, computer-assisted, image-guided navigation, and endobronchial ultrasound (EBUS) guided transtracheal and/or transbronchial sampling (e.g., aspiration[s]/biopsy[ies]) and all mediastinal and/or hilar lymph node stations or structures and therapeutic intervention(s) G2
CMS: 100-04,4,260.1; 100-04,4,260.1.1

C9752 ~~Destruction of intraosseous basivertebral nerve, first two vertebral bodies, including imaging guidance (e.g., fluoroscopy), lumbar/sacrum~~
To report, see ~64628

C9753 ~~Destruction of intraosseous basivertebral nerve, each additional vertebral body, including imaging guidance (e.g., fluoroscopy), lumbar/sacrum (list separately in addition to code for primary procedure)~~
To report, see ~64629

C9756 Intraoperative near-infrared fluorescence lymphatic mapping of lymph node(s) (sentinel or tumor draining) with administration of indocyanine green (ICG) (List separately in addition to code for primary procedure)

C9757 Laminotomy (hemilaminectomy), with decompression of nerve root(s), including partial facetectomy, foraminotomy and excision of herniated intervertebral disc, and repair of annular defect with implantation of bone anchored annular closure device, including annular defect measurement, alignment and sizing assessment, and image guidance; 1 interspace, lumbar J8

C9758 Blind procedure for NYHA Class III/IV heart failure; transcatheter implantation of interatrial shunt including right heart catheterization, transesophageal echocardiography (TEE)/intracardiac echocardiography (ICE), and all imaging with or without guidance (e.g., ultrasound, fluoroscopy), performed in an approved investigational device exemption (IDE) study E2

C9759 Transcatheter intraoperative blood vessel microinfusion(s) (e.g., intraluminal, vascular wall and/or perivascular) therapy, any vessel, including radiological supervision and interpretation, when performed N1

C9760 Nonrandomized, nonblinded procedure for NYHA Class II, III, IV heart failure; transcatheter implantation of interatrial shunt, including right and left heart catheterization, transseptal puncture, transesophageal echocardiography (TEE)/intracardiac echocardiography (ICE), and all imaging with or without guidance (e.g., ultrasound, fluoroscopy), performed in an approved investigational device exemption (IDE) study

▲ **C9761** Cystourethroscopy, with ureteroscopy and/or pyeloscopy, with lithotripsy, and ureteral catheterization for steerable vacuum aspiration of the kidney, collecting system, ureter, bladder, and urethra if applicable J8

C9762 Cardiac magnetic resonance imaging for morphology and function, quantification of segmental dysfunction; with strain imaging Z2

C9763 Cardiac magnetic resonance imaging for morphology and function, quantification of segmental dysfunction; with stress imaging Z2

C9764 Revascularization, endovascular, open or percutaneous, lower extremity artery(ies), except tibial/peroneal; with intravascular lithotripsy, includes angioplasty within the same vessel(s), when performed E2

C9765 Revascularization, endovascular, open or percutaneous, lower extremity artery(ies), except tibial/peroneal; with intravascular lithotripsy, and transluminal stent placement(s), includes angioplasty within the same vessel(s), when performed J8

C9766 Revascularization, endovascular, open or percutaneous, lower extremity artery(ies), except tibial/peroneal; with intravascular lithotripsy and atherectomy, includes angioplasty within the same vessel(s), when performed E2

C9767 Revascularization, endovascular, open or percutaneous, lower extremity artery(ies), except tibial/peroneal; with intravascular lithotripsy and transluminal stent placement(s), and atherectomy, includes angioplasty within the same vessel(s), when performed J8

C9768 Endoscopic ultrasound-guided direct measurement of hepatic portosystemic pressure gradient by any method (list separately in addition to code for primary procedure)

C9769 Cystourethroscopy, with insertion of temporary prostatic implant/stent with fixation/anchor and incisional struts ♂ J8

C9770 Vitrectomy, mechanical, pars plana approach, with subretinal injection of pharmacologic/biologic agent E2

C9771 Nasal/sinus endoscopy, cryoablation nasal tissue(s) and/or nerve(s), unilateral or bilateral J8

C9772 Revascularization, endovascular, open or percutaneous, tibial/peroneal artery(ies), with intravascular lithotripsy, includes angioplasty within the same vessel(s), when performed J8

C9773 Revascularization, endovascular, open or percutaneous, tibial/peroneal artery(ies); with intravascular lithotripsy, and transluminal stent placement(s), includes angioplasty within the same vessel(s), when performed J8

Special Coverage Instructions   Noncovered by Medicare   Carrier Discretion   ☑ Quantity Alert ● New Code ○ Recycled/Reinstated ▲ Revised Code

28 — C Codes   Ⓐ Age Edit   Ⓜ Maternity Edit   ♀ Female Only   ♂ Male Only   Ⓐ-Ⓨ OPPS Status Indicators   © 2021 Optum360, LLC

C9774 Revascularization, endovascular, open or percutaneous, tibial/peroneal artery(ies); with intravascular lithotripsy and atherectomy, includes angioplasty within the same vessel(s), when performed [J8]

C9775 Revascularization, endovascular, open or percutaneous, tibial/peroneal artery(ies); with intravascular lithotripsy and transluminal stent placement(s), and atherectomy, includes angioplasty within the same vessel(s), when performed [J8]

● **C9776** Intraoperative near-infrared fluorescence imaging of major extra-hepatic bile duct(s) (e.g., cystic duct, common bile duct and common hepatic duct) with intravenous administration of indocyanine green (ICG) (list separately in addition to code for primary procedure) [N1]

▲ **C9777** Esophageal mucosal integrity testing by electrical impedance, transoral, includes esophagoscopy or esophagogastroduodenoscopy [N1]

● **C9778** Colpopexy, vaginal; minimally invasive extraperitoneal approach (sacrospinous) [♀] [G2]

● **C9779** Endoscopic submucosal dissection (ESD), including endoscopy or colonoscopy, mucosal closure, when performed

● **C9780** Insertion of central venous catheter through central venous occlusion via inferior and superior approaches (e.g., inside-out technique), including imaging guidance

C9803 Hospital outpatient clinic visit specimen collection for Severe Acute Respiratory Syndrome Coronavirus 2 (SARS-CoV-2) (Coronavirus disease [COVID-19]), any specimen source [N1]

C9898 Radiolabeled product provided during a hospital inpatient stay [N]
CMS: 100-04,4,260.1; 100-04,4,260.1.1

C9899 Implanted prosthetic device, payable only for inpatients who do not have inpatient coverage [A]

Special Coverage Instructions   Noncovered by Medicare   Carrier Discretion   ☑ Quantity Alert   ● New Code   ○ Recycled/Reinstated   ▲ Revised Code

© 2021 Optum360, LLC   [A2]-[Z3] ASC Pmt   **CMS:** IOM   **AHA:** Coding Clinic   ♿ DMEPOS Paid   ⊘ SNF Excluded   **C Codes — 29**

Durable Medical Equipment E0100-E8002

E codes include durable medical equipment such as canes, crutches, walkers, commodes, decubitus care, bath and toilet aids, hospital beds, oxygen and related respiratory equipment, monitoring equipment, pacemakers, patient lifts, safety equipment, restraints, traction equipment, fracture frames, wheelchairs, and artificial kidney machines.

Canes

E0100   **Cane, includes canes of all materials, adjustable or fixed, with tip**   Y ⅙ (NU, RR, UE)

White canes for the blind are not covered under Medicare.

E0105   **Cane, quad or three-prong, includes canes of all materials, adjustable or fixed, with tips**   Y ⅙ (NU, RR, UE)

Crutches

E0110   **Crutches, forearm, includes crutches of various materials, adjustable or fixed, pair, complete with tips and handgrips**   Y ☑ ⅙ (NU, RR, UE)

Forearm cuff

Axilla pad

Standard underarm crutch (E0112-E0117)

Hand grip

Hand grip

Adjustment

Standard forearm crutch (E0110–E0111)

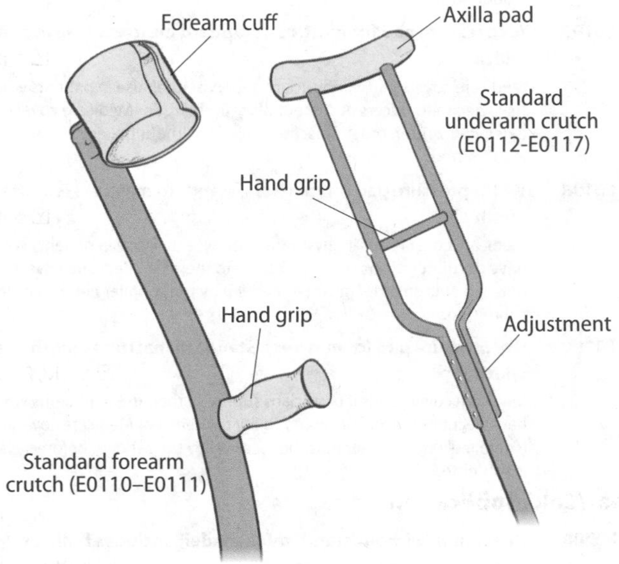

E0111   **Crutch, forearm, includes crutches of various materials, adjustable or fixed, each, with tip and handgrips**   Y ☑ ⅙ (NU, RR, UE)

E0112   **Crutches, underarm, wood, adjustable or fixed, pair, with pads, tips, and handgrips**   Y ☑ ⅙ (NU, RR, UE)

E0113   **Crutch, underarm, wood, adjustable or fixed, each, with pad, tip, and handgrip**   Y ☑ ⅙ (NU, RR, UE)

E0114   **Crutches, underarm, other than wood, adjustable or fixed, pair, with pads, tips, and handgrips**   Y ☑ ⅙ (NU, RR, UE)

AHA: 2Q, '02, 1-3

E0116   **Crutch, underarm, other than wood, adjustable or fixed, with pad, tip, handgrip, with or without shock absorber, each**   Y ☑ ⅙ (NU, RR, UE)

E0117   **Crutch, underarm, articulating, spring assisted, each**   Y ☑ ⅙ (RR)

E0118   **Crutch substitute, lower leg platform, with or without wheels, each**   E ☑

Medicare covers walkers if patient's ambulation is impaired.

Walkers

E0130   **Walker, rigid (pickup), adjustable or fixed height**   Y ⅙ (NU, RR, UE)

CMS: 100-04,36,50.15

E0135   **Walker, folding (pickup), adjustable or fixed height**   Y ⅙ (NU, RR, UE)

Medicare covers walkers if patient's ambulation is impaired.

CMS: 100-04,36,50.15

E0140   **Walker, with trunk support, adjustable or fixed height, any type**   Y ⅙ (RR)

CMS: 100-04,36,50.15

E0141   **Walker, rigid, wheeled, adjustable or fixed height**   Y ⅙ (NU, RR, UE)

Medicare covers walkers if patient's ambulation is impaired.

CMS: 100-04,36,50.15

E0143   **Walker, folding, wheeled, adjustable or fixed height**   Y ⅙ (NU, RR, UE)

Medicare covers walkers if patient's ambulation is impaired.

CMS: 100-04,36,50.15

E0144   **Walker, enclosed, four-sided framed, rigid or folding, wheeled with posterior seat**   Y ⅙ (RR)

CMS: 100-04,36,50.15

E0147   **Walker, heavy-duty, multiple braking system, variable wheel resistance**   Y ⅙ (NU, RR, UE)

Medicare covers safety roller walkers only in patients with severe neurological disorders or restricted use of one hand. In some cases, coverage will be extended to patients with a weight exceeding the limits of a standard wheeled walker.

CMS: 100-04,36,50.15

E0148   **Walker, heavy-duty, without wheels, rigid or folding, any type, each**   Y ☑ (NU, RR, UE)

CMS: 100-04,36,50.15

E0149   **Walker, heavy-duty, wheeled, rigid or folding, any type**   Y ⅙ (RR)

CMS: 100-04,36,50.15

Attachments

E0153   **Platform attachment, forearm crutch, each**   Y ☑ ⅙ (NU, RR, UE)

E0154   **Platform attachment, walker, each**   Y ☑ ⅙ (NU, RR, UE)

CMS: 100-04,36,50.14; 100-04,36,50.15

E0155   **Wheel attachment, rigid pick-up walker, per pair**   Y ☑ ⅙ (NU, RR, UE)

CMS: 100-04,36,50.15

E0156   **Seat attachment, walker**   Y ☑ (NU, RR, UE)

CMS: 100-04,36,50.14; 100-04,36,50.15

E0157   **Crutch attachment, walker, each**   Y ☑ ⅙ (NU, RR, UE)

CMS: 100-04,36,50.14; 100-04,36,50.15

E0158   **Leg extensions for walker, per set of four**   Y ☑ ⅙ (NU, RR, UE)

CMS: 100-04,36,50.14; 100-04,36,50.15

E0159   **Brake attachment for wheeled walker, replacement, each**   Y ☑ ⅙ (NU, RR, UE)

CMS: 100-04,36,50.15

Commodes

E0160   **Sitz type bath or equipment, portable, used with or without commode**   Y ⅙ (NU, RR, UE)

Medicare covers sitz baths if medical record indicates that the patient has an infection or injury of the perineal area and the sitz bath is prescribed by the physician.

Special Coverage Instructions   Noncovered by Medicare   Carrier Discretion   ☑ Quantity Alert   ● New Code   ○ Recycled/Reinstated   ▲ Revised Code

© 2021 Optum360, LLC   A2-Z3 ASC Pmt   CMS: IOM   AHA: Coding Clinic   ⅙ DMEPOS Paid   ⊘ SNF Excluded   E Codes — 31

Durable Medical Equipment

E0161 — E0235

E0161 Sitz type bath or equipment, portable, used with or without commode, with faucet attachment(s) ☑ & (NU, RR, UE)
Medicare covers sitz baths if medical record indicates that the patient has an infection or injury of the perineal area and the sitz bath is prescribed by the physician.

E0162 Sitz bath chair ☑ & (NU, RR, UE)
Medicare covers sitz baths if medical record indicates that the patient has an infection or injury of the perineal area and the sitz bath is prescribed by the physician.

E0163 Commode chair, mobile or stationary, with fixed arms ☑ & (NU, RR, UE)
Medicare covers commodes for patients confined to their beds or rooms, for patients without indoor bathroom facilities, and to patients who cannot climb or descend the stairs necessary to reach the bathrooms in their homes.

E0165 Commode chair, mobile or stationary, with detachable arms ☑ & (RR)
Medicare covers commodes for patients confined to their beds or rooms, for patients without indoor bathroom facilities, and to patients who cannot climb or descend the stairs necessary to reach the bathrooms in their homes.

E0167 Pail or pan for use with commode chair, replacement only ☑ & (NU, RR, UE)
Medicare covers commodes for patients confined to their beds or rooms, for patients without indoor bathroom facilities, and to patients who cannot climb or descend the stairs necessary to reach the bathrooms in their homes.

E0168 Commode chair, extra wide and/or heavy-duty, stationary or mobile, with or without arms, any type, each ☑ ☑ & (NU, RR, UE)

E0170 Commode chair with integrated seat lift mechanism, electric, any type ☑ & (RR)

E0171 Commode chair with integrated seat lift mechanism, nonelectric, any type ☑ & (RR)

E0172 Seat lift mechanism placed over or on top of toilet, any type ☑

E0175 Footrest, for use with commode chair, each ☑ ☑ & (NU, RR, UE)

Decubitus Care Equipment

E0181 Powered pressure reducing mattress overlay/pad, alternating, with pump, includes heavy-duty ☑ & (RR)
For Medicare coverage, a detailed written order must be received by the supplier before a claim is submitted.

E0182 Pump for alternating pressure pad, for replacement only ☑ & (RR)
For Medicare coverage, a detailed written order must be received by the supplier before a claim is submitted.

E0184 Dry pressure mattress ☑ & (NU, RR, UE)
For Medicare coverage, a detailed written order must be received by the supplier before a claim is submitted.

E0185 Gel or gel-like pressure pad for mattress, standard mattress length and width ☑ & (NU, RR, UE)
For Medicare coverage, a detailed written order must be received by the supplier before a claim is submitted.

E0186 Air pressure mattress ☑ & (RR)
For Medicare coverage, a detailed written order must be received by the supplier before a claim is submitted.

E0187 Water pressure mattress ☑ & (RR)
For Medicare coverage, a detailed written order must be received by the supplier before a claim is submitted.

E0188 Synthetic sheepskin pad ☑ & (NU, RR, UE)
For Medicare coverage, a detailed written order must be received by the supplier before a claim is submitted.

E0189 Lambswool sheepskin pad, any size ☑ & (NU, RR, UE)
For Medicare coverage, a detailed written order must be received by the supplier before a claim is submitted.

E0190 Positioning cushion/pillow/wedge, any shape or size, includes all components and accessories ☑

E0191 Heel or elbow protector, each ☑ ☑ & (NU, UE)

E0193 Powered air flotation bed (low air loss therapy) ☑ & (RR)

E0194 Air fluidized bed ☑ & (RR)
An air fluidized bed is covered by Medicare if the patient has a stage 3 or stage 4 pressure sore and, without the bed, would require institutionalization. For Medicare coverage, a detailed written order must be received by the supplier before a claim is submitted.

E0196 Gel pressure mattress ☑ & (RR)
Medicare covers pads if physicians supervise their use in patients who have decubitus ulcers or susceptibility to them. For Medicare coverage, a detailed written order must be received by the supplier before a claim is submitted.

E0197 Air pressure pad for mattress, standard mattress length and width ☑ & (RR)
Medicare covers pads if physicians supervise their use in patients who have decubitus ulcers or susceptibility to them. For Medicare coverage, a detailed written order must be received by the supplier before a claim is submitted.

E0198 Water pressure pad for mattress, standard mattress length and width ☑ & (RR)
Medicare covers pads if physicians supervise their use in patients who have decubitus ulcers or susceptibility to them.For Medicare coverage, a detailed written order must be received by the supplier before a claim is submitted.

E0199 Dry pressure pad for mattress, standard mattress length and width ☑ & (NU, RR, UE)
Medicare covers pads if physicians supervise their use in patients who have decubitus ulcers or susceptibility to them. For Medicare coverage, a detailed written order must be received by the supplier before a claim is submitted.

Heat/Cold Application

E0200 Heat lamp, without stand (table model), includes bulb, or infrared element ☑ & (NU, RR, UE)

E0202 Phototherapy (bilirubin) light with photometer ☑ & (RR)

E0203 Therapeutic lightbox, minimum 10,000 lux, table top model ☑

E0205 Heat lamp, with stand, includes bulb, or infrared element ☑ & (NU, RR, UE)

E0210 Electric heat pad, standard ☑ & (NU, RR, UE)

E0215 Electric heat pad, moist ☑ & (NU, RR, UE)

E0217 Water circulating heat pad with pump ☑ & (NU, RR, UE)

E0218 Fluid circulating cold pad with pump, any type ☑

E0221 Infrared heating pad system ☑
AHA: 1Q, '02, 5

E0225 Hydrocollator unit, includes pads ☑ & (NU, RR, UE)

E0231 Noncontact wound-warming device (temperature control unit, AC adapter and power cord) for use with warming card and wound cover ☑
AHA: 1Q, '02, 5

E0232 Warming card for use with the noncontact wound-warming device and noncontact wound-warming wound cover ☑
AHA: 1Q, '02, 5

E0235 Paraffin bath unit, portable (see medical supply code A4265 for paraffin) ☑ & (RR)

E0236	Pump for water circulating pad	Y & (RR)
E0239	Hydrocollator unit, portable	Y & (NU, RR, UE)

Bath and Toilet Aids

E0240	Bath/shower chair, with or without wheels, any size	E
E0241	Bathtub wall rail, each	E ☑
E0242	Bathtub rail, floor base	E
E0243	Toilet rail, each	E ☑
E0244	Raised toilet seat	E
E0245	Tub stool or bench	E
E0246	Transfer tub rail attachment	E
E0247	Transfer bench for tub or toilet with or without commode opening	E
E0248	Transfer bench, heavy-duty, for tub or toilet with or without commode opening	E
E0249	Pad for water circulating heat unit, for replacement only	Y & (NU, RR, UE)

Hospital Beds and Accessories

E0250	Hospital bed, fixed height, with any type side rails, with mattress	Y & (RR)
E0251	Hospital bed, fixed height, with any type side rails, without mattress	Y & (RR)
E0255	Hospital bed, variable height, hi-lo, with any type side rails, with mattress	Y & (RR)
E0256	Hospital bed, variable height, hi-lo, with any type side rails, without mattress	Y & (RR)
E0260	Hospital bed, semi-electric (head and foot adjustment), with any type side rails, with mattress	Y & (RR)
E0261	Hospital bed, semi-electric (head and foot adjustment), with any type side rails, without mattress	Y & (RR)
E0265	Hospital bed, total electric (head, foot, and height adjustments), with any type side rails, with mattress	Y & (RR)
E0266	Hospital bed, total electric (head, foot, and height adjustments), with any type side rails, without mattress	Y & (RR)
E0270	Hospital bed, institutional type includes: oscillating, circulating and Stryker frame, with mattress	E
E0271	Mattress, innerspring CMS: 100-04,36,50.14	Y & (NU, RR, UE)
E0272	Mattress, foam rubber CMS: 100-04,36,50.14	Y & (NU, RR, UE)
E0273	Bed board	E
E0274	Over-bed table	E
E0275	Bed pan, standard, metal or plastic Reusable, autoclavable bedpans are covered by Medicare for bed-confined patients.	Y & (NU, RR, UE)
E0276	Bed pan, fracture, metal or plastic Reusable, autoclavable bedpans are covered by Medicare for bed-confined patients.	Y & (NU, RR, UE)
E0277	Powered pressure-reducing air mattress	Y & (RR)
E0280	Bed cradle, any type CMS: 100-04,36,50.14	Y & (NU, RR, UE)
E0290	Hospital bed, fixed height, without side rails, with mattress	Y & (RR)
E0291	Hospital bed, fixed height, without side rails, without mattress	Y & (RR)
E0292	Hospital bed, variable height, hi-lo, without side rails, with mattress	Y & (RR)
E0293	Hospital bed, variable height, hi-lo, without side rails, without mattress	Y & (RR)
E0294	Hospital bed, semi-electric (head and foot adjustment), without side rails, with mattress	Y & (RR)
E0295	Hospital bed, semi-electric (head and foot adjustment), without side rails, without mattress	Y & (RR)
E0296	Hospital bed, total electric (head, foot, and height adjustments), without side rails, with mattress	Y & (RR)
E0297	Hospital bed, total electric (head, foot, and height adjustments), without side rails, without mattress	Y & (RR)
E0300	Pediatric crib, hospital grade, fully enclosed, with or without top enclosure	Y & (RR)
E0301	Hospital bed, heavy-duty, extra wide, with weight capacity greater than 350 pounds, but less than or equal to 600 pounds, with any type side rails, without mattress	Y & (RR)
E0302	Hospital bed, extra heavy-duty, extra wide, with weight capacity greater than 600 pounds, with any type side rails, without mattress	Y & (RR)
E0303	Hospital bed, heavy-duty, extra wide, with weight capacity greater than 350 pounds, but less than or equal to 600 pounds, with any type side rails, with mattress	Y & (RR)
E0304	Hospital bed, extra heavy-duty, extra wide, with weight capacity greater than 600 pounds, with any type side rails, with mattress	Y & (RR)
E0305	Bedside rails, half-length	Y & (RR)
E0310	Bedside rails, full-length CMS: 100-04,36,50.14	Y & (NU, RR, UE)
E0315	Bed accessory: board, table, or support device, any type	E
E0316	Safety enclosure frame/canopy for use with hospital bed, any type AHA: 1Q, '02, 5	Y & (RR)
E0325	Urinal; male, jug-type, any material	♂ Y & (NU, RR, UE)
E0326	Urinal; female, jug-type, any material	A ♀ Y & (NU, RR, UE)
E0328	Hospital bed, pediatric, manual, 360 degree side enclosures, top of headboard, footboard and side rails up to 24 in above the spring, includes mattress	Y
E0329	Hospital bed, pediatric, electric or semi-electric, 360 degree side enclosures, top of headboard, footboard and side rails up to 24 in above the spring, includes mattress	Y
E0350	Control unit for electronic bowel irrigation/evacuation system	E
E0352	Disposable pack (water reservoir bag, speculum, valving mechanism, and collection bag/box) for use with the electronic bowel irrigation/evacuation system	E
E0370	Air pressure elevator for heel	E
E0371	Nonpowered advanced pressure reducing overlay for mattress, standard mattress length and width	Y & (RR)
E0372	Powered air overlay for mattress, standard mattress length and width	Y & (RR)
E0373	Nonpowered advanced pressure reducing mattress	Y & (RR)

Special Coverage Instructions   Noncovered by Medicare   Carrier Discretion   ☑ Quantity Alert ● New Code ○ Recycled/Reinstated ▲ Revised Code

© 2021 Optum360, LLC   A2-Z3 ASC Pmt   CMS: IOM   AHA: Coding Clinic   & DMEPOS Paid   ⊘ SNF Excluded   E Codes — 33

Durable Medical Equipment

E0424 — E0487

Oxygen and Related Respiratory Equipment

E0424 Stationary compressed gaseous oxygen system, rental; includes container, contents, regulator, flowmeter, humidifier, nebulizer, cannula or mask, and tubing 　Ⓨ ♿ (RR)

For the first claim filed for home oxygen equipment or therapy, submit a certificate of medical necessity that includes the oxygen flow rate, anticipated frequency and duration of oxygen therapy, and physician signature. Medicare accepts oxygen therapy as medically necessary in cases documenting any of the following: erythocythemia with a hematocrit greater than 56 percent; a P pulmonale on EKG; or dependent edema consistent with congestive heart failure.
CMS: 100-04,20,130.6; 100-04,20,30.6

E0425 Stationary compressed gas system, purchase; includes regulator, flowmeter, humidifier, nebulizer, cannula or mask, and tubing 　Ⓔ

E0430 Portable gaseous oxygen system, purchase; includes regulator, flowmeter, humidifier, cannula or mask, and tubing 　Ⓔ

E0431 Portable gaseous oxygen system, rental; includes portable container, regulator, flowmeter, humidifier, cannula or mask, and tubing 　Ⓨ ♿ (RR)
CMS: 100-04,20,130.6

E0433 Portable liquid oxygen system, rental; home liquefier used to fill portable liquid oxygen containers, includes portable containers, regulator, flowmeter, humidifier, cannula or mask and tubing, with or without supply reservoir and contents gauge 　Ⓨ ♿ (RR)
CMS: 100-04,20,130.6

E0434 Portable liquid oxygen system, rental; includes portable container, supply reservoir, humidifier, flowmeter, refill adaptor, contents gauge, cannula or mask, and tubing 　Ⓨ ♿ (RR)
CMS: 100-04,20,130.6

E0435 Portable liquid oxygen system, purchase; includes portable container, supply reservoir, flowmeter, humidifier, contents gauge, cannula or mask, tubing and refill adaptor 　Ⓔ

E0439 Stationary liquid oxygen system, rental; includes container, contents, regulator, flowmeter, humidifier, nebulizer, cannula or mask, & tubing 　Ⓨ ♿ (RR)
CMS: 100-04,20,130.6

E0440 Stationary liquid oxygen system, purchase; includes use of reservoir, contents indicator, regulator, flowmeter, humidifier, nebulizer, cannula or mask, and tubing 　Ⓔ

E0441 Stationary oxygen contents, gaseous, 1 month's supply = 1 unit 　Ⓨ ☑ ♿
CMS: 100-04,20,30.6

E0442 Stationary oxygen contents, liquid, 1 month's supply = 1 unit 　Ⓨ ☑ ♿

E0443 Portable oxygen contents, gaseous, 1 month's supply = 1 unit 　Ⓨ ☑ ♿
CMS: 100-04,20,30.6

E0444 Portable oxygen contents, liquid, 1 month's supply = 1 unit 　Ⓨ ☑ ♿

E0445 Oximeter device for measuring blood oxygen levels noninvasively 　Ⓝ

E0446 Topical oxygen delivery system, not otherwise specified, includes all supplies and accessories 　Ⓐ

E0447 Portable oxygen contents, liquid, 1 month's supply = 1 unit, prescribed amount at rest or nighttime exceeds 4 liters per minute (LPM)

E0455 Oxygen tent, excluding croup or pediatric tents 　Ⓨ

E0457 Chest shell (cuirass) 　Ⓔ

E0459 Chest wrap 　Ⓔ

E0462 Rocking bed, with or without side rails 　Ⓨ ♿ (RR)

E0465 Home ventilator, any type, used with invasive interface, (e.g., tracheostomy tube) 　Ⓨ ♿ (RR)

E0466 Home ventilator, any type, used with noninvasive interface, (e.g., mask, chest shell) 　Ⓨ ♿ (RR)

E0467 Home ventilator, multi-function respiratory device, also performs any or all of the additional functions of oxygen concentration, drug nebulization, aspiration, and cough stimulation, includes all accessories, components and supplies for all functions 　(RR)

E0470 Respiratory assist device, bi-level pressure capability, without backup rate feature, used with noninvasive interface, e.g., nasal or facial mask (intermittent assist device with continuous positive airway pressure device) 　Ⓨ ♿ (RR)
CMS: 100-03,240.4

E0471 Respiratory assist device, bi-level pressure capability, with back-up rate feature, used with noninvasive interface, e.g., nasal or facial mask (intermittent assist device with continuous positive airway pressure device) 　Ⓨ ♿ (RR)
CMS: 100-03,240.4

E0472 Respiratory assist device, bi-level pressure capability, with backup rate feature, used with invasive interface, e.g., tracheostomy tube (intermittent assist device with continuous positive airway pressure device) 　Ⓨ ♿ (RR)
CMS: 100-03,240.4

E0480 Percussor, electric or pneumatic, home model 　Ⓨ ♿ (RR)

E0481 Intrapulmonary percussive ventilation system and related accessories 　Ⓔ
AHA: 1Q, '02, 5

E0482 Cough stimulating device, alternating positive and negative airway pressure 　Ⓨ ♿ (RR)
AHA: 1Q, '02, 5

E0483 High frequency chest wall oscillation system, includes all accessories and supplies, each 　Ⓨ ☑ ♿ (RR)

E0484 Oscillatory positive expiratory pressure device, nonelectric, any type, each 　Ⓨ ☑ (NU, RR, UE)

E0485 Oral device/appliance used to reduce upper airway collapsibility, adjustable or nonadjustable, prefabricated, includes fitting and adjustment 　Ⓨ ♿ (NU, RR, UE)

E0486 Oral device/appliance used to reduce upper airway collapsibility, adjustable or nonadjustable, custom fabricated, includes fitting and adjustment 　Ⓨ ♿ (NU, RR, UE)

E0487 Spirometer, electronic, includes all accessories 　Ⓝ

Special Coverage Instructions　　Noncovered by Medicare　　Carrier Discretion　　☑ Quantity Alert　● New Code　○ Recycled/Reinstated　▲ Revised Code

34 — E Codes　　Ⓐ Age Edit　Ⓜ Maternity Edit　♀ Female Only　♂ Male Only　Ⓐ-Ⓨ OPPS Status Indicators　　© 2021 Optum360, LLC

IPPB Machines

E0500 IPPB machine, all types, with built-in nebulization; manual or automatic valves; internal or external power source ☒ ⅄ ☖ (RR)

Intermittent Positive Pressure Breathing (IPPB) devices

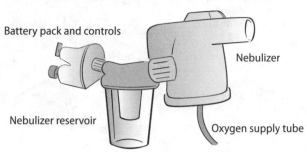

Battery pack and controls

Nebulizer

Nebulizer reservoir

Oxygen supply tube

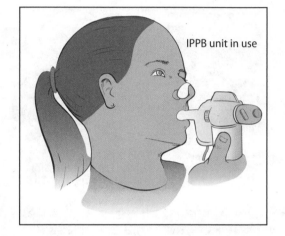

IPPB unit in use

Humidifiers/Compressors/Nebulizers

E0550 Humidifier, durable for extensive supplemental humidification during IPPB treatments or oxygen delivery ⅄ ☖ (RR)

E0555 Humidifier, durable, glass or autoclavable plastic bottle type, for use with regulator or flowmeter ⅄

E0560 Humidifier, durable for supplemental humidification during IPPB treatment or oxygen delivery ⅄ ☖ (NU, RR, UE)

E0561 Humidifier, nonheated, used with positive airway pressure device ⅄ ☖ (NU, RR, UE)
CMS: 100-03,240.4; 100-04,36,50.14

E0562 Humidifier, heated, used with positive airway pressure device ⅄ ☖ (NU, RR, UE)
CMS: 100-03,240.4; 100-04,36,50.14

E0565 Compressor, air power source for equipment which is not self-contained or cylinder driven ⅄ ☖ (RR)

E0570 Nebulizer, with compressor ⅄ ☖ (RR)

E0572 Aerosol compressor, adjustable pressure, light duty for intermittent use ⅄ ☖ (RR)

E0574 Ultrasonic/electronic aerosol generator with small volume nebulizer ⅄ ☖ (RR)

E0575 Nebulizer, ultrasonic, large volume ⅄ ☖ (RR)

E0580 Nebulizer, durable, glass or autoclavable plastic, bottle type, for use with regulator or flowmeter ⅄ ☖ (NU, RR, UE)

E0585 Nebulizer, with compressor and heater ⅄ ☖ (RR)

Pumps and Vaporizers

E0600 Respiratory suction pump, home model, portable or stationary, electric ⅄ ☖ (RR)

E0601 Continuous positive airway pressure (CPAP) device ⅄ ☖ (RR)
CMS: 100-03,240.4

E0602 Breast pump, manual, any type Ⓜ ♀ ⅄ ☖ (NU, RR, UE)

E0603 Breast pump, electric (AC and/or DC), any type Ⓜ ♀ Ⓝ
AHA: 1Q, '02, 5

E0604 Breast pump, hospital grade, electric (AC and/or DC), any type Ⓜ ♀ Ⓐ
AHA: 1Q, '02, 5

E0605 Vaporizer, room type ⅄ ☖ (NU, RR, UE)

E0606 Postural drainage board ⅄ ☖ (RR)

Monitoring Devices

E0607 Home blood glucose monitor ⅄ ☖ (NU, RR, UE)
Medicare covers home blood testing devices for diabetic patients when the devices are prescribed by the patients' physicians. Many commercial payers provide this coverage to noninsulin dependent diabetics as well.

E0610 Pacemaker monitor, self-contained, (checks battery depletion, includes audible and visible check systems) ⅄ ☖ (NU, RR, UE)

E0615 Pacemaker monitor, self-contained, checks battery depletion and other pacemaker components, includes digital/visible check systems ⅄ ☖ (NU, RR, UE)

E0616 Implantable cardiac event recorder with memory, activator, and programmer Ⓝ

E0617 External defibrillator with integrated electrocardiogram analysis ⅄ ☖ (RR)

E0618 Apnea monitor, without recording feature ⅄ ☖ (RR)

E0619 Apnea monitor, with recording feature ⅄ ☖ (RR)

E0620 Skin piercing device for collection of capillary blood, laser, each ⅄ ☖ (RR)
AHA: 1Q, '02, 5

Patient Lifts

E0621 Sling or seat, patient lift, canvas or nylon ⅄ ☖ (NU, RR, UE)

E0625 Patient lift, bathroom or toilet, not otherwise classified Ⓔ

E0627 Seat lift mechanism, electric, any type ⅄ ☖ (NU, RR, UE)
CMS: 100-04,20,100; 100-04,20,130.2; 100-04,20,130.3; 100-04,20,130.4; 100-04,20,130.5

E0629 Seat lift mechanism, nonelectric, any type ⅄ ☖ (NU, RR, UE)
CMS: 100-04,20,100; 100-04,20,130.2; 100-04,20,130.3; 100-04,20,130.4; 100-04,20,130.5

E0630 Patient lift, hydraulic or mechanical, includes any seat, sling, strap(s), or pad(s) ⅄ ☖ (RR)

E0635 Patient lift, electric, with seat or sling ⅄ ☖ (RR)

E0636 Multipositional patient support system, with integrated lift, patient accessible controls ⅄ ☖ (RR)

E0637 Combination sit-to-stand frame/table system, any size including pediatric, with seat lift feature, with or without wheels Ⓔ

E0638 Standing frame/table system, one position (e.g., upright, supine or prone stander), any size including pediatric, with or without wheels Ⓔ

E0639 Patient lift, moveable from room to room with disassembly and reassembly, includes all components/accessories Ⓔ ☖ (RR)

E0640 Patient lift, fixed system, includes all components/accessories Ⓔ ☖ (RR)

Special Coverage Instructions Noncovered by Medicare Carrier Discretion ☑ Quantity Alert ● New Code ○ Recycled/Reinstated ▲ Revised Code

© 2021 Optum360, LLC Ⓐ²–Ⓩ³ ASC Pmt CMS: IOM AHA: Coding Clinic ☖ DMEPOS Paid ⊘ SNF Excluded E Codes — 35

Durable Medical Equipment

E0641 — E0747

E0641	Standing frame/table system, multi-position (e.g., 3-way stander), any size including pediatric, with or without wheels	E
E0642	Standing frame/table system, mobile (dynamic stander), any size including pediatric	E

Compression Devices

E0650	Pneumatic compressor, nonsegmental home model	Y ♿ (NU, RR, UE)
E0651	Pneumatic compressor, segmental home model without calibrated gradient pressure	Y ♿ (NU, RR, UE)
E0652	Pneumatic compressor, segmental home model with calibrated gradient pressure	Y ♿ (NU, RR, UE)
E0655	Nonsegmental pneumatic appliance for use with pneumatic compressor, half arm	Y ♿ (NU, RR, UE)
E0656	Segmental pneumatic appliance for use with pneumatic compressor, trunk	Y ♿ (RR)
E0657	Segmental pneumatic appliance for use with pneumatic compressor, chest	Y ♿ (RR)
E0660	Nonsegmental pneumatic appliance for use with pneumatic compressor, full leg	Y ♿ (NU, RR, UE)
E0665	Nonsegmental pneumatic appliance for use with pneumatic compressor, full arm	Y ♿ (NU, RR, UE)
E0666	Nonsegmental pneumatic appliance for use with pneumatic compressor, half leg	Y ♿ (NU, RR, UE)
E0667	Segmental pneumatic appliance for use with pneumatic compressor, full leg	Y ♿ (NU, RR, UE)
E0668	Segmental pneumatic appliance for use with pneumatic compressor, full arm	Y ♿ (NU, RR, UE)
E0669	Segmental pneumatic appliance for use with pneumatic compressor, half leg	Y ♿ (NU, RR, UE)
E0670	Segmental pneumatic appliance for use with pneumatic compressor, integrated, two full legs and trunk	Y ♿ (NU, RR, UE)
E0671	Segmental gradient pressure pneumatic appliance, full leg	Y ♿ (NU, RR, UE)
E0672	Segmental gradient pressure pneumatic appliance, full arm	Y ♿ (NU, RR, UE)
E0673	Segmental gradient pressure pneumatic appliance, half leg	Y ♿ (NU, RR, UE)
E0675	Pneumatic compression device, high pressure, rapid inflation/deflation cycle, for arterial insufficiency (unilateral or bilateral system)	Y ♿ (RR)
E0676	Intermittent limb compression device (includes all accessories), not otherwise specified	Y

Ultraviolet Light

E0691	Ultraviolet light therapy system, includes bulbs/lamps, timer and eye protection; treatment area 2 sq ft or less	Y ♿ (NU, RR, UE)
E0692	Ultraviolet light therapy system panel, includes bulbs/lamps, timer and eye protection, 4 ft panel	Y ♿ (NU, RR, UE)
E0693	Ultraviolet light therapy system panel, includes bulbs/lamps, timer and eye protection, 6 ft panel	Y ♿ (NU, RR, UE)
E0694	Ultraviolet multidirectional light therapy system in 6 ft cabinet, includes bulbs/lamps, timer, and eye protection	Y ♿ (NU, RR, UE)

Safety Equipment

E0700	Safety equipment, device or accessory, any type	E

Restraints (E0710)

Fabric wrist restraint

Padded leather restraints may feature a locking device

Body restraint

Fabric gait belt for assistance in walking (E0700)

E0705	Transfer device, any type, each	B ☑ ♿ (NU, RR, UE)
E0710	Restraints, any type (body, chest, wrist, or ankle)	E

Nerve Stimulators and Devices

E0720	Transcutaneous electrical nerve stimulation (TENS) device, two-lead, localized stimulation	Y ♿ (NU)

A Certificate of Medical Necessity is required for the purchase of a TENS. It is not required for rentals.
CMS: 100-03,10.2; 100-03,160.27; 100-03,160.7.1; 100-04,20,30.1.2

E0730	Transcutaneous electrical nerve stimulation (TENS) device, four or more leads, for multiple nerve stimulation	Y ♿ (NU)

A Certificate of Medical Necessity is required for the purchase of a TENS. It is not required for rentals.
CMS: 100-03,10.2; 100-03,160.27; 100-03,160.7.1; 100-04,20,30.1.2

E0731	Form-fitting conductive garment for delivery of TENS or NMES (with conductive fibers separated from the patient's skin by layers of fabric)	Y ♿ (NU)

CMS: 100-03,10.2; 100-03,160.13

E0740	Nonimplanted pelvic floor electrical stimulator, complete system	Y ♿ (RR)
E0744	Neuromuscular stimulator for scoliosis	Y ♿ (RR)
E0745	Neuromuscular stimulator, electronic shock unit	Y ♿ (RR)
E0746	Electromyography (EMG), biofeedback device	N

Biofeedback therapy is covered by Medicare only for re-education of specific muscles or for treatment of incapacitating muscle spasm or weakness.

E0747	Osteogenesis stimulator, electrical, noninvasive, other than spinal applications	Y (NU, RR, UE)

Medicare covers noninvasive osteogenic stimulation for nonunion of long bone fractures, failed fusion, or congenital pseudoarthroses.

Special Coverage Instructions   Noncovered by Medicare   Carrier Discretion   ☑ Quantity Alert   ● New Code   ○ Recycled/Reinstated   ▲ Revised Code

36 — E Codes   A Age Edit   M Maternity Edit   ♀ Female Only   ♂ Male Only   A-Y OPPS Status Indicators   © 2021 Optum360, LLC

E0748 Osteogenesis stimulator, electrical, noninvasive, spinal applications Y (NU, RR, UE)

Medicare covers noninvasive osteogenic stimulation as an adjunct to spinal fusion surgery for patients at high risk of pseudoarthroses due to previously failed spinal fusion, or for those undergoing fusion of three or more vertebrae.

E0749 Osteogenesis stimulator, electrical, surgically implanted N (RR)

Medicare covers invasive osteogenic stimulation for nonunion of long bone fractures or as an adjunct to spinal fusion surgery for patients at high risk of pseudoarthroses due to previously failed spinal fusion, or for those undergoing fusion of three or more vertebrae.
CMS: 100-04,4,190

E0755 Electronic salivary reflex stimulator (intraoral/noninvasive) E

E0760 Osteogenesis stimulator, low intensity ultrasound, noninvasive Y (NU, RR, UE)
CMS: 100-04,32,110.5

E0761 Nonthermal pulsed high frequency radiowaves, high peak power electromagnetic energy treatment device E

E0762 Transcutaneous electrical joint stimulation device system, includes all accessories B & (RR)

E0764 Functional neuromuscular stimulation, transcutaneous stimulation of sequential muscle groups of ambulation with computer control, used for walking by spinal cord injured, entire system, after completion of training program Y (RR)

E0765 FDA approved nerve stimulator, with replaceable batteries, for treatment of nausea and vomiting Y & (NU, RR, UE)

E0766 Electrical stimulation device used for cancer treatment, includes all accessories, any type Y (RR)

E0769 Electrical stimulation or electromagnetic wound treatment device, not otherwise classified B
CMS: 100-04,32,11.1

E0770 Functional electrical stimulator, transcutaneous stimulation of nerve and/or muscle groups, any type, complete system, not otherwise specified Y

Infusion Supplies

E0776 IV pole Y & (NU, RR, UE)

E0779 Ambulatory infusion pump, mechanical, reusable, for infusion 8 hours or greater Y & (RR)

E0780 Ambulatory infusion pump, mechanical, reusable, for infusion less than 8 hours Y & (NU)

E0781 Ambulatory infusion pump, single or multiple channels, electric or battery operated, with administrative equipment, worn by patient Y & (RR)

E0782 Infusion pump, implantable, nonprogrammable (includes all components, e.g., pump, catheter, connectors, etc.) N (NU, RR, UE)
CMS: 100-04,4,190

E0783 Infusion pump system, implantable, programmable (includes all components, e.g., pump, catheter, connectors, etc.) N (NU, RR, UE)
CMS: 100-04,4,190

E0784 External ambulatory infusion pump, insulin Y & (RR)
Covered by some commercial payers with preauthorization.

E0785 Implantable intraspinal (epidural/intrathecal) catheter used with implantable infusion pump, replacement N & (KF)
CMS: 100-04,4,190

E0786 Implantable programmable infusion pump, replacement (excludes implantable intraspinal catheter) N (NU, RR, UE)

E0787 External ambulatory infusion pump, insulin, dosage rate adjustment using therapeutic continuous glucose sensing

E0791 Parenteral infusion pump, stationary, single, or multichannel Y & (RR)

Traction Equipment

E0830 Ambulatory traction device, all types, each N

E0840 Traction frame, attached to headboard, cervical traction Y & (NU, RR, UE)

E0849 Traction equipment, cervical, free-standing stand/frame, pneumatic, applying traction force to other than mandible Y & (RR)

E0850 Traction stand, freestanding, cervical traction Y & (NU, RR, UE)

E0855 Cervical traction equipment not requiring additional stand or frame Y & (RR)

E0856 Cervical traction device, with inflatable air bladder(s) Y & (RR)

E0860 Traction equipment, overdoor, cervical Y & (NU, RR, UE)

E0870 Traction frame, attached to footboard, extremity traction (e.g., Buck's) Y & (NU, RR, UE)

E0890 Traction frame, attached to footboard, pelvic traction Y & (NU, RR, UE)

E0900 Traction stand, freestanding, pelvic traction (e.g., Buck's) Y & (NU, RR, UE)

Orthopedic Devices

E0910 Trapeze bars, also known as Patient Helper, attached to bed, with grab bar Y & (RR)

E0911 Trapeze bar, heavy-duty, for patient weight capacity greater than 250 pounds, attached to bed, with grab bar Y & (RR)

E0912 Trapeze bar, heavy-duty, for patient weight capacity greater than 250 pounds, freestanding, complete with grab bar Y & (RR)

E0920 Fracture frame, attached to bed, includes weights Y & (RR)

E0930 Fracture frame, freestanding, includes weights Y & (RR)

E0935 Continuous passive motion exercise device for use on knee only Y & (RR)

E0936 Continuous passive motion exercise device for use other than knee E

E0940 Trapeze bar, freestanding, complete with grab bar Y & (RR)

E0941 Gravity assisted traction device, any type Y & (RR)

E0942 Cervical head harness/halter Y & (NU, RR, UE)

E0944 Pelvic belt/harness/boot Y & (NU, RR, UE)

E0945 Extremity belt/harness Y & (NU, RR, UE)

E0946 Fracture, frame, dual with cross bars, attached to bed, (e.g., Balken, four-poster) Y & (RR)

E0947 Fracture frame, attachments for complex pelvic traction Y & (NU, RR, UE)

E0948 Fracture frame, attachments for complex cervical traction Y & (NU, RR, UE)

Wheelchair Accessories

E0950 Wheelchair accessory, tray, each Y ☑ & (NU, RR, UE)

E0951 Heel loop/holder, any type, with or without ankle strap, each Y ☑ & (NU, RR, UE)

E0952 Toe loop/holder, any type, each Y ☑ & (NU, RR, UE)

Special Coverage Instructions   Noncovered by Medicare   Carrier Discretion   ☑ Quantity Alert ● New Code   ○ Recycled/Reinstated   ▲ Revised Code

© 2021 Optum360, LLC   A2-Z3 ASC Pmt   CMS: IOM   AHA: Coding Clinic   & DMEPOS Paid   ⊘ SNF Excluded   E Codes — 37

Durable Medical Equipment

E0953 — E1039

E0953 Wheelchair accessory, lateral thigh or knee support, any type including fixed mounting hardware, each Y &. (NU, RR, UE)

E0954 Wheelchair accessory, foot box, any type, includes attachment and mounting hardware, each foot Y &. (NU, RR, UE)

E0955 Wheelchair accessory, headrest, cushioned, any type, including fixed mounting hardware, each Y ☑ &. (RR)

E0956 Wheelchair accessory, lateral trunk or hip support, any type, including fixed mounting hardware, each Y ☑ &. (NU, RR, UE)

E0957 Wheelchair accessory, medial thigh support, any type, including fixed mounting hardware, each Y ☑ &. (NU, RR, UE)

E0958 Manual wheelchair accessory, one-arm drive attachment, each Y ☑ &. (RR)

E0959 Manual wheelchair accessory, adapter for amputee, each B ☑ &. (NU, RR, UE)

E0960 Wheelchair accessory, shoulder harness/straps or chest strap, including any type mounting hardware Y &. (NU, RR, UE)

E0961 Manual wheelchair accessory, wheel lock brake extension (handle), each B ☑ &. (NU, RR, UE)

E0966 Manual wheelchair accessory, headrest extension, each B ☑ &. (NU, RR, UE)

E0967 Manual wheelchair accessory, hand rim with projections, any type, replacement only, each Y ☑ &. (NU, RR, UE)

E0968 Commode seat, wheelchair Y &. (RR)

E0969 Narrowing device, wheelchair Y &. (NU, RR, UE)

E0970 No. 2 footplates, except for elevating legrest E
See code(s): K0037, K0042

E0971 Manual wheelchair accessory, antitipping device, each B ☑ &. (NU, RR, UE)

E0973 Wheelchair accessory, adjustable height, detachable armrest, complete assembly, each B ☑ &. (NU, RR, UE)

E0974 Manual wheelchair accessory, antirollback device, each B ☑ &. (NU, RR, UE)

E0978 Wheelchair accessory, positioning belt/safety belt/pelvic strap, each B ☑ &. (NU, RR, UE)

E0980 Safety vest, wheelchair Y ☑ &. (NU, RR, UE)

E0981 Wheelchair accessory, seat upholstery, replacement only, each Y ☑ &. (NU, RR, UE)

E0982 Wheelchair accessory, back upholstery, replacement only, each Y ☑ &. (NU, RR, UE)

E0983 Manual wheelchair accessory, power add-on to convert manual wheelchair to motorized wheelchair, joystick control Y &. (RR)

E0984 Manual wheelchair accessory, power add-on to convert manual wheelchair to motorized wheelchair, tiller control Y &. (RR)

E0985 Wheelchair accessory, seat lift mechanism Y &. (RR)

E0986 Manual wheelchair accessory, push-rim activated power assist system Y ☑ &. (RR)

E0988 Manual wheelchair accessory, lever-activated, wheel drive, pair Y ☑ &. (RR)

E0990 Wheelchair accessory, elevating legrest, complete assembly, each B ☑ &. (NU, RR, UE)

E0992 Manual wheelchair accessory, solid seat insert B &. (NU, RR, UE)

E0994 Armrest, each Y ☑ &. (NU, RR, UE)

E0995 Wheelchair accessory, calf rest/pad, replacement only, each B ☑ &. (NU, RR, UE)

E1002 Wheelchair accessory, power seating system, tilt only Y &. (RR)

E1003 Wheelchair accessory, power seating system, recline only, without shear reduction Y &. (RR)

E1004 Wheelchair accessory, power seating system, recline only, with mechanical shear reduction Y &. (RR)

E1005 Wheelchair accessory, power seating system, recline only, with power shear reduction Y &. (RR)

E1006 Wheelchair accessory, power seating system, combination tilt and recline, without shear reduction Y &. (RR)

E1007 Wheelchair accessory, power seating system, combination tilt and recline, with mechanical shear reduction Y &. (RR)

E1008 Wheelchair accessory, power seating system, combination tilt and recline, with power shear reduction Y &. (RR)

E1009 Wheelchair accessory, addition to power seating system, mechanically linked leg elevation system, including pushrod and legrest, each Y ☑ &. (NU, RR, UE)

E1010 Wheelchair accessory, addition to power seating system, power leg elevation system, including legrest, pair Y ☑ &. (RR)

E1011 Modification to pediatric size wheelchair, width adjustment package (not to be dispensed with initial chair) Y &. (NU, RR, UE)

E1012 Wheelchair accessory, addition to power seating system, center mount power elevating leg rest/platform, complete system, any type, each Y &. (RR)

E1014 Reclining back, addition to pediatric size wheelchair Y &. (RR)

E1015 Shock absorber for manual wheelchair, each Y ☑ &. (NU, RR, UE)

E1016 Shock absorber for power wheelchair, each Y ☑ &. (NU, RR, UE)

E1017 Heavy-duty shock absorber for heavy-duty or extra heavy-duty manual wheelchair, each Y ☑ &. (NU, RR, UE)

E1018 Heavy-duty shock absorber for heavy-duty or extra heavy-duty power wheelchair, each Y ☑ &. (NU, RR, UE)

E1020 Residual limb support system for wheelchair, any type Y &. (RR)

E1028 Wheelchair accessory, manual swingaway, retractable or removable mounting hardware for joystick, other control interface or positioning accessory Y &. (RR)

E1029 Wheelchair accessory, ventilator tray, fixed Y &. (RR)

E1030 Wheelchair accessory, ventilator tray, gimbaled Y &. (RR)

E1031 Rollabout chair, any and all types with castors 5 in or greater Y &. (RR)

E1035 Multi-positional patient transfer system, with integrated seat, operated by care giver, patient weight capacity up to and including 300 lbs Y &. (RR)
CMS: 100-02,15,110

E1036 Multi-positional patient transfer system, extra-wide, with integrated seat, operated by caregiver, patient weight capacity greater than 300 lbs Y &. (RR)

E1037 Transport chair, pediatric size Y &. (RR)

E1038 Transport chair, adult size, patient weight capacity up to and including 300 pounds Y &. (RR)

E1039 Transport chair, adult size, heavy-duty, patient weight capacity greater than 300 pounds Y &. (RR)

Special Coverage Instructions   Noncovered by Medicare   Carrier Discretion   ☑ Quantity Alert ● New Code   ○ Recycled/Reinstated ▲ Revised Code

38 — E Codes   A Age Edit   M Maternity Edit   ♀ Female Only   ♂ Male Only   A-Y OPPS Status Indicators   © 2021 Optum360, LLC

Wheelchairs

E1050 Fully-reclining wheelchair, fixed full-length arms, swing-away detachable elevating legrests ☑ ⅊ (RR)

E1060 Fully-reclining wheelchair, detachable arms, desk or full-length, swing-away detachable elevating legrests ☑ ⅊ (RR)

E1070 Fully-reclining wheelchair, detachable arms (desk or full-length) swing-away detachable footrest ☑ ⅊ (RR)

E1083 Hemi-wheelchair, fixed full-length arms, swing-away detachable elevating legrest ☑ ⅊ (RR)

E1084 Hemi-wheelchair, detachable arms desk or full-length arms, swing-away detachable elevating legrests ☑ ⅊ (RR)

E1085 Hemi-wheelchair, fixed full-length arms, swing-away detachable footrests ☑
See code(s): K0002

E1086 Hemi-wheelchair, detachable arms, desk or full-length, swing-away detachable footrests ☑
See code(s): K0002

E1087 High strength lightweight wheelchair, fixed full-length arms, swing-away detachable elevating legrests ☑ ⅊ (RR)

E1088 High strength lightweight wheelchair, detachable arms desk or full-length, swing-away detachable elevating legrests ☑ ⅊ (RR)

E1089 High-strength lightweight wheelchair, fixed-length arms, swing-away detachable footrest ☑
See code(s): K0004

E1090 High-strength lightweight wheelchair, detachable arms, desk or full-length, swing-away detachable footrests ☑
See code(s): K0004

E1092 Wide heavy-duty wheel chair, detachable arms (desk or full-length), swing-away detachable elevating legrests ☑ ⅊ (RR)

E1093 Wide heavy-duty wheelchair, detachable arms, desk or full-length arms, swing-away detachable footrests ☑ ⅊ (RR)

E1100 Semi-reclining wheelchair, fixed full-length arms, swing-away detachable elevating legrests ☑ ⅊ (RR)

E1110 Semi-reclining wheelchair, detachable arms (desk or full-length) elevating legrest ☑ ⅊ (RR)

E1130 Standard wheelchair, fixed full-length arms, fixed or swing-away detachable footrests ☑
See code(s): K0001

E1140 Wheelchair, detachable arms, desk or full-length, swing-away detachable footrests ☑
See code(s): K0001

E1150 Wheelchair, detachable arms, desk or full-length swing-away detachable elevating legrests ☑ ⅊ (RR)

E1160 Wheelchair, fixed full-length arms, swing-away detachable elevating legrests ☑ ⅊ (RR)

E1161 Manual adult size wheelchair, includes tilt in space ☑ ⅊ (RR)

E1170 Amputee wheelchair, fixed full-length arms, swing-away detachable elevating legrests ☑ ⅊ (RR)

E1171 Amputee wheelchair, fixed full-length arms, without footrests or legrest ☑ ⅊ (RR)

E1172 Amputee wheelchair, detachable arms (desk or full-length) without footrests or legrest ☑ ⅊ (RR)

E1180 Amputee wheelchair, detachable arms (desk or full-length) swing-away detachable footrests ☑ ⅊ (RR)

E1190 Amputee wheelchair, detachable arms (desk or full-length) swing-away detachable elevating legrests ☑ ⅊ (RR)

E1195 Heavy-duty wheelchair, fixed full-length arms, swing-away detachable elevating legrests ☑ ⅊ (RR)

E1200 Amputee wheelchair, fixed full-length arms, swing-away detachable footrest ☑ ⅊ (RR)

E1220 Wheelchair; specially sized or constructed, (indicate brand name, model number, if any) and justification ☑

E1221 Wheelchair with fixed arm, footrests ☑ ⅊ (RR)

E1222 Wheelchair with fixed arm, elevating legrests ☑ ⅊ (RR)

E1223 Wheelchair with detachable arms, footrests ☑ ⅊ (RR)

E1224 Wheelchair with detachable arms, elevating legrests ☑ ⅊ (RR)

E1225 Wheelchair accessory, manual semi-reclining back, (recline greater than 15 degrees, but less than 80 degrees), each ☑ ☑ ⅊ (RR)

E1226 Wheelchair accessory, manual fully reclining back, (recline greater than 80 degrees), each Ⓑ ☑ ⅊ (NU, RR, UE)
See also K0028

E1227 Special height arms for wheelchair ☑ ⅊ (NU, RR, UE)

E1228 Special back height for wheelchair ☑ ⅊ (RR)

E1229 Wheelchair, pediatric size, not otherwise specified ☑

E1230 Power operated vehicle (three- or four-wheel nonhighway), specify brand name and model number ☑ ⅊ (NU, RR, UE)
Prior authorization is required by Medicare for this item.

E1231 Wheelchair, pediatric size, tilt-in-space, rigid, adjustable, with seating system ☑ ⅊ (NU, RR, UE)

E1232 Wheelchair, pediatric size, tilt-in-space, folding, adjustable, with seating system ☑ ⅊ (RR)

E1233 Wheelchair, pediatric size, tilt-in-space, rigid, adjustable, without seating system ☑ ⅊ (RR)

E1234 Wheelchair, pediatric size, tilt-in-space, folding, adjustable, without seating system ☑ ⅊ (RR)

E1235 Wheelchair, pediatric size, rigid, adjustable, with seating system ☑ ⅊ (RR)

E1236 Wheelchair, pediatric size, folding, adjustable, with seating system ☑ ⅊ (RR)

E1237 Wheelchair, pediatric size, rigid, adjustable, without seating system ☑ ⅊ (RR)

E1238 Wheelchair, pediatric size, folding, adjustable, without seating system ☑ ⅊ (RR)

E1239 Power wheelchair, pediatric size, not otherwise specified ☑

E1240 Lightweight wheelchair, detachable arms, (desk or full-length) swing-away detachable, elevating legrest ☑ ⅊ (RR)

E1250 Lightweight wheelchair, fixed full-length arms, swing-away detachable footrest ☑
See code(s): K0003

E1260 Lightweight wheelchair, detachable arms (desk or full-length) swing-away detachable footrest ☑
See code(s): K0003

E1270 Lightweight wheelchair, fixed full-length arms, swing-away detachable elevating legrests ☑ ⅊ (RR)

E1280 Heavy-duty wheelchair, detachable arms (desk or full-length) elevating legrests ☑ ⅊ (RR)

Special Coverage Instructions   Noncovered by Medicare   Carrier Discretion   ☑ Quantity Alert   ● New Code   ○ Recycled/Reinstated   ▲ Revised Code

© 2021 Optum360, LLC   Ⓐ²-Ⓩ³ ASC Pmt   CMS: IOM   AHA: Coding Clinic   ⅊ DMEPOS Paid   ⊘ SNF Excluded   E Codes — 39

Durable Medical Equipment

E1285 — E1805

E1285	Heavy-duty wheelchair, fixed full-length arms, swing-away detachable footrest	E
	See code(s): K0006	
E1290	Heavy-duty wheelchair, detachable arms (desk or full-length) swing-away detachable footrest	E
	See code(s): K0006	
E1295	Heavy-duty wheelchair, fixed full-length arms, elevating legrest	Y 🦽 (RR)
E1296	Special wheelchair seat height from floor	Y 🦽 (NU, RR, UE)
E1297	Special wheelchair seat depth, by upholstery	Y 🦽 (NU, RR, UE)
E1298	Special wheelchair seat depth and/or width, by construction	Y 🦽 (NU, RR, UE)

Whirlpool - Equipment

E1300	Whirlpool, portable (overtub type)	E
E1310	Whirlpool, nonportable (built-in type)	Y 🦽 (NU, RR, UE)

Additional Oxygen Related Equipment

E1352	Oxygen accessory, flow regulator capable of positive inspiratory pressure	Y
E1353	Regulator	Y 🦽
E1354	Oxygen accessory, wheeled cart for portable cylinder or portable concentrator, any type, replacement only, each	Y ☑
E1355	Stand/rack	Y 🦽
E1356	Oxygen accessory, battery pack/cartridge for portable concentrator, any type, replacement only, each	Y ☑
E1357	Oxygen accessory, battery charger for portable concentrator, any type, replacement only, each	Y ☑
E1358	Oxygen accessory, DC power adapter for portable concentrator, any type, replacement only, each	Y ☑
E1372	Immersion external heater for nebulizer	Y 🦽 (NU, RR, UE)
E1390	Oxygen concentrator, single delivery port, capable of delivering 85 percent or greater oxygen concentration at the prescribed flow rate	Y 🦽 (RR)
	CMS: 100-04,20,130.6	
E1391	Oxygen concentrator, dual delivery port, capable of delivering 85 percent or greater oxygen concentration at the prescribed flow rate, each	Y ☑ 🦽 (RR)
	CMS: 100-04,20,130.6	
E1392	Portable oxygen concentrator, rental	Y 🦽 (RR)
	CMS: 100-04,20,130.6	
E1399	Durable medical equipment, miscellaneous	Y
	CMS: 100-04,20,30.9; 100-04,32,110.5	
E1405	Oxygen and water vapor enriching system with heated delivery	Y 🦽 (RR)
	CMS: 100-04,20,20; 100-04,20,20.4	
E1406	Oxygen and water vapor enriching system without heated delivery	Y 🦽 (RR)
	CMS: 100-04,20,20; 100-04,20,20.4	

Artificial Kidney Machines and Accessories

E1500	Centrifuge, for dialysis	A ⊘
	AHA: 1Q, '02, 5	
E1510	Kidney, dialysate delivery system kidney machine, pump recirculating, air removal system, flowrate meter, power off, heater and temperature control with alarm, IV poles, pressure gauge, concentrate container	A ⊘
E1520	Heparin infusion pump for hemodialysis	A ⊘

E1530	Air bubble detector for hemodialysis, each, replacement	A ☑ ⊘
E1540	Pressure alarm for hemodialysis, each, replacement	A ☑ ⊘
E1550	Bath conductivity meter for hemodialysis, each	A ☑ ⊘
E1560	Blood leak detector for hemodialysis, each, replacement	A ☑ ⊘
E1570	Adjustable chair, for ESRD patients	A ⊘
E1575	Transducer protectors/fluid barriers, for hemodialysis, any size, per 10	A ☑ ⊘
E1580	Unipuncture control system for hemodialysis	A ⊘
E1590	Hemodialysis machine	A ⊘
E1592	Automatic intermittent peritoneal dialysis system	A ⊘
E1594	Cycler dialysis machine for peritoneal dialysis	A ⊘
E1600	Delivery and/or installation charges for hemodialysis equipment	A ⊘
E1610	Reverse osmosis water purification system, for hemodialysis	A ⊘
E1615	Deionizer water purification system, for hemodialysis	A ⊘
E1620	Blood pump for hemodialysis, replacement	A ⊘
E1625	Water softening system, for hemodialysis	A ⊘
● E1629	Tablo hemodialysis system for the billable dialysis service	
E1630	Reciprocating peritoneal dialysis system	A ⊘
E1632	Wearable artificial kidney, each	A ☑ ⊘
E1634	Peritoneal dialysis clamps, each	B ☑
E1635	Compact (portable) travel hemodialyzer system	A ⊘
E1636	Sorbent cartridges, for hemodialysis, per 10	A ☑ ⊘
E1637	Hemostats, each	A ☑ ⊘
	AHA: 1Q, '02, 5	
E1639	Scale, each	A ☑ ⊘
	AHA: 1Q, '02, 5	
E1699	Dialysis equipment, not otherwise specified	A ⊘
	CMS: 100-04,8,20	

Jaw Motion Rehabilitation System and Accessories

E1700	Jaw motion rehabilitation system	Y 🦽 (RR)
	Medicare jurisdiction: local contractor.	
E1701	Replacement cushions for jaw motion rehabilitation system, package of 6	Y ☑ 🦽
	Medicare jurisdiction: local contractor.	
E1702	Replacement measuring scales for jaw motion rehabilitation system, package of 200	Y ☑ 🦽
	Medicare jurisdiction: local contractor.	

Flexion/Extension Device

E1800	Dynamic adjustable elbow extension/flexion device, includes soft interface material	Y 🦽 (RR)
E1801	Static progressive stretch elbow device, extension and/or flexion, with or without range of motion adjustment, includes all components and accessories	Y 🦽 (RR)
	AHA: 1Q, '02, 5	
E1802	Dynamic adjustable forearm pronation/supination device, includes soft interface material	Y 🦽 (RR)
E1805	Dynamic adjustable wrist extension/flexion device, includes soft interface material	Y 🦽 (RR)

Special Coverage Instructions   Noncovered by Medicare   Carrier Discretion   ☑ Quantity Alert ● New Code ○ Recycled/Reinstated ▲ Revised Code

40 — E Codes   A Age Edit   M Maternity Edit   ♀ Female Only   ♂ Male Only   A-Y OPPS Status Indicators   © 2021 Optum360, LLC

E1806 Static progressive stretch wrist device, flexion and/or extension, with or without range of motion adjustment, includes all components and accessories ☑ ൠ (RR)
AHA: 1Q, '02, 5

E1810 Dynamic adjustable knee extension/flexion device, includes soft interface material ☑ ൠ (RR)

E1811 Static progressive stretch knee device, extension and/or flexion, with or without range of motion adjustment, includes all components and accessories ☑ ൠ (RR)
AHA: 1Q, '02, 5

E1812 Dynamic knee, extension/flexion device with active resistance control ☑ ൠ (RR)

E1815 Dynamic adjustable ankle extension/flexion device, includes soft interface material ☑ ൠ (RR)

E1816 Static progressive stretch ankle device, flexion and/or extension, with or without range of motion adjustment, includes all components and accessories ☑ ൠ (RR)
AHA: 1Q, '02, 5

E1818 Static progressive stretch forearm pronation/supination device, with or without range of motion adjustment, includes all components and accessories ☑ ൠ (RR)
AHA: 1Q, '02, 5

E1820 Replacement soft interface material, dynamic adjustable extension/flexion device ☑ ൠ (NU, RR, UE)

E1821 Replacement soft interface material/cuffs for bi-directional static progressive stretch device ☑ ൠ (NU, RR, UE)
AHA: 1Q, '02, 5

E1825 Dynamic adjustable finger extension/flexion device, includes soft interface material ☑ ൠ (RR)

E1830 Dynamic adjustable toe extension/flexion device, includes soft interface material ☑ ൠ (RR)

E1831 Static progressive stretch toe device, extension and/or flexion, with or without range of motion adjustment, includes all components and accessories ☑ ൠ (RR)

E1840 Dynamic adjustable shoulder flexion/abduction/rotation device, includes soft interface material ☑ ൠ (RR)
AHA: 1Q, '02, 5

E1841 Static progressive stretch shoulder device, with or without range of motion adjustment, includes all components and accessories ☑ ൠ (RR)

Other Devices

E1902 Communication board, nonelectronic augmentative or alternative communication device ☑
AHA: 1Q, '02, 5

E2000 Gastric suction pump, home model, portable or stationary, electric ☑ ൠ (RR)
AHA: 1Q, '02, 5

E2100 Blood glucose monitor with integrated voice synthesizer ☑ ൠ (NU, RR, UE)
AHA: 1Q, '02, 5

E2101 Blood glucose monitor with integrated lancing/blood sample ☑ ൠ (NU, RR, UE)
AHA: 1Q, '02, 5

E2120 Pulse generator system for tympanic treatment of inner ear endolymphatic fluid ☑ ൠ (RR)

DME Wheelchair Accessory

E2201 Manual wheelchair accessory, nonstandard seat frame, width greater than or equal to 20 in and less than 24 in ☑ ☑ ൠ (NU, RR, UE)

E2202 Manual wheelchair accessory, nonstandard seat frame width, 24-27 in ☑ ☑ ൠ (NU, RR, UE)

E2203 Manual wheelchair accessory, nonstandard seat frame depth, 20 to less than 22 in ☑ ☑ ൠ (NU, RR, UE)

E2204 Manual wheelchair accessory, nonstandard seat frame depth, 22 to 25 in ☑ ☑ ൠ (NU, RR, UE)

E2205 Manual wheelchair accessory, handrim without projections (includes ergonomic or contoured), any type, replacement only, each ☑ ☑ ൠ (NU, RR, UE)

E2206 Manual wheelchair accessory, wheel lock assembly, complete, replacement only, each ☑ ☑ ൠ (NU, RR, UE)

E2207 Wheelchair accessory, crutch and cane holder, each ☑ ☑ ൠ (NU, RR, UE)

E2208 Wheelchair accessory, cylinder tank carrier, each ☑ ☑ ൠ (NU, RR, UE)

E2209 Accessory, arm trough, with or without hand support, each ☑ ☑ ൠ (NU, RR, UE)

E2210 Wheelchair accessory, bearings, any type, replacement only, each ☑ ☑ ൠ (NU, RR, UE)

E2211 Manual wheelchair accessory, pneumatic propulsion tire, any size, each ☑ ☑ ൠ (NU, RR, UE)

E2212 Manual wheelchair accessory, tube for pneumatic propulsion tire, any size, each ☑ ☑ ൠ (NU, UE)

E2213 Manual wheelchair accessory, insert for pneumatic propulsion tire (removable), any type, any size, each ☑ ☑ ൠ (NU, RR, UE)

E2214 Manual wheelchair accessory, pneumatic caster tire, any size, each ☑ ☑ ൠ (NU, RR, UE)

E2215 Manual wheelchair accessory, tube for pneumatic caster tire, any size, each ☑ ☑ ൠ (NU, RR, UE)

E2216 Manual wheelchair accessory, foam filled propulsion tire, any size, each ☑ ☑ ൠ (NU, RR, UE)

E2217 Manual wheelchair accessory, foam filled caster tire, any size, each ☑ ☑ ൠ (NU, RR, UE)

E2218 Manual wheelchair accessory, foam propulsion tire, any size, each ☑ ☑ ൠ (NU, RR, UE)

E2219 Manual wheelchair accessory, foam caster tire, any size, each ☑ ☑ ൠ (NU, RR, UE)

E2220 Manual wheelchair accessory, solid (rubber/plastic) propulsion tire, any size, replacement only, each ☑ ☑ ൠ (NU, RR, UE)

E2221 Manual wheelchair accessory, solid (rubber/plastic) caster tire (removable), any size, replacement only, each ☑ ☑ ൠ (NU, RR, UE)

E2222 Manual wheelchair accessory, solid (rubber/plastic) caster tire with integrated wheel, any size, replacement only, each ☑ ☑ ൠ (NU, RR, UE)

E2224 Manual wheelchair accessory, propulsion wheel excludes tire, any size, replacement only, each ☑ ☑ ൠ (NU, RR, UE)

E2225 Manual wheelchair accessory, caster wheel excludes tire, any size, replacement only, each ☑ ☑ ൠ (NU, RR, UE)

E2226 Manual wheelchair accessory, caster fork, any size, replacement only, each ☑ ☑ ൠ (NU, RR, UE)

E2227 Manual wheelchair accessory, gear reduction drive wheel, each ☑ ☑ ൠ (RR)

E2228 Manual wheelchair accessory, wheel braking system and lock, complete, each ☑ ☑ ൠ (RR)

E2230 Manual wheelchair accessory, manual standing system ☑

Special Coverage Instructions   Noncovered by Medicare   Carrier Discretion   ☑ Quantity Alert   ● New Code   ○ Recycled/Reinstated   ▲ Revised Code

© 2021 Optum360, LLC   A2-Z3 ASC Pmt   CMS: IOM   AHA: Coding Clinic   ൠ DMEPOS Paid   ⊘ SNF Excluded   E Codes — 41

Durable Medical Equipment

E2231 — E2373

E2231 Manual wheelchair accessory, solid seat support base (replaces sling seat), includes any type mounting hardware   Y & (NU, RR, UE)

E2291 Back, planar, for pediatric size wheelchair including fixed attaching hardware   Y

E2292 Seat, planar, for pediatric size wheelchair including fixed attaching hardware   Y

E2293 Back, contoured, for pediatric size wheelchair including fixed attaching hardware   Y

E2294 Seat, contoured, for pediatric size wheelchair including fixed attaching hardware   Y

E2295 Manual wheelchair accessory, for pediatric size wheelchair, dynamic seating frame, allows coordinated movement of multiple positioning features   Y

E2300 Wheelchair accessory, power seat elevation system, any type   Y
CMS: 100-04,20,30.9

E2301 Wheelchair accessory, power standing system, any type   Y

E2310 Power wheelchair accessory, electronic connection between wheelchair controller and one power seating system motor, including all related electronics, indicator feature, mechanical function selection switch, and fixed mounting hardware   Y & (RR)

E2311 Power wheelchair accessory, electronic connection between wheelchair controller and 2 or more power seating system motors, including all related electronics, indicator feature, mechanical function selection switch, and fixed mounting hardware   Y & (RR)

E2312 Power wheelchair accessory, hand or chin control interface, mini-proportional remote joystick, proportional, including fixed mounting hardware   Y & (RR)

E2313 Power wheelchair accessory, harness for upgrade to expandable controller, including all fasteners, connectors and mounting hardware, each   Y ☑ & (RR)

E2321 Power wheelchair accessory, hand control interface, remote joystick, nonproportional, including all related electronics, mechanical stop switch, and fixed mounting hardware   Y & (RR)

E2322 Power wheelchair accessory, hand control interface, multiple mechanical switches, nonproportional, including all related electronics, mechanical stop switch, and fixed mounting hardware   Y & (RR)

E2323 Power wheelchair accessory, specialty joystick handle for hand control interface, prefabricated   Y & (NU, RR, UE)

E2324 Power wheelchair accessory, chin cup for chin control interface   Y & (NU, RR, UE)

E2325 Power wheelchair accessory, sip and puff interface, nonproportional, including all related electronics, mechanical stop switch, and manual swingaway mounting hardware   Y & (RR)

E2326 Power wheelchair accessory, breath tube kit for sip and puff interface   Y & (RR)

E2327 Power wheelchair accessory, head control interface, mechanical, proportional, including all related electronics, mechanical direction change switch, and fixed mounting hardware   Y & (RR)

E2328 Power wheelchair accessory, head control or extremity control interface, electronic, proportional, including all related electronics and fixed mounting hardware   Y & (RR)

E2329 Power wheelchair accessory, head control interface, contact switch mechanism, nonproportional, including all related electronics, mechanical stop switch, mechanical direction change switch, head array, and fixed mounting hardware   Y & (RR)

E2330 Power wheelchair accessory, head control interface, proximity switch mechanism, nonproportional, including all related electronics, mechanical stop switch, mechanical direction change switch, head array, and fixed mounting hardware   Y & (RR)

E2331 Power wheelchair accessory, attendant control, proportional, including all related electronics and fixed mounting hardware   Y

E2340 Power wheelchair accessory, nonstandard seat frame width, 20-23 in   Y ☑ & (NU, RR, UE)

E2341 Power wheelchair accessory, nonstandard seat frame width, 24-27 in   Y ☑ & (NU, RR, UE)

E2342 Power wheelchair accessory, nonstandard seat frame depth, 20 or 21 in   Y ☑ & (NU, RR, UE)

E2343 Power wheelchair accessory, nonstandard seat frame depth, 22-25 in   Y ☑ & (NU, RR, UE)

E2351 Power wheelchair accessory, electronic interface to operate speech generating device using power wheelchair control interface   Y & (NU, RR, UE)

E2358 Power wheelchair accessory, group 34 nonsealed lead acid battery, each   Y ☑

E2359 Power wheelchair accessory, group 34 sealed lead acid battery, each (e.g., gel cell, absorbed glass mat)   Y & (NU, RR, UE)

E2360 Power wheelchair accessory, 22 NF nonsealed lead acid battery, each   Y ☑ & (NU, RR, UE)

E2361 Power wheelchair accessory, 22 NF sealed lead acid battery, each (e.g., gel cell, absorbed glassmat)   Y ☑ & (NU, RR, UE)

E2362 Power wheelchair accessory, group 24 nonsealed lead acid battery, each   Y ☑ & (NU, RR, UE)

E2363 Power wheelchair accessory, group 24 sealed lead acid battery, each (e.g., gel cell, absorbed glassmat)   Y ☑ & (NU, RR, UE)

E2364 Power wheelchair accessory, U-1 nonsealed lead acid battery, each   Y ☑ & (NU, RR, UE)

E2365 Power wheelchair accessory, U-1 sealed lead acid battery, each (e.g., gel cell, absorbed glassmat)   Y ☑ & (NU, RR, UE)

E2366 Power wheelchair accessory, battery charger, single mode, for use with only one battery type, sealed or nonsealed, each   Y ☑ & (NU, RR, UE)

E2367 Power wheelchair accessory, battery charger, dual mode, for use with either battery type, sealed or nonsealed, each   Y ☑ & (NU, RR, UE)

E2368 Power wheelchair component, drive wheel motor, replacement only   Y & (RR)

E2369 Power wheelchair component, drive wheel gear box, replacement only   Y & (RR)

E2370 Power wheelchair component, integrated drive wheel motor and gear box combination, replacement only   Y & (RR)

E2371 Power wheelchair accessory, group 27 sealed lead acid battery, (e.g., gel cell, absorbed glassmat), each   Y ☑ & (NU, RR, UE)

E2372 Power wheelchair accessory, group 27 nonsealed lead acid battery, each   Y ☑ & (NU, RR, UE)

E2373 Power wheelchair accessory, hand or chin control interface, compact remote joystick, proportional, including fixed mounting hardware   Y & (RR)

Special Coverage Instructions   Noncovered by Medicare   Carrier Discretion   ☑ Quantity Alert   ● New Code   ○ Recycled/Reinstated   ▲ Revised Code

E2374 Power wheelchair accessory, hand or chin control interface, standard remote joystick (not including controller), proportional, including all related electronics and fixed mounting hardware, replacement only Y & (RR)

E2375 Power wheelchair accessory, nonexpandable controller, including all related electronics and mounting hardware, replacement only Y & (RR)

E2376 Power wheelchair accessory, expandable controller, including all related electronics and mounting hardware, replacement only Y & (RR)

E2377 Power wheelchair accessory, expandable controller, including all related electronics and mounting hardware, upgrade provided at initial issue Y & (RR)

E2378 Power wheelchair component, actuator, replacement only Y & (RR)

E2381 Power wheelchair accessory, pneumatic drive wheel tire, any size, replacement only, each Y ☑ & (NU, RR, UE)

E2382 Power wheelchair accessory, tube for pneumatic drive wheel tire, any size, replacement only, each Y ☑ & (NU, RR, UE)

E2383 Power wheelchair accessory, insert for pneumatic drive wheel tire (removable), any type, any size, replacement only, each Y ☑ & (NU, RR, UE)

E2384 Power wheelchair accessory, pneumatic caster tire, any size, replacement only, each Y ☑ & (NU, RR, UE)

E2385 Power wheelchair accessory, tube for pneumatic caster tire, any size, replacement only, each Y ☑ & (NU, RR, UE)

E2386 Power wheelchair accessory, foam filled drive wheel tire, any size, replacement only, each Y ☑ & (NU, RR, UE)

E2387 Power wheelchair accessory, foam filled caster tire, any size, replacement only, each Y ☑ & (NU, RR, UE)

E2388 Power wheelchair accessory, foam drive wheel tire, any size, replacement only, each Y ☑ & (NU, RR, UE)

E2389 Power wheelchair accessory, foam caster tire, any size, replacement only, each Y ☑ & (NU, UE)

E2390 Power wheelchair accessory, solid (rubber/plastic) drive wheel tire, any size, replacement only, each Y ☑ & (NU, RR, UE)

E2391 Power wheelchair accessory, solid (rubber/plastic) caster tire (removable), any size, replacement only, each Y ☑ & (NU, RR, UE)

E2392 Power wheelchair accessory, solid (rubber/plastic) caster tire with integrated wheel, any size, replacement only, each Y ☑ & (NU, RR, UE)

E2394 Power wheelchair accessory, drive wheel excludes tire, any size, replacement only, each Y ☑ & (NU, RR, UE)

E2395 Power wheelchair accessory, caster wheel excludes tire, any size, replacement only, each Y ☑ & (NU, RR, UE)

E2396 Power wheelchair accessory, caster fork, any size, replacement only, each Y ☑ & (NU, RR, UE)

E2397 Power wheelchair accessory, lithium-based battery, each Y ☑ & (NU, RR, UE)

E2398 Wheelchair accessory, dynamic positioning hardware for back

Wound Therapy

E2402 Negative pressure wound therapy electrical pump, stationary or portable Y & (RR)
CMS: 100-02,7,40.1.2.8

Speech Generating Device

E2500 Speech generating device, digitized speech, using prerecorded messages, less than or equal to eight minutes recording time Y ☑ & (NU, RR, UE)

E2502 Speech generating device, digitized speech, using prerecorded messages, greater than eight minutes but less than or equal to 20 minutes recording time Y ☑ & (NU, RR, UE)

E2504 Speech generating device, digitized speech, using prerecorded messages, greater than 20 minutes but less than or equal to 40 minutes recording time Y ☑ & (NU, RR, UE)

E2506 Speech generating device, digitized speech, using prerecorded messages, greater than 40 minutes recording time Y ☑ & (NU, RR, UE)

E2508 Speech generating device, synthesized speech, requiring message formulation by spelling and access by physical contact with the device Y ☑ & (NU, RR, UE)

E2510 Speech generating device, synthesized speech, permitting multiple methods of message formulation and multiple methods of device access Y & (NU, RR, UE)

E2511 Speech generating software program, for personal computer or personal digital assistant Y & (NU, RR, UE)

E2512 Accessory for speech generating device, mounting system Y & (NU, RR, UE)

E2599 Accessory for speech generating device, not otherwise classified Y

Wheelchair Cushion

E2601 General use wheelchair seat cushion, width less than 22 in, any depth Y & (NU, RR, UE)

E2602 General use wheelchair seat cushion, width 22 in or greater, any depth Y & (NU, RR, UE)

E2603 Skin protection wheelchair seat cushion, width less than 22 in, any depth Y & (NU, RR, UE)

E2604 Skin protection wheelchair seat cushion, width 22 in or greater, any depth Y & (NU, RR, UE)

E2605 Positioning wheelchair seat cushion, width less than 22 in, any depth Y & (NU, RR, UE)

E2606 Positioning wheelchair seat cushion, width 22 in or greater, any depth Y & (NU, RR, UE)

E2607 Skin protection and positioning wheelchair seat cushion, width less than 22 in, any depth Y & (NU, RR, UE)

E2608 Skin protection and positioning wheelchair seat cushion, width 22 in or greater, any depth Y & (NU, RR, UE)

E2609 Custom fabricated wheelchair seat cushion, any size Y

E2610 Wheelchair seat cushion, powered B

E2611 General use wheelchair back cushion, width less than 22 in, any height, including any type mounting hardware Y & (NU, RR, UE)

E2612 General use wheelchair back cushion, width 22 in or greater, any height, including any type mounting hardware Y & (NU, RR, UE)

E2613 Positioning wheelchair back cushion, posterior, width less than 22 in, any height, including any type mounting hardware Y & (NU, RR, UE)

E2614 Positioning wheelchair back cushion, posterior, width 22 in or greater, any height, including any type mounting hardware Y & (NU, RR, UE)

Special Coverage Instructions   Noncovered by Medicare   Carrier Discretion   ☑ Quantity Alert ● New Code   ○ Recycled/Reinstated   ▲ Revised Code

© 2021 Optum360, LLC   A2 - Z3 ASC Pmt   CMS: IOM   AHA: Coding Clinic   & DMEPOS Paid   ⊘ SNF Excluded   E Codes — 43

Durable Medical Equipment

E2615 — E8002

E2615 Positioning wheelchair back cushion, posterior-lateral, width less than 22 in, any height, including any type mounting hardware ☑ 占 (NU, RR, UE)

E2616 Positioning wheelchair back cushion, posterior-lateral, width 22 in or greater, any height, including any type mounting hardware ☑ 占 (NU, RR, UE)

E2617 Custom fabricated wheelchair back cushion, any size, including any type mounting hardware ☑

E2619 Replacement cover for wheelchair seat cushion or back cushion, each ☑ ☑ 占 (NU, RR, UE)

E2620 Positioning wheelchair back cushion, planar back with lateral supports, width less than 22 in, any height, including any type mounting hardware ☑ 占 (NU, RR, UE)

E2621 Positioning wheelchair back cushion, planar back with lateral supports, width 22 in or greater, any height, including any type mounting hardware ☑ 占 (NU, RR, UE)

E2622 Skin protection wheelchair seat cushion, adjustable, width less than 22 in, any depth ☑ 占 (NU, RR, UE)

E2623 Skin protection wheelchair seat cushion, adjustable, width 22 in or greater, any depth ☑ 占 (NU, RR, UE)

E2624 Skin protection and positioning wheelchair seat cushion, adjustable, width less than 22 in, any depth ☑ 占 (NU, RR, UE)

E2625 Skin protection and positioning wheelchair seat cushion, adjustable, width 22 in or greater, any depth ☑ 占 (NU, RR, UE)

Wheelchair Arm Support

E2626 Wheelchair accessory, shoulder elbow, mobile arm support attached to wheelchair, balanced, adjustable ☑ 占 (NU, RR, UE)

E2627 Wheelchair accessory, shoulder elbow, mobile arm support attached to wheelchair, balanced, adjustable Rancho type ☑ 占 (NU, RR, UE)

E2628 Wheelchair accessory, shoulder elbow, mobile arm support attached to wheelchair, balanced, reclining ☑ 占 (NU, RR, UE)

E2629 Wheelchair accessory, shoulder elbow, mobile arm support attached to wheelchair, balanced, friction arm support (friction dampening to proximal and distal joints) ☑ 占 (NU, RR, UE)

E2630 Wheelchair accessory, shoulder elbow, mobile arm support, monosuspension arm and hand support, overhead elbow forearm hand sling support, yoke type suspension support ☑ 占 (NU, RR, UE)

E2631 Wheelchair accessory, addition to mobile arm support, elevating proximal arm ☑ 占 (NU, RR, UE)

E2632 Wheelchair accessory, addition to mobile arm support, offset or lateral rocker arm with elastic balance control ☑ 占 (NU, RR, UE)

E2633 Wheelchair accessory, addition to mobile arm support, supinator ☑ 占 (NU, RR, UE)

Gait Trainer

E8000 Gait trainer, pediatric size, posterior support, includes all accessories and components E

E8001 Gait trainer, pediatric size, upright support, includes all accessories and components E

E8002 Gait trainer, pediatric size, anterior support, includes all accessories and components E

Special Coverage Instructions   Noncovered by Medicare   Carrier Discretion   ☑ Quantity Alert ● New Code   ○ Recycled/Reinstated ▲ Revised Code

44 — E Codes   Ⓐ Age Edit   Ⓜ Maternity Edit   ♀ Female Only   ♂ Male Only   Ⓐ-Ⓨ OPPS Status Indicators   © 2021 Optum360, LLC

Procedures/Professional Services (Temporary) G0008-G9999

The G codes are used to identify professional health care procedures and services that would otherwise be coded in CPT but for which there are no CPT codes. Please refer to your CPT book for possible alternate code(s).

Immunization Administration

G0008   **Administration of influenza virus vaccine**   [S]
CMS: 100-02,12,40.11; 100-02,13,220; 100-02,13,220.1; 100-02,13,220.3; 100-02,15,50.4.4.2; 100-04,18,10.2.1; 100-04,18,10.2.2.1; 100-04,18,10.2.5.2; 100-04,18,10.3.1.1; 100-04,18,10.4; 100-04,18,10.4.1; 100-04,18,10.4.2; 100-04,18,10.4.3; 100-04,18,140.8; 1004-04,13,220.1
AHA: 4Q, '16, 1-3; 2Q, '09, 1; 2Q, '06, 5; 2Q, '03, 7

G0009   **Administration of pneumococcal vaccine**   [S]
CMS: 100-02,12,40.11; 100-02,13,220; 100-02,13,220.1; 100-02,13,220.3; 100-02,15,50.4.4.2; 100-04,18,10.2.1; 100-04,18,10.2.2.1; 100-04,18,10.2.5.2; 100-04,18,10.3.1.1; 100-04,18,10.4; 100-04,18,10.4.1; 100-04,18,10.4.2; 100-04,18,10.4.3; 100-04,18,140.8; 1004-04,13,220.1
AHA: 4Q, '16, 1-3; 2Q, '09, 1; 2Q, '03, 7

G0010   **Administration of hepatitis B vaccine**   [S]
CMS: 100-02,12,40.11; 100-02,13,220; 100-02,13,220.1; 100-02,13,220.3; 100-02,15,50.4.4.2; 100-04,18,10.2.1; 100-04,18,10.2.2.1; 100-04,18,10.2.5.2; 100-04,18,10.3.1.1; 100-04,18,140.8; 1004-04,13,220.1
AHA: 4Q, '16, 1-3

Semen Analysis

G0027   **Semen analysis; presence and/or motility of sperm excluding Huhner**   ♂ [Q]

Quality Measures

● **G0028**   Documentation of medical reason(s) for not screening for tobacco use (e.g., limited life expectancy, other medical reason)

● **G0029**   Tobacco screening not performed or tobacco cessation intervention not provided on the date of the encounter or within the previous 12 months, reason not otherwise specified

○ **G0030**   Patient screened for tobacco use and received tobacco cessation intervention on the date of the encounter or within the previous 12 months (counseling, pharmacotherapy, or both), if identified as a tobacco user

○ **G0031**   Palliative care services given to patient any time during the measurement period

○ **G0032**   Two or more antipsychotic prescriptions ordered for patients who had a diagnosis of schizophrenia, schizoaffective disorder, or bipolar disorder on or between January 1 of the year prior to the measurement period and the index prescription start date (IPSD) for antipsychotics

○ **G0033**   Two or more benzodiazepine prescriptions ordered for patients who had a diagnosis of seizure disorders, rapid eye movement sleep behavior disorder, benzodiazepine withdrawal, ethanol withdrawal, or severe generalized anxiety disorder on or between January 1 of the year prior to the measurement period and the IPSD for benzodiazepines

○ **G0034**   Patients receiving palliative care during the measurement period

○ **G0035**   Patient has any emergency department encounter during the performance period with place of service indicator 23

○ **G0036**   Patient or care partner decline assessment

○ **G0037**   On date of encounter, patient is not able to participate in assessment or screening, including nonverbal patients, delirious, severely aphasic, severely developmentally delayed, severe visual or hearing impairment and for those patients, no knowledgeable informant available

○ **G0038**   Clinician determines patient does not require referral

○ **G0039**   Patient not referred, reason not otherwise specified

○ **G0040**   Patient already receiving physical/occupational/speech/recreational therapy during the measurement period

○ **G0041**   Patient and/or care partner decline referral

○ **G0042**   Referral to physical, occupational, speech, or recreational therapy

○ **G0043**   Patients with mechanical prosthetic heart valve

○ **G0044**   Patients with moderate or severe mitral stenosis

○ **G0045**   Clinical follow-up and MRS score assessed at 90 days following endovascular stroke intervention

○ **G0046**   Clinical follow-up and MRS score not assessed at 90 days following endovascular stroke intervention

○ **G0047**   Pediatric patient with minor blunt head trauma and PECARN prediction criteria are not assessed

● **G0048**   Patients who receive palliative care services any time during the intake period through the end of the measurement year

● **G0049**   With maintenance hemodialysis (in-center and home HD) for the complete reporting month

○ **G0050**   Patients with a catheter that have limited life expectancy

○ **G0051**   Patients under hospice care in the current reporting month

○ **G0052**   Patients on peritoneal dialysis for any portion of the reporting month

○ **G0053**   Advancing rheumatology patient care MIPS value pathways

○ **G0054**   Coordinating stroke care to promote prevention and cultivate positive outcomes MIPS value pathways

○ **G0055**   Advancing care for heart disease MIPS value pathways

○ **G0056**   Optimizing chronic disease management MIPS value pathways

○ **G0057**   Proposed adopting best practices and promoting patient safety within emergency medicine MIPS value pathways

○ **G0058**   Improving care for lower extremity joint repair MIPS value pathways

○ **G0059**   Patient safety and support of positive experiences with anesthesia MIPS value pathways

○ **G0060**   Allergy/Immunology MIPS specialty set

○ **G0061**   Anesthesiology MIPS specialty set

○ **G0062**   Audiology MIPS specialty set

○ **G0063**   Cardiology MIPS specialty set

○ **G0064**   Certified Nurse Midwife MIPS specialty set

○ **G0065**   Chiropractic Medicine MIPS specialty set

○ **G0066**   Clinical Social Work MIPS specialty set

● **G0067**   Dentistry MIPS specialty set

Professional Services

G0068   Professional services for the administration of anti-infective, pain management, chelation, pulmonary hypertension, inotropic, or other intravenous infusion drug or biological (excluding chemotherapy or other highly complex drug or biological) for each infusion drug administration calendar day in the individual's home, each 15 min
CMS: 100-04,20,180; 100-04,32,411.3; 100-04,32,411.4; 100-04,32,411.5; 100-04,32,411.6

Special Coverage Instructions   Noncovered by Medicare   Carrier Discretion   ☑ Quantity Alert   ● New Code   ○ Recycled/Reinstated   ▲ Revised Code

© 2021 Optum360, LLC   [A2]-[Z3] ASC Pmt   CMS: IOM   AHA: Coding Clinic   � DMEPOS Paid   ⊘ SNF Excluded   G Codes — 45

G0069 Professional services for the administration of subcutaneous immunotherapy or other subcutaneous infusion drug or biological for each infusion drug administration calendar day in the individual's home, each 15 min
CMS: 100-04,20,180; 100-04,32,411.3; 100-04,32,411.4; 100-04,32,411.5; 100-04,32,411.6

G0070 Professional services for the administration of intravenous chemotherapy or other intravenous highly complex drug or biological infusion for each infusion drug administration calendar day in the individual's home, each 15 min
CMS: 100-04,20,180; 100-04,32,411.3; 100-04,32,411.4; 100-04,32,411.5; 100-04,32,411.6

G0071 Payment for communication technology-based services for 5 minutes or more of a virtual (nonface-to-face) communication between a rural health clinic (RHC) or federally qualified health center (FQHC) practitioner and RHC or FQHC patient, or 5 minutes or more of remote evaluation of recorded video and/or images by an RHC or FQHC practitioner, occurring in lieu of an office visit; RHC or FQHC only
CMS: 100-04,9,70.7

G0076 Brief (20 minutes) care management home visit for a new patient. For use only in a Medicare-approved CMMI model (services must be furnished within a beneficiary's home, domiciliary, rest home, assisted living and/or nursing facility)

G0077 Limited (30 minutes) care management home visit for a new patient. For use only in a Medicare-approved CMMI model (services must be furnished within a beneficiary's home, domiciliary, rest home, assisted living and/or nursing facility)

G0078 Moderate (45 minutes) care management home visit for a new patient. For use only in a Medicare-approved CMMI model (services must be furnished within a beneficiary's home, domiciliary, rest home, assisted living and/or nursing facility)

G0079 Comprehensive (60 minutes) care management home visit for a new patient. For use only in a Medicare-approved CMMI model (services must be furnished within a beneficiary's home, domiciliary, rest home, assisted living and/or nursing facility)

G0080 Extensive (75 minutes) care management home visit for a new patient. For use only in a Medicare-approved CMMI model (services must be furnished within a beneficiary's home, domiciliary, rest home, assisted living and/or nursing facility)

G0081 Brief (20 minutes) care management home visit for an existing patient. For use only in a Medicare-approved CMMI model (services must be furnished within a beneficiary's home, domiciliary, rest home, assisted living and/or nursing facility)

G0082 Limited (30 minutes) care management home visit for an existing patient. For use only in a Medicare-approved CMMI model (services must be furnished within a beneficiary's home, domiciliary, rest home, assisted living and/or nursing facility)

G0083 Moderate (45 minutes) care management home visit for an existing patient. For use only in a Medicare-approved CMMI model (services must be furnished within a beneficiary's home, domiciliary, rest home, assisted living and/or nursing facility)

G0084 Comprehensive (60 minutes) care management home visit for an existing patient. For use only in a Medicare-approved CMMI model (services must be furnished within a beneficiary's home, domiciliary, rest home, assisted living and/or nursing facility)

G0085 Extensive (75 minutes) care management home visit for an existing patient. For use only in a Medicare-approved CMMI model (services must be furnished within a beneficiary's home, domiciliary, rest home, assisted living and/or nursing facility)

G0086 Limited (30 minutes) care management home care plan oversight. For use only in a Medicare-approved CMMI model (services must be furnished within a beneficiary's home, domiciliary, rest home, assisted living and/or nursing facility)

G0087 Comprehensive (60 minutes) care management home care plan oversight. For use only in a Medicare-approved CMMI model (services must be furnished within a beneficiary's home, domiciliary, rest home, assisted living and/or nursing facility)

Screening Services

G0101 Cervical or vaginal cancer screening; pelvic and clinical breast examination A ♀ S ⊘
G0101 can be reported with an E/M code when a separately identifiable E/M service was provided.
CMS: 100-02,13,220; 100-02,13,220.1; 100-03,210.2; 1004-04,13,220.1
AHA: 4Q, '02, 8; 3Q, '01, 6; 3Q, '01, 3

G0102 Prostate cancer screening; digital rectal examination ♂ N ⊘
CMS: 100-02,13,220; 100-02,13,220.1; 100-02,13,220.3

G0103 Prostate cancer screening; prostate specific antigen test (PSA) ♂ A
CMS:

G0104 Colorectal cancer screening; flexible sigmoidoscopy T P3 ⊘
Medicare covers colorectal screening for cancer via flexible sigmoidoscopy once every four years for patients 50 years or older.
CMS: 100-02,15,280.2.2; 100-04,18,60; 100-04,18,60.1; 100-04,18,60.1.1; 100-04,18,60.2; 100-04,18,60.2.1; 100-04,18,60.6; 100-04,18,60.7
AHA: 2Q, '09, 1

G0105 Colorectal cancer screening; colonoscopy on individual at high risk T A2 ⊘
An individual with ulcerative enteritis or a history of a malignant neoplasm of the lower gastrointestinal tract is considered at high-risk for colorectal cancer, as defined by CMS.
CMS: 100-02,15,280.2.2; 100-04,12,30.1; 100-04,18,60; 100-04,18,60.1; 100-04,18,60.1.1; 100-04,18,60.2; 100-04,18,60.2.1; 100-04,18,60.2.2; 100-04,18,60.6; 100-04,18,60.7; 100-04,18,60.8; 100-04,23,30.2; 100-04,4,250.18
AHA: 2Q, '09, 1

G0106 Colorectal cancer screening; alternative to G0104, screening sigmoidoscopy, barium enema S
CMS: 100-02,15,280.2.2; 100-04,18,60; 100-04,18,60.1; 100-04,18,60.1.1; 100-04,18,60.2; 100-04,18,60.2.1; 100-04,18,60.6; 100-04,18,60.7
AHA: 2Q, '09, 1

G0108 Diabetes outpatient self-management training services, individual, per 30 minutes A ☑ ⊘
CMS: 100-02,13,220.3; 100-02,15,300; 100-02,15,300.2; 100-02,15,300.3; 100-02,15,300.4; 100-04,12,190.3; 100-04,12,190.3.6; 100-04,12,190.6; 100-04,12,190.6.1; 100-04,12,190.7; 100-04,18,120.1; 100-04,4,300.6

G0109 Diabetes outpatient self-management training services, group session (two or more), per 30 minutes A ☑ ⊘
CMS: 100-02,15,300.2; 100-02,15,300.3; 100-04,12,190.3; 100-04,12,190.3.6; 100-04,12,190.6; 100-04,12,190.6.1; 100-04,12,190.7; 100-04,4,300.6

G0117 Glaucoma screening for high risk patients furnished by an optometrist or ophthalmologist S ⊘
CMS: 100-02,13,220; 100-02,13,220.1; 100-02,13,220.3; 100-02,15,280.1; 100-04,18,70.1.1; 1004-04,13,220.1
AHA: 1Q, '02, 5; 1Q, '02, 4; 3Q, '01, 12

G0118 Glaucoma screening for high risk patient furnished under the direct supervision of an optometrist or ophthalmologist S ⊘
CMS: 100-02,13,220; 100-02,13,220.1; 100-02,13,220.3; 100-02,15,280.1; 100-04,18,70.1.1; 1004-04,13,220.1
AHA: 1Q, '02, 5; 1Q, '02, 4; 3Q, '01, 12

G0120 Colorectal cancer screening; alternative to G0105, screening colonoscopy, barium enema S
CMS: 100-02,15,280.2.2; 100-04,18,60; 100-04,18,60.1; 100-04,18,60.1.1; 100-04,18,60.2; 100-04,18,60.2.1; 100-04,18,60.6; 100-04,18,60.7; 100-04,18,60.8

G0121 Colorectal cancer screening; colonoscopy on individual not meeting criteria for high risk　T A2 ⊘
　　CMS: 100-02,15,280.2.2; 100-04,12,30.1; 100-04,18,60; 100-04,18,60.1; 100-04,18,60.1.1; 100-04,18,60.2; 100-04,18,60.2.1; 100-04,18,60.2.2; 100-04,18,60.5; 100-04,18,60.6; 100-04,23,30.2; 100-04,4,250.18
　　AHA: 3Q, '01, 12

G0122 Colorectal cancer screening; barium enema　E
　　CMS: 100-04,18,60; 100-04,18,60.2; 100-04,18,60.2.1; 100-04,18,60.5; 100-04,18,60.6; 100-04,18,60.7; 100-04,18,60.8

G0123 Screening cytopathology, cervical or vaginal (any reporting system), collected in preservative fluid, automated thin layer preparation, screening by cytotechnologist under physician supervision　A ♀ A
　　See also P3000-P3001.
　　CMS: 100-03,210.2.1; 100-04,18,30.2.1; 100-04,18,30.5; 100-04,18,30.6

G0124 Screening cytopathology, cervical or vaginal (any reporting system), collected in preservative fluid, automated thin layer preparation, requiring interpretation by physician　A ♀ B ⊘
　　See also P3000-P3001.
　　CMS: 100-03,210.2.1; 100-04,18,30.2.1; 100-04,18,30.5; 100-04,18,30.6

Miscellaneous Services

G0127 Trimming of dystrophic nails, any number　01 ⊘
　　CMS: 100-02,15,290

G0128 Direct (face-to-face with patient) skilled nursing services of a registered nurse provided in a comprehensive outpatient rehabilitation facility, each 10 minutes beyond the first 5 minutes　B ☑ ⊘
　　CMS: 100-02,12,30.1; 100-02,12,40.8; 100-04,5,100.3; 100-04,5,20.4

G0129 Occupational therapy services requiring the skills of a qualified occupational therapist, furnished as a component of a partial hospitalization treatment program, per session (45 minutes or more)　P ☑
　　CMS: 100-04,4,260.1; 100-04,4,260.1.1
　　AHA: 4Q, '12, 11-14

G0130 Single energy x-ray absorptiometry (SEXA) bone density study, one or more sites; appendicular skeleton (peripheral) (e.g., radius, wrist, heel)　S Z3

G0141 Screening cytopathology smears, cervical or vaginal, performed by automated system, with manual rescreening, requiring interpretation by physician　A ♀ B ⊘
　　CMS: 100-03,210.2.1; 100-04,18,30.2.1; 100-04,18,30.5; 100-04,18,30.6

G0143 Screening cytopathology, cervical or vaginal (any reporting system), collected in preservative fluid, automated thin layer preparation, with manual screening and rescreening by cytotechnologist under physician supervision　A ♀ A
　　CMS: 100-03,210.2.1; 100-04,18,30.2.1; 100-04,18,30.5; 100-04,18,30.6

G0144 Screening cytopathology, cervical or vaginal (any reporting system), collected in preservative fluid, automated thin layer preparation, with screening by automated system, under physician supervision　A ♀ A
　　CMS: 100-03,210.2.1; 100-04,18,30.2.1; 100-04,18,30.5; 100-04,18,30.6

G0145 Screening cytopathology, cervical or vaginal (any reporting system), collected in preservative fluid, automated thin layer preparation, with screening by automated system and manual rescreening under physician supervision　A ♀ A
　　CMS: 100-03,210.2.1; 100-04,18,30.2.1; 100-04,18,30.5; 100-04,18,30.6

G0147 Screening cytopathology smears, cervical or vaginal, performed by automated system under physician supervision　A ♀ A
　　CMS: 100-03,210.2.1; 100-04,18,30.2.1; 100-04,18,30.5; 100-04,18,30.6

G0148 Screening cytopathology smears, cervical or vaginal, performed by automated system with manual rescreening　A ♀ A
　　CMS: 100-03,210.2.1; 100-04,18,30.2.1; 100-04,18,30.5; 100-04,18,30.6

G0151 Services performed by a qualified physical therapist in the home health or hospice setting, each 15 minutes　B ☑
　　CMS: 100-01,3,30.3; 100-04,10,40.2; 100-04,11,10; 100-04,11,130.1; 100-04,11,30.3

G0152 Services performed by a qualified occupational therapist in the home health or hospice setting, each 15 minutes　B ☑
　　CMS: 100-01,3,30.3; 100-04,10,40.2; 100-04,11,10; 100-04,11,130.1; 100-04,11,30.3

G0153 Services performed by a qualified speech-language pathologist in the home health or hospice setting, each 15 minutes　B ☑
　　CMS: 100-01,3,30.3; 100-04,10,40.2; 100-04,11,10; 100-04,11,130.1; 100-04,11,30.3

G0155 Services of clinical social worker in home health or hospice settings, each 15 minutes　B ☑
　　CMS: 100-01,3,30.3; 100-04,10,40.2; 100-04,11,10; 100-04,11,130.1; 100-04,11,30.3

G0156 Services of home health/hospice aide in home health or hospice settings, each 15 minutes　B ☑
　　CMS: 100-01,3,30.3; 100-04,10,40.2; 100-04,11,10; 100-04,11,130.1; 100-04,11,30.3

G0157 Services performed by a qualified physical therapist assistant in the home health or hospice setting, each 15 minutes　B ☑
　　CMS: 100-04,10,40.2; 100-04,11,10

G0158 Services performed by a qualified occupational therapist assistant in the home health or hospice setting, each 15 minutes　B ☑
　　CMS: 100-04,10,40.2; 100-04,11,10

G0159 Services performed by a qualified physical therapist, in the home health setting, in the establishment or delivery of a safe and effective physical therapy maintenance program, each 15 minutes　B ☑
　　CMS: 100-04,10,40.2

G0160 Services performed by a qualified occupational therapist, in the home health setting, in the establishment or delivery of a safe and effective occupational therapy maintenance program, each 15 minutes　B ☑
　　CMS: 100-04,10,40.2

G0161 Services performed by a qualified speech-language pathologist, in the home health setting, in the establishment or delivery of a safe and effective speech-language pathology maintenance program, each 15 minutes　B ☑
　　CMS: 100-04,10,40.2

G0162 Skilled services by a registered nurse (RN) for management and evaluation of the plan of care; each 15 minutes (the patient's underlying condition or complication requires an RN to ensure that essential nonskilled care achieves its purpose in the home health or hospice setting)　B ☑
　　CMS: 100-04,10,40.2; 100-04,11,10

G0166 External counterpulsation, per treatment session　01 ☑ ⊘
　　CMS: 100-04,32,130; 100-04,32,130.1

G0168 Wound closure utilizing tissue adhesive(s) only　B ⊘
　　CMS: 100-04,10,40.2
　　AHA: 1Q, '05, 5; 4Q, '01, 10; 3Q, '01, 13

G0175 Scheduled interdisciplinary team conference (minimum of three exclusive of patient care nursing staff) with patient present　V
　　CMS: 100-04,4,160
　　AHA: 3Q, '01, 6; 3Q, '01, 3

Special Coverage Instructions　　Noncovered by Medicare　　Carrier Discretion　　☑ Quantity Alert　● New Code　○ Recycled/Reinstated　▲ Revised Code

© 2021 Optum360, LLC　　A2-Z3 ASC Pmt　　CMS: IOM　　AHA: Coding Clinic　　DMEPOS Paid　　⊘ SNF Excluded　　G Codes — 47

Procedures/Professional Services (Temporary)

G0176 — G0249

G0176 Activity therapy, such as music, dance, art or play therapies not for recreation, related to the care and treatment of patient's disabling mental health problems, per session (45 minutes or more) P
CMS: 100-04,4,260.1; 100-04,4,260.1.1; 100-04,4,260.5
AHA: 4Q, '12, 11-14

G0177 Training and educational services related to the care and treatment of patient's disabling mental health problems per session (45 minutes or more) N
CMS: 100-04,4,260.1; 100-04,4,260.1.1
AHA: 4Q, '12, 11-14

G0179 Physician or allowed practitioner re-certification for Medicare-covered home health services under a home health plan of care (patient not present), including contacts with home health agency and review of reports of patient status required by physicians and allowed practitioners to affirm the initial implementation of the plan of care M ⊘
CMS: 100-02,7,30.5.4; 100-04,10,20.1.2; 100-04,12,180; 100-04,12,180.1

G0180 Physician or allowed practitioner certification for Medicare-covered home health services under a home health plan of care (patient not present), including contacts with home health agency and review of reports of patient status required by physicians or allowed practitioners to affirm the initial implementation of the plan of care M ⊘
CMS: 100-02,7,30.5.4; 100-04,10,20.1.2; 100-04,12,180; 100-04,12,180.1

G0181 Physician or allowed practitioner supervision of a patient receiving Medicare-covered services provided by a participating home health agency (patient not present) requiring complex and multidisciplinary care modalities involving regular physician or allowed practitioner development and/or revision of care plans M ⊘
CMS: 100-04,12,180; 100-04,12,180.1
AHA: 2Q, '15, 10

G0182 Physician supervision of a patient under a Medicare-approved hospice (patient not present) requiring complex and multidisciplinary care modalities involving regular physician development and/or revision of care plans, review of subsequent reports of patient status, review of laboratory and other studies, communication (including telephone calls) with other health care professionals involved in the patient's care, integration of new information into the medical treatment plan and/or adjustment of medical therapy, within a calendar month, 30 minutes or more M ⊘
CMS: 100-04,11,40.1.3.1; 100-04,12,180; 100-04,12,180.1
AHA: 2Q, '15, 10

G0186 Destruction of localized lesion of choroid (for example, choroidal neovascularization); photocoagulation, feeder vessel technique (one or more sessions) T R2 ⊘

G0219 PET imaging whole body; melanoma for noncovered indications E
CMS: 100-03,220.6.10; 100-03,220.6.12; 100-03,220.6.17; 100-03,220.6.3; 100-03,220.6.4; 100-03,220.6.6; 100-03,220.6.7; 100-04,13,60; 100-04,13,60.16
AHA: 1Q, '02, 5; 1Q, '02, 10; 2Q, '01, 5

G0235 PET imaging, any site, not otherwise specified E Z2
CMS: 100-03,220.6.10; 100-03,220.6.12; 100-03,220.6.13; 100-03,220.6.17; 100-03,220.6.2; 100-03,220.6.3; 100-03,220.6.4; 100-03,220.6.5; 100-03,220.6.6; 100-03,220.6.7; 100-03,220.6.9; 100-04,13,60; 100-04,13,60.13; 100-04,13,60.14; 100-04,13,60.16; 100-04,13,60.17
AHA: 1Q, '07, 6

G0237 Therapeutic procedures to increase strength or endurance of respiratory muscles, face-to-face, one-on-one, each 15 minutes (includes monitoring) S ☑ ⊘
CMS: 100-02,12,30.1; 100-02,12,40.5
AHA: 1Q, '02, 5

G0238 Therapeutic procedures to improve respiratory function, other than described by G0237, one-on-one, face-to-face, per 15 minutes (includes monitoring) S ☑
CMS: 100-02,12,30.1; 100-02,12,40.5
AHA: 1Q, '02, 5

G0239 Therapeutic procedures to improve respiratory function or increase strength or endurance of respiratory muscles, two or more individuals (includes monitoring) S
CMS: 100-02,12,30.1; 100-02,12,40.5
AHA: 1Q, '02, 5

G0245 Initial physician evaluation and management of a diabetic patient with diabetic sensory neuropathy resulting in a loss of protective sensation (LOPS) which must include: (1) the diagnosis of LOPS, (2) a patient history, (3) a physical examination that consists of at least the following elements: (a) visual inspection of the forefoot, hindfoot, and toe web spaces, (b) evaluation of a protective sensation, (c) evaluation of foot structure and biomechanics, (d) evaluation of vascular status and skin integrity, and (e) evaluation and recommendation of footwear, and (4) patient education V ⊘
CMS: 100-04,32,80.2; 100-04,32,80.3; 100-04,32,80.6; 100-04,32,80.8
AHA: 4Q, '02, 9-10; 3Q, '02, 11

G0246 Follow-up physician evaluation and management of a diabetic patient with diabetic sensory neuropathy resulting in a loss of protective sensation (LOPS) to include at least the following: (1) a patient history, (2) a physical examination that includes: (a) visual inspection of the forefoot, hindfoot, and toe web spaces, (b) evaluation of protective sensation, (c) evaluation of foot structure and biomechanics, (d) evaluation of vascular status and skin integrity, and (e) evaluation and recommendation of footwear, and (3) patient education V ⊘
CMS: 100-03,70.2.1; 100-04,32,80; 100-04,32,80.2; 100-04,32,80.3; 100-04,32,80.6; 100-04,32,80.8
AHA: 4Q, '02, 9-10; 3Q, '02, 11

G0247 Routine foot care by a physician of a diabetic patient with diabetic sensory neuropathy resulting in a loss of protective sensation (LOPS) to include the local care of superficial wounds (i.e., superficial to muscle and fascia) and at least the following, if present: (1) local care of superficial wounds, (2) debridement of corns and calluses, and (3) trimming and debridement of nails 01 ⊘
CMS: 100-03,70.2.1; 100-04,32,80; 100-04,32,80.2; 100-04,32,80.3; 100-04,32,80.6; 100-04,32,80.8
AHA: 4Q, '02, 9-10; 3Q, '02, 11

G0248 Demonstration, prior to initiation of home INR monitoring, for patient with either mechanical heart valve(s), chronic atrial fibrillation, or venous thromboembolism who meets Medicare coverage criteria, under the direction of a physician; includes: face-to-face demonstration of use and care of the INR monitor, obtaining at least one blood sample, provision of instructions for reporting home INR test results, and documentation of patient's ability to perform testing and report results V
CMS: 100-03,190.11; 100-04,32,80
AHA: 4Q, '02, 9-10; 3Q, '02, 11

G0249 Provision of test materials and equipment for home INR monitoring of patient with either mechanical heart valve(s), chronic atrial fibrillation, or venous thromboembolism who meets Medicare coverage criteria; includes: provision of materials for use in the home and reporting of test results to physician; testing not occurring more frequently than once a week; testing materials, billing units of service include four tests V ☑
CMS: 100-03,190.11
AHA: 4Q, '02, 9-10; 3Q, '02, 11

Special Coverage Instructions   Noncovered by Medicare   Carrier Discretion   ☑ Quantity Alert   ● New Code   ○ Recycled/Reinstated   ▲ Revised Code

A Age Edit   M Maternity Edit   ♀ Female Only   ♂ Male Only   A-Y OPPS Status Indicators   © 2021 Optum360, LLC

G0250 Physician review, interpretation, and patient management of home INR testing for patient with either mechanical heart valve(s), chronic atrial fibrillation, or venous thromboembolism who meets Medicare coverage criteria; testing not occurring more frequently than once a week; billing units of service include four tests M ☑ ⊘
CMS: 100-03,190.11
AHA: 4Q, '02, 9-10; 3Q, '02, 11

G0252 PET imaging, full and partial-ring PET scanners only, for initial diagnosis of breast cancer and/or surgical planning for breast cancer (e.g., initial staging of axillary lymph nodes) E
CMS: 100-03,220.6.10; 100-03,220.6.3; 100-04,13,60; 100-04,13,60.16
AHA: 1Q, '07, 6; 4Q, '02, 9-10

G0255 Current perception threshold/sensory nerve conduction test, (SNCT) per limb, any nerve E
AHA: 4Q, '02, 9-10

G0257 Unscheduled or emergency dialysis treatment for an ESRD patient in a hospital outpatient department that is not certified as an ESRD facility S
CMS: 100-04,4,200.2; 100-04,8,60.4.7
AHA: 3Q, '14, 4; 1Q, '03, 7; 4Q, '02, 9-10

G0259 Injection procedure for sacroiliac joint; arthrography N
AHA: 4Q, '02, 9-10

G0260 Injection procedure for sacroiliac joint; provision of anesthetic, steroid and/or other therapeutic agent, with or without arthrography T A2
AHA: 4Q, '02, 9-10

G0268 Removal of impacted cerumen (one or both ears) by physician on same date of service as audiologic function testing N ⊘
AHA: 2Q, '16, 2-3; 1Q, '03, 11

G0269 Placement of occlusive device into either a venous or arterial access site, postsurgical or interventional procedure (e.g., angioseal plug, vascular plug) N ⊘
AHA: 4Q, '12, 10; 3Q, '11, 3; 4Q, '10, 6

G0270 Medical nutrition therapy; reassessment and subsequent intervention(s) following second referral in same year for change in diagnosis, medical condition or treatment regimen (including additional hours needed for renal disease), individual, face-to-face with the patient, each 15 minutes A ☑ ⊘
CMS: 100-04,12,190.3; 100-04,12,190.6; 100-04,12,190.6.1; 100-04,12,190.7

G0271 Medical nutrition therapy, reassessment and subsequent intervention(s) following second referral in same year for change in diagnosis, medical condition, or treatment regimen (including additional hours needed for renal disease), group (two or more individuals), each 30 minutes A ☑ ⊘

G0276 Blinded procedure for lumbar stenosis, percutaneous image-guided lumbar decompression (PILD) or placebo-control, performed in an approved coverage with evidence development (CED) clinical trial J G2
CMS: 100-03,150.13; 100-04,32,330.1; 100-04,32,330.2

G0277 Hyperbaric oxygen under pressure, full body chamber, per 30 minute interval S
AHA: 3Q, '15, 7

G0278 Iliac and/or femoral artery angiography, nonselective, bilateral or ipsilateral to catheter insertion, performed at the same time as cardiac catheterization and/or coronary angiography, includes positioning or placement of the catheter in the distal aorta or ipsilateral femoral or iliac artery, injection of dye, production of permanent images, and radiologic supervision and interpretation (List separately in addition to primary procedure) N ⊘
AHA: 3Q, '11, 3; 4Q, '06, 8

G0279 Diagnostic digital breast tomosynthesis, unilateral or bilateral (list separately in addition to 77065 or 77066) A
CMS: 100-04,18,20.2; 100-04,18,20.2.1; 100-04,18,20.2.2; 100-04,18,20.6

G0281 Electrical stimulation, (unattended), to one or more areas, for chronic Stage III and Stage IV pressure ulcers, arterial ulcers, diabetic ulcers, and venous stasis ulcers not demonstrating measurable signs of healing after 30 days of conventional care, as part of a therapy plan of care A
CMS: 100-02,15,220.4; 100-04,32,11.1; 100-04,5,10.3.2; 100-04,5,10.3.3
AHA: 2Q, '03, 7; 1Q, '03, 7

G0282 Electrical stimulation, (unattended), to one or more areas, for wound care other than described in G0281 E
CMS: 100-04,32,11.1
AHA: 2Q, '03, 7; 1Q, '03, 7

G0283 Electrical stimulation (unattended), to one or more areas for indication(s) other than wound care, as part of a therapy plan of care A
CMS: 100-02,15,220.4; 100-04,5,10.3.2; 100-04,5,10.3.3
AHA: 2Q, '09, 1; 2Q, '03, 7; 1Q, '03, 7

G0288 Reconstruction, computed tomographic angiography of aorta for surgical planning for vascular surgery N

G0289 Arthroscopy, knee, surgical, for removal of loose body, foreign body, debridement/shaving of articular cartilage (chondroplasty) at the time of other surgical knee arthroscopy in a different compartment of the same knee N ⊘
AHA: 2Q, '03, 9

G0293 Noncovered surgical procedure(s) using conscious sedation, regional, general, or spinal anesthesia in a Medicare qualifying clinical trial, per day Q1 ☑
AHA: 4Q, '02, 9-10

G0294 Noncovered procedure(s) using either no anesthesia or local anesthesia only, in a Medicare qualifying clinical trial, per day Q1 ☑
AHA: 4Q, '02, 9-10

G0295 Electromagnetic therapy, to one or more areas, for wound care other than described in G0329 or for other uses E
AHA: 1Q, '03, 7

G0296 Counseling visit to discuss need for lung cancer screening using low dose CT scan (LDCT) (service is for eligibility determination and shared decision making) S
CMS: 100-02,13,220; 100-02,13,220.1; 100-02,13,220.3; 100-04,18,220; 100-04,18,220.1; 100-04,18,220.2; 100-04,18,220.3; 100-04,18,220.4; 100-04,18,220.5; 1004-04,13,220.1

G0299 Direct skilled nursing services of a registered nurse (RN) in the home health or hospice setting, each 15 minutes B
CMS: 100-01,3,30.3; 100-04,10,40.2; 100-04,11,130.1; 100-04,11,30.3

G0300 Direct skilled nursing services of a licensed practical nurse (LPN) in the home health or hospice setting, each 15 minutes B
CMS: 100-01,3,30.3; 100-04,10,40.2; 100-04,11,130.1; 100-04,11,30.3

G0302 Preoperative pulmonary surgery services for preparation for LVRS, complete course of services, to include a minimum of 16 days of services S ☑

G0303 Preoperative pulmonary surgery services for preparation for LVRS, 10 to 15 days of services S ☑

G0304 Preoperative pulmonary surgery services for preparation for LVRS, 1 to 9 days of services S ☑

G0305 Postdischarge pulmonary surgery services after LVRS, minimum of 6 days of services S ☑

G0306 Complete CBC, automated (HgB, HCT, RBC, WBC, without platelet count) and automated WBC differential count Q
CMS: 100-02,11,20.2

Special Coverage Instructions   Noncovered by Medicare   Carrier Discretion   ☑ Quantity Alert ● New Code   ○ Recycled/Reinstated   ▲ Revised Code

Procedures/Professional Services (Temporary)

G0307 — G0383

G0307 Complete CBC, automated (HgB, HCT, RBC, WBC; without platelet count) ▫Q
CMS: 100-02,11,20.2

○ **G0327** Colorectal cancer screening; blood-based biomarker
CMS: 100-04,18,60; 100-04,18,60.1; 100-04,18,60.1.1; 100-04,18,60.2; 100-04,18,60.2.1; 100-04,18,60.6; 100-04,18,60.7; 100-04,18,60.8

G0328 Colorectal cancer screening; fecal occult blood test, immunoassay, one to three simultaneous determinations ▫A
CMS: 100-02,15,280.2.2; 100-04,16,70.8; 100-04,18,60; 100-04,18,60.1; 100-04,18,60.1.1; 100-04,18,60.2; 100-04,18,60.2.1; 100-04,18,60.6; 100-04,18,60.7
AHA: 2Q, '12, 9

G0329 Electromagnetic therapy, to one or more areas for chronic Stage III and Stage IV pressure ulcers, arterial ulcers, diabetic ulcers and venous stasis ulcers not demonstrating measurable signs of healing after 30 days of conventional care as part of a therapy plan of care ▫A
CMS: 100-02,15,220.4; 100-04,32,11.2; 100-04,5,10.3.2; 100-04,5,10.3.3

G0333 Pharmacy dispensing fee for inhalation drug(s); initial 30-day supply as a beneficiary ▫M

G0337 Hospice evaluation and counseling services, preelection ▫B
CMS: 100-04,11,10

G0339 Image guided robotic linear accelerator-based stereotactic radiosurgery, complete course of therapy in one session or first session of fractionated treatment ▫B ⊘
AHA: 4Q, '13, 8-10; 1Q, '04, 6

G0340 Image guided robotic linear accelerator-based stereotactic radiosurgery, delivery including collimator changes and custom plugging, fractionated treatment, all lesions, per session, second through fifth sessions, maximum five sessions per course of treatment ▫B ⊘
AHA: 4Q, '13, 8-10; 1Q, '04, 6

G0341 Percutaneous islet cell transplant, includes portal vein catheterization and infusion ▫C ⊘
CMS: 100-04,32,70

G0342 Laparoscopy for islet cell transplant, includes portal vein catheterization and infusion ▫C ⊘
CMS: 100-04,32,70

G0343 Laparotomy for islet cell transplant, includes portal vein catheterization and infusion ▫C ⊘
CMS: 100-04,32,70

G0372 Physician service required to establish and document the need for a power mobility device ▫M ⊘
CMS: 100-04,12,30.6.15.4

Observation/Emergency Department Services

G0378 Hospital observation service, per hour ▫N
CMS: 100-02,6,20.6; 100-04,01,50.3.2; 100-04,4,290.1; 100-04,4,290.2.2; 100-04,4,290.4.1; 100-04,4,290.4.2; 100-04,4,290.4.3; 100-04,4,290.5.1; 100-04,4,290.5.2; 100-04,4,290.5.3
AHA: 4Q, '05, 7, 9

G0379 Direct admission of patient for hospital observation care ▫J
CMS: 100-02,6,20.6; 100-04,4,290.4.1; 100-04,4,290.4.2; 100-04,4,290.4.3; 100-04,4,290.5.1; 100-04,4,290.5.2; 100-04,4,290.5.3
AHA: 4Q, '05, 7, 9

G0380 Level 1 hospital emergency department visit provided in a type B emergency department; (the ED must meet at least one of the following requirements: (1) it is licensed by the state in which it is located under applicable state law as an emergency room or emergency department; (2) it is held out to the public (by name, posted signs, advertising, or other means) as a place that provides care for emergency medical conditions on an urgent basis without requiring a previously scheduled appointment; or (3) during the calendar year immediately preceding the calendar year in which a determination under 42 CFR 489.24 is being made, based on a representative sample of patient visits that occurred during that calendar year, it provides at least one-third of all of its outpatient visits for the treatment of emergency medical conditions on an urgent basis without requiring a previously scheduled appointment) ▫J
CMS: 100-04,4,160
AHA: 4Q, '13, 7; 1Q, '09, 1; 4Q, '07, 1

G0381 Level 2 hospital emergency department visit provided in a type B emergency department; (the ED must meet at least one of the following requirements: (1) it is licensed by the state in which it is located under applicable state law as an emergency room or emergency department; (2) it is held out to the public (by name, posted signs, advertising, or other means) as a place that provides care for emergency medical conditions on an urgent basis without requiring a previously scheduled appointment; or (3) during the calendar year immediately preceding the calendar year in which a determination under 42 CFR 489.24 is being made, based on a representative sample of patient visits that occurred during that calendar year, it provides at least one-third of all of its outpatient visits for the treatment of emergency medical conditions on an urgent basis without requiring a previously scheduled appointment) ▫J
CMS: 100-04,4,160
AHA: 4Q, '13, 7; 1Q, '09, 1; 4Q, '07, 1

G0382 Level 3 hospital emergency department visit provided in a type B emergency department; (the ED must meet at least one of the following requirements: (1) it is licensed by the state in which it is located under applicable state law as an emergency room or emergency department; (2) it is held out to the public (by name, posted signs, advertising, or other means) as a place that provides care for emergency medical conditions on an urgent basis without requiring a previously scheduled appointment; or (3) during the calendar year immediately preceding the calendar year in which a determination under 42 CFR 489.24 is being made, based on a representative sample of patient visits that occurred during that calendar year, it provides at least one-third of all of its outpatient visits for the treatment of emergency medical conditions on an urgent basis without requiring a previously scheduled appointment) ▫J
CMS: 100-04,4,160
AHA: 4Q, '13, 7; 1Q, '09, 1; 4Q, '07, 1

G0383 Level 4 hospital emergency department visit provided in a type B emergency department; (the ED must meet at least one of the following requirements: (1) it is licensed by the state in which it is located under applicable state law as an emergency room or emergency department; (2) it is held out to the public (by name, posted signs, advertising, or other means) as a place that provides care for emergency medical conditions on an urgent basis without requiring a previously scheduled appointment; or (3) during the calendar year immediately preceding the calendar year in which a determination under 42 CFR 489.24 is being made, based on a representative sample of patient visits that occurred during that calendar year, it provides at least one-third of all of its outpatient visits for the treatment of emergency medical conditions on an urgent basis without requiring a previously scheduled appointment) ▫J
CMS: 100-04,4,160
AHA: 4Q, '13, 7; 1Q, '09, 1; 4Q, '07, 1

Special Coverage Instructions   Noncovered by Medicare   Carrier Discretion   ☑ Quantity Alert   ● New Code   ○ Recycled/Reinstated   ▲ Revised Code

▫A Age Edit   ▫M Maternity Edit   ♀ Female Only   ♂ Male Only   ▫A-▫Y OPPS Status Indicators   © 2021 Optum360, LLC

G0384 Level 5 hospital emergency department visit provided in a type B emergency department; (the ED must meet at least one of the following requirements: (1) it is licensed by the state in which it is located under applicable state law as an emergency room or emergency department; (2) it is held out to the public (by name, posted signs, advertising, or other means) as a place that provides care for emergency medical conditions on an urgent basis without requiring a previously scheduled appointment; or (3) during the calendar year immediately preceding the calendar year in which a determination under 42 CFR 489.24 is being made, based on a representative sample of patient visits that occurred during that calendar year, it provides at least one-third of all of its outpatient visits for the treatment of emergency medical conditions on an urgent basis without requiring a previously scheduled appointment) ☐J
CMS: 100-04,4,160; 100-04,4,290.5.1
AHA: 4Q, '13, 7; 1Q, '09, 1; 4Q, '07, 1

Other Services

G0390 Trauma response team associated with hospital critical care service ☐S
CMS: 100-04,4,160.1

Alcohol or Substance Abuse

G0396 Alcohol and/or substance (other than tobacco) misuse structured assessment (e.g., audit, dast), and brief intervention 15 to 30 minutes ☐S ☑ ☐
CMS: 100-04,12,190.3; 100-04,12,190.6; 100-04,12,190.6.1; 100-04,12,190.7; 100-04,4,200.6

G0397 Alcohol and/or substance (other than tobacco) misuse structured assessment (e.g., audit, dast), and intervention, greater than 30 minutes ☐S ☑ ☐
CMS: 100-04,12,190.3; 100-04,12,190.6; 100-04,12,190.6.1; 100-04,12,190.7; 100-04,4,200.6

Home Sleep Study

G0398 Home sleep study test (HST) with type II portable monitor, unattended; minimum of 7 channels: EEG, EOG, EMG, ECG/heart rate, airflow, respiratory effort and oxygen saturation ☐S
CMS: 100-03,240.4
AHA: 3Q, '08, 5

G0399 Home sleep test (HST) with type III portable monitor, unattended; minimum of 4 channels: 2 respiratory movement/airflow, 1 ECG/heart rate and 1 oxygen saturation ☐S
CMS: 100-03,240.4
AHA: 3Q, '08, 5

G0400 Home sleep test (HST) with type IV portable monitor, unattended; minimum of 3 channels ☐S
CMS: 100-03,240.4
AHA: 3Q, '08, 5

Initial Physical Exam

G0402 Initial preventive physical examination; face-to-face visit, services limited to new beneficiary during the first 12 months of Medicare enrollment ☐V ☐
CMS: 100-02,13,220; 100-02,13,220.1; 100-02,13,220.3; 100-04,12,100.1.1; 100-04,18,140.6; 100-04,18,80; 100-04,18,80.1; 100-04,18,80.2; 100-04,18,80.3.3; 100-04,18,80.4; 1004-04,13,220.1
AHA: 4Q, '09, 7

G0403 Electrocardiogram, routine ECG with 12 leads; performed as a screening for the initial preventive physical examination with interpretation and report ☐M
CMS: 100-04,18,80; 100-04,18,80.1; 100-04,18,80.2

G0404 Electrocardiogram, routine ECG with 12 leads; tracing only, without interpretation and report, performed as a screening for the initial preventive physical examination ☐S
CMS: 100-04,18,80; 100-04,18,80.1; 100-04,18,80.2; 100-04,18,80.3.3

G0405 Electrocardiogram, routine ECG with 12 leads; interpretation and report only, performed as a screening for the initial preventive physical examination ☐B ☐
CMS: 100-04,18,80; 100-04,18,80.1; 100-04,18,80.2

Follow-up Telehealth

G0406 Follow-up inpatient consultation, limited, physicians typically spend 15 minutes communicating with the patient via telehealth ☐B ☐
CMS: 100-04,12,190.3; 100-04,12,190.3.1; 100-04,12,190.3.3; 100-04,12,190.3.5; 100-04,12,190.6; 100-04,12,190.6.1; 100-04,12,190.7

G0407 Follow-up inpatient consultation, intermediate, physicians typically spend 25 minutes communicating with the patient via telehealth ☐B ☐
CMS: 100-04,12,190.3; 100-04,12,190.3.1; 100-04,12,190.3.3; 100-04,12,190.3.5; 100-04,12,190.6; 100-04,12,190.6.1; 100-04,12,190.7

G0408 Follow-up inpatient consultation, complex, physicians typically spend 35 minutes communicating with the patient via telehealth ☐B ☐
CMS: 100-04,12,190.3; 100-04,12,190.3.1; 100-04,12,190.3.3; 100-04,12,190.3.5; 100-04,12,190.6; 100-04,12,190.6.1; 100-04,12,190.7

Psychological Services

G0409 Social work and psychological services, directly relating to and/or furthering the patient's rehabilitation goals, each 15 minutes, face-to-face; individual (services provided by a CORF qualified social worker or psychologist in a CORF) ☐B ☑
CMS: 100-02,12,30.1; 100-04,5,100.11; 100-04,5,100.4

G0410 Group psychotherapy other than of a multiple-family group, in a partial hospitalization setting, approximately 45 to 50 minutes ☐P
CMS: 100-04,4,260.1; 100-04,4,260.1.1
AHA: 4Q, '12, 11-14; 4Q, '09, 9

G0411 Interactive group psychotherapy, in a partial hospitalization setting, approximately 45 to 50 minutes ☐P
CMS: 100-04,4,260.1; 100-04,4,260.1.1
AHA: 4Q, '12, 11-14; 4Q, '09, 9

Fracture Care

G0412 Open treatment of iliac spine(s), tuberosity avulsion, or iliac wing fracture(s), unilateral or bilateral for pelvic bone fracture patterns which do not disrupt the pelvic ring, includes internal fixation, when performed ☐C ☐

G0413 Percutaneous skeletal fixation of posterior pelvic bone fracture and/or dislocation, for fracture patterns which disrupt the pelvic ring, unilateral or bilateral, (includes ilium, sacroiliac joint and/or sacrum) ☐J ☐

G0414 Open treatment of anterior pelvic bone fracture and/or dislocation for fracture patterns which disrupt the pelvic ring, unilateral or bilateral, includes internal fixation when performed (includes pubic symphysis and/or superior/inferior rami) ☐C ☐

G0415 Open treatment of posterior pelvic bone fracture and/or dislocation, for fracture patterns which disrupt the pelvic ring, unilateral or bilateral, includes internal fixation, when performed (includes ilium, sacroiliac joint and/or sacrum) ☐C ☐

Surgical Pathology

G0416 Surgical pathology, gross and microscopic examinations, for prostate needle biopsy, any method ♂ ☐02
AHA: 2Q, '13, 6

Procedures/Professional Services (Temporary)

G0420 — G0453

Educational Services

G0420 Face-to-face educational services related to the care of chronic kidney disease; individual, per session, per 1 hour A ☑ ⊘
CMS: 100-02,15,200; 100-02,15,310; 100-02,15,310.1; 100-02,15,310.2; 100-02,15,310.4; 100-02,15,310.5; 100-04,12,190.3; 100-04,12,190.6; 100-04,12,190.6.1; 100-04,12,190.7

G0421 Face-to-face educational services related to the care of chronic kidney disease; group, per session, per 1 hour A ☑ ⊘
CMS: 100-02,15,200; 100-02,15,310; 100-02,15,310.1; 100-02,15,310.2; 100-02,15,310.4; 100-02,15,310.5; 100-04,12,190.3; 100-04,12,190.6; 100-04,12,190.6.1; 100-04,12,190.7

Cardiac and Pulmonary Rehabilitation

G0422 Intensive cardiac rehabilitation; with or without continuous ECG monitoring with exercise, per session S ☑ ⊘
CMS: 100-02,15,232; 100-04,32,140.2.2.1; 100-04,32,140.2.2.2; 100-04,32,140.3; 100-04,32,140.3.1; 100-08,15,4.2.8

G0423 Intensive cardiac rehabilitation; with or without continuous ECG monitoring; without exercise, per session S ☑ ⊘
CMS: 100-02,15,232; 100-04,32,140.2.2.1; 100-04,32,140.2.2.2; 100-04,32,140.3; 100-04,32,140.3.1; 100-08,15,4.2.8

G0424 ~~Pulmonary rehabilitation, including exercise (includes monitoring), 1 hour, per session, up to two sessions per day~~

Inpatient Telehealth

G0425 Telehealth consultation, emergency department or initial inpatient, typically 30 minutes communicating with the patient via telehealth B ☑ ⊘
CMS: 100-04,12,190.3; 100-04,12,190.3.1; 100-04,12,190.3.2; 100-04,12,190.6; 100-04,12,190.6.1; 100-04,12,190.7

G0426 Telehealth consultation, emergency department or initial inpatient, typically 50 minutes communicating with the patient via telehealth B ☑ ⊘
CMS: 100-04,12,190.3; 100-04,12,190.3.1; 100-04,12,190.3.2; 100-04,12,190.6; 100-04,12,190.6.1; 100-04,12,190.7

G0427 Telehealth consultation, emergency department or initial inpatient, typically 70 minutes or more communicating with the patient via telehealth B ☑ ⊘
CMS: 100-04,12,190.3; 100-04,12,190.3.1; 100-04,12,190.3.2; 100-04,12,190.6; 100-04,12,190.6.1; 100-04,12,190.7

Defect Fillers

G0428 Collagen meniscus implant procedure for filling meniscal defects (e.g., CMI, collagen scaffold, Menaflex) E
CMS: 100-03,150.12

G0429 Dermal filler injection(s) for the treatment of facial lipodystrophy syndrome (LDS) (e.g., as a result of highly active antiretroviral therapy) T P3
CMS: 100-03,250.5; 100-04,32,260.1; 100-04,32,260.2.1; 100-04,32,260.2.2

Laboratory Services

G0432 Infectious agent antibody detection by enzyme immunoassay (EIA) technique, HIV-1 and/or HIV-2, screening A
CMS: 100-03,190.14; 100-03,190.9; 100-03,210.7; 100-04,18,130.1; 100-04,18,130.2; 100-04,18,130.3; 100-04,18,130.4; 100-04,18,130.5

G0433 Infectious agent antibody detection by enzyme-linked immunosorbent assay (ELISA) technique, HIV-1 and/or HIV-2, screening A
CMS: 100-03,190.14; 100-03,190.9; 100-03,210.7; 100-04,16,70.8; 100-04,18,130.1; 100-04,18,130.2; 100-04,18,130.3; 100-04,18,130.4; 100-04,18,130.5

G0435 Infectious agent antibody detection by rapid antibody test, HIV-1 and/or HIV-2, screening A
CMS: 100-03,190.14; 100-03,190.9; 100-03,210.7; 100-04,18,130.1; 100-04,18,130.2; 100-04,18,130.3; 100-04,18,130.4; 100-04,18,130.5

Counseling and Wellness Visit

G0438 Annual wellness visit; includes a personalized prevention plan of service (PPS), initial visit A
CMS: 100-02,13,220; 100-02,13,220.1; 100-02,13,220.3; 100-02,15,280.5; 100-02,15,280.5.1; 100-04,12,100.1.1; 100-04,18,140; 100-04,18,140.1; 100-04,18,140.5; 100-04,18,140.6; 100-04,18,140.8; 100-04,4,200.11; 1004-04,13,220.1

G0439 Annual wellness visit, includes a personalized prevention plan of service (PPS), subsequent visit A
CMS: 100-02,13,220; 100-02,13,220.1; 100-02,13,220.3; 100-02,15,280.5; 100-02,15,280.5.1; 100-04,12,100.1.1; 100-04,18,140; 100-04,18,140.1; 100-04,18,140.5; 100-04,18,140.6; 100-04,18,140.8; 100-04,4,200.11; 1004-04,13,220.1

Other Services

G0442 Annual alcohol misuse screening, 15 minutes S ☑
CMS: 100-03,210.8; 100-04,12,190.3; 100-04,12,190.6; 100-04,12,190.6.1; 100-04,12,190.7; 100-04,18,180; 100-04,18,180.1; 100-04,18,180.2; 100-04,18,180.3; 100-04,18,180.4; 100-04,18,180.5; 100-04,32,180.4; 100-04,32,180.5

G0443 Brief face-to-face behavioral counseling for alcohol misuse, 15 minutes S ☑
CMS: 100-03,210.8; 100-04,12,190.3; 100-04,12,190.6; 100-04,12,190.6.1; 100-04,12,190.7; 100-04,18,180; 100-04,18,180.1; 100-04,18,180.2; 100-04,18,180.3; 100-04,18,180.4; 100-04,18,180.5; 100-04,32,180.4; 100-04,32,180.5

G0444 Annual depression screening, 15 minutes S ☑
CMS: 100-04,12,190.3; 100-04,12,190.6; 100-04,12,190.6.1; 100-04,12,190.7; 100-04,18,190; 100-04,18,190.1; 100-04,18,190.2; 100-04,18,190.3

G0445 Semiannual high intensity behavioral counseling to prevent STIs, individual, face-to-face, includes education skills training & guidance on how to change sexual behavior S ☑
CMS: 100-03,210.10; 100-04,12,190.3; 100-04,12,190.6; 100-04,12,190.6.1; 100-04,12,190.7; 100-04,18,170.1; 100-04,18,170.2; 100-04,18,170.3; 100-04,18,170.4; 100-04,18,170.4.1; 100-04,18,170.5

G0446 Annual, face-to-face intensive behavioral therapy for cardiovascular disease, individual, 15 minutes S ☑
CMS: 100-03,210.11; 100-04,12,190.3; 100-04,12,190.6; 100-04,12,190.6.1; 100-04,12,190.7; 100-04,18,160; 100-04,18,160.1; 100-04,18,160.2.1; 100-04,18,160.2.2; 100-04,18,160.3; 100-04,18,160.4; 100-04,18,160.5
AHA: 2Q, '12, 8

G0447 Face-to-face behavioral counseling for obesity, 15 minutes S ☑
CMS: 100-03,210.12; 100-04,12,190.3; 100-04,12,190.6; 100-04,12,190.6.1; 100-04,12,190.7; 100-04,18,200; 100-04,18,200.1; 100-04,18,200.2; 100-04,18,200.3; 100-04,18,200.4; 100-04,18,200.5

G0448 Insertion or replacement of a permanent pacing cardioverter-defibrillator system with transvenous lead(s), single or dual chamber with insertion of pacing electrode, cardiac venous system, for left ventricular pacing B
CMS: 100-04,32,270; 100-04,32,270.1; 100-04,32,270.2; 100-04,32,270.3

G0451 Development testing, with interpretation and report, per standardized instrument form 03
CMS: 100-02,15,220.4; 100-04,5,10.3.2; 100-04,5,10.3.3

Molecular Pathology

G0452 Molecular pathology procedure; physician interpretation and report B

Neurophysiology Monitoring

G0453 Continuous intraoperative neurophysiology monitoring, from outside the operating room (remote or nearby), per patient, (attention directed exclusively to one patient) each 15 minutes (list in addition to primary procedure) N

Special Coverage Instructions   Noncovered by Medicare   Carrier Discretion   ☑ Quantity Alert ● New Code   ○ Recycled/Reinstated ▲ Revised Code

52 — G Codes   A Age Edit   M Maternity Edit ♀ Female Only ♂ Male Only A-Y OPPS Status Indicators   © 2021 Optum360, LLC

Documentation and Preparation

G0454 Physician documentation of face-to-face visit for durable medical equipment determination performed by nurse practitioner, physician assistant or clinical nurse specialist ☒B

G0455 Preparation with instillation of fecal microbiota by any method, including assessment of donor specimen ☒Q1
AHA: 3Q, '13, 8

Prostate Brachytherapy

G0458 Low dose rate (LDR) prostate brachytherapy services, composite rate ♂B

Inpatient Telehealth Pharmacologic Management

G0459 Inpatient telehealth pharmacologic management, including prescription, use, and review of medication with no more than minimal medical psychotherapy ☒B
CMS: 100-04,12,190.3; 100-04,12,190.6; 100-04,12,190.6.1; 100-04,12,190.7
AHA: 2Q, '13, 9

Other Wound/Ulcer Care

▲ **G0460** Autologous platelet rich plasma for nondiabetic chronic wounds/ulcers, including phlebotomy, centrifugation, and all other preparatory procedures, administration and dressings, per treatment ☒T
CMS: 100-03,270.3; 100-04,32,11.3.1; 100-04,32,11.3.2; 100-04,32,11.3.3; 100-04,32,11.3.5; 100-04,32,11.3.6

Hospital Outpatient Visit

G0463 Hospital outpatient clinic visit for assessment and management of a patient ☒J
CMS: 100-04,4,160.2; 100-04,4,260.1; 100-04,4,260.1.1; 100-04,4,290.5.1; 100-04,4,290.5.3; 100-04,6,20.1.1.2; 100-04,6,30.4.1
AHA: 4Q, '14, 2

Platelet Rich Plasma

● **G0465** Autologous platelet rich plasma (PRP) for diabetic chronic wounds/ulcers, using an FDA-cleared device (includes administration, dressings, phlebotomy, centrifugation, and all other preparatory procedures, per treatment)

Federally Qualified Health Center Visits

G0466 Federally qualified health center (FQHC) visit, new patient ☒A
CMS: 100-04,9,60.6

G0467 Federally qualified health center (FQHC) visit, established patient ☒A
CMS: 100-04,9,60.6

G0468 Federally qualified health center (FQHC) visit, initial preventive physical exam (IPPE) or annual wellness visit (AWV) ☒A
CMS: 100-04,9,60.6

G0469 Federally qualified health center (FQHC) visit, mental health, new patient ☒A
CMS: 100-04,9,60.6

G0470 Federally qualified health center (FQHC) visit, mental health, established patient ☒A
CMS: 100-04,9,60.6

HHA and SNF Specimen Collection

G0471 Collection of venous blood by venipuncture or urine sample by catheterization from an individual in a skilled nursing facility (SNF) or by a laboratory on behalf of a home health agency (HHA) ☒A
CMS: 100-04,16,60.1.4

Hepatitis C Screening

G0472 Hepatitis C antibody screening for individual at high risk and other covered indication(s) ☒A
CMS: 100-02,13,220; 100-02,13,220.1; 100-02,13,220.3; 100-03,210.13; 100-04,18,210; 100-04,18,210.2; 100-04,18,210.3; 100-04,18,210.4; 1004-04,13,220.1

Behavioral Counseling

G0473 Face-to-face behavioral counseling for obesity, group (2-10), 30 minutes ☒S
CMS: 100-04,18,200.1; 100-04,18,200.2; 100-04,18,200.3; 100-04,18,200.4; 100-04,18,200.5

Screening Measures

G0475 HIV antigen/antibody, combination assay, screening ☒A
CMS: 100-03,210.7; 100-04,18,130.1; 100-04,18,130.2; 100-04,18,130.3; 100-04,18,130.5

G0476 Infectious agent detection by nucleic acid (DNA or RNA); human papillomavirus HPV), high-risk types (e.g., 16, 18, 31, 33, 35, 39, 45, 51, 52, 56, 58, 59, 68) for cervical cancer screening, must be performed in addition to pap test ♀A
CMS: 100-03,210.2.1; 100-04,18,30.2.1; 100-04,18,30.5; 100-04,18,30.6

Drug Testing

G0480 Drug test(s), definitive, utilizing (1) drug identification methods able to identify individual drugs and distinguish between structural isomers (but not necessarily stereoisomers), including, but not limited to, GC/MS (any type, single or tandem) and LC/MS (any type, single or tandem and excluding immunoassays (e.g., IA, EIA, ELISA, EMIT, FPIA) and enzymatic methods (e.g., alcohol dehydrogenase)), (2) stable isotope or other universally recognized internal standards in all samples (e.g., to control for matrix effects, interferences and variations in signal strength), and (3) method or drug-specific calibration and matrix-matched quality control material (e.g., to control for instrument variations and mass spectral drift); qualitative or quantitative, all sources, includes specimen validity testing, per day; 1-7 drug class(es), including metabolite(s) if performed ☒Q

G0481 Drug test(s), definitive, utilizing (1) drug identification methods able to identify individual drugs and distinguish between structural isomers (but not necessarily stereoisomers), including, but not limited to, GC/MS (any type, single or tandem) and LC/MS (any type, single or tandem and excluding immunoassays (e.g., IA, EIA, ELISA, EMIT, FPIA) and enzymatic methods (e.g., alcohol dehydrogenase)), (2) stable isotope or other universally recognized internal standards in all samples (e.g., to control for matrix effects, interferences and variations in signal strength), and (3) method or drug-specific calibration and matrix-matched quality control material (e.g., to control for instrument variations and mass spectral drift); qualitative or quantitative, all sources, includes specimen validity testing, per day; 8-14 drug class(es), including metabolite(s) if performed ☒Q

G0482 Drug test(s), definitive, utilizing (1) drug identification methods able to identify individual drugs and distinguish between structural isomers (but not necessarily stereoisomers), including, but not limited to, GC/MS (any type, single or tandem) and LC/MS (any type, single or tandem and excluding immunoassays (e.g., IA, EIA, ELISA, EMIT, FPIA) and enzymatic methods (e.g., alcohol dehydrogenase)), (2) stable isotope or other universally recognized internal standards in all samples (e.g., to control for matrix effects, interferences and variations in signal strength), and (3) method or drug-specific calibration and matrix-matched quality control material (e.g., to control for instrument variations and mass spectral drift); qualitative or quantitative, all sources, includes specimen validity testing, per day; 15-21 drug class(es), including metabolite(s) if performed ☒Q

Special Coverage Instructions   Noncovered by Medicare   Carrier Discretion   ☑ Quantity Alert   ● New Code   ○ Recycled/Reinstated   ▲ Revised Code

© 2021 Optum360, LLC   A2-Z3 ASC Pmt   CMS: IOM   AHA: Coding Clinic   ⅃ DMEPOS Paid   ⊘ SNF Excluded   G Codes — 53

Procedures/Professional Services (Temporary)

G0483 — G0513

G0483 Drug test(s), definitive, utilizing (1) drug identification methods able to identify individual drugs and distinguish between structural isomers (but not necessarily stereoisomers), including, but not limited to, GC/MS (any type, single or tandem) and LC/MS (any type, single or tandem and excluding immunoassays (e.g., IA, EIA, ELISA, EMIT, FPIA) and enzymatic methods (e.g., alcohol dehydrogenase)), (2) stable isotope or other universally recognized internal standards in all samples (e.g., to control for matrix effects, interferences and variations in signal strength), and (3) method or drug-specific calibration and matrix-matched quality control material (e.g., to control for instrument variations and mass spectral drift); qualitative or quantitative, all sources, includes specimen validity testing, per day; 22 or more drug class(es), including metabolite(s) if performed Q

Home Health Nursing Visit

G0490 Face-to-face home health nursing visit by a rural health clinic (RHC) or federally qualified health center (FQHC) in an area with a shortage of home health agencies; (services limited to RN or LPN only) A

Dialysis Procedures

G0491 Dialysis procedure at a Medicare certified ESRD facility for acute kidney injury without ESRD B
CMS: 100-04,8,40; 100-04,8,50.2

G0492 Dialysis procedure with single evaluation by a physician or other qualified health care professional for acute kidney injury without ESRD B

Skilled Nursing Services

G0493 Skilled services of a registered nurse (RN) for the observation and assessment of the patient's condition, each 15 minutes (the change in the patient's condition requires skilled nursing personnel to identify and evaluate the patient's need for possible modification of treatment in the home health or hospice setting) B
CMS: 100-04,10,40.2

G0494 Skilled services of a licensed practical nurse (LPN) for the observation and assessment of the patient's condition, each 15 minutes (the change in the patient's condition requires skilled nursing personnel to identify and evaluate the patient's need for possible modification of treatment in the home health or hospice setting) B
CMS: 100-04,10,40.2

G0495 Skilled services of a registered nurse (RN), in the training and/or education of a patient or family member, in the home health or hospice setting, each 15 minutes B
CMS: 100-04,10,40.2

G0496 Skilled services of a licensed practical nurse (LPN), in the training and/or education of a patient or family member, in the home health or hospice setting, each 15 minutes B
CMS: 100-04,10,40.2

Chemotherapy Infusion

G0498 Chemotherapy administration, intravenous infusion technique; initiation of infusion in the office/clinic setting using office/clinic pump/supplies, with continuation of the infusion in the community setting (e.g., home, domiciliary, rest home or assisted living) using a portable pump provided by the office/clinic, includes follow up office/clinic visit at the conclusion of the infusion S

Hepatitis B Screening

G0499 Hepatitis B screening in nonpregnant, high-risk individual includes hepatitis B surface antigen (HBSAG), antibodies to HBSAG (anti-HBS) and antibodies to hepatitis B core antigen (anti-HBC), and is followed by a neutralizing confirmatory test, when performed, only for an initially reactive HBSAG result A
CMS: 100-03,1,210.6; 100-04,18,230; 100-04,18,230.1; 100-04,18,230.2; 100-04,18,230.3

Moderate Sedation

G0500 Moderate sedation services provided by the same physician or other qualified health care professional performing a gastrointestinal endoscopic service that sedation supports, requiring the presence of an independent trained observer to assist in the monitoring of the patient's level of consciousness and physiological status; initial 15 minutes of intra-service time; patient age 5 years or older (additional time may be reported with 99153, as appropriate) N
CMS: 100-04,18,60.1.1

Mobility-Assistive Technology

G0501 Resource-intensive services for patients for whom the use of specialized mobility-assistive technology (such as adjustable height chairs or tables, patient lift, and adjustable padded leg supports) is medically necessary and used during the provision of an office/outpatient, evaluation and management visit (list separately in addition to primary service) N

Care Management Services

G0506 Comprehensive assessment of and care planning for patients requiring chronic care management services (list separately in addition to primary monthly care management service) N

Telehealth Consultation

G0508 Telehealth consultation, critical care, initial, physicians typically spend 60 minutes communicating with the patient and providers via telehealth B

G0509 Telehealth consultation, critical care, subsequent, physicians typically spend 50 minutes communicating with the patient and providers via telehealth B

RHC or FQHC General Care Management

G0511 Rural health clinic or federally qualified health center (RHC or FQHC) only, general care management, 20 minutes or more of clinical staff time for chronic care management services or behavioral health integration services directed by an RHC or FQHC practitioner (physician, NP, PA, or CNM), per calendar month A
CMS: 100-02,13,230.2; 100-04,9,70.8

G0512 Rural health clinic or federally qualified health center (RHC/FQHC) only, psychiatric collaborative care model (psychiatric COCM), 60 minutes or more of clinical staff time for psychiatric COCM services directed by an RHC or FQHC practitioner (physician, NP, PA, or CNM) and including services furnished by a behavioral health care manager and consultation with a psychiatric consultant, per calendar month A
CMS: 100-02,13,230.2; 100-02,13,230.3; 100-04,9,70.8

Prolonged Services

G0513 Prolonged preventive service(s) (beyond the typical service time of the primary procedure), in the office or other outpatient setting requiring direct patient contact beyond the usual service; first 30 minutes (list separately in addition to code for preventive service) N

Special Coverage Instructions   Noncovered by Medicare   Carrier Discretion   ☑ Quantity Alert ● New Code ○ Recycled/Reinstated ▲ Revised Code

54 — G Codes   A Age Edit   M Maternity Edit   ♀ Female Only   ♂ Male Only   A-Y OPPS Status Indicators   © 2021 Optum360, LLC

G0514 Prolonged preventive service(s) (beyond the typical service time of the primary procedure), in the office or other outpatient setting requiring direct patient contact beyond the usual service; each additional 30 minutes (list separately in addition to code G0513 for additional 30 minutes of preventive service) N

Drug Delivery Implants

G0516 Insertion of nonbiodegradable drug delivery implants, four or more (services for subdermal rod implant) Q1 N1

G0517 Removal of nonbiodegradable drug delivery implants, four or more (services for subdermal implants) Q1 N1

G0518 Removal with reinsertion, nonbiodegradable drug delivery implants, four or more (services for subdermal implants) Q1 N1

Drug Test(s)

G0659 Drug test(s), definitive, utilizing drug identification methods able to identify individual drugs and distinguish between structural isomers (but not necessarily stereoisomers), including but not limited to GC/MS (any type, single or tandem) and LC/MS (any type, single or tandem), excluding immunoassays (e.g., IA, EIA, ELISA, EMIT, FPIA) and enzymatic methods (e.g., alcohol dehydrogenase), performed without method or drug-specific calibration, without matrix-matched quality control material, or without use of stable isotope or other universally recognized internal standard(s) for each drug, drug metabolite or drug class per specimen; qualitative or quantitative, all sources, includes specimen validity testing, per day, any number of drug classes Q

Quality Measures

G0913 Improvement in visual function achieved within 90 days following cataract surgery M

G0914 Patient care survey was not completed by patient M

G0915 Improvement in visual function not achieved within 90 days following cataract surgery M

G0916 Satisfaction with care achieved within 90 days following cataract surgery M

G0917 Patient satisfaction survey was not completed by patient M

G0918 Satisfaction with care not achieved within 90 days following cataract surgery M

Clinical Decision Support Mechanism

G1001 Clinical Decision Support Mechanism eviCore, as defined by the Medicare Appropriate Use Criteria Program

G1002 Clinical Decision Support Mechanism MedCurrent, as defined by the Medicare Appropriate Use Criteria Program

G1003 Clinical Decision Support Mechanism Medicalis, as defined by the Medicare Appropriate Use Criteria Program

G1004 Clinical Decision Support Mechanism National Decision Support Company, as defined by the Medicare Appropriate Use Criteria Program

G1007 Clinical Decision Support Mechanism AIM Specialty Health, as defined by the Medicare Appropriate Use Criteria Program

G1008 Clinical Decision Support Mechanism Cranberry Peak, as defined by the Medicare Appropriate Use Criteria Program

G1009 Clinical Decision Support Mechanism Sage Health Management Solutions, as defined by the Medicare Appropriate Use Criteria Program

G1010 Clinical Decision Support Mechanism Stanson, as defined by the Medicare Appropriate Use Criteria Program

G1011 Clinical Decision Support Mechanism, qualified tool not otherwise specified, as defined by the Medicare Appropriate Use Criteria Program

G1012 Clinical Decision Support Mechanism AgileMD, as defined by the Medicare Appropriate Use Criteria Program

▲ **G1013** Clinical Decision Support Mechanism EvidenceCare ImagingCare, as defined by the Medicare Appropriate Use Criteria Program

G1014 Clinical Decision Support Mechanism InveniQA Semantic Answers in Medicine, as defined by the Medicare Appropriate Use Criteria Program

G1015 Clinical Decision Support Mechanism Reliant Medical Group, as defined by the Medicare Appropriate Use Criteria Program

G1016 Clinical Decision Support Mechanism Speed of Care, as defined by the Medicare Appropriate Use Criteria Program

G1017 Clinical Decision Support Mechanism HealthHelp, as defined by the Medicare Appropriate Use Criteria Program

G1018 Clinical Decision Support Mechanism INFINX, as defined by the Medicare Appropriate Use Criteria Program

G1019 Clinical Decision Support Mechanism LogicNets, as defined by the Medicare Appropriate Use Criteria Program

G1020 Clinical Decision Support Mechanism Curbside Clinical Augmented Workflow, as defined by the Medicare Appropriate Use Criteria Program

G1021 Clinical Decision Support Mechanism EHealthLine Clinical Decision Support Mechanism, as defined by the Medicare Appropriate Use Criteria Program

G1022 Clinical Decision Support Mechanism Intermountain Clinical Decision Support Mechanism, as defined by the Medicare Appropriate Use Criteria Program

G1023 Clinical Decision Support Mechanism Persivia Clinical Decision Support, as defined by the Medicare Appropriate Use Criteria Program

● **G1024** Clinical decision support mechanism Radrite, as defined by the Medicare Appropriate Use Criteria Program

Patient-Month Quality Measures

● **G1025** Patient-months where there are more than one Medicare capitated payment (MCP) provider listed for the month

● **G1026** The number of adult patient-months in the denominator who were on maintenance hemodialysis using a catheter continuously for 3 months or longer under the care of the same practitioner or group partner as of the last hemodialysis session of the reporting month

● **G1027** The number of adult patient-months in the denominator who were on maintenance hemodialysis under the care of the same practitioner or group partner as of the last hemodialysis session of the reporting month using a catheter continuously for less than 3 months

Nasal Naloxone

● **G1028** Take-home supply of nasal naloxone; 2-pack of 8 mg per 0.1 ml nasal spray (provision of the services by a Medicare-enrolled Opioid Treatment Program); list separately in addition to code for primary procedure

Convulsive Therapy Procedure

G2000 Blinded administration of convulsive therapy procedure, either electroconvulsive therapy (ECT, current covered gold standard) or magnetic seizure therapy (MST, noncovered experimental therapy), performed in an approved IDE-based clinical trial, per treatment session

Special Coverage Instructions   Noncovered by Medicare   Carrier Discretion   ☑ Quantity Alert   ● New Code   ○ Recycled/Reinstated   ▲ Revised Code

© 2021 Optum360, LLC   A2-Z3 ASC Pmt   CMS: IOM   AHA: Coding Clinic   ⅃ DMEPOS Paid   ⊘ SNF Excluded   G Codes — 55

Assessments, Evaluations, and CMMI Home Visits

G2001 Brief (20 minutes) in-home visit for a new patient postdischarge. For use only in a Medicare-approved CMMI model. (Services must be furnished within a beneficiary's home, domiciliary, rest home, assisted living and/or nursing facility within 90 days following discharge from an inpatient facility and no more than nine times.)

G2002 Limited (30 minutes) in-home visit for a new patient postdischarge. For use only in a Medicare-approved CMMI model. (Services must be furnished within a beneficiary's home, domiciliary, rest home, assisted living and/or nursing facility within 90 days following discharge from an inpatient facility and no more than nine times.)

G2003 Moderate (45 minutes) in-home visit for a new patient postdischarge. For use only in a Medicare-approved CMMI model. (Services must be furnished within a beneficiary's home, domiciliary, rest home, assisted living and/or nursing facility within 90 days following discharge from an inpatient facility and no more than nine times.)

G2004 Comprehensive (60 minutes) in-home visit for a new patient postdischarge. For use only in a Medicare-approved CMMI model. (Services must be furnished within a beneficiary's home, domiciliary, rest home, assisted living and/or nursing facility within 90 days following discharge from an inpatient facility and no more than nine times.)

G2005 Extensive (75 minutes) in-home visit for a new patient postdischarge. For use only in a Medicare-approved CMMI model. (Services must be furnished within a beneficiary's home, domiciliary, rest home, assisted living and/or nursing facility within 90 days following discharge from an inpatient facility and no more than nine times.)

G2006 Brief (20 minutes) in-home visit for an existing patient postdischarge. For use only in a Medicare-approved CMMI model. (Services must be furnished within a beneficiary's home, domiciliary, rest home, assisted living and/or nursing facility within 90 days following discharge from an inpatient facility and no more than nine times.)

G2007 Limited (30 minutes) in-home visit for an existing patient postdischarge. For use only in a Medicare-approved CMMI model. (Services must be furnished within a beneficiary's home, domiciliary, rest home, assisted living and/or nursing facility within 90 days following discharge from an inpatient facility and no more than nine times.)

G2008 Moderate (45 minutes) in-home visit for an existing patient postdischarge. For use only in a Medicare-approved CMMI model. (Services must be furnished within a beneficiary's home, domiciliary, rest home, assisted living and/or nursing facility within 90 days following discharge from an inpatient facility and no more than nine times.)

G2009 Comprehensive (60 minutes) in-home visit for an existing patient postdischarge. For use only in a Medicare-approved CMMI model. (Services must be furnished within a beneficiary's home, domiciliary, rest home, assisted living and/or nursing facility within 90 days following discharge from an inpatient facility and no more than nine times.)

G2010 Remote evaluation of recorded video and/or images submitted by an established patient (e.g., store and forward), including interpretation with follow-up with the patient within 24 business hours, not originating from a related E/M service provided within the previous 7 days nor leading to an E/M service or procedure within the next 24 hours or soonest available appointment

G2011 Alcohol and/or substance (other than tobacco) misuse structured assessment (e.g., audit, dast), and brief intervention, 5-14 minutes

G2012 Brief communication technology-based service, e.g., virtual check-in, by a physician or other qualified health care professional who can report evaluation and management services, provided to an established patient, not originating from a related E/M service provided within the previous 7 days nor leading to an E/M service or procedure within the next 24 hours or soonest available appointment; 5-10 minutes of medical discussion

G2013 Extensive (75 minutes) in-home visit for an existing patient postdischarge. For use only in a Medicare-approved CMMI model. (Services must be furnished within a beneficiary's home, domiciliary, rest home, assisted living and/or nursing facility within 90 days following discharge from an inpatient facility and no more than nine times.)

G2014 Limited (30 minutes) care plan oversight. For use only in a Medicare-approved CMMI model. (Services must be furnished within a beneficiary's home, domiciliary, rest home, assisted living and/or nursing facility within 90 days following discharge from an inpatient facility and no more than nine times.)

G2015 Comprehensive (60 minutes) home care plan oversight. For use only in a Medicare-approved CMMI model. (Services must be furnished within a beneficiary's home, domiciliary, rest home, assisted living and/or nursing facility within 90 days following discharge from an inpatient facility.)

Treatment in Place

● **G2020** Services for high intensity clinical services associated with the initial engagement and outreach of beneficiaries assigned to the SIP component of the PCF model (do not bill with chronic care management codes)

G2021 Health care practitioners rendering treatment in place (TIP)

G2022 A model participant (ambulance supplier/provider), the beneficiary refuses services covered under the model (transport to an alternate destination/treatment in place)

COVID-19 Specimen Collection

May be reported by clinical diagnostic laboratories.

G2023 Specimen collection for Severe Acute Respiratory Syndrome Coronavirus 2 (SARS-CoV-2) (Coronavirus disease [COVID-19]), any specimen source

G2024 Specimen collection for Severe Acute Respiratory Syndrome Coronavirus 2 (SARS-CoV-2) (Coronavirus disease [COVID-19]) from an individual in a SNF or by a laboratory on behalf of a HHA, any specimen source

G2025 Payment for a telehealth distant site service furnished by a Rural Health Clinic (RHC) or Federally Qualified Health Center (FQHC) only

Comprehensive Care Management Service

G2064 ~~Comprehensive care management services for a single high risk disease, e.g., principal care management, at least 30 minutes of physician or other qualified health care professional time per calendar month with the following elements: one complex chronic condition lasting at least 3 months, which is the focus of the care plan, the condition is of sufficient severity to place patient at risk of hospitalization or have been the cause of a recent hospitalization, the condition requires development or revision of disease specific care plan, the condition requires frequent adjustments in the medication regimen, and/or the management of the condition is unusually complex due to comorbidities~~

Special Coverage Instructions   Noncovered by Medicare   Carrier Discretion   ☑ Quantity Alert ● New Code   ○ Recycled/Reinstated   ▲ Revised Code

56 — G Codes   Ⓐ Age Edit   Ⓜ Maternity Edit   ♀ Female Only   ♂ Male Only   Ⓐ-Ⓨ OPPS Status Indicators   © 2021 Optum360, LLC

G2065 ~~Comprehensive care management for a single high risk disease services, e.g., principal care management, at least 30 minutes of clinical staff time directed by a physician or other qualified health care professional, per calendar month with the following elements: one complex chronic condition lasting at least 3 months, which is the focus of the care plan, the condition is of sufficient severity to place patient at risk of hospitalization or have been cause of a recent hospitalization, the condition requires development or revision of disease-specific care plan, the condition requires frequent adjustments in the medication regimen, and/or the management of the condition is unusually complex due to comorbidities~~

Device Evaluation/Interrogation

G2066 Interrogation device evaluation(s), (remote) up to 30 days; implantable cardiovascular physiologic monitor system, implantable loop recorder system, or subcutaneous cardiac rhythm monitor system, remote data acquisition(s), receipt of transmissions and technician review, technical support and distribution of results

Medication Assisted Treatment and Other Services

G2067 Medication assisted treatment, methadone; weekly bundle including dispensing and/or administration, substance use counseling, individual and group therapy, and toxicology testing, if performed (provision of the services by a Medicare-enrolled opioid treatment program)

CMS: 100-02,17,20; 100-02,17,40.1.1; 100-04,26,10.5; 100-04,39,30.6; 100-04,39,30.6.1; 100-04,39,30.7; 100-04,39,30.8; 100-04,39,30.9; 100-04,39,40; 100-04,39,40.2; 100-04,39,50; 100-04,39,50.1

G2068 Medication assisted treatment, buprenorphine (oral); weekly bundle including dispensing and/or administration, substance use counseling, individual and group therapy, and toxicology testing if performed (provision of the services by a Medicare-enrolled opioid treatment program)

CMS: 100-02,17,20; 100-02,17,40.1.1; 100-04,26,10.5; 100-04,39,30.6; 100-04,39,30.6.1; 100-04,39,30.7; 100-04,39,30.8; 100-04,39,30.9; 100-04,39,40; 100-04,39,40.2; 100-04,39,50; 100-04,39,50.1

G2069 Medication assisted treatment, buprenorphine (injectable); weekly bundle including dispensing and/or administration, substance use counseling, individual and group therapy, and toxicology testing if performed (provision of the services by a Medicare-enrolled opioid treatment program)

CMS: 100-02,17,20; 100-02,17,40.1.1; 100-04,26,10.5; 100-04,39,30.6; 100-04,39,30.6.1; 100-04,39,30.7; 100-04,39,30.8; 100-04,39,30.9; 100-04,39,40; 100-04,39,40.2; 100-04,39,50; 100-04,39,50.1

G2070 Medication assisted treatment, buprenorphine (implant insertion); weekly bundle including dispensing and/or administration, substance use counseling, individual and group therapy, and toxicology testing if performed (provision of the services by a Medicare-enrolled opioid treatment program)

CMS: 100-02,17,20; 100-02,17,40.1.1; 100-04,26,10.5; 100-04,39,30.6; 100-04,39,30.6.1; 100-04,39,30.7; 100-04,39,30.8; 100-04,39,30.9; 100-04,39,40; 100-04,39,40.2; 100-04,39,50; 100-04,39,50.1

G2071 Medication assisted treatment, buprenorphine (implant removal); weekly bundle including dispensing and/or administration, substance use counseling, individual and group therapy, and toxicology testing if performed (provision of the services by a Medicare-enrolled opioid treatment program)

CMS: 100-02,17,20; 100-02,17,40.1.1; 100-04,26,10.5; 100-04,39,30.6; 100-04,39,30.6.1; 100-04,39,30.7; 100-04,39,30.8; 100-04,39,30.9; 100-04,39,40; 100-04,39,40.2; 100-04,39,50; 100-04,39,50.1

G2072 Medication assisted treatment, buprenorphine (implant insertion and removal); weekly bundle including dispensing and/or administration, substance use counseling, individual and group therapy, and toxicology testing if performed (provision of the services by a Medicare-enrolled opioid treatment program)

CMS: 100-02,17,20; 100-02,17,40.1.1; 100-04,26,10.5; 100-04,39,30.6; 100-04,39,30.6.1; 100-04,39,30.7; 100-04,39,30.8; 100-04,39,30.9; 100-04,39,40; 100-04,39,40.2; 100-04,39,50; 100-04,39,50.1

G2073 Medication assisted treatment, naltrexone; weekly bundle including dispensing and/or administration, substance use counseling, individual and group therapy, and toxicology testing if performed (provision of the services by a Medicare-enrolled opioid treatment program)

CMS: 100-02,17,20; 100-02,17,40.1.1; 100-04,26,10.5; 100-04,39,30.6; 100-04,39,30.6.1; 100-04,39,30.7; 100-04,39,30.8; 100-04,39,30.9; 100-04,39,40; 100-04,39,40.2; 100-04,39,50; 100-04,39,50.1

G2074 Medication assisted treatment, weekly bundle not including the drug, including substance use counseling, individual and group therapy, and toxicology testing if performed (provision of the services by a Medicare-enrolled opioid treatment program)

CMS: 100-02,17,20; 100-02,17,40.1.1; 100-04,26,10.5; 100-04,39,30.2; 100-04,39,30.3; 100-04,39,30.6; 100-04,39,30.6.1; 100-04,39,30.7; 100-04,39,30.8; 100-04,39,30.9; 100-04,39,40; 100-04,39,40.2; 100-04,39,50; 100-04,39,50.1

G2075 Medication assisted treatment, medication not otherwise specified; weekly bundle including dispensing and/or administration, substance use counseling, individual and group therapy, and toxicology testing, if performed (provision of the services by a Medicare-enrolled opioid treatment program)

CMS: 100-02,17,20; 100-02,17,40.1.1; 100-04,26,10.5; 100-04,39,30.4; 100-04,39,30.6; 100-04,39,30.6.1; 100-04,39,30.7; 100-04,39,30.8; 100-04,39,30.9; 100-04,39,40; 100-04,39,40.2; 100-04,39,50; 100-04,39,50.1

G2076 Intake activities, including initial medical examination that is a complete, fully documented physical evaluation and initial assessment by a program physician or a primary care physician, or an authorized health care professional under the supervision of a program physician qualified personnel that includes preparation of a treatment plan that includes the patient's short-term goals and the tasks the patient must perform to complete the short-term goals; the patient's requirements for education, vocational rehabilitation, and employment; and the medical, psycho-social, economic, legal, or other supportive services that a patient needs, conducted by qualified personnel (provision of the services by a Medicare-enrolled opioid treatment program); list separately in addition to code for primary procedure

CMS: 100-02,17,20; 100-02,17,40.1.1; 100-04,26,10.5; 100-04,39,30.6; 100-04,39,30.6.1; 100-04,39,30.7; 100-04,39,30.8; 100-04,39,30.9; 100-04,39,40; 100-04,39,40.2; 100-04,39,50; 100-04,39,50.1

G2077 Periodic assessment; assessing periodically by qualified personnel to determine the most appropriate combination of services and treatment (provision of the services by a Medicare-enrolled opioid treatment program); list separately in addition to code for primary procedure

CMS: 100-02,17,20; 100-02,17,40.1.1; 100-04,26,10.5; 100-04,39,30.6; 100-04,39,30.6.1; 100-04,39,30.7; 100-04,39,30.8; 100-04,39,30.9; 100-04,39,40; 100-04,39,40.2; 100-04,39,50; 100-04,39,50.1

G2078 Take home supply of methadone; up to 7 additional day supply (provision of the services by a Medicare-enrolled opioid treatment program); list separately in addition to code for primary procedure

CMS: 100-02,17,20; 100-02,17,40.1.1; 100-04,26,10.5; 100-04,39,30.6; 100-04,39,30.6.1; 100-04,39,30.7; 100-04,39,30.9; 100-04,39,40; 100-04,39,40.2; 100-04,39,50; 100-04,39,50.1

Special Coverage Instructions   Noncovered by Medicare   Carrier Discretion   ☑ Quantity Alert ● New Code   ○ Recycled/Reinstated ▲ Revised Code

© 2021 Optum360, LLC   A2-Z3 ASC Pmt   CMS: IOM   AHA: Coding Clinic   DMEPOS Paid   SNF Excluded   G Codes — 57

Procedures/Professional Services (Temporary)

G2079 — G2109

G2079 Take home supply of buprenorphine (oral); up to 7 additional day supply (provision of the services by a Medicare-enrolled opioid treatment program); list separately in addition to code for primary procedure
CMS: 100-02,17,20; 100-02,17,40.1.1; 100-04,26,10.5; 100-04,39,30.6; 100-04,39,30.6.1; 100-04,39,30.7; 100-04,39,30.9; 100-04,39,40; 100-04,39,40.2; 100-04,39,50; 100-04,39,50.1

G2080 Each additional 30 minutes of counseling in a week of medication assisted treatment, (provision of the services by a Medicare-enrolled opioid treatment program); list separately in addition to code for primary procedure
CMS: 100-02,17,20; 100-02,17,40.1.1; 100-04,26,10.5; 100-04,39,30.6; 100-04,39,30.6.1; 100-04,39,30.7; 100-04,39,30.8; 100-04,39,30.9; 100-04,39,40; 100-04,39,40.2; 100-04,39,50; 100-04,39,50.1

▲ **G2081** Patients age 66 and older in institutional special needs plans (SNP) or residing in long-term care with a POS code 32, 33, 34, 54 or 56 for more than 90 consecutive days during the measurement period   Ⓐ

G2082 Office or other outpatient visit for the evaluation and management of an established patient that requires the supervision of a physician or other qualified health care professional and provision of up to 56 mg of esketamine nasal self administration, includes 2 hours post administration observation

G2083 Office or other outpatient visit for the evaluation and management of an established patient that requires the supervision of a physician or other qualified health care professional and provision of greater than 56 mg esketamine nasal self administration, includes 2 hours post administration observation

G2086 Office-based treatment for opioid use disorder, including development of the treatment plan, care coordination, individual therapy and group therapy and counseling; at least 70 minutes in the first calendar month

G2087 Office-based treatment for opioid use disorder, including care coordination, individual therapy and group therapy and counseling; at least 60 minutes in a subsequent calendar month

G2088 Office-based treatment for opioid use disorder, including care coordination, individual therapy and group therapy and counseling; each additional 30 minutes beyond the first 120 minutes (list separately in addition to code for primary procedure)

G2090 Patients 66 years of age and older with at least one claim/encounter for frailty during the measurement period and a dispensed medication for dementia during the measurement period or the year prior to the measurement period   Ⓐ

G2091 Patients 66 years of age and older with at least one claim/encounter for frailty during the measurement period and either one acute inpatient encounter with a diagnosis of advanced illness or two outpatient, observation, ED or nonacute inpatient encounters on different dates of service with an advanced illness diagnosis during the measurement period or the year prior to the measurement period   Ⓐ

G2092 Angiotensin converting enzyme (ACE) inhibitor or angiotensin receptor blocker (ARB) or angiotensin receptor-neprilysin inhibitor (ARNI) therapy prescribed or currently being taken

G2093 Documentation of medical reason(s) for not prescribing ACE inhibitor or ARB or ARNI therapy (e.g., hypotensive patients who are at immediate risk of cardiogenic shock, hospitalized patients who have experienced marked azotemia, allergy, intolerance, other medical reasons)

G2094 Documentation of patient reason(s) for not prescribing ACE inhibitor or ARB or ARNI therapy (e.g., patient declined, other patient reasons)

G2095 Documentation of system reason(s) for not prescribing ACE inhibitor or ARB or ARNI therapy (e.g., other system reasons)

G2096 Angiotensin converting enzyme (ACE) inhibitor or angiotensin receptor blocker (ARB) or angiotensin receptor-neprilysin inhibitor (ARNI) therapy was not prescribed, reason not given

▲ **G2097** Episodes where the patient had a competing diagnosis on or within 3 days after the episode date (e.g., intestinal infection, pertussis, bacterial infection, Lyme disease, otitis media, acute sinusitis, chronic sinusitis, infection of the adenoids, prostatitis, cellulitis, mastoiditis, or bone infections, acute lymphadenitis, impetigo, skin staph infections, pneumonia/gonococcal infections, venereal disease (syphilis, chlamydia, inflammatory diseases [female reproductive organs]), infections of the kidney, cystitis or UTI)

G2098 Patients 66 years of age and older with at least one claim/encounter for frailty during the measurement period and a dispensed medication for dementia during the measurement period or the year prior to the measurement period   Ⓐ

G2099 Patients 66 years of age and older with at least one claim/encounter for frailty during the measurement period and either one acute inpatient encounter with a diagnosis of advanced illness or two outpatient, observation, ED or nonacute inpatient encounters on different dates of service with an advanced illness diagnosis during the measurement period or the year prior to the measurement period   Ⓐ

G2100 Patients 66 years of age and older with at least one claim/encounter for frailty during the measurement period and a dispensed medication for dementia during the measurement period or the year prior to the measurement period   Ⓐ

G2101 Patients 66 years of age and older with at least one claim/encounter for frailty during the measurement period and either one acute inpatient encounter with a diagnosis of advanced illness or two outpatient, observation, ED or nonacute inpatient encounters on different dates of service with an advanced illness diagnosis during the measurement period or the year prior to the measurement period   Ⓐ

G2105 Patient age 66 or older in institutional special needs plans (SNP) or residing in long-term care with POS code 32, 33, 34, 54 or 56 for more than 90 consecutive days during the measurement period   Ⓐ

G2106 Patients 66 years of age and older with at least one claim/encounter for frailty during the measurement period and a dispensed medication for dementia during the measurement period or the year prior to the measurement period   Ⓐ

G2107 Patients 66 years of age and older with at least one claim/encounter for frailty during the measurement period and either one acute inpatient encounter with a diagnosis of advanced illness or two outpatient, observation, ED or nonacute inpatient encounters on different dates of service with an advanced illness diagnosis during the measurement period or the year prior to the measurement period   Ⓐ

G2108 Patient age 66 or older in institutional special needs plans (SNP) or residing in long-term care with POS code 32, 33, 34, 54 or 56 for more than 90 consecutive days during the measurement period   Ⓐ

G2109 Patients 66 years of age and older with at least one claim/encounter for frailty during the measurement period and a dispensed medication for dementia during the measurement period or the year prior to the measurement period   Ⓐ

Special Coverage Instructions   Noncovered by Medicare   Carrier Discretion   ☑ Quantity Alert ● New Code   ○ Recycled/Reinstated ▲ Revised Code

58 — G Codes   Ⓐ Age Edit   Ⓜ Maternity Edit   ♀ Female Only   ♂ Male Only   Ⓐ-Ⓨ OPPS Status Indicators   © 2021 Optum360, LLC

Procedures/Professional Services (Temporary)

G2110 — G2148

G2110 Patients 66 years of age and older with at least one claim/encounter for frailty during the measurement period and either one acute inpatient encounter with a diagnosis of advanced illness or two outpatient, observation, ED or nonacute inpatient encounters on different dates of service with an advanced illness diagnosis during the measurement period or the year prior to the measurement period Ⓐ

G2112 Patient receiving <=5 mg daily prednisone (or equivalent), or RA activity is worsening, or glucocorticoid use is for less than 6 months

G2113 Patient receiving >5 mg daily prednisone (or equivalent) for longer than 6 months, and improvement or no change in disease activity

G2115 Patients 66 - 80 years of age with at least one claim/encounter for frailty during the measurement period and a dispensed medication for dementia during the measurement period or the year prior to the measurement period Ⓐ

G2116 Patients 66 - 80 years of age with at least one claim/encounter for frailty during the measurement period and either one acute inpatient encounter with a diagnosis of advanced illness or two outpatient, observation, ED or nonacute inpatient encounters on different dates of service with an advanced illness diagnosis during the measurement period or the year prior to the measurement period Ⓐ

G2118 Patients 81 years of age and older with at least one claim/encounter for frailty during the measurement period Ⓐ

▲ **G2121** Depression, anxiety, apathy, and psychosis assessed

▲ **G2122** Depression, anxiety, apathy, and psychosis not assessed

G2125 Patients 81 years of age and older with at least one claim/encounter for frailty during the six months prior to the measurement period through December 31 of the measurement period Ⓐ

G2126 Patients 66 - 80 years of age with at least one claim/encounter for frailty during the measurement period and either one acute inpatient encounter with a diagnosis of advanced illness or two outpatient, observation, ED or nonacute inpatient encounters on different dates of service with an advanced illness diagnosis during the measurement period or the year prior to the measurement period Ⓐ

G2127 Patients 66 - 80 years of age with at least one claim/encounter for frailty during the measurement period and a dispensed medication for dementia during the measurement period or the year prior to the measurement period Ⓐ

G2128 Documentation of medical reason(s) for not on a daily aspirin or other antiplatelet (e.g., history of gastrointestinal bleed, intracranial bleed, blood disorders, idiopathic thrombocytopenic purpura (ITP), gastric bypass or documentation of active anticoagulant use during the measurement period)

G2129 Procedure related BP's not taken during an outpatient visit. Examples include same day surgery, ambulatory service center, GI, lab, dialysis, infusion center, chemotherapy

G2136 Back pain measured by the visual analog scale (VAS) at 3 months (6 to 20 weeks) postoperatively was less than or equal to 3.0 or back pain measured by the visual analog scale (VAS) within 3 months preoperatively and at 3 months (6 to 20 weeks) postoperatively demonstrated an improvement of 5.0 points or greater

G2137 Back pain measured by the visual analog scale (vas) at three months (6 - 20 weeks) postoperatively was greater than 3.0 and back pain measured by the visual analog scale (vas) within three months (6 - 20 weeks) preoperatively and at three months (6 - 20 weeks) postoperatively demonstrated a change of less than an improvement of 5.0 points

G2138 Back pain as measured by the visual analog scale (VAS) at 1 year (9 to 15 months) postoperatively was less than or equal to 3.0 or back pain measured by the visual analog scale (VAS) within 3 months preoperatively and at 1 year (9 to 15 months) postoperatively demonstrated a change of 5.0 points or greater

G2139 Back pain measured by the visual analog scale (VAS) pain at 1 year (9 to 15 months) postoperatively was greater than 3.0 and back pain measured by the visual analog scale (VAS) within 3 months preoperatively and at 1 year (9 to 15 months) postoperatively demonstrated a change of less than 5.0

▲ **G2140** Leg pain measured by the visual analog scale (VAS) at three months (6 to 20 weeks) postoperatively was less than or equal to 3.0 or leg pain measured by the visual analog scale (VAS) within three months preoperatively and at three months (6 to 20 weeks) postoperatively demonstrated an improvement of 5.0 points or greater

G2141 Leg pain measured by the visual analog scale (vas) at three months (6 - 20 weeks) postoperatively was greater than 3.0 and leg pain measured by the visual analog scale (vas) within three months preoperatively and at three months (6 - 20 weeks) postoperatively demonstrated less than an improvement of 5.0 points

▲ **G2142** Functional status measured by the Oswestry Disability Index (ODI version 2.1a) at 1 year (9 to 15 months) postoperatively was less than or equal to 22 or functional status measured by the ODI version 2.1a within 3 months preoperatively and at 1 year (9 to 15 months) postoperatively demonstrated an improvement of 30 points or greater

▲ **G2143** Functional status measured by the Oswestry Disability Index (ODI version 2.1a) at 1 year (9 to 15 months) postoperatively was greater than 22 and functional status measured by the ODI version 2.1a within 3 months preoperatively and at 1 year (9 to 15 months) postoperatively demonstrated an improvement of less than 30 points

▲ **G2144** Functional status measured by the Oswestry Disability Index (ODI version 2.1a) at 3 months (6 to 20 weeks) postoperatively was less than or equal to 22 or functional status measured by the ODI version 2.1a within 3 months preoperatively and at 3 months (6 to 20 weeks) postoperatively demonstrated an improvement of 30 points or greater

▲ **G2145** Functional status measured by the Oswestry Disability Index (ODI version 2.1a) at 3 months (6 to 20 weeks) postoperatively was greater than 22 and functional status measured by the ODI version 2.1a within 3 months preoperatively and at 3 months (6 to 20 weeks) postoperatively demonstrated an improvement of less than 30 points

G2146 Leg pain as measured by the visual analog scale (VAS) at 1 year (9 to 15 months) postoperatively was less than or equal to 3.0 or leg pain measured by the visual analog scale (VAS) within 3 months preoperatively and at 1 year (9 to 15 months) postoperatively demonstrated an improvement of 5.0 points or greater

G2147 Leg pain measured by the visual analog scale (VAS) at 1 year (9 to 15 months) postoperatively was greater than 3.0 and leg pain measured by the visual analog scale (VAS) within 3 months preoperatively and at 1 year (9 to 15 months) postoperatively demonstrated less than an improvement of 5.0 points

▲ **G2148** Multimodal pain management was used

G2149 Documentation of medical reason(s) for not using multimodal pain management (e.g., allergy to multiple classes of analgesics, intubated patient, hepatic failure, patient reports no pain during PACU stay, other medical reason(s))

▲ **G2150** Multimodal pain management was not used

G2151 Documentation stating patient has a diagnosis of a degenerative neurological condition such as ALS, MS, or Parkinson's diagnosed at any time before or during the episode of care

G2152 Risk-adjusted functional status change residual score for the neck impairment successfully calculated and the score was equal to zero (0) or greater than zero (> 0)

G2167 Risk-adjusted functional status change residual score for the neck impairment successfully calculated and the score was less than zero (< 0)

Home Health

G2168 Services performed by a physical therapist assistant in the home health setting in the delivery of a safe and effective physical therapy maintenance program, each 15 minutes

G2169 Services performed by an occupational therapist assistant in the home health setting in the delivery of a safe and effective occupational therapy maintenance program, each 15 minutes

Arteriovenous Fistual Creation

G2170 Percutaneous arteriovenous fistula creation (AVF), direct, any site, by tissue approximation using thermal resistance energy, and secondary procedures to redirect blood flow (e.g., transluminal balloon angioplasty, coil embolization) when performed, and includes all imaging and radiologic guidance, supervision and interpretation, when performed

G2171 Percutaneous arteriovenous fistula creation (AVF), direct, any site, using magnetic-guided arterial and venous catheters and radiofrequency energy, including flow-directing procedures (e.g., vascular coil embolization with radiologic supervision and interpretation, when performed) and fistulogram(s), angiography, venography, and/or ultrasound, with radiologic supervision and interpretation, when performed

Quality Measures

● **G2172** All inclusive payment for services related to highly coordinated and integrated opioid use disorder (OUD) treatment services furnished for the demonstration project

▲ **G2173** URI episodes where the patient had a comorbid condition during the 12 months prior to or on the episode date (e.g., tuberculosis, neutropenia, cystic fibrosis, chronic bronchitis, pulmonary edema, respiratory failure, rheumatoid lung disease)

▲ **G2174** URI episodes when the patient had an active prescription of antibiotics (table 1) in the 30 days prior to the episode date

▲ **G2175** Episodes where the patient had a comorbid condition during the 12 months prior to or on the episode date (e.g., tuberculosis, neutropenia, cystic fibrosis, chronic bronchitis, pulmonary edema, respiratory failure, rheumatoid lung disease)

G2176 Outpatient, ED, or observation visits that result in an inpatient admission

▲ **G2177** Acute bronchitis/bronchiolitis episodes when the patient had a new or refill prescription of antibiotics (table 1) in the 30 days prior to the episode date

G2178 Clinician documented that patient was not an eligible candidate for lower extremity neurological exam measure, for example patient bilateral amputee; patient has condition that would not allow them to accurately respond to a neurological exam (dementia, Alzheimer's, etc.); patient has previously documented diabetic peripheral neuropathy with loss of protective sensation

G2179 Clinician documented that patient had medical reason for not performing lower extremity neurological exam

G2180 Clinician documented that patient was not an eligible candidate for evaluation of footwear as patient is bilateral lower extremity amputee

G2181 BMI not documented due to medical reason or patient refusal of height or weight measurement

G2182 Patient receiving first-time biologic disease modifying antirheumatic drug therapy

G2183 Documentation patient unable to communicate and informant not available

G2184 Patient does not have a caregiver

G2185 Documentation caregiver is trained and certified in dementia care

G2186 Patient /caregiver dyad has been referred to appropriate resources and connection to those resources is confirmed

G2187 Patients with clinical indications for imaging of the head: head trauma

G2188 Patients with clinical indications for imaging of the head: new or change in headache above 50 years of age

G2189 Patients with clinical indications for imaging of the head: abnormal neurologic exam

G2190 Patients with clinical indications for imaging of the head: headache radiating to the neck

G2191 Patients with clinical indications for imaging of the head: positional headaches

G2192 Patients with clinical indications for imaging of the head: temporal headaches in patients over 55 years of age

G2193 Patients with clinical indications for imaging of the head: new onset headache in preschool children or younger (<6 years of age)

G2194 Patients with clinical indications for imaging of the head: new onset headache in pediatric patients with disabilities for which headache is a concern as inferred from behavior

G2195 Patients with clinical indications for imaging of the head: occipital headache in children

G2196 Patient identified as an unhealthy alcohol user when screened for unhealthy alcohol use using a systematic screening method

G2197 Patient screened for unhealthy alcohol use using a systematic screening method and not identified as an unhealthy alcohol user

G2198 Documentation of medical reason(s) for not screening for unhealthy alcohol use using a systematic screening method (e.g., limited life expectancy, other medical reasons)

G2199 Patient not screened for unhealthy alcohol use using a systematic screening method, reason not given

G2200 Patient identified as an unhealthy alcohol user received brief counseling

G2201 Documentation of medical reason(s) for not providing brief counseling (e.g., limited life expectancy, other medical reasons)

G2202 Patient did not receive brief counseling if identified as an unhealthy alcohol user, reason not given

G2203 Documentation of medical reason(s) for not providing brief counseling if identified as an unhealthy alcohol user (e.g., limited life expectancy, other medical reasons)

G2204 Patients between 50 and 85 years of age who received a screening colonoscopy during the performance period

Special Coverage Instructions   Noncovered by Medicare   Carrier Discretion   ☑ Quantity Alert ● New Code ○ Recycled/Reinstated ▲ Revised Code

60 — G Codes   Ⓐ Age Edit Ⓜ Maternity Edit ♀ Female Only ♂ Male Only Ⓐ-Ⓨ OPPS Status Indicators   © 2021 Optum360, LLC

G2205 Patients with pregnancy during adjuvant treatment course

G2206 Patient received adjuvant treatment course including both chemotherapy and HER2-targeted therapy

G2207 Reason for not administering adjuvant treatment course including both chemotherapy and HER2-targeted therapy (e.g. poor performance status (ECOG 3-4; Karnofsky =50), cardiac contraindications, insufficient renal function, insufficient hepatic function, other active or secondary cancer diagnoses, other medical contraindications, patients who died during initial treatment course or transferred during or after initial treatment course)

G2208 Patient did not receive adjuvant treatment course including both chemotherapy and HER2-targeted therapy

G2209 Patient refused to participate

G2210 Risk-adjusted functional status change residual score for the neck impairment not measured because the patient did not complete the neck FS PROM at initial evaluation and/or near discharge, reason not given

G2211 Visit complexity inherent to evaluation and management associated with medical care services that serve as the continuing focal point for all needed health care services and/or with medical care services that are part of ongoing care related to a patient's single, serious condition or a complex condition. (add-on code, list separately in addition to office/outpatient evaluation and management visit, new or established)

G2212 Prolonged office or other outpatient evaluation and management service(s) beyond the maximum required time of the primary procedure which has been selected using total time on the date of the primary service; each additional 15 minutes by the physician or qualified healthcare professional, with or without direct patient contact (list separately in addition to CPT codes 99205, 99215 for office or other outpatient evaluation and management services) (Do not report G2212 on the same date of service as 99354, 99355, 99358, 99359, 99415, 99416). (Do not report G2212 for any time unit less than 15 minutes)

G2213 Initiation of medication for the treatment of opioid use disorder in the emergency department setting, including assessment, referral to ongoing care, and arranging access to supportive services (list separately in addition to code for primary procedure)

G2214 Initial or subsequent psychiatric collaborative care management, first 30 minutes in a month of behavioral health care manager activities, in consultation with a psychiatric consultant, and directed by the treating physician or other qualified health care professional

▲ **G2215** Take home supply of nasal naloxone; 2-pack of 4 mg per 0.1 ml nasal spray (provision of the services by a Medicare-enrolled Opioid Treatment Program); list separately in addition to code for primary procedure
CMS: 100-02,17,20; 100-02,17,40.1.1; 100-04,39,30.6; 100-04,39,30.6.1; 100-04,39,30.7; 100-04,39,30.8; 100-04,39,40

G2216 Take home supply of injectable naloxone (provision of the services by a Medicare-enrolled opioid treatment program); list separately in addition to code for primary procedure
CMS: 100-02,17,20; 100-02,17,40.1.1; 100-04,39,30.6; 100-04,39,30.6.1; 100-04,39,30.7; 100-04,39,30.8; 100-04,39,40

G2250 Remote assessment of recorded video and/or images submitted by an established patient (e.g., store and forward), including interpretation with follow-up with the patient within 24 business hours, not originating from a related service provided within the previous 7 days nor leading to a service or procedure within the next 24 hours or soonest available appointment

G2251 Brief communication technology-based service, e.g. virtual check-in, by a qualified health care professional who cannot report evaluation and management services, provided to an established patient, not originating from a related service provided within the previous 7 days nor leading to a service or procedure within the next 24 hours or soonest available appointment; 5-10 minutes of clinical discussion

G2252 Brief communication technology-based service, e.g. virtual check-in, by a physician or other qualified health care professional who can report evaluation and management services, provided to an established patient, not originating from a related EM service provided within the previous 7 days nor leading to an EM service or procedure within the next 24 hours or soonest available appointment; 11-20 minutes of medical discussion

MIPS Specialty Sets

● **G4000** Dermatology MIPS specialty set
● **G4001** Diagnostic Radiology MIPS specialty set
● **G4002** Electrophysiology Cardiac Specialist MIPS specialty set
● **G4003** Emergency Medicine MIPS specialty set
● **G4004** Endocrinology MIPS specialty set
● **G4005** Family Medicine MIPS specialty set
● **G4006** Gastroenterology MIPS specialty set
● **G4007** General Surgery MIPS specialty set
● **G4008** Geriatrics MIPS specialty set
● **G4009** Hospitalists MIPS specialty set
● **G4010** Infectious Disease MIPS specialty set
● **G4011** Internal Medicine MIPS specialty set
● **G4012** Interventional Radiology MIPS specialty set
● **G4013** Mental/Behavioral Health MIPS specialty set
● **G4014** Nephrology MIPS specialty set
● **G4015** Neurology MIPS specialty set
● **G4016** Neurosurgical MIPS specialty set
● **G4017** Nutrition/Dietician MIPS specialty set
● **G4018** Obstetrics/Gynecology MIPS specialty set
● **G4019** Oncology/Hematology MIPS specialty set
● **G4020** Ophthalmology MIPS specialty set
● **G4021** Orthopedic surgery MIPS specialty set
● **G4022** Otolaryngology MIPS specialty set
● **G4023** Pathology MIPS specialty set
● **G4024** Pediatrics MIPS specialty set
● **G4025** Physical Medicine MIPS specialty set
● **G4026** Physical Therapy/Occupational Therapy MIPS specialty set
● **G4027** Plastic Surgery MIPS specialty set
● **G4028** Podiatry MIPS specialty set
● **G4029** Preventive Medicine MIPS specialty set
● **G4030** Pulmonology MIPS specialty set
● **G4031** Radiation Oncology MIPS specialty set
● **G4032** Rheumatology MIPS specialty set
● **G4033** Skilled Nursing Facility MIPS specialty set
● **G4034** Speech Language Pathology MIPS specialty set

Special Coverage Instructions   Noncovered by Medicare   Carrier Discretion   ☑ Quantity Alert ● New Code   ○ Recycled/Reinstated ▲ Revised Code

© 2021 Optum360, LLC   A2-Z3 ASC Pmt   CMS: IOM   AHA: Coding Clinic   DMEPOS Paid   ⊘ SNF Excluded   G Codes — 61

Procedures/Professional Services (Temporary)

G4035 — G8473

- ● **G4035** Thoracic Surgery MIPS specialty set
- ● **G4036** Urgent Care MIPS specialty set
- ● **G4037** Urology MIPS specialty set
- ● **G4038** Vascular Surgery MIPS specialty set

Radiation Therapy

G6001 Ultrasonic guidance for placement of radiation therapy fields Ⓑ

G6002 Stereoscopic x-ray guidance for localization of target volume for the delivery of radiation therapy Ⓑ

G6003 Radiation treatment delivery, single treatment area, single port or parallel opposed ports, simple blocks or no blocks: up to 5 mev Ⓑ

G6004 Radiation treatment delivery, single treatment area, single port or parallel opposed ports, simple blocks or no blocks: 6-10 mev Ⓑ

G6005 Radiation treatment delivery, single treatment area, single port or parallel opposed ports, simple blocks or no blocks: 11-19 mev Ⓑ

G6006 Radiation treatment delivery, single treatment area, single port or parallel opposed ports, simple blocks or no blocks: 20 mev or greater Ⓑ

G6007 Radiation treatment delivery, two separate treatment areas, three or more ports on a single treatment area, use of multiple blocks: up to 5 mev Ⓑ

G6008 Radiation treatment delivery, two separate treatment areas, three or more ports on a single treatment area, use of multiple blocks: 6-10 mev Ⓑ

G6009 Radiation treatment delivery, two separate treatment areas, three or more ports on a single treatment area, use of multiple blocks: 11-19 mev Ⓑ

G6010 Radiation treatment delivery, two separate treatment areas, three or more ports on a single treatment area, use of multiple blocks: 20 mev or greater Ⓑ

G6011 Radiation treatment delivery, three or more separate treatment areas, custom blocking, tangential ports, wedges, rotational beam, compensators, electron beam; up to 5 mev Ⓑ

G6012 Radiation treatment delivery, three or more separate treatment areas, custom blocking, tangential ports, wedges, rotational beam, compensators, electron beam; 6-10 mev Ⓑ

G6013 Radiation treatment delivery, three or more separate treatment areas, custom blocking, tangential ports, wedges, rotational beam, compensators, electron beam; 11-19 mev Ⓑ

G6014 Radiation treatment delivery, three or more separate treatment areas, custom blocking, tangential ports, wedges, rotational beam, compensators, electron beam; 20 mev or greater Ⓑ

G6015 Intensity modulated treatment delivery, single or multiple fields/arcs, via narrow spatially and temporally modulated beams, binary, dynamic MLC, per treatment session Ⓑ

G6016 Compensator-based beam modulation treatment delivery of inverse planned treatment using three or more high resolution (milled or cast) compensator, convergent beam modulated fields, per treatment session Ⓑ

G6017 Intra-fraction localization and tracking of target or patient motion during delivery of radiation therapy (e.g., 3D positional tracking, gating, 3D surface tracking), each fraction of treatment Ⓑ

Quality Measures

G8395 Left ventricular ejection fraction (LVEF) ≥ 40% or documentation as normal or mildly depressed left ventricular systolic function Ⓜ

G8396 Left ventricular ejection fraction (LVEF) not performed or documented Ⓜ

G8397 Dilated macular or fundus exam performed, including documentation of the presence or absence of macular edema and level of severity of retinopathy Ⓜ

G8399 Patient with documented results of a central dual-energy x-ray absorptiometry (DXA) ever being performed Ⓜ

G8400 Patient with central dual-energy x-ray absorptiometry (DXA) results not documented, reason not given Ⓜ

G8404 Lower extremity neurological exam performed and documented Ⓜ

G8405 Lower extremity neurological exam not performed Ⓜ

G8410 Footwear evaluation performed and documented Ⓜ

G8415 Footwear evaluation was not performed Ⓜ

G8416 Clinician documented that patient was not an eligible candidate for footwear evaluation measure Ⓜ

G8417 BMI is documented above normal parameters and a follow-up plan is documented Ⓜ

G8418 BMI is documented below normal parameters and a follow-up plan is documented Ⓜ

G8419 BMI documented outside normal parameters, no follow-up plan documented, no reason given Ⓜ

G8420 BMI is documented within normal parameters and no follow-up plan is required Ⓜ

G8421 BMI not documented and no reason is given Ⓜ

G8422 ~~BMI not documented, documentation the patient is not eligible for BMI calculation~~

G8427 Eligible clinician attests to documenting in the medical record they obtained, updated, or reviewed the patient's current medications Ⓜ

G8428 Current list of medications not documented as obtained, updated, or reviewed by the eligible clinician, reason not given Ⓜ

G8430 Documentation of a medical reason(s) for not documenting, updating, or reviewing the patient's current medications list (e.g., patient is in an urgent or emergent medical situation) Ⓜ

G8431 Screening for depression is documented as being positive and a follow-up plan is documented Ⓜ

G8432 Depression screening not documented, reason not given Ⓜ

▲ **G8433** Screening for depression not completed, documented patient or medical reason Ⓜ

G8450 Beta-blocker therapy prescribed Ⓜ

G8451 Beta-blocker therapy for LVEF < 40% not prescribed for reasons documented by the clinician (e.g., low blood pressure, fluid overload, asthma, patients recently treated with an intravenous positive inotropic agent, allergy, intolerance, other medical reasons, patient declined, other patient reasons, or other reasons attributable to the health care system) Ⓜ

G8452 Beta-blocker therapy not prescribed Ⓜ

G8465 High or very high risk of recurrence of prostate cancer Ⓜ

G8473 Angiotensin converting enzyme (ACE) inhibitor or angiotensin receptor blocker (ARB) therapy prescribed Ⓜ

Special Coverage Instructions   Noncovered by Medicare   Carrier Discretion   ☑ Quantity Alert ● New Code   ○ Recycled/Reinstated ▲ Revised Code

G8474 Angiotensin converting enzyme (ACE) inhibitor or angiotensin receptor blocker (ARB) therapy not prescribed for reasons documented by the clinician (e.g., allergy, intolerance, pregnancy, renal failure due to ACE inhibitor, diseases of the aortic or mitral valve, other medical reasons) or (e.g., patient declined, other patient reasons) or (e.g., lack of drug availability, other reasons attributable to the health care system) M

G8475 Angiotensin converting enzyme (ACE) inhibitor or angiotensin receptor blocker (ARB) therapy not prescribed, reason not given M

G8476 Most recent blood pressure has a systolic measurement of < 140 mm Hg and a diastolic measurement of < 90 mm Hg M

G8477 Most recent blood pressure has a systolic measurement of >=140 mm Hg and/or a diastolic measurement of >=90 mm Hg M

G8478 Blood pressure measurement not performed or documented, reason not given M

G8482 Influenza immunization administered or previously received M

G8483 Influenza immunization was not administered for reasons documented by clinician (e.g., patient allergy or other medical reasons, patient declined or other patient reasons, vaccine not available or other system reasons) M

G8484 Influenza immunization was not administered, reason not given M

G8506 Patient receiving angiotensin converting enzyme (ACE) inhibitor or angiotensin receptor blocker (ARB) therapy M

G8510 Screening for depression is documented as negative, a follow-up plan is not required M

G8511 Screening for depression documented as positive, follow-up plan not documented, reason not given M

G8535 Elder maltreatment screen not documented; documentation that patient is not eligible for the elder maltreatment screen at the time of the encounter M

G8536 No documentation of an elder maltreatment screen, reason not given M

G8539 Functional outcome assessment documented as positive using a standardized tool and a care plan based on identified deficiencies on the date of functional outcome assessment, is documented M

G8540 Functional outcome assessment not documented as being performed, documentation the patient is not eligible for a functional outcome assessment using a standardized tool at the time of the encounter M

G8541 Functional outcome assessment using a standardized tool, not documented, reason not given M

G8542 Functional outcome assessment using a standardized tool is documented; no functional deficiencies identified, care plan not required M

G8543 Documentation of a positive functional outcome assessment using a standardized tool; care plan not documented, reason not given M

G8559 Patient referred to a physician (preferably a physician with training in disorders of the ear) for an otologic evaluation M

G8560 Patient has a history of active drainage from the ear within the previous 90 days M

G8561 Patient is not eligible for the referral for otologic evaluation for patients with a history of active drainage measure M

G8562 Patient does not have a history of active drainage from the ear within the previous 90 days M

G8563 Patient not referred to a physician (preferably a physician with training in disorders of the ear) for an otologic evaluation, reason not given M

G8564 Patient was referred to a physician (preferably a physician with training in disorders of the ear) for an otologic evaluation, reason not specified) M

G8565 Verification and documentation of sudden or rapidly progressive hearing loss M

G8566 Patient is not eligible for the "referral for otologic evaluation for sudden or rapidly progressive hearing loss" measure M

G8567 Patient does not have verification and documentation of sudden or rapidly progressive hearing loss M

G8568 Patient was not referred to a physician (preferably a physician with training in disorders of the ear) for an otologic evaluation, reason not given M

G8569 Prolonged postoperative intubation (> 24 hrs) required M

G8570 Prolonged postoperative intubation (> 24 hrs) not required M

G8575 Developed postoperative renal failure or required dialysis M

G8576 No postoperative renal failure/dialysis not required M

G8577 Re-exploration required due to mediastinal bleeding with or without tamponade, graft occlusion, valve dysfunction or other cardiac reason M

G8578 Re-exploration not required due to mediastinal bleeding with or without tamponade, graft occlusion, valve dysfunction or other cardiac reason M

G8598 Aspirin or another antiplatelet therapy used M

G8599 Aspirin or another antiplatelet therapy not used, reason not given M

G8600 IV tPA initiated within 3 hours (≤ 180 minutes) of time last known well M

G8601 IV tPA not initiated within 3 hours (≤ 180 minutes) of time last known well for reasons documented by clinician M

G8602 IV tPA not initiated within 3 hours (≤ 180 minutes) of time last known well, reason not given M

G8633 Pharmacologic therapy (other than minerals/vitamins) for osteoporosis prescribed M

G8635 Pharmacologic therapy for osteoporosis was not prescribed, reason not given M

G8647 Risk-adjusted functional status change residual score for the knee impairment successfully calculated and the score was equal to zero (0) or greater than zero (> 0) M ☑

G8648 Risk-adjusted functional status change residual score for the knee impairment successfully calculated and the score was less than zero (< 0) M ☑

G8650 Risk-adjusted functional status change residual score for the knee impairment not measured because the patient did not complete the LEPF PROM at initial evaluation and/or near discharge, reason not given M

G8651 Risk-adjusted functional status change residual score for the hip impairment successfully calculated and the score was equal to zero (0) or greater than zero (> 0) M ☑

G8652 Risk-adjusted functional status change residual score for the hip impairment successfully calculated and the score was less than zero (< 0) M ☑

Special Coverage Instructions   Noncovered by Medicare   Carrier Discretion   ☑ Quantity Alert   ● New Code   ○ Recycled/Reinstated   ▲ Revised Code

© 2021 Optum360, LLC   A2-Z3 ASC Pmt   CMS: IOM   AHA: Coding Clinic   ᕲ DMEPOS Paid   ⊘ SNF Excluded   G Codes — 63

G8654 Risk-adjusted functional status change residual score for the hip impairment not measured because the patient did not complete the LEPF PROM at initial evaluation and/or near discharge, reason not given Ⓜ

G8655 Risk-adjusted functional status change residual score for the foot or ankle successfully calculated and the score was equal to zero (0) or greater than zero (> 0) Ⓜ ☑

G8656 Risk-adjusted functional status change residual score for the lower leg, foot or ankle impairment successfully calculated and the score was less than zero (< 0) Ⓜ ☑

G8658 Risk-adjusted functional status change residual score for the lower leg, foot or ankle impairment not measured because the patient did not complete the LEPF PROM at initial evaluation and/or near discharge, reason not given Ⓜ

G8659 Risk-adjusted functional status change residual score for the low back impairment successfully calculated and the score was equal to zero (0) or greater than zero (> 0) Ⓜ ☑

G8660 Risk-adjusted functional status change residual score for the low back impairment successfully calculated and the score was less than zero (< 0) Ⓜ ☑

G8661 Risk-adjusted functional status change residual score for the low back impairment not measured because the patient did not complete the FS status survey near discharge, patient not appropriate Ⓜ

G8662 Risk-adjusted functional status change residual score for the low back impairment not measured because the patient did not complete the low back FS PROM at initial evaluation and/or near discharge, reason not given Ⓜ

G8663 Risk-adjusted functional status change residual score for the shoulder impairment successfully calculated and the score was equal to zero (0) or greater than zero (> 0) Ⓜ ☑

G8664 Risk-adjusted functional status change residual score for the shoulder impairment successfully calculated and the score was less than zero (< 0) Ⓜ ☑

G8666 Risk-adjusted functional status change residual score for the shoulder impairment not measured because the patient did not complete the shoulder FS PROM at initial evaluation and/or near discharge, reason not given Ⓜ

G8667 Risk-adjusted functional status change residual score for the elbow, wrist or hand impairment successfully calculated and the score was equal to zero (0) or greater than zero (> 0) Ⓜ ☑

G8668 Risk-adjusted functional status change residual score for the elbow, wrist or hand impairment successfully calculated and the score was less than zero (< 0) Ⓜ ☑

G8670 Risk-adjusted functional status change residual score for the elbow, wrist or hand impairment not measured because the patient did not complete the elbow/wrist/hand FS PROM at initial evaluation and/or near discharge, reason not given Ⓜ

G8694 Left ventricular ejection fraction (LVEF) < 40% or documentation of moderate or severe LVSD Ⓜ ☑

G8708 Patient not prescribed or dispensed antibiotic Ⓜ

G8709 URI episodes when the patient had competing diagnoses on or three days after the episode date (e.g., intestinal infection, pertussis, bacterial infection, Lyme disease, otitis media, acute sinusitis, acute pharyngitis, acute tonsillitis, chronic sinusitis, infection of the pharynx/larynx/tonsils/adenoids, prostatitis, cellulitis, mastoiditis, or bone infections, acute lymphadenitis, impetigo, skin staph infections, pneumonia/gonococcal infections, venereal disease (syphilis, chlamydia, inflammatory diseases [female reproductive organs]), infections of the kidney, cystitis or UTI, and acne) Ⓜ

G8710 Patient prescribed or dispensed antibiotic Ⓜ

▲ **G8711** Prescribed or dispensed antibiotic on or within 3 days after the episode date Ⓜ

G8712 Antibiotic not prescribed or dispensed Ⓜ

G8721 PT category (primary tumor), PN category (regional lymph nodes), and histologic grade were documented in pathology report Ⓜ

G8722 Documentation of medical reason(s) for not including the PT category, the PN category or the histologic grade in the pathology report (e.g., re-excision without residual tumor; noncarcinomasanal canal) Ⓜ

G8723 Specimen site is other than anatomic location of primary tumor Ⓜ

G8724 PT category, PN category and histologic grade were not documented in the pathology report, reason not given Ⓜ

G8733 Elder maltreatment screen documented as positive and a follow-up plan is documented Ⓜ

G8734 Elder maltreatment screen documented as negative, no follow-up required Ⓜ

G8735 Elder maltreatment screen documented as positive, follow-up plan not documented, reason not given Ⓜ

G8749 Absence of signs of melanoma (tenderness, jaundice, localized neurologic signs such as weakness, or any other sign suggesting systemic spread) or absence of symptoms of melanoma (cough, dyspnea, pain, paresthesia, or any other symptom suggesting the possibility of systemic spread of melanoma) Ⓜ

G8752 Most recent systolic blood pressure < 140 mm Hg Ⓜ ☑

G8753 Most recent systolic blood pressure ≥ 140 mm Hg Ⓜ ☑

G8754 Most recent diastolic blood pressure < 90 mm Hg Ⓜ ☑

G8755 Most recent diastolic blood pressure ≥ 90 mm Hg Ⓜ ☑

G8756 No documentation of blood pressure measurement, reason not given Ⓜ

G8783 Normal blood pressure reading documented, follow-up not required Ⓜ

G8785 Blood pressure reading not documented, reason not given Ⓜ

G8797 Specimen site other than anatomic location of esophagus Ⓜ

G8798 Specimen site other than anatomic location of prostate Ⓜ

G8806 Performance of trans-abdominal or trans-vaginal ultrasound and pregnancy location documented Ⓐ ♀ Ⓜ

G8807 Transabdominal or transvaginal ultrasound not performed for reasons documented by clinician (e.g., patient has visited the ED multiple times within 72 hours, patient has a documented intrauterine pregnancy (IUP)) Ⓐ ♀ Ⓜ

G8808 Transabdominal or transvaginal ultrasound not performed, reason not given Ⓐ ♀ Ⓜ

G8815 Documented reason in the medical records for why the statin therapy was not prescribed (i.e., lower extremity bypass was for a patient with nonartherosclerotic disease) Ⓜ

G8816 Statin medication prescribed at discharge Ⓜ

G8817 Statin therapy not prescribed at discharge, reason not given Ⓜ

G8818 Patient discharge to home no later than postoperative day #7 Ⓜ

G8825 Patient not discharged to home by postoperative day #7 Ⓜ

Special Coverage Instructions   Noncovered by Medicare   Carrier Discretion   ☑ Quantity Alert   ● New Code   ○ Recycled/Reinstated   ▲ Revised Code

64 — G Codes   Ⓐ Age Edit   Ⓜ Maternity Edit   ♀ Female Only   ♂ Male Only   Ⓐ-Ⓨ OPPS Status Indicators   © 2021 Optum360, LLC

G8826	Patient discharged to home no later than postoperative day #2 following EVAR Ⓜ
G8833	Patient not discharged to home by postoperative day #2 following EVAR ⓂＭ
G8834	Patient discharged to home no later than postoperative day #2 following CEA ⓂＭ
G8838	Patient not discharged to home by postoperative day #2 following CEA ⓂＭ
G8839	Sleep apnea symptoms assessed, including presence or absence of snoring and daytime sleepiness ⓂＭ
G8840	Documentation of reason(s) for not documenting an assessment of sleep symptoms (e.g., patient didn't have initial daytime sleepiness, patient visited between initial testing and initiation of therapy) ⓂＭ
G8841	Sleep apnea symptoms not assessed, reason not given ⓂＭ
G8842	Apnea hypopnea index (AHI) or respiratory disturbance index (RDI) measured at the time of initial diagnosis ⓂＭ
G8843	Documentation of reason(s) for not measuring an apnea hypopnea index (AHI) or a respiratory disturbance index (RDI) at the time of initial diagnosis (e.g., psychiatric disease, dementia, patient declined, financial, insurance coverage, test ordered but not yet completed) ⓂＭ
G8844	Apnea hypopna index (AHI) or respiratory disturbance index (RDI) not measured at the time of initial diagnosis, reason not given ⓂＭ
G8845	Positive airway pressure therapy prescribed ⓂＭ
G8846	Moderate or severe obstructive sleep apnea (apnea hypopnea index (AHI) or respiratory disturbance index (RDI) of 15 or greater) ⓂＭ ☑
G8849	Documentation of reason(s) for not prescribing positive airway pressure therapy (e.g., patient unable to tolerate, alternative therapies use, patient declined, financial, insurance coverage) ⓂＭ
G8850	Positive airway pressure therapy not prescribed, reason not given ⓂＭ
G8851	Objective measurement of adherence to positive airway pressure therapy, documented ⓂＭ
G8852	Positive airway pressure therapy prescribed ⓂＭ
G8854	Documentation of reason(s) for not objectively measuring adherence to positive airway pressure therapy (e.g., patient did not bring data from continuous positive airway pressure (CPAP), therapy not yet initiated, not available on machine) ⓂＭ
G8855	Objective measurement of adherence to positive airway pressure therapy not performed, reason not given ⓂＭ
G8856	Referral to a physician for an otologic evaluation performed ⓂＭ
G8857	Patient is not eligible for the referral for otologic evaluation measure (e.g., patients who are already under the care of a physician for acute or chronic dizziness) ⓂＭ
G8858	Referral to a physician for an otologic evaluation not performed, reason not given ⓂＭ
G8863	Patients not assessed for risk of bone loss, reason not given ⓂＭ
G8864	Pneumococcal vaccine administered or previously received ⓂＭ
G8865	Documentation of medical reason(s) for not administering or previously receiving pneumococcal vaccine (e.g., patient allergic reaction, potential adverse drug reaction) ⓂＭ
G8866	Documentation of patient reason(s) for not administering or previously receiving pneumococcal vaccine (e.g., patient refusal) ⓂＭ
G8867	Pneumococcal vaccine not administered or previously received, reason not given ⓂＭ
G8869	Patient has documented immunity to hepatitis B and initiating anti-TNF therapy ⓂＭ
G8875	Clinician diagnosed breast cancer preoperatively by a minimally invasive biopsy method ⓂＭ
G8876	Documentation of reason(s) for not performing minimally invasive biopsy to diagnose breast cancer preoperatively (e.g., lesion too close to skin, implant, chest wall, etc., lesion could not be adequately visualized for needle biopsy, patient condition prevents needle biopsy [weight, breast thickness, etc.], duct excision without imaging abnormality, prophylactic mastectomy, reduction mammoplasty, excisional biopsy performed by another physician) ⓂＭ
G8877	Clinician did not attempt to achieve the diagnosis of breast cancer preoperatively by a minimally invasive biopsy method, reason not given ⓂＭ
G8878	Sentinel lymph node biopsy procedure performed ⓂＭ
G8880	Documentation of reason(s) sentinel lymph node biopsy not performed (e.g., reasons could include but not limited to: noninvasive cancer, incidental discovery of breast cancer on prophylactic mastectomy, incidental discovery of breast cancer on reduction mammoplasty, preoperative biopsy proven lymph node (LN) metastases, inflammatory carcinoma, Stage III locally advanced cancer, recurrent invasive breast cancer, clinically node positive after neoadjuvant systemic therapy, patient refusal after informed consent, patient with significant age, comorbidities, or limited life expectancy and favorable tumor; adjuvant systemic therapy unlikely to change) ⓂＭ
G8881	Stage of breast cancer is greater than T1N0M0 or T2N0M0 ⓂＭ
G8882	Sentinel lymph node biopsy procedure not performed, reason not given ⓂＭ
G8883	Biopsy results reviewed, communicated, tracked and documented ⓂＭ
G8884	Clinician documented reason that patient's biopsy results were not reviewed ⓂＭ
G8885	Biopsy results not reviewed, communicated, tracked or documented ⓂＭ
G8907	Patient documented not to have experienced any of the following events: a burn prior to discharge; a fall within the facility; wrong site/side/patient/procedure/implant event; or a hospital transfer or hospital admission upon discharge from the facility ⓂＭ
G8908	Patient documented to have received a burn prior to discharge ⓂＭ
G8909	Patient documented not to have received a burn prior to discharge ⓂＭ
G8910	Patient documented to have experienced a fall within ASC ⓂＭ
G8911	Patient documented not to have experienced a fall within ASC ⓂＭ
G8912	Patient documented to have experienced a wrong site, wrong side, wrong patient, wrong procedure or wrong implant event ⓂＭ
G8913	Patient documented not to have experienced a wrong site, wrong side, wrong patient, wrong procedure or wrong implant event ⓂＭ

Special Coverage Instructions   Noncovered by Medicare   Carrier Discretion   ☑ Quantity Alert   ● New Code   ○ Recycled/Reinstated   ▲ Revised Code

© 2021 Optum360, LLC   Ａ2-Ｚ3 ASC Pmt   CMS: IOM   AHA: Coding Clinic   ⅃ DMEPOS Paid   ⊘ SNF Excluded   G Codes — 65

G8914	Patient documented to have experienced a hospital transfer or hospital admission upon discharge from ASC	M
G8915	Patient documented not to have experienced a hospital transfer or hospital admission upon discharge from ASC	M
G8916	Patient with preoperative order for IV antibiotic surgical site infection (SSI) prophylaxis, antibiotic initiated on time	M
G8917	Patient with preoperative order for IV antibiotic surgical site infection (SSI) prophylaxis, antibiotic not initiated on time	M
G8918	Patient without preoperative order for IV antibiotic surgical site infection (SSI) prophylaxis	M
G8923	Left ventricular ejection fraction (LVEF) < 40% or documentation of moderately or severely depressed left ventricular systolic function	M
G8924	Spirometry test results demonstrate FEV1/FVC < 70%, FEV1 < 60% predicted and patient has COPD symptoms (e.g., dyspnea, cough/sputum, wheezing)	M
G8925	~~Spirometry test results demonstrate FEV1 >= 60%, FEV1/FVC >= 70%, predicted or patient does not have COPD symptoms~~	
G8926	~~Spirometry test not performed or documented, reason not given~~	
G8934	Left ventricular ejection fraction (LVEF) < 40% or documentation of moderately or severely depressed left ventricular systolic function	M
G8935	Clinician prescribed angiotensin converting enzyme (ACE) inhibitor or angiotensin receptor blocker (ARB) therapy	M
G8936	Clinician documented that patient was not an eligible candidate for angiotensin converting enzyme (ACE) inhibitor or angiotensin receptor blocker (ARB) therapy (e.g., allergy, intolerance, pregnancy, renal failure due to ACE inhibitor, diseases of the aortic or mitral valve, other medical reasons) or (e.g., patient declined, other patient reasons) or (e.g., lack of drug availability, other reasons attributable to the health care system)	M
G8937	Clinician did not prescribe angiotensin converting enzyme (ACE) inhibitor or angiotensin receptor blocker (ARB) therapy, reason not given	M
G8938	~~BMI is documented as being outside of normal parameters, follow-up plan is not documented, documentation the patient is not eligible~~	
G8941	Elder maltreatment screen documented as positive, follow-up plan not documented, documentation the patient is not eligible for follow-up plan at the time of the encounter	M
G8942	Functional outcomes assessment using a standardized tool is documented within the previous 30 days and care plan, based on identified deficiencies on the date of the functional outcome assessment, is documented	M
G8944	AJCC melanoma cancer stage 0 through IIC melanoma	M
G8946	Minimally invasive biopsy method attempted but not diagnostic of breast cancer (e.g., high risk lesion of breast such as atypical ductal hyperplasia, lobular neoplasia, atypical lobular hyperplasia, lobular carcinoma in situ, atypical columnar hyperplasia, flat epithelial atypia, radial scar, complex sclerosing lesion, papillary lesion, or any lesion with spindle cells)	M
▲ G8950	Elevated or hypertensive blood pressure reading documented, and the indicated follow-up is documented	M
▲ G8952	Elevated or hypertensive blood pressure reading documented, indicated follow-up not documented, reason not given	M
G8955	Most recent assessment of adequacy of volume management documented	
G8956	Patient receiving maintenance hemodialysis in an outpatient dialysis facility	M
G8958	Assessment of adequacy of volume management not documented, reason not given	M
G8961	Cardiac stress imaging test primarily performed on low-risk surgery patient for preoperative evaluation within 30 days preceding this surgery	M
G8962	Cardiac stress imaging test performed on patient for any reason including those who did not have low risk surgery or test that was performed more than 30 days preceding low risk surgery	M
G8963	Cardiac stress imaging performed primarily for monitoring of asymptomatic patient who had PCI wihin 2 years	M
G8964	Cardiac stress imaging test performed primarily for any other reason than monitoring of asymptomatic patient who had PCI wthin 2 years (e.g., symptomatic patient, patient greater than 2 years since PCI, initial evaluation, etc.)	M
G8965	Cardiac stress imaging test primarily performed on low CHD risk patient for initial detection and risk assessment	M
G8966	Cardiac stress imaging test performed on symptomatic or higher than low CHD risk patient or for any reason other than initial detection and risk assessment	M
▲ G8967	FDA-approved oral anticoagulant is prescribed	M
▲ G8968	Documentation of medical reason(s) for not prescribing an FDA-approved anticoagulant to a patient with a CHA2DS-VASc score of 0 or 1 for men; or 0, 1, or 2 for women (e.g., present or planned atrial appendage occlusion or ligation)	M
▲ G8969	Documentation of patient reason(s) for not prescribing an oral anticoagulant that is FDA-approved for the prevention of thromboembolism (e.g., patient preference for not receiving anticoagulation)	M
G8970	No risk factors or one moderate risk factor for thromboembolism	M

Coordinated Care

G9001	Coordinated care fee, initial rate	B
G9002	Coordinated care fee	B
G9003	Coordinated care fee, risk adjusted high, initial	B
G9004	Coordinated care fee, risk adjusted low, initial	B
G9005	Coordinated care fee risk adjusted maintenance	B
G9006	Coordinated care fee, home monitoring	B
G9007	Coordinated care fee, scheduled team conference	B
G9008	Coordinated care fee, physician coordinated care oversight services	B
G9009	Coordinated care fee, risk adjusted maintenance, Level 3	B
G9010	Coordinated care fee, risk adjusted maintenance, Level 4	B
G9011	Coordinated care fee, risk adjusted maintenance, Level 5	B
G9012	Other specified case management service not elsewhere classified	B

Demonstration Project

G9013	ESRD demo basic bundle Level I	E
G9014	ESRD demo expanded bundle including venous access and related services	E

Special Coverage Instructions   Noncovered by Medicare   Carrier Discretion   ☑ Quantity Alert ● New Code ○ Recycled/Reinstated ▲ Revised Code

66 — G Codes   A Age Edit   M Maternity Edit   ♀ Female Only   ♂ Male Only   A-Y OPPS Status Indicators   © 2021 Optum360, LLC

G9016 Smoking cessation counseling, individual, in the absence of or in addition to any other evaluation and management service, per session (6-10 minutes) [demo project code only] E ☑
CMS: 100-03,210.4.1

G9050 Oncology; primary focus of visit; work-up, evaluation, or staging at the time of cancer diagnosis or recurrence (for use in a Medicare-approved demonstration project) E

G9051 Oncology; primary focus of visit; treatment decision-making after disease is staged or restaged, discussion of treatment options, supervising/coordinating active cancer-directed therapy or managing consequences of cancer-directed therapy (for use in a Medicare-approved demonstration project) E

G9052 Oncology; primary focus of visit; surveillance for disease recurrence for patient who has completed definitive cancer-directed therapy and currently lacks evidence of recurrent disease; cancer-directed therapy might be considered in the future (for use in a Medicare-approved demonstration project) E

G9053 Oncology; primary focus of visit; expectant management of patient with evidence of cancer for whom no cancer-directed therapy is being administered or arranged at present; cancer-directed therapy might be considered in the future (for use in a Medicare-approved demonstration project) E

G9054 Oncology; primary focus of visit; supervising, coordinating or managing care of patient with terminal cancer or for whom other medical illness prevents further cancer treatment; includes symptom management, end-of-life care planning, management of palliative therapies (for use in a Medicare-approved demonstration project) E

G9055 Oncology; primary focus of visit; other, unspecified service not otherwise listed (for use in a Medicare-approved demonstration project) E

G9056 Oncology; practice guidelines; management adheres to guidelines (for use in a Medicare-approved demonstration project) E

G9057 Oncology; practice guidelines; management differs from guidelines as a result of patient enrollment in an institutional review board-approved clinical trial (for use in a Medicare-approved demonstration project) E

G9058 Oncology; practice guidelines; management differs from guidelines because the treating physician disagrees with guideline recommendations (for use in a Medicare-approved demonstration project) E

G9059 Oncology; practice guidelines; management differs from guidelines because the patient, after being offered treatment consistent with guidelines, has opted for alternative treatment or management, including no treatment (for use in a Medicare-approved demonstration project) E

G9060 Oncology; practice guidelines; management differs from guidelines for reason(s) associated with patient comorbid illness or performance status not factored into guidelines (for use in a Medicare-approved demonstration project) E

G9061 Oncology; practice guidelines; patient's condition not addressed by available guidelines (for use in a Medicare-approved demonstration project) E

G9062 Oncology; practice guidelines; management differs from guidelines for other reason(s) not listed (for use in a Medicare-approved demonstration project) E

G9063 Oncology; disease status; limited to nonsmall cell lung cancer; extent of disease initially established as Stage I (prior to neoadjuvant therapy, if any) with no evidence of disease progression, recurrence, or metastases (for use in a Medicare-approved demonstration project) M

G9064 Oncology; disease status; limited to nonsmall cell lung cancer; extent of disease initially established as Stage II (prior to neoadjuvant therapy, if any) with no evidence of disease progression, recurrence, or metastases (for use in a Medicare-approved demonstration project) M

G9065 Oncology; disease status; limited to nonsmall cell lung cancer; extent of disease initially established as Stage III a (prior to neoadjuvant therapy, if any) with no evidence of disease progression, recurrence, or metastases (for use in a Medicare-approved demonstration project) M

G9066 Oncology; disease status; limited to nonsmall cell lung cancer; Stage III B-IV at diagnosis, metastatic, locally recurrent, or progressive (for use in a Medicare-approved demonstration project) M

G9067 Oncology; disease status; limited to nonsmall cell lung cancer; extent of disease unknown, staging in progress, or not listed (for use in a Medicare-approved demonstration project) M

G9068 Oncology; disease status; limited to small cell and combined small cell/nonsmall cell; extent of disease initially established as limited with no evidence of disease progression, recurrence, or metastases (for use in a Medicare-approved demonstration project) M

G9069 Oncology; disease status; small cell lung cancer, limited to small cell and combined small cell/nonsmall cell; extensive Stage at diagnosis, metastatic, locally recurrent, or progressive (for use in a Medicare-approved demonstration project) M

G9070 Oncology; disease status; small cell lung cancer, limited to small cell and combined small cell/nonsmall; extent of disease unknown, staging in progress, or not listed (for use in a Medicare-approved demonstration project) M

G9071 Oncology; disease status; invasive female breast cancer (does not include ductal carcinoma in situ); adenocarcinoma as predominant cell type; Stage I or Stage IIA-IIB; or T3, N1, M0; and ER and/or PR positive; with no evidence of disease progression, recurrence, or metastases (for use in a Medicare-approved demonstration project) ♀ M

G9072 Oncology; disease status; invasive female breast cancer (does not include ductal carcinoma in situ); adenocarcinoma as predominant cell type; Stage I, or Stage IIA-IIB; or T3, N1, M0; and ER and PR negative; with no evidence of disease progression, recurrence, or metastases (for use in a Medicare-approved demonstration project) ♀ M

G9073 Oncology; disease status; invasive female breast cancer (does not include ductal carcinoma in situ); adenocarcinoma as predominant cell type; Stage IIIA-IIIB; and not T3, N1, M0; and ER and/or PR positive; with no evidence of disease progression, recurrence, or metastases (for use in a Medicare-approved demonstration project) ♀ M

G9074 Oncology; disease status; invasive female breast cancer (does not include ductal carcinoma in situ); adenocarcinoma as predominant cell type; Stage IIIA-IIIB; and not T3, N1, M0; and ER and PR negative; with no evidence of disease progression, recurrence, or metastases (for use in a Medicare-approved demonstration project) ♀ M

G9075 Oncology; disease status; invasive female breast cancer (does not include ductal carcinoma in situ); adenocarcinoma as predominant cell type; M1 at diagnosis, metastatic, locally recurrent, or progressive (for use in a Medicare-approved demonstration project) ♀ M

G9077 Oncology; disease status; prostate cancer, limited to adenocarcinoma as predominant cell type; T1-T2c and Gleason 2-7 and PSA < or equal to 20 at diagnosis with no evidence of disease progression, recurrence, or metastases (for use in a Medicare-approved demonstration project) ♂ M

Special Coverage Instructions · · · Noncovered by Medicare · · · Carrier Discretion · · · ☑ Quantity Alert · ● New Code · ○ Recycled/Reinstated · ▲ Revised Code

© 2021 Optum360, LLC · · · A2-Z3 ASC Pmt · · · CMS: IOM · · · AHA: Coding Clinic · · · ⅃ DMEPOS Paid · · · ⊘ SNF Excluded · · · G Codes — 67

Procedures/Professional Services (Temporary)

G9078 — G9103

G9078 Oncology; disease status; prostate cancer, limited to adenocarcinoma as predominant cell type; T2 or T3a Gleason 8-10 or PSA > 20 at diagnosis with no evidence of disease progression, recurrence, or metastases (for use in a Medicare-approved demonstration project) ♂ M

G9079 Oncology; disease status; prostate cancer, limited to adenocarcinoma as predominant cell type; T3b-T4, any N; any T, N1 at diagnosis with no evidence of disease progression, recurrence, or metastases (for use in a Medicare-approved demonstration project) ♂ M

G9080 Oncology; disease status; prostate cancer, limited to adenocarcinoma; after initial treatment with rising PSA or failure of PSA decline (for use in a Medicare-approved demonstration project) ♂ M

G9083 Oncology; disease status; prostate cancer, limited to adenocarcinoma; extent of disease unknown, staging in progress, or not listed (for use in a Medicare-approved demonstration project) ♂ M

G9084 Oncology; disease status; colon cancer, limited to invasive cancer, adenocarcinoma as predominant cell type; extent of disease initially established as T1-3, N0, M0 with no evidence of disease progression, recurrence or metastases (for use in a Medicare-approved demonstration project) M

G9085 Oncology; disease status; colon cancer, limited to invasive cancer, adenocarcinoma as predominant cell type; extent of disease initially established as T4, N0, M0 with no evidence of disease progression, recurrence, or metastases (for use in a Medicare-approved demonstration project) M

G9086 Oncology; disease status; colon cancer, limited to invasive cancer, adenocarcinoma as predominant cell type; extent of disease initially established as T1-4, N1-2, M0 with no evidence of disease progression, recurrence, or metastases (for use in a Medicare-approved demonstration project) M

G9087 Oncology; disease status; colon cancer, limited to invasive cancer, adenocarcinoma as predominant cell type; M1 at diagnosis, metastatic, locally recurrent, or progressive with current clinical, radiologic, or biochemical evidence of disease (for use in a Medicare-approved demonstration project) M

G9088 Oncology; disease status; colon cancer, limited to invasive cancer, adenocarcinoma as predominant cell type; M1 at diagnosis, metastatic, locally recurrent, or progressive without current clinical, radiologic, or biochemical evidence of disease (for use in a Medicare-approved demonstration project) M

G9089 Oncology; disease status; colon cancer, limited to invasive cancer, adenocarcinoma as predominant cell type; extent of disease unknown, staging in progress or not listed (for use in a Medicare-approved demonstration project) M

G9090 Oncology; disease status; rectal cancer, limited to invasive cancer, adenocarcinoma as predominant cell type; extent of disease initially established as T1-2, N0, M0 (prior to neoadjuvant therapy, if any) with no evidence of disease progression, recurrence, or metastases (for use in a Medicare-approved demonstration project) M

G9091 Oncology; disease status; rectal cancer, limited to invasive cancer, adenocarcinoma as predominant cell type; extent of disease initially established as T3, N0, M0 (prior to neoadjuvant therapy, if any) with no evidence of disease progression, recurrence, or metastases (for use in a Medicare-approved demonstration project) M

G9092 Oncology; disease status; rectal cancer, limited to invasive cancer, adenocarcinoma as predominant cell type; extent of disease initially established as T1-3, N1-2, M0 (prior to neoadjuvant therapy, if any) with no evidence of disease progression, recurrence or metastases (for use in a Medicare-approved demonstration project) M

G9093 Oncology; disease status; rectal cancer, limited to invasive cancer, adenocarcinoma as predominant cell type; extent of disease initially established as T4, any N, M0 (prior to neoadjuvant therapy, if any) with no evidence of disease progression, recurrence, or metastases (for use in a Medicare-approved demonstration project) M

G9094 Oncology; disease status; rectal cancer, limited to invasive cancer, adenocarcinoma as predominant cell type; M1 at diagnosis, metastatic, locally recurrent, or progressive (for use in a Medicare-approved demonstration project) M

G9095 Oncology; disease status; rectal cancer, limited to invasive cancer, adenocarcinoma as predominant cell type; extent of disease unknown, staging in progress or not listed (for use in a Medicare-approved demonstration project) M

G9096 Oncology; disease status; esophageal cancer, limited to adenocarcinoma or squamous cell carcinoma as predominant cell type; extent of disease initially established as T1-T3, N0-N1 or NX (prior to neoadjuvant therapy, if any) with no evidence of disease progression, recurrence, or metastases (for use in a Medicare-approved demonstration project) M

G9097 Oncology; disease status; esophageal cancer, limited to adenocarcinoma or squamous cell carcinoma as predominant cell type; extent of disease initially established as T4, any N, M0 (prior to neoadjuvant therapy, if any) with no evidence of disease progression, recurrence, or metastases (for use in a Medicare-approved demonstration project) M

G9098 Oncology; disease status; esophageal cancer, limited to adenocarcinoma or squamous cell carcinoma as predominant cell type; M1 at diagnosis, metastatic, locally recurrent, or progressive (for use in a Medicare-approved demonstration project) M

G9099 Oncology; disease status; esophageal cancer, limited to adenocarcinoma or squamous cell carcinoma as predominant cell type; extent of disease unknown, staging in progress, or not listed (for use in a Medicare-approved demonstration project) M

G9100 Oncology; disease status; gastric cancer, limited to adenocarcinoma as predominant cell type; post R0 resection (with or without neoadjuvant therapy) with no evidence of disease recurrence, progression, or metastases (for use in a Medicare-approved demonstration project) M

G9101 Oncology; disease status; gastric cancer, limited to adenocarcinoma as predominant cell type; post R1 or R2 resection (with or without neoadjuvant therapy) with no evidence of disease progression, or metastases (for use in a Medicare-approved demonstration project) M

G9102 Oncology; disease status; gastric cancer, limited to adenocarcinoma as predominant cell type; clinical or pathologic M0, unresectable with no evidence of disease progression, or metastases (for use in a Medicare-approved demonstration project) M

G9103 Oncology; disease status; gastric cancer, limited to adenocarcinoma as predominant cell type; clinical or pathologic M1 at diagnosis, metastatic, locally recurrent, or progressive (for use in a Medicare-approved demonstration project) M

Special Coverage Instructions   Noncovered by Medicare   Carrier Discretion   ☑ Quantity Alert ● New Code   ○ Recycled/Reinstated ▲ Revised Code

G9104 Oncology; disease status; gastric cancer, limited to adenocarcinoma as predominant cell type; extent of disease unknown, staging in progress, or not listed (for use in a Medicare-approved demonstration project) Ⓜ

G9105 Oncology; disease status; pancreatic cancer, limited to adenocarcinoma as predominant cell type; post R0 resection without evidence of disease progression, recurrence, or metastases (for use in a Medicare-approved demonstration project) Ⓜ

G9106 Oncology; disease status; pancreatic cancer, limited to adenocarcinoma; post R1 or R2 resection with no evidence of disease progression, or metastases (for use in a Medicare-approved demonstration project) Ⓜ

G9107 Oncology; disease status; pancreatic cancer, limited to adenocarcinoma; unresectable at diagnosis, M1 at diagnosis, metastatic, locally recurrent, or progressive (for use in a Medicare-approved demonstration project) Ⓜ

G9108 Oncology; disease status; pancreatic cancer, limited to adenocarcinoma; extent of disease unknown, staging in progress, or not listed (for use in a Medicare-approved demonstration project) Ⓜ

G9109 Oncology; disease status; head and neck cancer, limited to cancers of oral cavity, pharynx and larynx with squamous cell as predominant cell type; extent of disease initially established as T1-T2 and N0, M0 (prior to neoadjuvant therapy, if any) with no evidence of disease progression, recurrence, or metastases (for use in a Medicare-approved demonstration project) Ⓜ

G9110 Oncology; disease status; head and neck cancer, limited to cancers of oral cavity, pharynx and larynx with squamous cell as predominant cell type; extent of disease initially established as T3-4 and/or N1-3, M0 (prior to neoadjuvant therapy, if any) with no evidence of disease progression, recurrence, or metastases (for use in a Medicare-approved demonstration project) Ⓜ

G9111 Oncology; disease status; head and neck cancer, limited to cancers of oral cavity, pharynx and larynx with squamous cell as predominant cell type; M1 at diagnosis, metastatic, locally recurrent, or progressive (for use in a Medicare-approved demonstration project) Ⓜ

G9112 Oncology; disease status; head and neck cancer, limited to cancers of oral cavity, pharynx and larynx with squamous cell as predominant cell type; extent of disease unknown, staging in progress, or not listed (for use in a Medicare-approved demonstration project) Ⓜ

G9113 Oncology; disease status; ovarian cancer, limited to epithelial cancer; pathologic Stage IA-B (Grade 1) without evidence of disease progression, recurrence, or metastases (for use in a Medicare-approved demonstration project) ♀ Ⓜ

G9114 Oncology; disease status; ovarian cancer, limited to epithelial cancer; pathologic Stage IA-B (Grade 2-3); or Stage IC (all grades); or Stage II; without evidence of disease progression, recurrence, or metastases (for use in a Medicare-approved demonstration project) ♀ Ⓜ

G9115 Oncology; disease status; ovarian cancer, limited to epithelial cancer; pathologic Stage III-IV; without evidence of progression, recurrence, or metastases (for use in a Medicare-approved demonstration project) ♀ Ⓜ

G9116 Oncology; disease status; ovarian cancer, limited to epithelial cancer; evidence of disease progression, or recurrence, and/or platinum resistance (for use in a Medicare-approved demonstration project) ♀ Ⓜ

G9117 Oncology; disease status; ovarian cancer, limited to epithelial cancer; extent of disease unknown, staging in progress, or not listed (for use in a Medicare-approved demonstration project) ♀ Ⓜ

G9123 Oncology; disease status; chronic myelogenous leukemia, limited to Philadelphia chromosome positive and/or BCR-ABL positive; chronic phase not in hematologic, cytogenetic, or molecular remission (for use in a Medicare-approved demonstration project) Ⓜ

G9124 Oncology; disease status; chronic myelogenous leukemia, limited to Philadelphia chromosome positive and /or BCR-ABL positive; accelerated phase not in hematologic cytogenetic, or molecular remission (for use in a Medicare-approved demonstration project) Ⓜ

G9125 Oncology; disease status; chronic myelogenous leukemia, limited to Philadelphia chromosome positive and/or BCR-ABL positive; blast phase not in hematologic, cytogenetic, or molecular remission (for use in a Medicare-approved demonstration project) Ⓜ

G9126 Oncology; disease status; chronic myelogenous leukemia, limited to Philadelphia chromosome positive and/or BCR-ABL positive; in hematologic, cytogenetic, or molecular remission (for use in a Medicare-approved demonstration project) Ⓜ

G9128 Oncology; disease status; limited to multiple myeloma, systemic disease; smoldering, Stage I (for use in a Medicare-approved demonstration project) Ⓜ

G9129 Oncology; disease status; limited to multiple myeloma, systemic disease; Stage II or higher (for use in a Medicare-approved demonstration project) Ⓜ

G9130 Oncology; disease status; limited to multiple myeloma, systemic disease; extent of disease unknown, staging in progress, or not listed (for use in a Medicare-approved demonstration project) Ⓜ

G9131 Oncology; disease status; invasive female breast cancer (does not include ductal carcinoma in situ); adenocarcinoma as predominant cell type; extent of disease unknown, staging in progress, or not listed (for use in a Medicare-approved demonstration project) ♀ Ⓜ

G9132 Oncology; disease status; prostate cancer, limited to adenocarcinoma; hormone-refractory/androgen-independent (e.g., rising PSA on antiandrogen therapy or postorchiectomy); clinical metastases (for use in a Medicare-approved demonstration project) ♂ Ⓜ

G9133 Oncology; disease status; prostate cancer, limited to adenocarcinoma; hormone-responsive; clinical metastases or M1 at diagnosis (for use in a Medicare-approved demonstration project) ♂ Ⓜ

G9134 Oncology; disease status; non-Hodgkin's lymphoma, any cellular classification; Stage I, II at diagnosis, not relapsed, not refractory (for use in a Medicare-approved demonstration project) Ⓜ

G9135 Oncology; disease status; non-Hodgkin's lymphoma, any cellular classification; Stage III, IV, not relapsed, not refractory (for use in a Medicare-approved demonstration project) Ⓜ

G9136 Oncology; disease status; non-Hodgkin's lymphoma, transformed from original cellular diagnosis to a second cellular classification (for use in a Medicare-approved demonstration project) Ⓜ

G9137 Oncology; disease status; non-Hodgkin's lymphoma, any cellular classification; relapsed/refractory (for use in a Medicare-approved demonstration project) Ⓜ

Special Coverage Instructions Noncovered by Medicare Carrier Discretion ☑ Quantity Alert ● New Code ○ Recycled/Reinstated ▲ Revised Code

© 2021 Optum360, LLC A2-Z3 ASC Pmt CMS: IOM AHA: Coding Clinic ⚲ DMEPOS Paid ⊘ SNF Excluded G Codes — 69

Procedures/Professional Services (Temporary)

G9138 — G9246

G9138 Oncology; disease status; non-Hodgkin's lymphoma, any cellular classification; diagnostic evaluation, stage not determined, evaluation of possible relapse or nonresponse to therapy, or not listed (for use in a Medicare-approved demonstration project) Ⓜ

G9139 Oncology; disease status; chronic myelogenous leukemia, limited to Philadelphia chromosome positive and/or BCR-ABL positive; extent of disease unknown, staging in progress, not listed (for use in a Medicare-approved demonstration project) Ⓜ

G9140 Frontier Extended Stay Clinic demonstration; for a patient stay in a clinic approved for the CMS demonstration project; the following measures should be present: the stay must be equal to or greater than 4 hours; weather or other conditions must prevent transfer or the case falls into a category of monitoring and observation cases that are permitted by the rules of the demonstration; there is a maximum Frontier Extended Stay Clinic (FESC) visit of 48 hours, except in the case when weather or other conditions prevent transfer; payment is made on each period up to 4 hours, after the first 4 hours Ⓐ ☑

Warfarin Testing

G9143 Warfarin responsiveness testing by genetic technique using any method, any number of specimen(s) Ⓝ
CMS: 100-03,90.1; 100-04,32,250.1; 100-04,32,250.2

Outpatient IV Insulin TX

G9147 Outpatient Intravenous Insulin Treatment (OIVIT) either pulsatile or continuous, by any means, guided by the results of measurements for: respiratory quotient; and/or, urine urea nitrogen (UUN); and/or, arterial, venous or capillary glucose; and/or potassium concentration Ⓔ
CMS: 100-03,40.7; 100-04,4,320.1; 100-04,4,320.2

Quality Assurance

G9148 National Committee for Quality Assurance-Level 1 Medical Home Ⓜ

G9149 National Committee for Quality Assurance-Level 2 Medical Home Ⓜ

G9150 National Committee for Quality Assurance-Level 3 Medical Home Ⓜ

G9151 MAPCP Demonstration-state provided services Ⓜ

G9152 MAPCP Demonstration-Community Health Teams Ⓜ

G9153 MAPCP Demonstration-Physician Incentive Pool Ⓜ

Wheelchair Evaluation

G9156 Evaluation for wheelchair requiring face-to-face visit with physician Ⓜ

Monitor

G9157 Transesophageal Doppler used for cardiac monitoring Ⓑ
CMS: 100-04,32,310; 100-04,32,310.2; 100-04,32,310.3

BPCI Services

G9187 Bundled payments for care improvement initiative home visit for patient assessment performed by a qualified health care professional for individuals not considered homebound including, but not limited to, assessment of safety, falls, clinical status, fluid status, medication reconciliation/management, patient compliance with orders/plan of care, performance of activities of daily living, appropriateness of care setting; (for use only in the Medicare-approved bundled payments for care improvement initiative); may not be billed for a 30-day period covered by a transitional care management code Ⓔ

Miscellaneous Quality Measures

G9188 Beta-blocker therapy not prescribed, reason not given Ⓜ

G9189 Beta-blocker therapy prescribed or currently being taken Ⓜ

G9190 Documentation of medical reason(s) for not prescribing beta-blocker therapy (e.g., allergy, intolerance, other medical reasons) Ⓜ

G9191 Documentation of patient reason(s) for not prescribing beta-blocker therapy (e.g., patient declined, other patient reasons) Ⓜ

G9192 Documentation of system reason(s) for not prescribing beta-blocker therapy (e.g., other reasons attributable to the health care system) Ⓜ

G9196 Documentation of medical reason(s) for not ordering a first or second generation cephalosporin for antimicrobial prophylaxis (e.g., patients enrolled in clinical trials, patients with documented infection prior to surgical procedure of interest, patients who were receiving antibiotics more than 24 hours prior to surgery [except colon surgery patients taking oral prophylactic antibiotics], patients who were receiving antibiotics within 24 hours prior to arrival [except colon surgery patients taking oral prophylactic antibiotics], other medical reason(s)) Ⓜ

G9197 Documentation of order for first or second generation cephalosporin for antimicrobial prophylaxis Ⓜ

G9198 Order for first or second generation cephalosporin for antimicrobial prophylaxis was not documented, reason not given Ⓜ

G9212 DSM-IVTM criteria for major depressive disorder documented at the initial evaluation Ⓜ

G9213 DSM-IV-TR criteria for major depressive disorder not documented at the initial evaluation, reason not otherwise specified Ⓜ

G9223 Pneumocystis jiroveci pneumonia prophylaxis prescribed within 3 months of low CD4+ cell count below 500 cells/mm3 or a CD4 percentage below 15% Ⓜ

G9225 Foot exam was not performed, reason not given Ⓜ

G9226 Foot examination performed (includes examination through visual inspection, sensory exam with 10-g monofilament plus testing any one of the following: vibration using 128-Hz tuning fork, pinprick sensation, ankle reflexes, or vibration perception threshold, and pulse exam; report when all of the three components are completed) Ⓜ

G9227 Functional outcome assessment documented, care plan not documented, documentation the patient is not eligible for a care plan at the time of the encounter Ⓜ

G9228 Chlamydia, gonorrhea and syphilis screening results documented (report when results are present for all of the three screenings) Ⓜ

G9229 Chlamydia, gonorrhea, and syphilis screening results not documented (patient refusal is the only allowed exception) Ⓜ

G9230 Chlamydia, gonorrhea, and syphilis not screened, reason not given Ⓜ

G9231 Documentation of end stage renal disease (ESRD), dialysis, renal transplant before or during the measurement period or pregnancy during the measurement period Ⓜ

G9242 Documentation of viral load equal to or greater than 200 copies/ml or viral load not performed Ⓜ

G9243 Documentation of viral load less than 200 copies/ml Ⓜ

G9246 Patient did not have at least one medical visit in each 6 month period of the 24 month measurement period, with a minimum of 60 days between medical visits Ⓜ

Special Coverage Instructions   Noncovered by Medicare   Carrier Discretion   ☑ Quantity Alert   ● New Code   ○ Recycled/Reinstated   ▲ Revised Code

70 — G Codes   Ⓐ Age Edit   Ⓜ Maternity Edit   ♀ Female Only   ♂ Male Only   Ⓐ-Ⓨ OPPS Status Indicators   © 2021 Optum360, LLC

G9247 Patient had at least one medical visit in each 6 month period of the 24 month measurement period, with a minimum of 60 days between medical visits ☒

G9250 Documentation of patient pain brought to a comfortable level within 48 hours from initial assessment ☒

G9251 Documentation of patient with pain not brought to a comfortable level within 48 hours from initial assessment ☒

G9254 Documentation of patient discharged to home later than post-operative day 2 following CAS ☒

G9255 Documentation of patient discharged to home no later than post operative day 2 following CAS ☒

G9267 ~~Documentation of patient with one or more complications or mortality within 30 days~~

G9268 ~~Documentation of patient with one or more complications within 90 days~~

G9269 ~~Documentation of patient without one or more complications and without mortality within 30 days~~

G9270 ~~Documentation of patient without one or more complications within 90 days~~

G9273 Blood pressure has a systolic value of < 140 and a diastolic value of < 90 ☒

G9274 Blood pressure has a systolic value of = 140 and a diastolic value of = 90 or systolic value < 140 and diastolic value = 90 or systolic value = 140 and diastolic value < 90 ☒

G9275 Documentation that patient is a current nontobacco user ☒

G9276 Documentation that patient is a current tobacco user ☒

G9277 Documentation that the patient is on daily aspirin or antiplatelet or has documentation of a valid contraindication or exception to aspirin/antiplatelet; contraindications/exceptions include anticoagulant use, allergy to aspirin or antiplatelets, history of gastrointestinal bleed and bleeding disorder. Additionally, the following exceptions documented by the physician as a reason for not taking daily aspirin or antiplatelet are acceptable (use of nonsteroidal anti-inflammatory agents, documented risk for drug interaction, uncontrolled hypertension defined as > 180 systolic or > 110 diastolic or gastroesophageal reflux) ☒

G9278 Documentation that the patient is not on daily aspirin or antiplatelet regimen ☒

G9279 Pneumococcal screening performed and documentation of vaccination received prior to discharge ☒

G9280 Pneumococcal vaccination not administered prior to discharge, reason not specified ☒

G9281 Screening performed and documentation that vaccination not indicated/patient refusal ☒

G9282 Documentation of medical reason(s) for not reporting the histological type or NSCLC-NOS classification with an explanation (e.g., biopsy taken for other purposes in a patient with a history of nonsmall cell lung cancer or other documented medical reasons) ☒

G9283 Nonsmall cell lung cancer biopsy and cytology specimen report documents classification into specific histologic type or classified as NSCLC-NOS with an explanation ☒

G9284 Nonsmall cell lung cancer biopsy and cytology specimen report does not document classification into specific histologic type or classified as NSCLC-NOS with an explanation ☒

G9285 Specimen site other than anatomic location of lung or is not classified as nonsmall cell lung cancer ☒

G9286 Antibiotic regimen prescribed within 10 days after onset of symptoms ☒

G9287 Antibiotic regimen not prescribed within 10 days after onset of symptoms ☒

G9288 Documentation of medical reason(s) for not reporting the histological type or NSCLC-NOS classification with an explanation (e.g., a solitary fibrous tumor in a person with a history of nonsmall cell carcinoma or other documented medical reasons) ☒

G9289 Nonsmall cell lung cancer biopsy and cytology specimen report documents classification into specific histologic type or classified as NSCLC-NOS with an explanation ☒

G9290 Nonsmall cell lung cancer biopsy and cytology specimen report does not document classification into specific histologic type or classified as NSCLC-NOS with an explanation ☒

G9291 Specimen site other than anatomic location of lung, is not classified as nonsmall cell lung cancer or classified as NSCLC-NOS ☒

G9292 Documentation of medical reason(s) for not reporting PT category and a statement on thickness and ulceration and for PT1, mitotic rate (e.g., negative skin biopsies in a patient with a history of melanoma or other documented medical reasons) ☒

G9293 Pathology report does not include the PT category and a statement on thickness and ulceration and for PT1, mitotic rate ☒

G9294 Pathology report includes the PT category and a statement on thickness and ulceration and for PT1, mitotic rate ☒

G9295 Specimen site other than anatomic cutaneous location ☒

G9296 Patients with documented shared decision-making including discussion of conservative (nonsurgical) therapy (e.g., NSAIDs, analgesics, weight loss, exercise, injections) prior to the procedure ☒

G9297 Shared decision-making including discussion of conservative (nonsurgical) therapy (e.g., NSAIDs, analgesics, weight loss, exercise, injections) prior to the procedure, not documented, reason not given ☒

G9298 Patients who are evaluated for venous thromboembolic and cardiovascular risk factors within 30 days prior to the procedure (e.g., history of DVT, PE, MI, arrhythmia and stroke) ☒

G9299 Patients who are not evaluated for venous thromboembolic and cardiovascular risk factors within 30 days prior to the procedure (e.g., history of DVT, PE, MI, arrhythmia and stroke, reason not given) ☒

G9305 Intervention for presence of leak of endoluminal contents through an anastomosis not required ☒

G9306 Intervention for presence of leak of endoluminal contents through an anastomosis required ☒

G9307 No return to the operating room for a surgical procedure, for complications of the principal operative procedure, within 30 days of the principal operative procedure ☒

G9308 Unplanned return to the operating room for a surgical procedure, for complications of the principal operative procedure, within 30 days of the principal operative procedure ☒

G9309 No unplanned hospital readmission within 30 days of principal procedure ☒

G9310 Unplanned hospital readmission within 30 days of principal procedure ☒

G9311 No surgical site infection ☒

G9312 Surgical site infection ☒

Special Coverage Instructions   Noncovered by Medicare   Carrier Discretion   ☑ Quantity Alert   ● New Code   ○ Recycled/Reinstated   ▲ Revised Code

© 2021 Optum360, LLC   A2–Z3 ASC Pmt   CMS: IOM   AHA: Coding Clinic   ⅀ DMEPOS Paid   ⊘ SNF Excluded   G Codes — 71

G9313 Amoxicillin, with or without clavulanate, not prescribed as first line antibiotic at the time of diagnosis for documented reason Ⓜ

G9314 Amoxicillin, with or without clavulanate, not prescribed as first line antibiotic at the time of diagnosis, reason not given Ⓜ

G9315 Documentation amoxicillin, with or without clavulanate, prescribed as a first line antibiotic at the time of diagnosis Ⓜ

G9316 Documentation of patient-specific risk assessment with a risk calculator based on multi-institutional clinical data, the specific risk calculator used, and communication of risk assessment from risk calculator with the patient or family Ⓜ

G9317 Documentation of patient-specific risk assessment with a risk calculator based on multi-institutional clinical data, the specific risk calculator used, and communication of risk assessment from risk calculator with the patient or family not completed Ⓜ

G9318 Imaging study named according to standardized nomenclature Ⓜ

G9319 Imaging study not named according to standardized nomenclature, reason not given Ⓜ

G9321 Count of previous CT (any type of CT) and cardiac nuclear medicine (myocardial perfusion) studies documented in the 12-month period prior to the current study Ⓜ

G9322 Count of previous CT and cardiac nuclear medicine (myocardial perfusion) studies not documented in the 12-month period prior to the current study, reason not given Ⓜ

G9341 Search conducted for prior patient CT studies completed at nonaffiliated external health care facilities or entities within the past 12-months and are available through a secure, authorized, media-free, shared archive prior to an imaging study being performed Ⓜ

G9342 Search not conducted prior to an imaging study being performed for prior patient CT studies completed at nonaffiliated external health care facilities or entities within the past 12 months and are available through a secure, authorized, media-free, shared archive, reason not given Ⓜ

G9344 Due to system reasons search not conducted for DICOM format images for prior patient CT imaging studies completed at nonaffiliated external health care facilities or entities within the past 12 months that are available through a secure, authorized, media-free, shared archive (e.g., nonaffiliated external health care facilities or entities does not have archival abilities through a shared archival system) Ⓜ

G9345 Follow-up recommendations documented according to recommended guidelines for incidentally detected pulmonary nodules (e.g., follow-up CT imaging studies needed or that no follow-up is needed) based at a minimum on nodule size and patient risk factors Ⓜ

G9347 Follow-up recommendations not documented according to recommended guidelines for incidentally detected pulmonary nodules, reason not given Ⓜ

G9348 ~~CT scan of the paranasal sinuses ordered at the time of diagnosis for documented reasons~~

G9349 ~~CT scan of the paranasal sinuses ordered at the time of diagnosis or received within 28 days after date of diagnosis~~

G9350 ~~CT scan of the paranasal sinuses not ordered at the time of diagnosis or received within 28 days after date of diagnosis~~

G9351 More than one CT scan of the paranasal sinuses ordered or received within 90 days after diagnosis Ⓜ

G9352 More than one CT scan of the paranasal sinuses ordered or received within 90 days after the date of diagnosis, reason not given Ⓜ

G9353 More than one CT scan of the paranasal sinuses ordered or received within 90 days after the date of diagnosis for documented reasons (e.g., patients with complications, second CT obtained prior to surgery, other medical reasons) Ⓜ

G9354 One CT scan or no CT scan of the paranasal sinuses ordered within 90 days after the date of diagnosis Ⓜ

▲ **G9355** Elective delivery (without medical indication) by Cesarean birth or induction of labor not performed (<39 weeks of gestation) Ⓜ

▲ **G9356** Elective delivery (without medical indication) by Cesarean birth or induction of labor performed (<39 weeks of gestation) Ⓜ

G9357 Post-partum screenings, evaluations and education performed Ⓜ

G9358 Post-partum screenings, evaluations and education not performed Ⓜ

▲ **G9359** Documentation of negative or managed positive TB screen with further evidence that TB is not active prior to treatment with a biologic immune response modifier Ⓜ

G9360 No documentation of negative or managed positive TB screen Ⓜ

▲ **G9361** Medical indication for delivery by Cesarean birth or induction of labor (<39 weeks of gestation) [documentation of reason(s) for elective delivery (e.g., hemorrhage and placental complications, hypertension, preeclampsia and eclampsia, rupture of membranes (premature or prolonged), maternal conditions complicating pregnancy/delivery, fetal conditions complicating pregnancy/delivery, late pregnancy, prior uterine surgery, or participation in clinical trial)] Ⓜ

G9364 Sinusitis caused by, or presumed to be caused by, bacterial infection Ⓜ

▲ **G9367** At least two orders for high risk medications from the same drug class Ⓜ

▲ **G9368** At least two orders for high risk medications from the same drug class not ordered Ⓜ

G9380 Patient offered assistance with end of life issues during the measurement period Ⓜ

G9382 Patient not offered assistance with end of life issues during the measurement period Ⓜ

G9383 Patient received screening for HCV infection within the 12 month reporting period Ⓜ

G9384 Documentation of medical reason(s) for not receiving annual screening for HCV infection (e.g., decompensated cirrhosis indicating advanced disease [i.e., ascites, esophageal variceal bleeding, hepatic encephalopathy], hepatocellular carcinoma, waitlist for organ transplant, limited life expectancy, other medical reasons) Ⓜ

G9385 Documentation of patient reason(s) for not receiving annual screening for HCV infection (e.g., patient declined, other patient reasons) Ⓜ

G9386 Screening for HCV infection not received within the twelve-month reporting period, reason not given Ⓜ

G9393 Patient with an initial PHQ-9 score greater than nine who achieves remission at twelve months as demonstrated by a twelve-month (+/- 30 days) PHQ-9 score of less than five Ⓜ

G9394 Patient who had a diagnosis of bipolar disorder or personality disorder, death, permanent nursing home resident or receiving hospice or palliative care any time during the measurement or assessment period Ⓜ

Special Coverage Instructions   Noncovered by Medicare   Carrier Discretion   ☑ Quantity Alert ● New Code   ○ Recycled/Reinstated   ▲ Revised Code

72 — G Codes   Ⓐ Age Edit   Ⓜ Maternity Edit   ♀ Female Only   ♂ Male Only   Ⓐ-Ⓨ OPPS Status Indicators   © 2021 Optum360, LLC

G9395 Patient with an initial PHQ-9 score greater than nine who did not achieve remission at twelve months as demonstrated by a twelve-month (+/- 30 days) PHQ-9 score greater than or equal to five Ⓜ

G9396 Patient with an initial PHQ-9 score greater than nine who was not assessed for remission at twelve months (+/- 30 days) Ⓜ

G9399 ~~Documentation in the patient record of a discussion between the physician/clinician and the patient that includes all of the following: treatment choices appropriate to genotype, risks and benefits, evidence of effectiveness, and patient preferences toward the outcome of the treatment~~

G9400 ~~Documentation of medical or patient reason(s) for not discussing treatment options; medical reasons: patient is not a candidate for treatment due to advanced physical or mental health comorbidity (including active substance use); currently receiving antiviral treatment; successful antiviral treatment (with sustained virologic response) prior to reporting period; other documented medical reasons; patient reasons: patient unable or unwilling to participate in the discussion or other patient reasons~~

G9401 ~~No documentation in the patient record of a discussion between the physician or other qualfied healthcare professional and the patient that includes all of the following: treatment choices appropriate to genotype, risks and benefits, evidence of effectiveness, and patient preferences toward treatment~~

G9402 Patient received follow-up within 30 days after discharge Ⓜ

G9403 Clinician documented reason patient was not able to complete 30-day follow-up from acute inpatient setting discharge (e.g., patient death prior to follow-up visit, patient noncompliant for visit follow-up) Ⓜ

G9404 Patient did not receive follow-up on the date of discharge or within 30 days after discharge Ⓜ

G9405 Patient received follow up within 7 days after discharge Ⓜ

G9406 Clinician documented reason patient was not able to complete 7-day follow-up from acute inpatient setting discharge (i.e., patient death prior to follow-up visit, patient noncompliance for visit follow-up) Ⓜ

G9407 Patient did not receive follow-up on or within 7 days after discharge Ⓜ

G9408 Patients with cardiac tamponade and/or pericardiocentesis occurring within 30 days Ⓜ

G9409 Patients without cardiac tamponade and/or pericardiocentesis occurring within 30 days Ⓜ

G9410 Patient admitted within 180 days, status post CIED implantation, replacement, or revision with an infection requiring device removal or surgical revision Ⓜ

G9411 Patient not admitted within 180 days, status post CIED implantation, replacement, or revision with an infection requiring device removal or surgical revision Ⓜ

G9412 Patient admitted within 180 days, status post CIED implantation, replacement, or revision with an infection requiring device removal or surgical revision Ⓜ

G9413 Patient not admitted within 180 days, status post CIED implantation, replacement, or revision with an infection requiring device removal or surgical revision Ⓜ

G9414 Patient had one dose of meningococcal vaccine (serogroups A, C, W, Y) on or between the patient's 11th and 13th birthdays Ⓜ

G9415 Patient did not have one dose of meningococcal vaccine (serogroups A, C, W, Y) on or between the patient's 11th and 13th birthdays Ⓜ

G9416 Patient had one tetanus, diphtheria toxoids and acellular pertussis vaccine (TDaP) on or between the patient's 10th and 13th birthdays Ⓜ

G9417 Patient did not have one tetanus, diphtheria toxoids and acellular pertussis vaccine (TDaP) on or between the patient's 10th and 13th birthdays Ⓜ

▲ **G9418** Primary nonsmall cell lung cancer biopsy and cytology specimen report documents classification into specific histologic type following IASLC guidance or classified as NSCLC-NOS with an explanation Ⓜ

▲ **G9419** Documentation of medical reason(s) for not including the histological type or NSCLC-NOS classification with an explanation (e.g. specimen insufficient or non-diagnostic, specimen does not contain cancer, or other documented medical reasons) Ⓜ

G9420 Specimen site other than anatomic location of lung or is not classified as primary nonsmall cell lung cancer Ⓜ

▲ **G9421** Primary nonsmall cell lung cancer lung biopsy and cytology specimen report does not document classification into specific histologic type or histologic type does not follow IASLC guidance or is classified as NSCLC-NOS but without an explanation Ⓜ

▲ **G9422** Primary lung carcinoma resection report documents PT category, PN category and for nonsmall cell lung cancer, histologic type (e.g., squamous cell carcinoma, adenocarcinoma and not NSCLC-NOS) Ⓜ

G9423 Documentation of medical reason for not including PT category, PN category and histologic type (for patient with appropriate exclusion criteria [e.g., metastatic disease, benign tumors, malignant tumors other than carcinomas, inadequate surgical specimens]) Ⓜ

G9424 Specimen site other than anatomic location of lung, or classified as NSCLC-NOS Ⓜ

▲ **G9425** Primary lung carcinoma resection report does not document PT category, PN category and for nonsmall cell lung cancer, histologic type (e.g., squamous cell carcinoma, adenocarcinoma) Ⓜ

G9426 Improvement in median time from ED arrival to initial ED oral or parenteral pain medication administration performed for ED admitted patients Ⓜ

G9427 Improvement in median time from ED arrival to initial ED oral or parenteral pain medication administration not performed for ED admitted patients Ⓜ

▲ **G9428** Pathology report includes the PT category, thickness, ulceration and mitotic rate, peripheral and deep margin status and presence or absence of microsatellitosis for invasive tumors Ⓜ

▲ **G9429** Documentation of medical reason(s) for not including PT category, thickness, ulceration and mitotic rate, peripheral and deep margin status and presence or absence of microsatellitosis for invasive tumors (e.g., negative skin biopsies, insufficient tissue, or other documented medical reasons) Ⓜ

G9430 Specimen site other than anatomic cutaneous location Ⓜ

▲ **G9431** Pathology report does not include the PT category, thickness, ulceration and mitotic rate, peripheral and deep margin status and presence or absence of microsatellitosis for invasive tumors Ⓜ

G9432 Asthma well-controlled based on the ACT, C-ACT, ACQ, or ATAQ score and results documented Ⓜ

G9434 Asthma not well-controlled based on the ACT, C-ACT, ACQ, or ATAQ score, or specified asthma control tool not used, reason not given Ⓜ

G9448 ~~Patients who were born in the years 1945 to 1965~~

Special Coverage Instructions Noncovered by Medicare Carrier Discretion ☑ Quantity Alert ● New Code ○ Recycled/Reinstated ▲ Revised Code

G9449 ~~History of receiving blood transfusions prior to 1992~~

G9450 ~~History of injection drug use~~

G9451 Patient received one-time screening for HCV infection Ⓜ

G9452 Documentation of medical reason(s) for not receiving one-time screening for HCV infection (e.g., decompensated cirrhosis indicating advanced disease [i.e., ascites, esophageal variceal bleeding, hepatic encephalopathy], hepatocellular carcinoma, waitlist for organ transplant, limited life expectancy, other medical reasons) Ⓜ

G9453 Documentation of patient reason(s) for not receiving one-time screening for HCV infection (e.g., patient declined, other patient reasons) Ⓜ

G9454 One-time screening for HCV infection not received within 12-month reporting period and no documentation of prior screening for HCV infection, reason not given Ⓜ

G9455 Patient underwent abdominal imaging with ultrasound, contrast enhanced CT or contrast MRI for HCC Ⓜ

G9456 Documentation of medical or patient reason(s) for not ordering or performing screening for HCC. Medical reason: comorbid medical conditions with expected survival < 5 years, hepatic decompensation and not a candidate for liver transplantation, or other medical reasons; patient reasons: patient declined or other patient reasons (e.g., cost of tests, time related to accessing testing equipment) Ⓜ

G9457 Patient did not undergo abdominal imaging and did not have a documented reason for not undergoing abdominal imaging in the submission period Ⓜ

G9458 Patient documented as tobacco user and received tobacco cessation intervention (must include at least one of the following: advice given to quit smoking or tobacco use, counseling on the benefits of quitting smoking or tobacco use, assistance with or referral to external smoking or tobacco cessation support programs, or current enrollment in smoking or tobacco use cessation program) if identified as a tobacco user Ⓜ

G9459 Currently a tobacco nonuser Ⓜ

G9460 Tobacco assessment or tobacco cessation intervention not performed, reason not given Ⓜ

G9468 Patient not receiving corticosteroids greater than or equal to 10 mg/day of prednisone equivalents for 60 or greater consecutive days or a single prescription equating to 600 mg prednisone or greater for all fills Ⓜ

G9470 Patients not receiving corticosteroids greater than or equal to 10 mg/day of prednisone equivalents for 60 or greater consecutive days or a single prescription equating to 600 mg prednisone or greater for all fills Ⓜ

G9471 Within the past 2 years, central dual-energy x-ray absorptiometry (DXA) not ordered or documented Ⓜ

Hospice Services

G9473 Services performed by chaplain in the hospice setting, each 15 minutes Ⓑ

G9474 Services performed by dietary counselor in the hospice setting, each 15 minutes Ⓑ

G9475 Services performed by other counselor in the hospice setting, each 15 minutes Ⓑ

G9476 Services performed by volunteer in the hospice setting, each 15 minutes Ⓑ

G9477 Services performed by care coordinator in the hospice setting, each 15 minutes Ⓑ

G9478 Services performed by other qualified therapist in the hospice setting, each 15 minutes Ⓑ

G9479 Services performed by qualified pharmacist in the hospice setting, each 15 minutes Ⓑ

Medicare Care Choice Model Program

G9480 Admission to Medicare Care Choice Model Program (MCCM) Ⓑ

CMS Innovation Center Demonstration Project

G9481 Remote in-home visit for the evaluation and management of a new patient for use only in a Medicare-approved CMS Innovation Center Demonstration Project, which requires these three key components: a problem focused history; a problem focused examination; straightforward medical decision making, furnished in real time using interactive audio and video technology. Counseling and coordination of care with other physicians, other qualified health care professionals or agencies are provided consistent with the nature of the problem(s) and the needs of the patient or the family or both. Usually, the presenting problem(s) are self limited or minor. Typically, 10 minutes are spent with the patient or family or both via real time, audio and video intercommunications technology Ⓑ

G9482 Remote in-home visit for the evaluation and management of a new patient for use only in a Medicare-approved CMS Innovation Center Demonstration Project, which requires these three key components: an expanded problem focused history; an expanded problem focused examination; straightforward medical decision making, furnished in real time using interactive audio and video technology. Counseling and coordination of care with other physicians, other qualified health care professionals or agencies are provided consistent with the nature of the problem(s) and the needs of the patient or the family or both. Usually, the presenting problem(s) are of low to moderate severity. Typically, 20 minutes are spent with the patient or family or both via real time, audio and video intercommunications technology Ⓑ

G9483 Remote in-home visit for the evaluation and management of a new patient for use only in a Medicare-approved CMS Innovation Center Demonstration Project, which requires these three key components: a detailed history; a detailed examination; medical decision making of low complexity, furnished in real time using interactive audio and video technology. Counseling and coordination of care with other physicians, other qualified health care professionals or agencies are provided consistent with the nature of the problem(s) and the needs of the patient or the family or both. Usually, the presenting problem(s) are of moderate severity. Typically, 30 minutes are spent with the patient or family or both via real time, audio and video intercommunications technology Ⓑ

G9484 Remote in-home visit for the evaluation and management of a new patient for use only in a Medicare-approved CMS Innovation Center Demonstration Project, which requires these three key components: a comprehensive history; a comprehensive examination; medical decision making of moderate complexity, furnished in real time using interactive audio and video technology. Counseling and coordination of care with other physicians, other qualified health care professionals or agencies are provided consistent with the nature of the problem(s) and the needs of the patient or the family or both. Usually, the presenting problem(s) are of moderate to high severity. Typically, 45 minutes are spent with the patient or family or both via real time, audio and video intercommunications technology Ⓑ

Special Coverage Instructions   Noncovered by Medicare   Carrier Discretion   ☑ Quantity Alert   ● New Code   ○ Recycled/Reinstated   ▲ Revised Code

74 — G Codes   Ⓐ Age Edit   Ⓜ Maternity Edit   ♀ Female Only   ♂ Male Only   Ⓐ-Ⓨ OPPS Status Indicators   © 2021 Optum360, LLC

G9485 Remote in-home visit for the evaluation and management of a new patient for use only in a Medicare-approved CMS Innovation Center Demonstration Project, which requires these three key components: a comprehensive history; a comprehensive examination; medical decision making of high complexity, furnished in real time using interactive audio and video technology. Counseling and coordination of care with other physicians, other qualified health care professionals or agencies are provided consistent with the nature of the problem(s) and the needs of the patient or the family or both. Usually, the presenting problem(s) are of moderate to high severity. Typically, 60 minutes are spent with the patient or family or both via real time, audio and video intercommunications technology ☐B

G9486 Remote in-home visit for the evaluation and management of an established patient for use only in a Medicare-approved CMS Innovation Center Demonstration Project, which requires at least two of the following three key components: a problem focused history; a problem focused examination; straightforward medical decision making, furnished in real time using interactive audio and video technology. Counseling and coordination of care with other physicians, other qualified health care professionals or agencies are provided consistent with the nature of the problem(s) and the needs of the patient or the family or both. Usually, the presenting problem(s) are self limited or minor. Typically, 10 minutes are spent with the patient or family or both via real time, audio and video intercommunications technology ☐B

G9487 Remote in-home visit for the evaluation and management of an established patient for use only in a Medicare-approved CMS Innovation Center Demonstration Project, which requires at least two of the following three key components: an expanded problem focused history; an expanded problem focused examination; medical decision making of low complexity, furnished in real time using interactive audio and video technology. Counseling and coordination of care with other physicians, other qualified health care professionals or agencies are provided consistent with the nature of the problem(s) and the needs of the patient or the family or both. Usually, the presenting problem(s) are of low to moderate severity. Typically, 15 minutes are spent with the patient or family or both via real time, audio and video intercommunications technology ☐B

G9488 Remote in-home visit for the evaluation and management of an established patient for use only in a Medicare-approved CMS Innovation Center Demonstration Project, which requires at least two of the following three key components: a detailed history; a detailed examination; medical decision making of moderate complexity, furnished in real time using interactive audio and video technology. Counseling and coordination of care with other physicians, other qualified health care professionals or agencies are provided consistent with the nature of the problem(s) and the needs of the patient or the family or both. Usually, the presenting problem(s) are of moderate to high severity. Typically, 25 minutes are spent with the patient or family or both via real time, audio and video intercommunications technology ☐B

G9489 Remote in-home visit for the evaluation and management of an established patient for use only in a Medicare-approved CMS Innovation Center Demonstration Project, which requires at least two of the following three key components: a comprehensive history; a comprehensive examination; medical decision making of high complexity, furnished in real time using interactive audio and video technology. Counseling and coordination of care with other physicians, other qualified health care professionals or agencies are provided consistent with the nature of the problem(s) and the needs of the patient or the family or both. Usually, the presenting problem(s) are of moderate to high severity. Typically, 40 minutes are spent with the patient or family or both via real time, audio and video intercommunications technology ☐B

G9490 CMS Innovation Center Models, home visit for patient assessment performed by clinical staff for an individual not considered homebound, including, but not necessarily limited to patient assessment of clinical status, safety/fall prevention, functional status/ambulation, medication reconciliation/management, compliance with orders/plan of care, performance of activities of daily living, and ensuring beneficiary connections to community and other services. (For use only in Medicare-approved CMS Innovation Center Models); may not be billed for a 30 day period covered by a transitional care management code ☐B

Quality Measures

G9497 Received instruction from the anesthesiologist or proxy prior to the day of surgery to abstain from smoking on the day of surgery Ⓜ

G9498 Antibiotic regimen prescribed Ⓜ

G9500 Radiation exposure indices, or exposure time and number of fluorographic images in final report for procedures using fluoroscopy, documented Ⓜ

G9501 Radiation exposure indices, or exposure time and number of fluorographic images not documented in final report for procedure using fluoroscopy, reason not given Ⓜ

G9502 Documentation of medical reason for not performing foot exam (i.e., patients who have had either a bilateral amputation above or below the knee, or both a left and right amputation above or below the knee before or during the measurement period) Ⓜ

G9504 Documented reason for not assessing hepatitis B virus (HBV) status (e.g., patient not initiating anti-TNF therapy, patient declined) prior to initiating anti-TNF therapy Ⓜ

G9505 Antibiotic regimen prescribed within 10 days after onset of symptoms for documented medical reason Ⓜ

G9506 Biologic immune response modifier prescribed Ⓜ

G9507 Documentation that the patient is on a statin medication or has documentation of a valid contraindication or exception to statin medications; contraindications/exceptions that can be defined by diagnosis codes include pregnancy during the measurement period, active liver disease, rhabdomyolysis, end stage renal disease on dialysis and heart failure; provider documented contraindications/exceptions include breastfeeding during the measurement period, woman of child-bearing age not actively taking birth control, allergy to statin, drug interaction (HIV protease inhibitors, nefazodone, cyclosporine, gemfibrozil, and danazol) and intolerance (with supporting documentation of trying a statin at least once within the last 5 years or diagnosis codes for myostitis or toxic myopathy related to drugs) Ⓜ

G9508 Documentation that the patient is not on a statin medication Ⓜ

Special Coverage Instructions   Noncovered by Medicare   Carrier Discretion   ☑ Quantity Alert ● New Code ○ Recycled/Reinstated ▲ Revised Code

© 2021 Optum360, LLC   A2-Z3 ASC Pmt   CMS: IOM   AHA: Coding Clinic   DMEPOS Paid   ⊘ SNF Excluded   G Codes — 75

Procedures/Professional Services (Temporary)

G9509 — G9582

G9509 Adult patients 18 years of age or older with major depression or dysthymia who reached remission at twelve months as demonstrated by a twelve-month (+/-60 days) PHQ-9 or PHQ-9M score of less than 5

G9510 Adult patients 18 years of age or older with major depression or dysthymia who did not reach remission at 12 months as demonstrated by a 12 month (+/-60 days) PHQ-9 or PHQ-9M score of less than 5. Either PHQ-9 or PHQ-9M score was not assessed or is greater than or equal to 5 Ⓜ

G9511 Index PHQ-9 or PHQ-9M score greater than 9 documented during the twelve-month denominator identification period Ⓜ

G9512 Individual had a PDC of 0.8 or greater Ⓜ

G9513 Individual did not have a PDC of 0.8 or greater Ⓜ

G9514 Patient required a return to the operating room within 90 days of surgery Ⓜ

G9515 Patient did not require a return to the operating room within 90 days of surgery Ⓜ

G9516 Patient achieved an improvement in visual acuity, from their preoperative level, within 90 days of surgery Ⓜ

G9517 Patient did not achieve an improvement in visual acuity, from their preoperative level, within 90 days of surgery, reason not given Ⓜ

G9518 Documentation of active injection drug use Ⓜ

G9519 Patient achieves final refraction (spherical equivalent) +/- 1.0 diopters of their planned refraction within 90 days of surgery Ⓜ

G9520 Patient does not achieve final refraction (spherical equivalent) +/- 1.0 diopters of their planned refraction within 90 days of surgery Ⓜ

G9521 Total number of emergency department visits and inpatient hospitalizations less than two in the past 12 months Ⓜ

G9522 Total number of emergency department visits and inpatient hospitalizations equal to or greater than two in the past 12 months or patient not screened, reason not given Ⓜ

Blunt Head Trauma

G9529 Patient with minor blunt head trauma had an appropriate indication(s) for a head CT Ⓜ

G9530 Patient presented with a minor blunt head trauma and had a head CT ordered for trauma by an emergency care provider Ⓜ

G9531 Patient has documentation of ventricular shunt, brain tumor, multisystem trauma, or is currently taking an antiplatelet medication including: abciximab, anagrelide, cangrelor, cilostazol, clopidogrel, dipyridamole, eptifibatide, prasugrel, ticlopidine, ticagrelor, tirofiban, or vorapaxar Ⓜ

G9533 Patient with minor blunt head trauma did not have an appropriate indication(s) for a head CT Ⓜ

Miscellaneous Quality Measures

G9537 Imaging needed as part of a clinical trial; or other clinician ordered the study Ⓜ

G9539 Intent for potential removal at time of placement Ⓜ

G9540 Patient alive 3 months post procedure Ⓜ

G9541 Filter removed within 3 months of placement Ⓜ

G9542 Documented reassessment for the appropriateness of filter removal within 3 months of placement Ⓜ

G9543 Documentation of at least two attempts to reach the patient to arrange a clinical reassessment for the appropriateness of filter removal within 3 months of placement Ⓜ

G9544 Patients that do not have the filter removed, documented reassessment for the appropriateness of filter removal, or documentation of at least two attempts to reach the patient to arrange a clinical reassessment for the appropriateness of filter removal within 3 months of placement Ⓜ

G9547 Cystic renal lesion that is simple appearing (Bosniak I or II), or adrenal lesion less than or equal to 1.0 cm or adrenal lesion greater than 1.0 cm but less than or equal to 4.0 cm classified as likely benign by unenhanced CT or washout protocol CT, or MRI with in- and opposed-phase sequences or other equivalent institutional imaging protocols Ⓜ

G9548 Final reports for imaging studies stating no follow up imaging is recommended Ⓜ

G9549 Documentation of medical reason(s) that follow up imaging is indicated (e.g., patient has lymphadenopathy, signs of metastasis or an active diagnosis or history of cancer, and other medical reason(s)) Ⓜ

G9550 Final reports for imaging studies with follow-up imaging recommended, or final reports that do not include a specific recommendation of no follow-up Ⓜ

G9551 Final reports for imaging studies without an incidentally found lesion noted Ⓜ

G9552 Incidental thyroid nodule < 1.0 cm noted in report Ⓜ

G9553 Prior thyroid disease diagnosis Ⓜ

▲ **G9554** Final reports for CT, CTA, MRI or MRA of the chest or neck with follow-up imaging recommended Ⓜ

G9555 Documentation of medical reason(s) for recommending follow up imaging (e.g., patient has multiple endocrine neoplasia, patient has cervical lymphadenopathy, other medical reason(s)) Ⓜ

▲ **G9556** Final reports for CT, CTA, MRI or MRA of the chest or neck with follow-up imaging not recommended Ⓜ

▲ **G9557** Final reports for CT, CTA, MRI or MRA studies of the chest or neck without an incidentally found thyroid nodule < 1.0 cm noted or no nodule found Ⓜ

Opiate Therapy

G9561 ~~Patients prescribed opiates for longer than six weeks~~

G9562 ~~Patients who had a follow-up evaluation conducted at least every three months during opioid therapy~~

G9563 ~~Patients who did not have a follow-up evaluation conducted at least every three months during opioid therapy~~

G9577 ~~Patients prescribed opiates for longer than six weeks~~

G9578 ~~Documentation of signed opioid treatment agreement at least once during opioid therapy~~

G9579 ~~No documentation of a signed opioid treatment agreement at least once during opioid therapy~~

Stroke Therapy

▲ **G9580** Door to puncture time of 90 minutes or less Ⓜ

▲ **G9582** Door to puncture time of greater than 90 minutes, no reason given Ⓜ

Opiate Therapy

G9583 ~~Patients prescribed opiates for longer than six weeks~~

G9584 ~~Patient evaluated for risk of misuse of opiates by using a brief validated instrument (e.g., opioid risk tool, SOAPP-R) or patient interviewed at least once during opioid therapy~~

G9585 ~~Patient not evaluated for risk of misuse of opiates by using a brief validated instrument (e.g., opioid risk tool, SOAAP-R) or patient not interviewed at least once during opioid therapy~~

Blunt Head Trauma

G9593 Pediatric patient with minor blunt head trauma classified as low risk according to the PECARN prediction rules ☒

G9594 Patient presented with a minor blunt head trauma and had a head CT ordered for trauma by an emergency care provider ☒

G9595 Patient has documentation of ventricular shunt, brain tumor, or coagulopathy ☒

G9596 Pediatric patient had a head CT for trauma ordered by someone other than an emergency care provider or was ordered for a reason other than trauma ☒

G9597 Pediatric patient with minor blunt head trauma not classified as low risk according to the PECARN prediction rules ☒

Aortic Aneurysm

G9598 Aortic aneurysm 5.5-5.9 cm maximum diameter on centerline formatted CT or minor diameter on axial formatted CT ☒

G9599 Aortic aneurysm 6.0 cm or greater maximum diameter on centerline formatted CT or minor diameter on axial formatted CT ☒

Patient Survey

G9603 Patient survey score improved from baseline following treatment ☒

G9604 Patient survey results not available ☒

G9605 Patient survey score did not improve from baseline following treatment ☒

Intraoperative Cystoscopy

G9606 Intraoperative cystoscopy performed to evaluate for lower tract injury ☒

G9607 Documented medical reasons for not performing intraoperative cystoscopy (e.g., urethral pathology precluding cystoscopy, any patient who has a congenital or acquired absence of the urethra) or in the case of patient death ☒

G9608 Intraoperative cystoscopy not performed to evaluate for lower tract injury ☒

Aspirin/Antiplatelet Therapy

G9609 Documentation of an order for antiplatelet agents ☒

G9610 Documentation of medical reason(s) in the patient's record for not ordering antiplatelet agents ☒

G9611 Order for antiplatelet agents was not documented in the patient's record, reason not given ☒

Colonoscopy Documentation

G9612 Photodocumentation of two or more cecal landmarks to establish a complete examination ☒

G9613 Documentation of postsurgical anatomy (e.g., right hemicolectomy, ileocecal resection, etc.) ☒

G9614 Photodocumentation of less than two cecal landmarks (i.e., no cecal landmarks or only one cecal landmark) to establish a complete examination ☒

Uterine Malignancy Screening

G9618 Documentation of screening for uterine malignancy or those that had an ultrasound and/or endometrial sampling of any kind ♀☒

G9620 Patient not screened for uterine malignancy, or those that have not had an ultrasound and/or endometrial sampling of any kind, reason not given ♀☒

Alcohol Use

G9621 Patient identified as an unhealthy alcohol user when screened for unhealthy alcohol use using a systematic screening method and received brief counseling ☒

G9622 Patient not identified as an unhealthy alcohol user when screened for unhealthy alcohol use using a systematic screening method ☒

G9623 Documentation of medical reason(s) for not screening for unhealthy alcohol use (e.g., limited life expectancy, other medical reasons) ☒

G9624 Patient not screened for unhealthy alcohol use using a systematic screening method or patient did not receive brief counseling if identified as an unhealthy alcohol user, reason not given ☒

Bladder/Ureter Injury

G9625 Patient sustained bladder injury at the time of surgery or discovered subsequently up to 30 days post-surgery ☒

G9626 Documented medical reason for not reporting bladder injury (e.g., gynecologic or other pelvic malignancy documented, concurrent surgery involving bladder pathology, injury that occurs during urinary incontinence procedure, patient death from nonmedical causes not related to surgery, patient died during procedure without evidence of bladder injury) ☒

G9627 Patient did not sustain bladder injury at the time of surgery nor discovered subsequently up to 30 days post-surgery ☒

G9628 Patient sustained bowel injury at the time of surgery or discovered subsequently up to 30 days post-surgery ☒

G9629 Documented medical reasons for not reporting bowel injury (e.g., gynecologic or other pelvic malignancy documented, planned (e.g., not due to an unexpected bowel injury) resection and/or re-anastomosis of bowel, or patient death from nonmedical causes not related to surgery, patient died during procedure without evidence of bowel injury) ☒

G9630 Patient did not sustain a bowel injury at the time of surgery nor discovered subsequently up to 30 days post-surgery ☒

G9631 Patient sustained ureter injury at the time of surgery or discovered subsequently up to 30 days postsurgery ☒

G9632 Documented medical reasons for not reporting ureter injury (e.g., gynecologic or other pelvic malignancy documented, concurrent surgery involving bladder pathology, injury that occurs during a urinary incontinence procedure, patient death from nonmedical causes not related to surgery, patient died during procedure without evidence of ureter injury) ☒

G9633 Patient did not sustain ureter injury at the time of surgery nor discovered subsequently up to 30 days postsurgery ☒

Health-Related Quality of Life

G9634 ~~Health-related quality of life assessed with tool during at least two visits and quality of life score remained the same or improved~~

G9635 ~~Health-related quality of life not assessed with tool for documented reason(s) (e.g., patient has a cognitive or neuropsychiatric impairment that impairs his/her ability to complete the HRQOL survey, patient has the inability to read and/or write in order to complete the HRQOL questionnaire)~~

G9636 ~~Health-related quality of life not assessed with tool during at least two visits or quality of life score declined~~

Procedures/Professional Services (Temporary)

G9637 — G9684

Quality Measures

G9637 Final reports with documentation of one or more dose reduction techniques (e.g., automated exposure control, adjustment of the mA and/or kV according to patient size, use of iterative reconstruction technique) M

G9638 Final reports without documentation of one or more dose reduction techniques (e.g., automated exposure control, adjustment of the mA and/or kV according to patient size, use of iterative reconstruction technique) M

G9639 ~~Major amputation or open surgical bypass not required within 48 hours of the index endovascular lower extremity revascularization procedure~~

G9640 ~~Documentation of planned hybrid or staged procedure~~

G9641 ~~Major amputation or open surgical bypass required within 48 hours of the index endovascular lower extremity revascularization procedure~~

G9642 Current smoker (e.g., cigarette, cigar, pipe, e-cigarette or marijuana) M

G9643 Elective surgery M

G9644 Patients who abstained from smoking prior to anesthesia on the day of surgery or procedure M

G9645 Patients who did not abstain from smoking prior to anesthesia on the day of surgery or procedure M

G9646 Patients with 90 day MRS score of 0 to 2 M

G9647 ~~Patients in whom MRS score could not be obtained at 90 day follow-up~~

G9648 Patients with 90 day MRS score greater than 2 M

Psoriasis Therapy

G9649 Psoriasis assessment tool documented meeting any one of the specified benchmarks (e.g., (PGA; 5-point or 6-point scale), body surface area (BSA), psoriasis area and severity index (PASI) and/or dermatology life quality index (DLQI)) M

G9651 Psoriasis assessment tool documented not meeting any one of the specified benchmarks (e.g., (PGA; 5-point or 6-point scale), body surface area (BSA), psoriasis area and severity index (PASI) and/or dermatology life quality index (DLQI)) or psoriasis assessment tool not documented M

Anesthesia Services

G9654 Monitored anesthesia care (MAC) M

G9655 A transfer of care protocol or handoff tool/checklist that includes the required key handoff elements is used M

G9656 Patient transferred directly from anesthetizing location to PACU or other non-ICU location M

G9658 A transfer of care protocol or handoff tool/checklist that includes the required key handoff elements is not used M

Reason for Colonoscopy

G9659 Patients greater than or equal to 86 years of age who underwent a screening colonoscopy and did not have a history of colorectal cancer or other valid medical reason for the colonoscopy, including: iron deficiency anemia, lower gastrointestinal bleeding, Crohn's disease (i.e., regional enteritis), familial adenomatous polyposis, Lynch syndrome (i.e., hereditary nonpolyposis colorectal cancer), inflammatory bowel disease, ulcerative colitis, abnormal finding of gastrointestinal tract, or changes in bowel habits M

G9660 Documentation of medical reason(s) for a colonoscopy performed on a patient greater than or equal to 86 years of age (e.g., iron deficiency anemia, lower gastrointestinal bleeding, Crohn's disease (i.e., regional enteritis), familial history of adenomatous polyposis, Lynch syndrome (i.e., hereditary nonpolyposis colorectal cancer), inflammatory bowel disease, ulcerative colitis, abnormal finding of gastrointestinal tract, or changes in bowel habits) M

G9661 Patients greater than or equal to 86 years of age who received a colonoscopy for an assessment of signs/symptoms of GI tract illness, and/or because the patient meets high risk criteria, and/or to follow-up on previously diagnosed advanced lesions M

Statin Therapy

▲ **G9662** Previously diagnosed or have an active diagnosis of clinical ASCVD, including ASCVD procedure M

▲ **G9663** Any LDL-C laboratory test result >= 190 mg/dl M

G9664 Patients who are currently statin therapy users or received an order (prescription) for statin therapy M

G9665 Patients who are not currently statin therapy users or did not receive an order (prescription) for statin therapy M

G9666 ~~Patient's highest fasting or direct LDL-C laboratory test result in the measurement period or two years prior to the beginning of the measurement period is 70-189 mg/dl~~

Cardiovascular Measures

G9674 Patients with clinical ASCVD diagnosis M

G9675 Patients who have ever had a fasting or direct laboratory result of LDL-C = 190 mg/dl M

G9676 Patients aged 40 to 75 years at the beginning of the measurement period with type 1 or type 2 diabetes and with an ldl-c result of 70-189 mg/dl recorded as the highest fasting or direct laboratory test result in the measurement year or during the two years prior to the beginning of the measurement period M

Oncology Demonstration Project

G9678 Oncology Care Model (OCM) Monthly Enhanced Oncology Services (MEOS) payment for OCM-enhanced services. G9678 payments may only be made to OCM practitioners for OCM beneficiaries for the furnishing of enhanced services as defined in the OCM participation agreement B

G9678 may only be billed for OCM beneficiaries by OCM practitioners.

Nursing Facility Care

G9679 Onsite acute care treatment of a nursing facility resident with pneumonia. May only be billed once per day per beneficiary B

G9680 Onsite acute care treatment of a nursing facility resident with CHF. May only be billed once per day per beneficiary B

G9681 Onsite acute care treatment of a nursing facility resident with COPD or asthma. May only be billed once per day per beneficiary B

G9682 Onsite acute care treatment of a nursing facility resident with a skin infection. May only be billed once per day per beneficiary B

G9683 Facility service(s) for the onsite acute care treatment of a nursing facility resident with fluid or electrolyte disorder. (May only be billed once per day per beneficiary.) This service is for a demonstration project B

G9684 Onsite acute care treatment of a nursing facility resident for a UTI. May only be billed once per day per beneficiary B

Special Coverage Instructions   Noncovered by Medicare   Carrier Discretion   ☑ Quantity Alert ● New Code   ○ Recycled/Reinstated   ▲ Revised Code

Ⓐ Age Edit   M Maternity Edit   ♀ Female Only   ♂ Male Only   Ⓐ-Ⓨ OPPS Status Indicators   © 2021 Optum360, LLC

G9685　Physician service or other qualified health care professional for the evaluation and management of a beneficiary's acute change in condition in a nursing facility. This service is for a demonstration project　Ⓜ

Other Quality Measures

G9687　Hospice services provided to patient any time during the measurement period　Ⓜ

G9688　Patients using hospice services any time during the measurement period　Ⓜ

G9689　Patient admitted for performance of elective carotid intervention　Ⓜ

G9690　Patient receiving hospice services any time during the measurement period　Ⓜ

G9691　Patient had hospice services any time during the measurement period　Ⓜ

G9692　Hospice services received by patient any time during the measurement period　Ⓜ

G9693　Patient use of hospice services any time during the measurement period　Ⓜ

G9694　Hospice services utilized by patient any time during the measurement period　Ⓜ

G9695　Long-acting inhaled bronchodilator prescribed　Ⓜ

G9696　Documentation of medical reason(s) for not prescribing a long-acting inhaled bronchodilator　Ⓜ

G9697　Documentation of patient reason(s) for not prescribing a long-acting inhaled bronchodilator　Ⓜ

G9698　Documentation of system reason(s) for not prescribing a long-acting inhaled bronchodilator　Ⓜ

G9699　Long-acting inhaled bronchodilator not prescribed, reason not otherwise specified　Ⓜ

G9700　Patients who use hospice services any time during the measurement period　Ⓜ

G9702　Patients who use hospice services any time during the measurement period　Ⓜ

▲ G9703　Episodes where the patient is taking antibiotics (table 1) in the 30 days prior to the episode date, or had an active prescription on the episode date　Ⓜ

G9704　AJCC breast cancer Stage I: T1 mic or T1a documented　Ⓜ

G9705　AJCC breast cancer Stage I: T1b (tumor > 0.5 cm but <= 1 cm in greatest dimension) documented　Ⓜ

G9706　Low (or very low) risk of recurrence, prostate cancer　Ⓜ

G9707　Patient received hospice services any time during the measurement period　Ⓜ

G9708　Women who had a bilateral mastectomy or who have a history of a bilateral mastectomy or for whom there is evidence of a right and a left unilateral mastectomy　Ⓜ

G9709　Hospice services used by patient any time during the measurement period　Ⓜ

G9710　Patient was provided hospice services any time during the measurement period　Ⓜ

G9711　Patients with a diagnosis or past history of total colectomy or colorectal cancer　Ⓜ

G9712　Documentation of medical reason(s) for prescribing or dispensing antibiotic (e.g., intestinal infection, pertussis, bacterial infection, lyme disease, otitis media, acute sinusitis, acute pharyngitis, acute tonsillitis, chronic sinusitis, infection of the pharynx/larynx/tonsils/adenoids, prostatitis, cellulitis/mastoiditis/bone infections, acute lymphadenitis, impetigo, skin staph infections, pneumonia, gonococcal infections/venereal disease (syphilis, chlamydia, inflammatory diseases [female reproductive organs]), infections of the kidney, cystitis/UTI, acne, HIV disease/asymptomatic HIV, cystic fibrosis, disorders of the immune system, malignancy neoplasms, chronic bronchitis, emphysema, bronchiectasis, extrinsic allergic alveolitis, chronic airway obstruction, chronic obstructive asthma, pneumoconiosis and other lung disease due to external agents, other diseases of the respiratory system, and tuberculosis　Ⓜ

G9713　Patients who use hospice services any time during the measurement period　Ⓜ

G9714　Patient is using hospice services any time during the measurement period　Ⓜ

G9715　Patients who use hospice services any time during the measurement period　Ⓜ

▲ G9716　BMI is documented as being outside of normal parameters, follow-up plan is not completed for documented medical reason　Ⓜ

G9717　Documentation stating the patient has had a diagnosis of depression or has had a diagnosis of bipolar disorder　Ⓜ

G9718　Hospice services for patient provided any time during the measurement period　Ⓜ

G9719　Patient is not ambulatory, bed ridden, immobile, confined to chair, wheelchair bound, dependent on helper pushing wheelchair, independent in wheelchair or minimal help in wheelchair　Ⓜ

G9720　Hospice services for patient occurred any time during the measurement period　Ⓜ

G9721　Patient not ambulatory, bed ridden, immobile, confined to chair, wheelchair bound, dependent on helper pushing wheelchair, independent in wheelchair or minimal help in wheelchair　Ⓜ

G9722　Documented history of renal failure or baseline serum creatinine >= 4.0 mg/dl; renal transplant recipients are not considered to have preoperative renal failure, unless, since transplantation the CR has been or is 4.0 or higher　Ⓜ

G9723　Hospice services for patient received any time during the measurement period　Ⓜ

G9724　Patients who had documentation of use of anticoagulant medications overlapping the measurement year　Ⓜ

G9725　Patients who use hospice services any time during the measurement period　Ⓜ

G9726　Patient refused to participate　Ⓜ

G9727　Patient unable to complete the LEPF PROM at initial evaluation and/or discharge due to blindness, illiteracy, severe mental incapacity or language incompatibility and an adequate proxy is not available　Ⓜ

G9728　Patient refused to participate　Ⓜ

G9729　Patient unable to complete the LEPF PROM at initial evaluation and/or discharge due to blindness, illiteracy, severe mental incapacity or language incompatibility and an adequate proxy is not available　Ⓜ

G9730　Patient refused to participate　Ⓜ

Special Coverage Instructions　　Noncovered by Medicare　　Carrier Discretion　　☑ Quantity Alert　　● New Code　　○ Recycled/Reinstated　　▲ Revised Code

G9731 Patient unable to complete the LEPF PROM at initial evaluation and/or discharge due to blindness, illiteracy, severe mental incapacity or language incompatibility and an adequate proxy is not available M

G9732 Patient refused to participate M

G9733 Patient unable to complete the low back FS PROM at initial evaluation and/or discharge due to blindness, illiteracy, severe mental incapacity or language incompatibility and an adequate proxy is not available M

G9734 Patient refused to participate M

G9735 Patient unable to complete the shoulder FS PROM at initial evaluation and/or discharge due to blindness, illiteracy, severe mental incapacity or language incompatibility and an adequate proxy is not available M

G9736 Patient refused to participate M

G9737 Patient unable to complete the elbow/wrist/hand FS PROM at initial evaluation and/or discharge due to blindness, illiteracy, severe mental incapacity or language incompatibility and an adequate proxy is not available M

G9740 Hospice services given to patient any time during the measurement period M

G9741 Patients who use hospice services any time during the measurement period M

G9744 Patient not eligible due to active diagnosis of hypertension M

G9745 Documented reason for not screening or recommending a follow-up for high blood pressure M

G9746 Patient has mitral stenosis or prosthetic heart valves or patient has transient or reversible cause of AF (e.g., pneumonia, hyperthyroidism, pregnancy, cardiac surgery) M

G9751 Patient died at any time during the 24-month measurement period M

G9752 Emergency surgery M

G9753 Documentation of medical reason for not conducting a search for DICOM format images for prior patient CT imaging studies completed at nonaffiliated external healthcare facilities or entities within the past 12 months that are available through a secure, authorized, media-free, shared archive (e.g., trauma, acute myocardial infarction, stroke, aortic aneurysm where time is of the essence) M

G9754 A finding of an incidental pulmonary nodule M

G9755 Documentation of medical reason(s) for not including a recommended interval and modality for follow-up or for no follow-up, and source of recommendations (e.g., patients with unexplained fever, immunocompromised patients who are at risk for infection) M

G9756 Surgical procedures that included the use of silicone oil M

G9757 Surgical procedures that included the use of silicone oil M

G9758 Patient in hospice at any time during the measurement period M

G9760 Patients who use hospice services any time during the measurement period M

G9761 Patients who use hospice services any time during the measurement period M

G9762 Patient had at least two HPV vaccines (with at least 146 days between the two) or three HPV vaccines on or between the patient's 9th and 13th birthdays M

G9763 Patient did not have at least two HPV vaccines (with at least 146 days between the two) or three HPV vaccines on or between the patient's 9th and 13th birthdays M

G9764 Patient has been treated with a systemic medication for psoriasis vulgaris M

G9765 Documentation that the patient declined change in medication or alternative therapies were unavailable, has documented contraindications, or has not been treated with a systemic medication for at least six consecutive months (e.g., experienced adverse effects or lack of efficacy with all other therapy options) in order to achieve better disease control as measured by PGA, BSA, PASI, or DLQI M

G9766 Patients who are transferred from one institution to another with a known diagnosis of CVA for endovascular stroke treatment M

G9767 Hospitalized patients with newly diagnosed CVA considered for endovascular stroke treatment M

G9768 Patients who utilize hospice services any time during the measurement period M

G9769 Patient had a bone mineral density test in the past two years or received osteoporosis medication or therapy in the past 12 months M

G9770 Peripheral nerve block (PNB) M

G9771 At least one body temperature measurement equal to or greater than 35.5 degrees celsius (or 95.9 degrees fahrenheit) achieved within the 30 minutes immediately before or the 15 minutes immediately after anesthesia end time M

G9772 Documentation of medical reason(s) for not achieving at least one body temperature measurement equal to or greater than 35.5 degrees Celsius (or 95.9 degrees Fahrenheit) within the 30 minutes immediately before or the 15 minutes immediately after anesthesia end time (e.g., emergency cases, intentional hypothermia, etc.) M

G9773 At least one body temperature measurement equal to or greater than 35.5 degrees celsius (or 95.9 degrees fahrenheit) not achieved within the 30 minutes immediately before or the 15 minutes immediately after anesthesia end time, reason not given M

G9774 Patients who have had a hysterectomy M

G9775 Patient received at least two prophylactic pharmacologic antiemetic agents of different classes preoperatively and/or intraoperatively M

G9776 Documentation of medical reason for not receiving at least two prophylactic pharmacologic antiemetic agents of different classes preoperatively and/or intraoperatively (e.g., intolerance or other medical reason) M

G9777 Patient did not receive at least two prophylactic pharmacologic antiemetic agents of different classes preoperatively and/or intraoperatively M

▲ **G9778** Patients who have a diagnosis of pregnancy at any time during the measurement period M

▲ **G9779** Patients who are breastfeeding at any time during the measurement period M

▲ **G9780** Patients who have a diagnosis of rhabdomyolysis at any time during the measurement period M

Special Coverage Instructions   Noncovered by Medicare   Carrier Discretion   ☑ Quantity Alert ● New Code   ○ Recycled/Reinstated   ▲ Revised Code

80 — G Codes   Ⓐ Age Edit   Ⓜ Maternity Edit   ♀ Female Only   ♂ Male Only   Ⓐ-Ⓨ OPPS Status Indicators   © 2021 Optum360, LLC

▲ **G9781** Documentation of medical reason(s) for not currently being a statin therapy user or receiving an order (prescription) for statin therapy (e.g., patients with statin-associated muscle symptoms or an allergy to statin medication therapy, patients who are receiving palliative or hospice care, patients with active liver disease or hepatic disease or insufficiency, and patients with end stage renal disease [ESRD]) Ⓜ

▲ **G9782** History of or active diagnosis of familial hypercholesterolemia Ⓜ

G9783 ~~Documentation of patients with diabetes who have a most recent fasting or direct LDL-C laboratory test result <70 mg/dl and are not taking statin therapy~~

G9784 Pathologists/dermatopathologists providing a second opinion on a biopsy Ⓜ

G9785 Pathology report diagnosing cutaneous basal cell carcinoma, squamous cell carcinoma, or melanoma (to include in situ disease) sent from the pathologist/dermatopathologist to the biopsying clinician for review within 7 days from the time when the tissue specimen was received by the pathologist Ⓜ

G9786 Pathology report diagnosing cutaneous basal cell carcinoma, squamous cell carcinoma, or melanoma (to include in situ disease) was not sent from the pathologist/dermatopathologist to the biopsying clinician for review within 7 days from the time when the tissue specimen was received by the pathologist Ⓜ

G9787 Patient alive as of the last day of the measurement year Ⓜ

G9788 Most recent BP is less than or equal to 140/90 mm Hg Ⓜ

G9789 Blood pressure recorded during inpatient stays, emergency room visits, urgent care visits, and patient self-reported BP's (home and health fair BP results) Ⓜ

G9790 Most recent BP is greater than 140/90 mm Hg, or blood pressure not documented Ⓜ

G9791 Most recent tobacco status is tobacco free Ⓜ

G9792 Most recent tobacco status is not tobacco free Ⓜ

G9793 Patient is currently on a daily aspirin or other antiplatelet Ⓜ

G9794 Documentation of medical reason(s) for not on a daily aspirin or other antiplatelet (e.g., history of gastrointestinal bleed, intracranial bleed, idiopathic thrombocytopenic purpura (ITP), gastric bypass or documentation of active anticoagulant use during the measurement period) Ⓜ

G9795 Patient is not currently on a daily aspirin or other antiplatelet Ⓜ

G9796 Patient is currently on a statin therapy Ⓜ

G9797 Patient is not on a statin therapy Ⓜ

G9805 Patients who use hospice services any time during the measurement period Ⓜ

G9806 Patients who received cervical cytology or an HPV test Ⓜ

G9807 Patients who did not receive cervical cytology or an HPV test Ⓜ

G9808 Any patients who had no asthma controller medications dispensed during the measurement year Ⓜ

G9809 Patients who use hospice services any time during the measurement period Ⓜ

G9810 Patient achieved a PDC of at least 75% for their asthma controller medication Ⓜ

G9811 Patient did not achieve a PDC of at least 75% for their asthma controller medication Ⓜ

G9812 Patient died including all deaths occurring during the hospitalization in which the operation was performed, even if after 30 days, and those deaths occurring after discharge from the hospital, but within 30 days of the procedure Ⓜ

G9813 Patient did not die within 30 days of the procedure or during the index hospitalization Ⓜ

G9818 Documentation of sexual activity Ⓜ

G9819 Patients who use hospice services any time during the measurement period Ⓜ

G9820 Documentation of a chlamydia screening test with proper follow-up Ⓜ

G9821 No documentation of a chlamydia screening test with proper follow-up Ⓜ

▲ **G9822** Patients who had an endometrial ablation procedure during the 12 months prior to the index date (exclusive of the index date) Ⓜ

▲ **G9823** Endometrial sampling or hysteroscopy with biopsy and results documented during the 12 months prior to the index date (exclusive of the index date) of the endometrial ablation Ⓜ

▲ **G9824** Endometrial sampling or hysteroscopy with biopsy and results not documented during the 12 months prior to the index date (exclusive of the index date) of the endometrial ablation Ⓜ

G9830 HER2/neu positive Ⓜ

G9831 AJCC Stage at breast cancer diagnosis = II or III Ⓜ

G9832 AJCC Stage at breast cancer diagnosis = I (Ia or Ib) and T-Stage at breast cancer diagnosis does not equal = T1, T1a, T1b Ⓜ

G9838 Patient has metastatic disease at diagnosis Ⓜ

G9839 Anti-EGFR monoclonal antibody therapy Ⓜ

G9840 RAS (KRAS and NRAS) gene mutation testing performed before initiation of anti-EGFR MoAb Ⓜ

G9841 RAS (KRAS and NRAS) gene mutation testing not performed before initiation of anti-EGFR MoAb Ⓜ

G9842 Patient has metastatic disease at diagnosis Ⓜ

G9843 RAS (KRAS or NRAS) gene mutation Ⓜ

G9844 Patient did not receive anti-EGFR monoclonal antibody therapy Ⓜ

G9845 Patient received anti-EGFR monoclonal antibody therapy Ⓜ

G9846 Patients who died from cancer Ⓜ

G9847 Patient received chemotherapy in the last 14 days of life Ⓜ

G9848 Patient did not receive chemotherapy in the last 14 days of life Ⓜ

G9852 Patients who died from cancer Ⓜ

G9853 Patient admitted to the ICU in the last 30 days of life Ⓜ

G9854 Patient was not admitted to the ICU in the last 30 days of life Ⓜ

G9858 Patient enrolled in hospice Ⓜ

G9859 Patients who died from cancer Ⓜ

G9860 Patient spent less than three days in hospice care Ⓜ

G9861 Patient spent greater than or equal to three days in hospice care Ⓜ

Special Coverage Instructions   Noncovered by Medicare   Carrier Discretion   ☑ Quantity Alert   ● New Code   ○ Recycled/Reinstated   ▲ Revised Code

© 2021 Optum360, LLC   A2-Z3 ASC Pmt   CMS: IOM   AHA: Coding Clinic   DMEPOS Paid   ⊘ SNF Excluded   G Codes — 81

Procedures/Professional Services (Temporary)

G9862 — G9883

G9862 Documentation of medical reason(s) for not recommending at least a 10 year follow-up interval (e.g., inadequate prep, familial or personal history of colonic polyps, patient had no adenoma and age is = 66 years old, or life expectancy < 10 years old, other medical reasons) Ⓜ

▲ **G9868** Receipt and analysis of remote, asynchronous images for dermatologic and/or ophthalmologic evaluation, for use only in a Medicare-approved CMMI model, less than 10 minutes Ⓑ

▲ **G9869** Receipt and analysis of remote, asynchronous images for dermatologic and/or ophthalmologic evaluation, for use only in a Medicare-approved CMMI model, 10 to 20 minutes Ⓑ

▲ **G9870** Receipt and analysis of remote, asynchronous images for dermatologic and/or ophthalmologic evaluation, for use only in a Medicare-approved CMMI model, more than 20 minutes Ⓑ

G9873 First Medicare Diabetes Prevention Program (MDPP) core session was attended by an MDPP beneficiary under the MDPP Expanded Model (EM). A core session is an MDPP service that: (1) is furnished by an MDPP supplier during months 1 through 6 of the MDPP services period; (2) is approximately 1 hour in length; and (3) adheres to a CDC-approved DPP curriculum for core sessions Ⓜ

G9874 Four total Medicare Diabetes Prevention Program (MDPP) core sessions were attended by an MDPP beneficiary under the MDPP Expanded Model (EM). A core session is an MDPP service that: (1) is furnished by an MDPP supplier during months 1 through 6 of the MDPP services period; (2) is approximately 1 hour in length; and (3) adheres to a CDC-approved DPP curriculum for core sessions Ⓜ

G9875 Nine total Medicare Diabetes Prevention Program (MDPP) core sessions were attended by an MDPP beneficiary under the MDPP Expanded Model (EM). A core session is an MDPP service that: (1) is furnished by an MDPP supplier during months 1 through 6 of the MDPP services period; (2) is approximately 1 hour in length; and (3) adheres to a CDC-approved DPP curriculum for core sessions Ⓜ

G9876 Two Medicare Diabetes Prevention Program (MDPP) core maintenance sessions (MS) were attended by an MDPP beneficiary in months (mo) 7-9 under the MDPP Expanded Model (EM). A core maintenance session is an MDPP service that: (1) is furnished by an MDPP supplier during months 7 through 12 of the MDPP services period; (2) is approximately 1 hour in length; and (3) adheres to a CDC-approved DPP curriculum for maintenance sessions. The beneficiary did not achieve at least 5% weight loss (WL) from his/her baseline weight, as measured by at least one in-person weight measurement at a core maintenance session in months 7-9 Ⓜ

G9877 Two Medicare Diabetes Prevention Program (MDPP) core maintenance sessions (MS) were attended by an MDPP beneficiary in months (mo) 10-12 under the MDPP Expanded Model (EM). A core maintenance session is an MDPP service that: (1) is furnished by an MDPP supplier during months 7 through 12 of the MDPP services period; (2) is approximately 1 hour in length; and (3) adheres to a CDC-approved DPP curriculum for maintenance sessions. The beneficiary did not achieve at least 5% weight loss (WL) from his/her baseline weight, as measured by at least one in-person weight measurement at a core maintenance session in months 10-12 Ⓜ

G9878 Two Medicare Diabetes Prevention Program (MDPP) core maintenance sessions (MS) were attended by an MDPP beneficiary in months (mo) 7-9 under the MDPP Expanded Model (EM). A core maintenance session is an MDPP service that: (1) is furnished by an MDPP supplier during months 7 through 12 of the MDPP services period; (2) is approximately 1 hour in length; and (3) adheres to a CDC-approved DPP curriculum for maintenance sessions. The beneficiary achieved at least 5% weight loss (WL) from his/her baseline weight, as measured by at least one in-person weight measurement at a core maintenance session in months 7-9 Ⓜ

G9879 Two Medicare Diabetes Prevention Program (MDPP) core maintenance sessions (MS) were attended by an MDPP beneficiary in months (mo) 10-12 under the MDPP Expanded Model (EM). A core maintenance session is an MDPP service that: (1) is furnished by an MDPP supplier during months 7 through 12 of the MDPP services period; (2) is approximately 1 hour in length; and (3) adheres to a CDC-approved DPP curriculum for maintenance sessions. The beneficiary achieved at least 5% weight loss (WL) from his/her baseline weight, as measured by at least one in-person weight measurement at a core maintenance session in months 10-12 Ⓜ

G9880 The MDPP beneficiary achieved at least 5% weight loss (WL) from his/her baseline weight in months 1-12 of the MDPP services period under the MDPP Expanded Model (EM). This is a one-time payment available when a beneficiary first achieves at least 5% weight loss from baseline as measured by an in-person weight measurement at a core session or core maintenance session Ⓜ

G9881 The MDPP beneficiary achieved at least 9% weight loss (WL) from his/her baseline weight in months 1-24 under the MDPP Expanded Model (EM). This is a one-time payment available when a beneficiary first achieves at least 9% weight loss from baseline as measured by an in-person weight measurement at a core session, core maintenance session, or ongoing maintenance session Ⓜ

G9882 Two Medicare Diabetes Prevention Program (MDPP) ongoing maintenance sessions (MS) were attended by an MDPP beneficiary in months (mo) 13-15 under the MDPP Expanded Model (EM). An ongoing maintenance session is an MDPP service that: (1) is furnished by an MDPP supplier during months 13 through 24 of the MDPP services period; (2) is approximately 1 hour in length; and (3) adheres to a CDC-approved DPP curriculum for maintenance sessions. The beneficiary maintained at least 5% weight loss (WL) from his/her baseline weight, as measured by at least one in-person weight measurement at an ongoing maintenance session in months 13-15 Ⓜ

G9883 Two Medicare Diabetes Prevention Program (MDPP) ongoing maintenance sessions (MS) were attended by an MDPP beneficiary in months (mo) 16-18 under the MDPP Expanded Model (EM). An ongoing maintenance session is an MDPP service that: (1) is furnished by an MDPP supplier during months 13 through 24 of the MDPP services period; (2) is approximately 1 hour in length; and (3) adheres to a CDC-approved DPP curriculum for maintenance sessions. The beneficiary maintained at least 5% weight loss (WL) from his/her baseline weight, as measured by at least one in-person weight measurement at an ongoing maintenance session in months 16-18 Ⓜ

Special Coverage Instructions   Noncovered by Medicare   Carrier Discretion   ☑ Quantity Alert   ● New Code   ○ Recycled/Reinstated   ▲ Revised Code

82 — G Codes   Ⓐ Age Edit   Ⓜ Maternity Edit   ♀ Female Only   ♂ Male Only   Ⓐ-Ⓨ OPPS Status Indicators   © 2021 Optum360, LLC

G9884 Two Medicare Diabetes Prevention Program (MDPP) ongoing maintenance sessions (MS) were attended by an MDPP beneficiary in months (mo) 19-21 under the MDPP Expanded Model (EM). An ongoing maintenance session is an MDPP service that: (1) is furnished by an MDPP supplier during months 13 through 24 of the MDPP services period; (2) is approximately 1 hour in length; and (3) adheres to a CDC-approved DPP curriculum for maintenance sessions. The beneficiary maintained at least 5% weight loss (WL) from his/her baseline weight, as measured by at least one in-person weight measurement at an ongoing maintenance session in months 19-21 Ⓜ

G9885 Two Medicare Diabetes Prevention Program (MDPP) ongoing maintenance sessions (MS) were attended by an MDPP beneficiary in months (mo) 22-24 under the MDPP Expanded Model (EM). An ongoing maintenance session is an MDPP service that: (1) is furnished by an MDPP supplier during months 13 through 24 of the MDPP services period; (2) is approximately 1 hour in length; and (3) adheres to a CDC-approved DPP curriculum for maintenance sessions. The beneficiary maintained at least 5% weight loss (WL) from his/her baseline weight, as measured by at least one in-person weight measurement at an ongoing maintenance session in months 22-24 Ⓜ

G9890 Bridge Payment: A one-time payment for the first Medicare Diabetes Prevention Program (MDPP) core session, core maintenance session, or ongoing maintenance session furnished by an MDPP supplier to an MDPP beneficiary during months 1-24 of the MDPP Expanded Model (EM) who has previously received MDPP services from a different MDPP supplier under the MDPP Expanded Model. A supplier may only receive one bridge payment per MDPP beneficiary Ⓜ

G9891 MDPP session reported as a line-item on a claim for a payable MDPP Expanded Model (EM) HCPCS code for a session furnished by the billing supplier under the MDPP Expanded Model and counting toward achievement of the attendance performance goal for the payable MDPP Expanded Model HCPCS code. (This code is for reporting purposes only) Ⓜ

G9892 Documentation of patient reason(s) for not performing a dilated macular examination Ⓜ

G9893 Dilated macular exam was not performed, reason not otherwise specified Ⓜ

G9894 Androgen deprivation therapy prescribed/administered in combination with external beam radiotherapy to the prostate Ⓜ

G9895 Documentation of medical reason(s) for not prescribing/administering androgen deprivation therapy in combination with external beam radiotherapy to the prostate (e.g., salvage therapy) Ⓜ

G9896 Documentation of patient reason(s) for not prescribing/administering androgen deprivation therapy in combination with external beam radiotherapy to the prostate Ⓜ

G9897 Patients who were not prescribed/administered androgen deprivation therapy in combination with external beam radiotherapy to the prostate, reason not given Ⓜ

G9898 Patients age 66 or older in institutional special needs plans (SNP) or residing in long-term care with POS code 32, 33, 34, 54, or 56 for more than 90 consecutive days during the measurement period Ⓜ

G9899 Screening, diagnostic, film, digital or digital breast tomosynthesis (3D) mammography results documented and reviewed Ⓜ

G9900 Screening, diagnostic, film, digital or digital breast tomosynthesis (3D) mammography results were not documented and reviewed, reason not otherwise specified Ⓜ

G9901 Patient age 66 or older in institutional special needs plans (SNP) or residing in long-term care with POS code 32, 33, 34, 54, or 56 for more than 90 consecutive days during the measurement period Ⓜ

G9902 Patient screened for tobacco use and identified as a tobacco user Ⓜ

G9903 Patient screened for tobacco use and identified as a tobacco nonuser Ⓜ

G9904 Documentation of medical reason(s) for not screening for tobacco use (e.g., limited life expectancy, other medical reason) Ⓜ

G9905 Patient not screened for tobacco use, reason not given Ⓜ

▲ **G9906** Patient identified as a tobacco user received tobacco cessation intervention on the date of the encounter or within the previous 12 months (counseling and/or pharmacotherapy) Ⓜ

▲ **G9907** Documentation of medical reason(s) for not providing tobacco cessation intervention on the date of the encounter or within the previous 12 months (e.g., limited life expectancy, other medical reason) Ⓜ

▲ **G9908** Patient identified as tobacco user did not receive tobacco cessation intervention on the date of the encounter or within the previous 12 months (counseling and/or pharmacotherapy), reason not given Ⓜ

▲ **G9909** Documentation of medical reason(s) for not providing tobacco cessation intervention on the date of the encounter or within the previous 12 months if identified as a tobacco user (e.g., limited life expectancy, other medical reason) Ⓜ

G9910 Patients age 66 or older in institutional special needs plans (SNP) or residing in long-term care with POS code 32, 33, 34, 54 or 56 for more than 90 consecutive days during the measurement period Ⓜ

G9911 Clinically node negative (T1N0M0 or T2N0M0) invasive breast cancer before or after neoadjuvant systemic therapy Ⓜ

G9912 Hepatitis B virus (HBV) status assessed and results interpreted prior to initiating anti-TNF (tumor necrosis factor) therapy Ⓜ

G9913 Hepatitis B virus (HBV) status not assessed and results interpreted prior to initiating anti-TNF (tumor necrosis factor) therapy, reason not given Ⓜ

G9914 Patient receiving an anti-TNF agent Ⓜ

G9915 No record of HBV results documented Ⓜ

G9916 Functional status performed once in the last 12 months Ⓜ

G9917 Documentation of advanced stage dementia and caregiver knowledge is limited Ⓜ

G9918 Functional status not performed, reason not otherwise specified Ⓜ

G9919 Screening performed and positive and provision of recommendations Ⓜ

G9920 Screening performed and negative Ⓜ

G9921 No screening performed, partial screening performed or positive screen without recommendations and reason is not given or otherwise specified Ⓜ

G9922 Safety concerns screen provided and if positive then documented mitigation recommendations Ⓜ

G9923 Safety concerns screen provided and negative Ⓜ

G9925 Safety concerns screening not provided, reason not otherwise specified Ⓜ

Special Coverage Instructions   Noncovered by Medicare   Carrier Discretion   ☑ Quantity Alert ● New Code ○ Recycled/Reinstated ▲ Revised Code

© 2021 Optum360, LLC   A2-Z3 ASC Pmt   CMS: IOM   AHA: Coding Clinic   DMEPOS Paid   ⊘ SNF Excluded   G Codes — 83

Procedures/Professional Services (Temporary)

G9926 — G9979

G9926 Safety concerns screening positive screen is without provision of mitigation recommendations, including but not limited to referral to other resources M

▲ **G9927** Documentation of system reason(s) for not prescribing an FDA-approved anticoagulation due to patient being currently enrolled in a clinical trial related to AF/atrial flutter treatment M

▲ **G9928** FDA-approved anticoagulant not prescribed, reason not given M

G9929 Patient with transient or reversible cause of AF (e.g., pneumonia, hyperthyroidism, pregnancy, cardiac surgery) M

G9930 Patients who are receiving comfort care only M

G9931 Documentation of CHA2DS2-VASc risk score of 0 or 1 for men; or 0, 1, or 2 for women M

G9932 Documentation of patient reason(s) for not having records of negative or managed positive TB screen (e.g., patient does not return for Mantoux (PPD) skin test evaluation) M

G9938 Patients age 66 or older in institutional special needs plans (SNP) or residing in long-term care with POS code 32, 33, 34, 54, or 56 for more than 90 consecutive days during the six months prior to the measurement period through December 31 of the measurement period M

G9939 Pathologist(s)/dermatopathologist(s) is the same clinician who performed the biopsy M

G9940 Documentation of medical reason(s) for not on a statin (e.g., pregnancy, in vitro fertilization, clomiphene Rx, ESRD, cirrhosis, muscular pain and disease during the measurement period or prior year) M

G9942 Patient had any additional spine procedures performed on the same date as the lumbar discectomy/laminectomy M

G9943 Back pain was not measured by the visual analog scale (VAS) within three months preoperatively and at three months (6 - 20 weeks) postoperatively M

G9945 Patient had cancer, acute fracture or infection related to the lumbar spine or patient had neuromuscular, idiopathic or congenital lumbar scoliosis M

G9946 Back pain was not measured by the visual analog scale (VAS) within three months preoperatively and at one year (9 - 15 months) postoperatively M

G9948 Patient had any additional spine procedures performed on the same date as the lumbar discectomy/laminectomy M

G9949 Leg pain was not measured by the visual analog scale (vas) at three months (6 - 20 weeks) postoperatively M

G9954 Patient exhibits 2 or more risk factors for postoperative vomiting M

G9955 Cases in which an inhalational anesthetic is used only for induction M

G9956 Patient received combination therapy consisting of at least two prophylactic pharmacologic antiemetic agents of different classes preoperatively and/or intraoperatively M

G9957 Documentation of medical reason for not receiving combination therapy consisting of at least two prophylactic pharmacologic antiemetic agents of different classes preoperatively and/or intraoperatively (e.g., intolerance or other medical reason) M

G9958 Patient did not receive combination therapy consisting of at least two prophylactic pharmacologic antiemetic agents of different classes preoperatively and/or intraoperatively M

G9959 Systemic antimicrobials not prescribed M

G9960 Documentation of medical reason(s) for prescribing systemic antimicrobials M

G9961 Systemic antimicrobials prescribed M

G9962 Embolization endpoints are documented separately for each embolized vessel and ovarian artery angiography or embolization performed in the presence of variant uterine artery anatomy M

G9963 Embolization endpoints are not documented separately for each embolized vessel or ovarian artery angiography or embolization not performed in the presence of variant uterine artery anatomy M

G9964 Patient received at least one well-child visit with a PCP during the performance period M

G9965 Patient did not receive at least one well-child visit with PCP during the performance period M

G9968 Patient was referred to another provider or specialist during the performance period M

G9969 Provider who referred the patient to another provider received a report from the provider to whom the patient was referred M

G9970 Provider who referred the patient to another provider did not receive a report from the provider to whom the patient was referred M

G9974 Dilated macular exam performed, including documentation of the presence or absence of macular thickening or geographic atrophy or hemorrhage and the level of macular degeneration severity M

G9975 Documentation of medical reason(s) for not performing a dilated macular examination M

G9976 Documentation of patient reason(s) for not performing a dilated macular examination

G9977 Dilated macular exam was not performed, reason not otherwise specified

G9978 Remote in-home visit for the evaluation and management of a new patient for use only in a Medicare-approved Bundled Payments for Care Improvement Advanced (BPCI Advanced) model episode of care, which requires these three key components: a problem focused history; a problem focused examination; straightforward medical decision making, furnished in real time using interactive audio and video technology. Counseling and coordination of care with other physicians, other qualified health care professionals or agencies are provided consistent with the nature of the problem(s) and the needs of the patient or the family or both. Usually, the presenting problem(s) are self limited or minor. Typically, 10 minutes are spent with the patient or family or both via real time, audio and video intercommunications technology

G9979 Remote in-home visit for the evaluation and management of a new patient for use only in a Medicare-approved Bundled Payments for Care Improvement Advanced (BPCI Advanced) model episode of care, which requires these three key components: an expanded problem focused history; an expanded problem focused examination; straightforward medical decision making, furnished in real time using interactive audio and video technology. Counseling and coordination of care with other physicians, other qualified health care professionals or agencies are provided consistent with the nature of the problem(s) and the needs of the patient or the family or both. Usually, the presenting problem(s) are of low to moderate severity. Typically, 20 minutes are spent with the patient or family or both via real time, audio and video intercommunications technology

Special Coverage Instructions   Noncovered by Medicare   Carrier Discretion   ☑ Quantity Alert ● New Code   ○ Recycled/Reinstated   ▲ Revised Code

84 — G Codes   Ⓐ Age Edit   Ⓜ Maternity Edit   ♀ Female Only   ♂ Male Only   Ⓐ–Ⓨ OPPS Status Indicators   © 2021 Optum360, LLC

Procedures/Professional Services (Temporary)

G9980 — G9992

G9980 Remote in-home visit for the evaluation and management of a new patient for use only in a Medicare-approved Bundled Payments for Care Improvement Advanced (BPCI Advanced) model episode of care, which requires these three key components: a detailed history; a detailed examination; medical decision making of low complexity, furnished in real time using interactive audio and video technology. Counseling and coordination of care with other physicians, other qualified health care professionals or agencies are provided consistent with the nature of the problem(s) and the needs of the patient or the family or both. Usually, the presenting problem(s) are of moderate severity. Typically, 30 minutes are spent with the patient or family or both via real time, audio and video intercommunications technology

G9981 Remote in-home visit for the evaluation and management of a new patient for use only in a Medicare-approved Bundled Payments for Care Improvement Advanced (BPCI Advanced) model episode of care, which requires these three key components: a comprehensive history; a comprehensive examination; medical decision making of moderate complexity, furnished in real time using interactive audio and video technology. Counseling and coordination of care with other physicians, other qualified health care professionals or agencies are provided consistent with the nature of the problem(s) and the needs of the patient or the family or both. Usually, the presenting problem(s) are of moderate to high severity. Typically, 45 minutes are spent with the patient or family or both via real time, audio and video intercommunications technology

G9982 Remote in-home visit for the evaluation and management of a new patient for use only in a Medicare-approved Bundled Payments for Care Improvement Advanced (BPCI Advanced) model episode of care, which requires these three key components: a comprehensive history; a comprehensive examination; medical decision making of high complexity, furnished in real time using interactive audio and video technology. Counseling and coordination of care with other physicians, other qualified health care professionals or agencies are provided consistent with the nature of the problem(s) and the needs of the patient or the family or both. Usually, the presenting problem(s) are of moderate to high severity. Typically, 60 minutes are spent with the patient or family or both via real time, audio and video intercommunications technology

G9983 Remote in-home visit for the evaluation and management of an established patient for use only in a Medicare-approved Bundled Payments for Care Improvement Advanced (BPCI Advanced) model episode of care, which requires at least two of the following three key components: a problem focused history; a problem focused examination; straightforward medical decision making, furnished in real time using interactive audio and video technology. Counseling and coordination of care with other physicians, other qualified health care professionals or agencies are provided consistent with the nature of the problem(s) and the needs of the patient or the family or both. Usually, the presenting problem(s) are self limited or minor. Typically, 10 minutes are spent with the patient or family or both via real time, audio and video intercommunications technology

G9984 Remote in-home visit for the evaluation and management of an established patient for use only in a Medicare-approved Bundled Payments for Care Improvement Advanced (BPCI Advanced) model episode of care, which requires at least two of the following three key components: an expanded problem focused history; an expanded problem focused examination; medical decision making of low complexity, furnished in real time using interactive audio and video technology. Counseling and coordination of care with other physicians, other qualified health care professionals or agencies are provided consistent with the nature of the problem(s) and the needs of the patient or the family or both. Usually, the presenting problem(s) are of low to moderate severity. Typically, 15 minutes are spent with the patient or family or both via real time, audio and video intercommunications technology

G9985 Remote in-home visit for the evaluation and management of an established patient for use only in a Medicare-approved Bundled Payments for Care Improvement Advanced (BPCI Advanced) model episode of care, which requires at least two of the following three key components: a detailed history; a detailed examination; medical decision making of moderate complexity, furnished in real time using interactive audio and video technology. Counseling and coordination of care with other physicians, other qualified health care professionals or agencies are provided consistent with the nature of the problem(s) and the needs of the patient or the family or both. Usually, the presenting problem(s) are of moderate to high severity. Typically, 25 minutes are spent with the patient or family or both via real time, audio and video intercommunications technology

G9986 Remote in-home visit for the evaluation and management of an established patient for use only in a Medicare-approved Bundled Payments for Care Improvement Advanced (BPCI Advanced) model episode of care, which requires at least two of the following three key components: a comprehensive history; a comprehensive examination; medical decision making of high complexity, furnished in real time using interactive audio and video technology. Counseling and coordination of care with other physicians, other qualified health care professionals or agencies are provided consistent with the nature of the problem(s) and the needs of the patient or the family or both. Usually, the presenting problem(s) are of moderate to high severity. Typically, 40 minutes are spent with the patient or family or both via real time, audio and video intercommunications technology

G9987 Bundled Payments for Care Improvement Advanced (BPCI Advanced) model home visit for patient assessment performed by clinical staff for an individual not considered homebound, including, but not necessarily limited to patient assessment of clinical status, safety/fall prevention, functional status/ambulation, medication reconciliation/management, compliance with orders/plan of care, performance of activities of daily living, and ensuring beneficiary connections to community and other services; for use only for a BPCI Advanced model episode of care; may not be billed for a 30-day period covered by a transitional care management code

● **G9988** Palliative care services provided to patient any time during the measurement period

● **G9989** Documentation of medical reason(s) for not administering pneumococcal vaccine (e.g., adverse reaction to vaccine)

● **G9990** Pneumococcal vaccine was not administered on or after patient's 60th birthday and before the end of the measurement period, reason not otherwise specified

● **G9991** Pneumococcal vaccine administered on or after patient's 60th birthday and before the end of the measurement period

● **G9992** Palliative care services used by patient any time during the measurement period

Special Coverage Instructions   Noncovered by Medicare   Carrier Discretion   ☑ Quantity Alert ● New Code   ○ Recycled/Reinstated   ▲ Revised Code

© 2021 Optum360, LLC   A2-Z3 ASC Pmt   CMS: IOM   AHA: Coding Clinic   ⅃ DMEPOS Paid   ⊘ SNF Excluded   G Codes — 85

● **G9993** Patient was provided pallative care services any time during the measurement period

● **G9994** Patient is using palliative care services any time during the measurement period

● **G9995** Patients who use palliative care services any time during the measurement period

● **G9996** Documentation stating the patient has received or is currently receiving palliative or hospice care

● **G9997** Documentation of patient pregnancy anytime during the measurement period prior to and including the current encounter

● **G9998** Documentation of medical reason(s) for an interval of less than 3 years since the last colonoscopy (e.g., last colonoscopy incomplete, last colonoscopy had inadequate prep, piecemeal removal of adenomas, last colonoscopy found greater than 10 adenomas, or patient at high risk for colon cancer [Crohn's disease, ulcerative colitis, lower gastrointestinal bleeding, personal or family history of colon cancer, hereditary colorectal cancer syndromes])

● **G9999** Documentation of system reason(s) for an interval of less than 3 years since the last colonoscopy (e.g., unable to locate previous colonoscopy report, previous colonoscopy report was incomplete)

Special Coverage Instructions   Noncovered by Medicare   Carrier Discretion   ☑ Quantity Alert ● New Code   ○ Recycled/Reinstated ▲ Revised Code

86 — G Codes   Ⓐ Age Edit   Ⓜ Maternity Edit   ♀ Female Only   ♂ Male Only   Ⓐ-Ⓨ OPPS Status Indicators   © 2021 Optum360, LLC

Alcohol and Drug Abuse Treatment Services H0001-H2037

The H codes are used by those state Medicaid agencies that are mandated by state law to establish separate codes for identifying mental health services that include alcohol and drug treatment services.

H0001   **Alcohol and/or drug assessment**

H0002   **Behavioral health screening to determine eligibility for admission to treatment program**

H0003   **Alcohol and/or drug screening; laboratory analysis of specimens for presence of alcohol and/or drugs**

H0004   **Behavioral health counseling and therapy, per 15 minutes** ☑

H0005   **Alcohol and/or drug services; group counseling by a clinician**

H0006   **Alcohol and/or drug services; case management**

H0007   **Alcohol and/or drug services; crisis intervention (outpatient)**

H0008   **Alcohol and/or drug services; subacute detoxification (hospital inpatient)**

H0009   **Alcohol and/or drug services; acute detoxification (hospital inpatient)**

H0010   **Alcohol and/or drug services; subacute detoxification (residential addiction program inpatient)**

H0011   **Alcohol and/or drug services; acute detoxification (residential addiction program inpatient)**

H0012   **Alcohol and/or drug services; subacute detoxification (residential addiction program outpatient)**

H0013   **Alcohol and/or drug services; acute detoxification (residential addiction program outpatient)**

H0014   **Alcohol and/or drug services; ambulatory detoxification**

H0015   **Alcohol and/or drug services; intensive outpatient (treatment program that operates at least 3 hours/day and at least 3 days/week and is based on an individualized treatment plan), including assessment, counseling; crisis intervention, and activity therapies or education**

H0016   **Alcohol and/or drug services; medical/somatic (medical intervention in ambulatory setting)**

H0017   **Behavioral health; residential (hospital residential treatment program), without room and board, per diem** ☑

H0018   **Behavioral health; short-term residential (nonhospital residential treatment program), without room and board, per diem** ☑

H0019   **Behavioral health; long-term residential (nonmedical, nonacute care in a residential treatment program where stay is typically longer than 30 days), without room and board, per diem** ☑

H0020   **Alcohol and/or drug services; methadone administration and/or service (provision of the drug by a licensed program)**

H0021   **Alcohol and/or drug training service (for staff and personnel not employed by providers)**

H0022   **Alcohol and/or drug intervention service (planned facilitation)**

H0023   **Behavioral health outreach service (planned approach to reach a targeted population)**

H0024   **Behavioral health prevention information dissemination service (one-way direct or nondirect contact with service audiences to affect knowledge and attitude)**

H0025   **Behavioral health prevention education service (delivery of services with target population to affect knowledge, attitude and/or behavior)**

H0026   **Alcohol and/or drug prevention process service, community-based (delivery of services to develop skills of impactors)**

H0027   **Alcohol and/or drug prevention environmental service (broad range of external activities geared toward modifying systems in order to mainstream prevention through policy and law)**

H0028   **Alcohol and/or drug prevention problem identification and referral service (e.g., student assistance and employee assistance programs), does not include assessment**

H0029   **Alcohol and/or drug prevention alternatives service (services for populations that exclude alcohol and other drug use e.g., alcohol free social events)**

H0030   **Behavioral health hotline service**

H0031   **Mental health assessment, by nonphysician**

H0032   **Mental health service plan development by nonphysician**

H0033   **Oral medication administration, direct observation**

H0034   **Medication training and support, per 15 minutes** ☑

H0035   **Mental health partial hospitalization, treatment, less than 24 hours** ☑

H0036   **Community psychiatric supportive treatment, face-to-face, per 15 minutes** ☑

H0037   **Community psychiatric supportive treatment program, per diem** ☑

H0038   **Self-help/peer services, per 15 minutes** ☑

H0039   **Assertive community treatment, face-to-face, per 15 minutes** ☑

H0040   **Assertive community treatment program, per diem** ☑

H0041   **Foster care, child, nontherapeutic, per diem** A ☑

H0042   **Foster care, child, nontherapeutic, per month** A ☑

H0043   **Supported housing, per diem** ☑

H0044   **Supported housing, per month** ☑

H0045   **Respite care services, not in the home, per diem** ☑

H0046   **Mental health services, not otherwise specified**

H0047   **Alcohol and/or other drug abuse services, not otherwise specified**

H0048   **Alcohol and/or other drug testing: collection and handling only, specimens other than blood**

H0049   **Alcohol and/or drug screening**

H0050   **Alcohol and/or drug services, brief intervention, per 15 minutes** ☑

H1000   **Prenatal care, at-risk assessment** M ♀
     AHA: 1Q, '02, 5

H1001   **Prenatal care, at-risk enhanced service; antepartum management** M ♀
     AHA: 1Q, '02, 5

H1002   **Prenatal care, at risk enhanced service; care coordination** M ♀
     AHA: 1Q, '02, 5

H1003   **Prenatal care, at-risk enhanced service; education** M ♀
     AHA: 1Q, '02, 5

H1004   **Prenatal care, at-risk enhanced service; follow-up home visit** M ♀
     AHA: 1Q, '02, 5

H1005   **Prenatal care, at-risk enhanced service package (includes H1001-H1004)** M ♀
     AHA: 1Q, '02, 5

H1010   **Nonmedical family planning education, per session** ☑

Special Coverage Instructions   Noncovered by Medicare   Carrier Discretion   ☑ Quantity Alert ● New Code ○ Recycled/Reinstated ▲ Revised Code

Alcohol and Drug Abuse Treatment Services

H1011 — H2037

H1011	Family assessment by licensed behavioral health professional for state defined purposes	
H2000	Comprehensive multidisciplinary evaluation	
H2001	Rehabilitation program, per 1/2 day	☑
H2010	Comprehensive medication services, per 15 minutes	☑
H2011	Crisis intervention service, per 15 minutes	☑
H2012	Behavioral health day treatment, per hour	☑
H2013	Psychiatric health facility service, per diem	☑
H2014	Skills training and development, per 15 minutes	☑
H2015	Comprehensive community support services, per 15 minutes	☑
H2016	Comprehensive community support services, per diem	☑
H2017	Psychosocial rehabilitation services, per 15 minutes	☑
H2018	Psychosocial rehabilitation services, per diem	☑
H2019	Therapeutic behavioral services, per 15 minutes	☑
H2020	Therapeutic behavioral services, per diem	☑
H2021	Community-based wrap-around services, per 15 minutes	☑
H2022	Community-based wrap-around services, per diem	☑
H2023	Supported employment, per 15 minutes	☑
H2024	Supported employment, per diem	☑
H2025	Ongoing support to maintain employment, per 15 minutes	☑
H2026	Ongoing support to maintain employment, per diem	☑
H2027	Psychoeducational service, per 15 minutes	☑
H2028	Sexual offender treatment service, per 15 minutes	☑
H2029	Sexual offender treatment service, per diem	☑
H2030	Mental health clubhouse services, per 15 minutes	☑
H2031	Mental health clubhouse services, per diem	☑
H2032	Activity therapy, per 15 minutes	☑
H2033	Multisystemic therapy for juveniles, per 15 minutes	☑
H2034	Alcohol and/or drug abuse halfway house services, per diem	☑
H2035	Alcohol and/or other drug treatment program, per hour	☑
H2036	Alcohol and/or other drug treatment program, per diem	☑
H2037	Developmental delay prevention activities, dependent child of client, per 15 minutes	Ⓐ ☑

J Codes Drugs J0120-J8499

J codes include drugs that ordinarily cannot be self-administered, chemotherapy drugs, immunosuppressive drugs, inhalation solutions, and other miscellaneous drugs and solutions.

Miscellaneous Drugs

J0120 Injection, tetracycline, up to 250 mg N N1 ☑

J0121 Injection, omadacycline, 1 mg K2
Use this code for Nuzyra.

J0122 Injection, eravacycline, 1 mg N1
Use this code for Xerava.

J0129 Injection, abatacept, 10 mg (code may be used for Medicare when drug administered under the direct supervision of a physician, not for use when drug is self-administered) K K2 ☑
Use this code for Orencia.
CMS: 100-02,15,50.5

J0130 Injection abciximab, 10 mg N N1 ☑
Use this code for ReoPro.

J0131 Injection, acetaminophen, 10 mg N N1 ☑
Use this code for OFIRMEV.

J0132 Injection, acetylcysteine, 100 mg N N1 ☑
Use this code for Acetadote.

J0133 Injection, acyclovir, 5 mg N N1 ☑
Use this code for Zovirax.
CMS: 100-04,20,180; 100-04,32,411.3

J0135 Injection, adalimumab, 20 mg K K2 ☑
Use this code for Humira.
CMS: 100-02,15,50.5
AHA: 3Q, '05, 7, 9; 2Q, '05, 11

J0153 Injection, adenosine, 1 mg (not to be used to report any adenosine phosphate compounds) N N1 ☑
Use this code for Adenocard, Adenoscan.
AHA: 1Q, '15, 6

J0171 Injection, adrenalin, epinephrine, 0.1 mg N N1 ☑

● **J0172** Injection, aducanumab-avwa, 2 mg
Use this code for Aduhelm.

J0178 Injection, aflibercept, 1 mg K K2 ☑
Use this code for Eylea.

J0179 Injection, brolucizumab-dbll, 1 mg K2
Use this code for Beovu.

J0180 Injection, agalsidase beta, 1 mg K K2 ☑
Use this code for Fabrazyme.
AHA: 2Q, '05, 11

J0185 Injection, aprepitant, 1 mg K2
Use this code for Cinvanti.

J0190 Injection, biperiden lactate, per 5 mg E ☑

J0200 Injection, alatrofloxacin mesylate, 100 mg E ☑

J0202 Injection, alemtuzumab, 1 mg K K2 ☑
Use this code for Lemtrada.
AHA: 1Q, '16, 6-8

J0205 Injection, alglucerase, per 10 units E ☑
Use this code for Ceredase.
AHA: 2Q, '05, 11

J0207 Injection, amifostine, 500 mg K K2 ☑
Use this code for Ethyol.

J0210 Injection, methyldopa HCl, up to 250 mg N ☑
Use this code for Aldomet.

J0215 Injection, alefacept, 0.5 mg E ☑
Use this for Amevive.

J0220 Injection, alglucosidase alfa, 10 mg, not otherwise specified K K2 ☑
Use this code for Myozyme.
AHA: 2Q, '13, 5; 1Q, '08, 6

J0221 Injection, alglucosidase alfa, (Lumizyme), 10 mg K K2 ☑
AHA: 2Q, '13, 5

J0222 Injection, patisiran, 0.1 mg K2
Use this code for Onpattro.

J0223 Injection, givosiran, 0.5 mg K2
Use this code for Givlaari.

● **J0224** Injection, lumasiran, 0.5 mg K2

J0256 Injection, alpha 1-proteinase inhibitor (human), not otherwise specified, 10 mg K K2 ☑
Use this code for Aralast, Aralast NP, Prolastin C, Zemira.
AHA: 2Q, '13, 5; 2Q, '05, 11

J0257 Injection, alpha 1 proteinase inhibitor (human), (GLASSIA), 10 mg K K2 ☑

J0270 Injection, alprostadil, 1.25 mcg (code may be used for Medicare when drug administered under the direct supervision of a physician, not for use when drug is self-administered) B ☑
Use this code for Alprostadil, Caverject, Edex, Prostin VR Pediatric.

J0275 Alprostadil urethral suppository (code may be used for Medicare when drug administered under the direct supervision of a physician, not for use when drug is self-administered) B ☑
Use this code for Muse.

J0278 Injection, amikacin sulfate, 100 mg N N1 ☑
Use this code for Amikin.

J0280 Injection, aminophyllin, up to 250 mg N N1 ☑
AHA: 4Q, '05, 1-6

J0282 Injection, amiodarone HCl, 30 mg N N1 ☑
Use this code for Cordarone IV.

J0285 Injection, amphotericin B, 50 mg N N1 ☑
Use this for Amphocin, Fungizone.
CMS: 100-04,20,180; 100-04,32,411.3

J0287 Injection, amphotericin B lipid complex, 10 mg K K2 ☑
Use this code for Abelcet.
CMS: 100-04,20,180; 100-04,32,411.3

J0288 Injection, amphotericin B cholesteryl sulfate complex, 10 mg E ☑
Use this code for Amphotec.
CMS: 100-04,20,180; 100-04,32,411.3

J0289 Injection, amphotericin B liposome, 10 mg K K2 ☑
Use this code for Ambisome.
CMS: 100-04,20,180; 100-04,32,411.3

J0290 Injection, ampicillin sodium, 500 mg N N1 ☑

J0291 Injection, plazomicin, 5 mg K2
Use this code for Zemdri.

J0295 Injection, ampicillin sodium/sulbactam sodium, per 1.5 g N N1 ☑
Use this code for Unasyn.

J0300 Injection, amobarbital, up to 125 mg K K2 ☑
Use this code for Amytal.

J0330 Injection, succinylcholine chloride, up to 20 mg N N1 ☑
Use this code for Anectine, Quelicin.

J0348 Injection, anidulafungin, 1 mg N N1 ☑
Use this code for Eraxis.

Special Coverage Instructions   Noncovered by Medicare   Carrier Discretion   ☑ Quantity Alert ● New Code   ○ Recycled/Reinstated   ▲ Revised Code

© 2021 Optum360, LLC   A2 - Z3 ASC Pmt   CMS: IOM   AHA: Coding Clinic   DMEPOS Paid   ⊘ SNF Excluded   J Codes — 89

Drugs Administered Other Than Oral Method

J0350 — J0600

Code	Description	Indicators
J0350	**Injection, anistreplase, per 30 units** Use this code for Eminase.	E ☑
J0360	**Injection, hydralazine HCl, up to 20 mg**	N N1 ☑
J0364	**Injection, apomorphine HCl, 1 mg** Use this code for Apokyn. **CMS:** 100-02,15,50.5	E ☑
J0365	**Injection, aprotinin, 10,000 kiu** Use this code for Trasylol.	E ☑
J0380	**Injection, metaraminol bitartrate, per 10 mg** Use this code for Aramine.	N ☑
J0390	**Injection, chloroquine HCl, up to 250 mg** Use this code for Aralen.	N K2 ☑
J0395	**Injection, arbutamine HCl, 1 mg**	E ☑
J0400	**Injection, aripiprazole, intramuscular, 0.25 mg** Use this code for Abilify. **AHA:** 1Q, '08, 6	K N1 ☑
J0401	**Injection, aripiprazole, extended release, 1 mg** Use this code for the Abilify Maintena kit. **AHA:** 1Q, '14, 6	K K2 ☑
J0456	**Injection, azithromycin, 500 mg** Use this code for Zithromax.	N N1 ☑
J0461	**Injection, atropine sulfate, 0.01 mg** Use this code for AtroPen.	N N1 ☑
J0470	**Injection, dimercaprol, per 100 mg** Use this code for BAL.	K N1 ☑
J0475	**Injection, baclofen, 10 mg** Use this code for Lioresal, Gablofen.	K K2 ☑
J0476	**Injection, baclofen, 50 mcg for intrathecal trial** Use this code for Lioresal, Gablofen.	K N1 ☑
J0480	**Injection, basiliximab, 20 mg** Use this code for Simulect.	K K2 ☑
J0485	**Injection, belatacept, 1 mg** Use this code for Nulojix.	K K2 ☑
J0490	**Injection, belimumab, 10 mg** Use this code for BENLYSTA.	K K2 ☑
J0500	**Injection, dicyclomine HCl, up to 20 mg** Use this code for Bentyl.	N N1 ☑
J0515	**Injection, benztropine mesylate, per 1 mg** Use this code for Cogentin.	N N1 ☑
J0517	**Injection, benralizumab, 1 mg** Use this code for Fasenra.	K2
J0520	**Injection, bethanechol chloride, Myotonachol or Urecholine, up to 5 mg**	E ☑
J0558	**Injection, penicillin G benzathine and penicillin G procaine, 100,000 units** Use this code for Bicillin CR, Bicillin CR 900/300, Bicillin CR Tubex.	N K2 ☑
J0561	**Injection, penicillin G benzathine, 100,000 units** **AHA:** 2Q, '13, 5	K K2 ☑
J0565	**Injection, bezlotoxumab, 10 mg** Use this code for Zinplava.	G K2
J0567	**Injection, cerliponase alfa, 1 mg** Use this code for Brineura.	N1
J0570	**Buprenorphine implant, 74.2 mg** Use this code for Probuphine. **AHA:** 1Q, '17, 9-10	G K2 ☑
J0571	**Buprenorphine, oral, 1 mg** Use this code for Subutex. **AHA:** 1Q, '15, 6	E ☑
J0572	**Buprenorphine/naloxone, oral, less than or equal to 3 mg buprenorphine** Use this code for Bunavail, Suboxone, Zubsolv. **AHA:** 1Q, '15, 6	E ☑
J0573	**Buprenorphine/naloxone, oral, greater than 3 mg, but less than or equal to 6 mg buprenorphine** Use this code for Bunavail, Suboxone, Zubsolv. **AHA:** 1Q, '16, 6-8; 1Q, '15, 6	E ☑
J0574	**Buprenorphine/naloxone, oral, greater than 6 mg, but less than or equal to 10 mg buprenorphine** Use this code for Bunavail, Suboxone. **AHA:** 1Q, '16, 6-8; 1Q, '15, 6	E ☑
J0575	**Buprenorphine/naloxone, oral, greater than 10 mg buprenorphine** Use this code for Suboxone. **AHA:** 1Q, '16, 6-8; 1Q, '15, 6	E ☑
J0583	**Injection, bivalirudin, 1 mg** Use this code for Angiomax.	N N1 ☑
J0584	**Injection, burosumab-twza, 1 mg** Use this code for Crysvita. **CMS:** 100-04,4,260.1; 100-04,4,260.1.1	K2
J0585	**Injection, onabotulinumtoxinA, 1 unit** Use this code for Botox, Botox Cosmetic.	K K2 ☑
J0586	**Injection, abobotulinumtoxinA, 5 units** Use this code for Dysport.	K K2 ☑
J0587	**Injection, rimabotulinumtoxinB, 100 units** Use this code for Myobloc. **AHA:** 2Q, '02, 8-9; 1Q, '02, 5	K K2 ☑
J0588	**Injection, incobotulinumtoxinA, 1 unit** Use this code for XEOMIN.	K K2 ☑
J0591	**Injection, deoxycholic acid, 1 mg** Use this code for Kybella.	
J0592	**Injection, buprenorphine HCl, 0.1 mg** Use this code for Buprenex.	N N1 ☑
J0593	**Injection, lanadelumab-flyo, 1 mg (code may be used for Medicare when drug administered under direct supervision of a physician, not for use when drug is self-administered)** Use this code for Takhzyro.	N1
J0594	**Injection, busulfan, 1 mg** Use this code for Busulfex.	K K2 ☑
J0595	**Injection, butorphanol tartrate, 1 mg** Use this code for Stadol. **AHA:** 2Q, '05, 11	N N1 ☑
J0596	**Injection, C1 esterase inhibitor (recombinant), Ruconest, 10 units** **CMS:** 100-02,15,50.5	K K2 ☑
J0597	**Injection, C1 esterase inhibitor (human), Berinert, 10 units**	K K2 ☑
J0598	**Injection, C1 esterase inhibitor (human), Cinryze, 10 units**	K K2 ☑
J0599	**Injection, C1 esterase inhibitor (human), (Haegarda), 10 units**	K2
J0600	**Injection, edetate calcium disodium, up to 1,000 mg** Use this code for Calcium Disodium Versenate, Calcium EDTA.	K K2 ☑

☑ Special Coverage Instructions   Noncovered by Medicare   Carrier Discretion   ☑ Quantity Alert   ● New Code   ○ Recycled/Reinstated   ▲ Revised Code

   A Age Edit   M Maternity Edit   ♀ Female Only   ♂ Male Only   A-Y OPPS Status Indicators   © 2021 Optum360, LLC

J0604   Cinacalcet, oral, 1 mg, (for ESRD on dialysis)   `B`
Use this code for Sensipar.

J0606   Injection, etelcalcetide, 0.1 mg   `K` `N1`
Use this code for Parsabiv.

J0610   Injection, calcium gluconate, per 10 ml   `N1` ☑

J0620   Injection, calcium glycerophosphate and calcium lactate, per 10 ml   `N` `N1` ☑

J0630   Injection, calcitonin salmon, up to 400 units   `K` `K2` ☑
Use this code for Calcimar, Miacalcin.
CMS: 100-04,10,90.1

J0636   Injection, calcitriol, 0.1 mcg   `N` `N1` ☑
Use this code for Calcijex.

J0637   Injection, caspofungin acetate, 5 mg   `K` `N1` ☑
Use this code for Cancidas.

J0638   Injection, canakinumab, 1 mg   `K` `K2` ☑
Use this code for ILARIS.

J0640   Injection, leucovorin calcium, per 50 mg   `N` `N1` ☑
AHA: 1Q, '09, 10

J0641   Injection, levoleucovorin, not otherwise specified, 0.5 mg   `K` `K2` ☑

J0642   Injection, levoleucovorin (Khapzory), 0.5 mg   `K2`

J0670   Injection, mepivacaine HCl, per 10 ml   `N` `N1` ☑
Use this code for Carbocaine, Polocaine, Isocaine HCl, Scandonest

J0690   Injection, cefazolin sodium, 500 mg   `N` `N1` ☑

J0691   Injection, lefamulin, 1 mg   `K2`
Use this code for Xenleta.

J0692   Injection, cefepime HCl, 500 mg   `N` `N1` ☑
AHA: 1Q, '02, 5

J0693   ~~Injection, cefiderocol, 5 mg~~
To report, see ~J0699

J0694   Injection, cefoxitin sodium, 1 g   `N` `N1` ☑

J0695   Injection, ceftolozane 50 mg and tazobactam 25 mg   `K` `K2` ☑
Use this code for Zerbaxa.

J0696   Injection, ceftriaxone sodium, per 250 mg   `N` `N1` ☑

J0697   Injection, sterile cefuroxime sodium, per 750 mg   `N` `N1` ☑

J0698   Injection, cefotaxime sodium, per g   `N` `N1` ☑

● **J0699**   Injection, cefiderocol, 10 mg   `K2`
Use this code for Fetroja.

J0702   Injection, betamethasone acetate 3 mg and betamethasone sodium phosphate 3 mg   `N` `N1` ☑

J0706   Injection, caffeine citrate, 5 mg   `N` `N1` ☑
AHA: 2Q, '02, 8-9; 1Q, '02, 5

J0710   Injection, cephapirin sodium, up to 1 g   `E` ☑

J0712   Injection, ceftaroline fosamil, 10 mg   `K` `K2` ☑

J0713   Injection, ceftazidime, per 500 mg   `N` `N1` ☑

J0714   Injection, ceftazidime and avibactam, 0.5 g/0.125 g   `K` `K2` ☑
Use this code for Avycaz.
AHA: 1Q, '16, 6-8

J0715   Injection, ceftizoxime sodium, per 500 mg   `N` `N1` ☑

J0716   Injection, Centruroides immune f(ab)2, up to 120 mg   `K` `K2` ☑
Use this code for Anascorp.

J0717   Injection, certolizumab pegol, 1 mg (code may be used for Medicare when drug administered under the direct supervision of a physician, not for use when drug is self-administered)   `K` `K2` ☑
CMS: 100-02,15,50.5
AHA: 1Q, '14, 7

J0720   Injection, chloramphenicol sodium succinate, up to 1 g   `N` `N1` ☑

J0725   Injection, chorionic gonadotropin, per 1,000 USP units   `N` `N1` ☑
CMS: 100-02,15,50.5

J0735   Injection, clonidine HCl, 1 mg   `N` `N1` ☑

J0740   Injection, cidofovir, 375 mg   `K` `K2` ☑

● **J0741**   Injection, cabotegravir and rilpivirine, 2 mg/3 mg   `K2`
Use this code for Cabenuva.

J0742   Injection, imipenem 4 mg, cilastatin 4 mg and relebactam 2 mg   `K2`
Use this code for Recarbrio.

J0743   Injection, cilastatin sodium; imipenem, per 250 mg   `N` `N1` ☑

J0744   Injection, ciprofloxacin for intravenous infusion, 200 mg   `N` `N1` ☑
AHA: 1Q, '02, 5

J0745   Injection, codeine phosphate, per 30 mg   `N` `K2` ☑

J0770   Injection, colistimethate sodium, up to 150 mg   `N` `N1` ☑

J0775   Injection, collagenase, clostridium histolyticum, 0.01 mg   `K` `K2` ☑

J0780   Injection, prochlorperazine, up to 10 mg   `N` `N1` ☑

J0791   Injection, crizanlizumab-tmca, 5 mg   `K2`
Use this code for ADAKVEO.

J0795   Injection, corticorelin ovine triflutate, 1 mcg   `K` `K2` ☑

J0800   Injection, corticotropin, up to 40 units   `K` `N1` ☑
CMS: 100-02,15,50.5

J0834   Injection, cosyntropin, 0.25 mg   `N` `N1` ☑
Use this code for Cortrosyn.

J0840   Injection, crotalidae polyvalent immune fab (ovine), up to 1 g   `K` `K2` ☑

J0841   Injection, crotalidae immune F(ab')2 (equine), 120 mg   `K2`
Use this code for Anavip.
CMS: 100-04,4,260.1; 100-04,4,260.1.1

J0850   Injection, cytomegalovirus immune globulin intravenous (human), per vial   `K` `K2` ☑

J0875   Injection, dalbavancin, 5 mg   `K` `K2` ☑
Use this code for Dalvance.

J0878   Injection, daptomycin, 1 mg   `K` `N1` ☑
Use this code for Cubicin.
AHA: 2Q, '05, 11

J0881   Injection, darbepoetin alfa, 1 mcg (non-ESRD use)   `K` `K2` ☑
Use this code for Aranesp.
CMS: 100-03,110.21; 100-04,17,80.12

J0882   Injection, darbepoetin alfa, 1 mcg (for ESRD on dialysis)   `K` `K2` ☑ ⊘
Use this code for Aranesp.
CMS: 100-04,8,60.4; 100-04,8,60.4.1; 100-04,8,60.4.2; 100-04,8,60.4.5.1; 100-04,8,60.4.6.3; 100-04,8,60.4.6.4; 100-04,8,60.4.6.5

J0883   Injection, argatroban, 1 mg (for non-ESRD use)   `K` `K2` ☑

J0884   Injection, argatroban, 1 mg (for ESRD on dialysis)   `K` `K2` ☑

Special Coverage Instructions   Noncovered by Medicare   Carrier Discretion   ☑ Quantity Alert   ● New Code   ○ Recycled/Reinstated   ▲ Revised Code

© 2021 Optum360, LLC   `A2`-`Z3` ASC Pmt   **CMS:** IOM   **AHA:** Coding Clinic   ⚕ DMEPOS Paid   ⊘ SNF Excluded   **J Codes — 91**

Drugs Administered Other Than Oral Method

J0885   **Injection, epoetin alfa, (for non-ESRD use), 1000 units**   K K2 ☑
Use this code for Epogen/Procrit.
CMS: 100-03,110.21; 100-04,17,80.12
AHA: 2Q, '06, 4, 5

J0887   **Injection, epoetin beta, 1 mcg, (for ESRD on dialysis)**   N M1 ☑
Use this code for Mircera.
AHA: 1Q, '15, 6

J0888   **Injection, epoetin beta, 1 mcg, (for non-ESRD use)**   K K2 ☑
Use this code for Mircera.
AHA: 1Q, '15, 6

J0890   **Injection, peginesatide, 0.1 mg (for ESRD on dialysis)**   E ☑
Use this code for Omontys.
CMS: 100-04,8,60.4; 100-04,8,60.4.1; 100-04,8,60.4.2; 100-04,8,60.4.5.1; 100-04,8,60.4.7

J0894   **Injection, decitabine, 1 mg**   K K2 ☑ ⊘
Use this code for Dacogen.

J0895   **Injection, deferoxamine mesylate, 500 mg**   N M1 ☑
Use this code for Desferal.
CMS: 100-04,20,180; 100-04,32,411.3

J0896   **Injection, luspatercept-aamt, 0.25 mg**   K2
Use this code for REBLOZYL.

J0897   **Injection, denosumab, 1 mg**   K K2 ☑
Use this code for XGEVA, Prolia.
CMS: 100-04,10,90.1
AHA: 1Q, '16, 5

J0945   **Injection, brompheniramine maleate, per 10 mg**   N M1 ☑

J1000   **Injection, depo-estradiol cypionate, up to 5 mg**   N M1 ☑
Use this code for depGynogen, Depogen, Estradiol Cypionate.

J1020   **Injection, methylprednisolone acetate, 20 mg**   N M1 ☑
Use this code for Depo-Medrol.
AHA: 2Q, '09, 9; 3Q, '05, 10

J1030   **Injection, methylprednisolone acetate, 40 mg**   N M1 ☑
Use this code for DepoMedalone40, Depo-Medrol, Sano-Drol.
AHA: 2Q, '09, 9; 3Q, '05, 10

J1040   **Injection, methylprednisolone acetate, 80 mg**   N M1 ☑
Use this code for Cortimed, DepMedalone, DepoMedalone 80, Depo-Medrol, Duro Cort, Methylcotolone, Pri-Methylate, Sano-Drol.
AHA: 2Q, '09, 9

J1050   **Injection, medroxyprogesterone acetate, 1 mg**   N M1 ☑

J1071   **Injection, testosterone cypionate, 1 mg**   N M1 ☑
Use this code for Depo-testostrone.
AHA: 2Q, '15, 7; 1Q, '15, 6

J1094   **Injection, dexamethasone acetate, 1 mg**   N M1 ☑
Use this code for Cortastat LA, Dalalone L.A., Dexamethasone Acetate Anhydrous, Dexone LA.

J1095   **Injection, dexamethasone 9%, intraocular, 1 mcg**   K2

J1096   **Dexamethasone, lacrimal ophthalmic insert, 0.1 mg**   K2
Use this code for Dextenza.

J1097   **Phenylephrine 10.16 mg/ml and ketorolac 2.88 mg/ml ophthalmic irrigation solution, 1 ml**   K2
Use this code for Omidria.

J1100   **Injection, dexamethasone sodium phosphate, 1 mg**   N M1 ☑
Use this code for Cortastat, Dalalone, Decaject, Dexone, Solurex, Adrenocort, Primethasone, Dexasone, Dexim, Medidex, Spectro-Dex.

J1110   **Injection, dihydroergotamine mesylate, per 1 mg**   K M1 ☑
Use this code for D.H.E. 45.

J1120   **Injection, acetazolamide sodium, up to 500 mg**   N M1 ☑
Use this code for Diamox.
AHA: 4Q, '05, 1-6; 3Q, '04, 1-10

J1130   **Injection, diclofenac sodium, 0.5 mg**   K M1 ☑
Use this code for Dyloject.
AHA: 1Q, '17, 9-10

J1160   **Injection, digoxin, up to 0.5 mg**   N M1 ☑
Use this code for Lanoxin.
AHA: 4Q, '05, 1-6

J1162   **Injection, digoxin immune fab (ovine), per vial**   K K2 ☑
Use this code for Digibind, Digifab.

J1165   **Injection, phenytoin sodium, per 50 mg**   N M1 ☑
Use this code for Dilantin.

J1170   **Injection, hydromorphone, up to 4 mg**   N M1 ☑
Use this code for Dilaudid, Dilaudid-HP.
CMS: 100-04,20,180; 100-04,32,411.3

J1180   **Injection, dyphylline, up to 500 mg**   E ☑

J1190   **Injection, dexrazoxane HCl, per 250 mg**   K K2 ☑
Use this code for Zinecard.

J1200   **Injection, diphenhydramine HCl, up to 50 mg**   N M1 ☑
Use this code for Benadryl, Benahist 10, Benahist 50, Benoject-10, Benoject-50, Bena-D 10, Bena-D 50, Nordryl, Dihydrex, Dimine, Diphenacen-50, Hyrexin-50, Truxadryl, Wehdryl.
AHA: 1Q, '02, 1-2

J1201   **Injection, cetirizine HCl, 0.5 mg**   K2
Use this code for Quzyttir.

J1205   **Injection, chlorothiazide sodium, per 500 mg**   N M1 ☑
Use this code for Diuril Sodium.

J1212   **Injection, DMSO, dimethyl sulfoxide, 50%, 50 ml**   K K2 ☑
Use this code for Rimso 50. DMSO is covered only as a treatment of interstitial cystitis.

J1230   **Injection, methadone HCl, up to 10 mg**   N M1 ☑
Use this code for Dolophine HCl.

J1240   **Injection, dimenhydrinate, up to 50 mg**   N M1 ☑
Use this code for Dramamine, Dinate, Dommanate, Dramanate, Dramilin, Dramocen, Dramoject, Dymenate, Hydrate, Marmine, Wehamine.

J1245   **Injection, dipyridamole, per 10 mg**   N M1 ☑
Use this code for Persantine IV.
AHA: 4Q, '05, 1-6; 3Q, '04, 1-10

J1250   **Injection, dobutamine HCl, per 250 mg**   N M1 ☑
CMS: 100-04,20,180; 100-04,32,411.3
AHA: 4Q, '05, 1-6; 3Q, '04, 1-10

J1260   **Injection, dolasetron mesylate, 10 mg**   N M1 ☑
Use this code for Anzemet.

J1265   **Injection, dopamine HCl, 40 mg**   N M1 ☑
CMS: 100-04,20,180; 100-04,32,411.3
AHA: 4Q, '05, 1-6

J1267   **Injection, doripenem, 10 mg**   N M1 ☑
Use this code for Doribax.

J1270   **Injection, doxercalciferol, 1 mcg**   N M1 ☑
Use this code for Hectorol.
AHA: 1Q, '02, 5

J1290   **Injection, ecallantide, 1 mg**   K K2 ☑
Use this code for KALBITOR.

J1300   **Injection, eculizumab, 10 mg**   K K2 ☑
Use this code for Soliris.
AHA: 1Q, '08, 6

Special Coverage Instructions   Noncovered by Medicare   Carrier Discretion   ☑ Quantity Alert   ● New Code   ○ Recycled/Reinstated   ▲ Revised Code

A Age Edit   M Maternity Edit   ♀ Female Only   ♂ Male Only   A-Y OPPS Status Indicators   © 2021 Optum360, LLC

J1301 **Injection, edaravone, 1 mg** ☒K2
Use this code for Radicava.

J1303 **Injection, ravulizumab-cwvz, 10 mg** ☒K2
Use this code for Ultomiris.

● **J1305** **Injection, evinacumab-dgnb, 5 mg** ☒K2
Use this code for Evkeeza.

J1320 **Injection, amitriptyline HCl, up to 20 mg** N N1 ☑
Use this code for Elavil.

J1322 **Injection, elosulfase alfa, 1 mg** K K2 ☑
Use this code for Vimizim.
AHA: 1Q, '15, 6

J1324 **Injection, enfuvirtide, 1 mg** E ☑
Use this code for Fuzeon.
CMS: 100-02,15,50.5

J1325 **Injection, epoprostenol, 0.5 mg** N N1 ☑
Use this code for Flolan and Veletri. See K0455 for infusion pump for epoprosterol.
CMS: 100-04,20,180; 100-04,32,411.3

J1327 **Injection, eptifibatide, 5 mg** K N1 ☑
Use this code for Integrilin.

J1330 **Injection, ergonovine maleate, up to 0.2 mg** N ☑
Medicare jurisdiction: local contractor. Use this code for Ergotrate Maleate.

J1335 **Injection, ertapenem sodium, 500 mg** N N1 ☑
Use this code for Invanz.

J1364 **Injection, erythromycin lactobionate, per 500 mg** K K2 ☑

J1380 **Injection, estradiol valerate, up to 10 mg** N N1 ☑
Use this code for Delestrogen, Dioval, Dioval XX, Dioval 40, Duragen-10, Duragen-20, Duragen-40, Estradiol L.A., Estradiol L.A. 20, Estradiol L.A. 40, Gynogen L.A. 10, Gynogen L.A. 20, Gynogen L.A. 40, Valergen 10, Valergen 20, Valergen 40, Estra-L 20, Estra-L 40, L.A.E. 20.

J1410 **Injection, estrogen conjugated, per 25 mg** K K2 ☑
Use this code for Natural Estrogenic Substance, Premarin Intravenous, Primestrin Aqueous.

● **J1426** **Injection, casimersen, 10 mg** ☒K2
Use this code for Amondys 45.

● **J1427** **Injection, viltolarsen, 10 mg** ☒K2
Use this code for Viltepso.

J1428 **Injection, eteplirsen, 10 mg** G N1
Use this code for Exondys 51.

J1429 **Injection, golodirsen, 10 mg** ☒K2
Use this code for Vyondys 53.

J1430 **Injection, ethanolamine oleate, 100 mg** K K2 ☑
Use this code for Ethamolin.

J1435 **Injection, estrone, per 1 mg** E ☑
Use this code for Estone Aqueous, Estragyn, Estro-A, Estrone, Estronol, Theelin Aqueous, Estone 5, Kestrone 5.

J1436 **Injection, etidronate disodium, per 300 mg** E ☑
Use this code for Didronel.

J1437 **Injection, ferric derisomaltose, 10 mg** ☒K2
Use this code for Monoferric.

J1438 **Injection, etanercept, 25 mg (code may be used for Medicare when drug administered under the direct supervision of a physician, not for use when drug is self-administered)** K K2 ☑
Use this code for Enbrel.
CMS: 100-02,15,50.5

J1439 **Injection, ferric carboxymaltose, 1 mg** K K2 ☑
Use this code for Injectafer.
AHA: 1Q, '15, 6

J1442 **Injection, filgrastim (G-CSF), excludes biosimilars, 1 mcg** K K2 ☑
Use this code for Neupogen.
AHA: 1Q, '14, 7

▲ **J1443** **Injection, ferric pyrophosphate citrate solution (Triferic), 0.1 mg of iron** N ☑
Use this code for Triferic solution.
AHA: 1Q, '16, 6-8

J1444 **Injection, ferric pyrophosphate citrate powder, 0.1 mg of iron**
Use this code for Triferic powder.

● **J1445** **Injection, ferric pyrophosphate citrate solution (Triferic AVNU), 0.1 mg of iron**

J1447 **Injection, tbo-filgrastim, 1 mcg** K K2 ☑
Use this code for Granix.
AHA: 1Q, '16, 6-8

● **J1448** **Injection, trilaciclib, 1 mg** ☒K2
Use this code for Cosela.

J1450 **Injection, fluconazole, 200 mg** N N1 ☑
Use this code for Diflucan.
CMS: 100-02,15,50.6

J1451 **Injection, fomepizole, 15 mg** K K2 ☑
Use this code for Antizol.
CMS: 100-02,15,50.6

J1452 **Injection, fomivirsen sodium, intraocular, 1.65 mg** E ☑
Use this code for Vitravene.
CMS: 100-02,15,50.4.2; 100-02,15,50.6

J1453 **Injection, fosaprepitant, 1 mg** K K2 ☑
Use this code for Emend.
CMS: 100-02,15,50.6

J1454 **Injection, fosnetupitant 235 mg and palonosetron 0.25 mg** ☒K2
Use this code for Akynzeo.
CMS: 100-02,15,50.6

J1455 **Injection, foscarnet sodium, per 1,000 mg** K K2 ☑
Use this code for Foscavir.
CMS: 100-02,15,50.6; 100-04,20,180; 100-04,32,411.3

J1457 **Injection, gallium nitrate, 1 mg** E ☑
Use this code for Ganite.
CMS: 100-02,15,50.6; 100-04,20,180; 100-04,32,411.3
AHA: 2Q, '05, 11

J1458 **Injection, galsulfase, 1 mg** K K2 ☑
Use this code for Naglazyme.
CMS: 100-02,15,50.6

J1459 **Injection, immune globulin (Privigen), intravenous, nonlyophilized (e.g., liquid), 500 mg** K K2 ☑
CMS: 100-02,15,50.6

J1460 **Injection, gamma globulin, intramuscular, 1 cc** K K2 ☑
Use this code for GamaSTAN SD.
CMS: 100-02,15,50.6; 100-04,17,80.6

● **J1554** **Injection, immune globulin (Asceniv), 500 mg** ☒K2
CMS: 100-02,15,50.6

J1555 **Injection, immune globulin (Cuvitru), 100 mg** K K2 ☑
CMS: 100-02,15,50.6; 100-04,20,180; 100-04,32,411.3

J1556 **Injection, immune globulin (Bivigam), 500 mg** K K2 ☑
CMS: 100-02,15,50.6

J1557 **Injection, immune globulin, (Gammaplex), intravenous, nonlyophilized (e.g., liquid), 500 mg** K K2 ☑
CMS: 100-02,15,50.6

J1558 **Injection, immune globulin (xembify), 100 mg** ☒K2
CMS: 100-02,15,50.6; 100-04,32,411.3

Special Coverage Instructions   Noncovered by Medicare   Carrier Discretion   ☑ Quantity Alert   ● New Code   ○ Recycled/Reinstated   ▲ Revised Code

© 2021 Optum360, LLC   A2-Z3 ASC Pmt   CMS: IOM   AHA: Coding Clinic   ♿ DMEPOS Paid   ⊘ SNF Excluded   J Codes — 93

Drugs Administered Other Than Oral Method

J1559 — J1726

Code	Description	Indicators
J1559	Injection, immune globulin (Hizentra), 100 mg CMS: 100-02,15,50.6; 100-04,20,180; 100-04,32,411.3	K K2 ☑
J1560	Injection, gamma globulin, intramuscular, over 10 cc Use this code for GamaSTAN SD. CMS: 100-02,15,50.6; 100-04,17,80.6	K K2 ☑
J1561	Injection, immune globulin, (Gamunex/Gamunex-C/Gammaked), nonlyophilized (e.g., liquid), 500 mg CMS: 100-02,15,50.6; 100-04,20,180; 100-04,32,411.3 AHA: 1Q, '08, 6	K K2 ☑
J1562	Injection, immune globulin (Vivaglobin), 100 mg CMS: 100-02,15,50.6; 100-04,20,180; 100-04,32,411.3	E ☑
J1566	Injection, immune globulin, intravenous, lyophilized (e.g., powder), not otherwise specified, 500 mg Use this code for Carimune, Gammagard S/D, Iveegam, Polygam, Polygam S/D. CMS: 100-02,15,50.6 AHA: 2Q, '13, 5	K K2 ☑
J1568	Injection, immune globulin, (Octagam), intravenous, nonlyophilized (e.g., liquid), 500 mg CMS: 100-02,15,50.6 AHA: 1Q, '08, 6	K K2 ☑
J1569	Injection, immune globulin, (Gammagard liquid), nonlyophilized, (e.g., liquid), 500 mg CMS: 100-02,15,50.6; 100-04,20,180; 100-04,32,411.3 AHA: 1Q, '08, 6	K K2 ☑
J1570	Injection, ganciclovir sodium, 500 mg Use this code for Cytovene. CMS: 100-04,20,180; 100-04,32,411.3	N N1 ☑
J1571	Injection, hepatitis B immune globulin (Hepagam B), intramuscular, 0.5 ml AHA: 3Q, '08, 7, 8; 1Q, '08, 6	K K2 ☑
J1572	Injection, immune globulin, (Flebogamma/Flebogamma Dif), intravenous, nonlyophilized (e.g., liquid), 500 mg AHA: 1Q, '08, 6	K K2 ☑
J1573	Injection, hepatitis B immune globulin (Hepagam B), intravenous, 0.5 ml AHA: 3Q, '08, 7, 8; 1Q, '08, 6	K K2 ☑
J1575	Injection, immune globulin/hyaluronidase, 100 mg immuneglobulin Use this code for HyQvia. CMS: 100-04,20,180; 100-04,32,411.3 AHA: 1Q, '16, 6-8	K K2 ☑
J1580	Injection, garamycin, gentamicin, up to 80 mg Use this code for Gentamicin Sulfate, Jenamicin.	N N1 ☑
J1595	Injection, glatiramer acetate, 20 mg Use this code for Copaxone. CMS: 100-02,15,50.5	K K2 ☑
J1599	Injection, immune globulin, intravenous, nonlyophilized (e.g., liquid), not otherwise specified, 500 mg AHA: 2Q, '13, 5	N N1 ☑
J1600	Injection, gold sodium thiomalate, up to 50 mg Use this code for Myochrysine. CMS: 100-04,4,20.6.4	E ☑
J1602	Injection, golimumab, 1 mg, for intravenous use Use this code for Simponi. AHA: 1Q, '14, 6	K K2 ☑
J1610	Injection, glucagon HCl, per 1 mg Use this code for Glucagen. AHA: 4Q, '05, 1-6	K K2 ☑
J1620	Injection, gonadorelin HCl, per 100 mcg Use this code for Factrel, Lutrepulse.	E ☑
J1626	Injection, granisetron HCl, 100 mcg Use this code for Kytril. CMS: 100-04,4,20.6.4	N N1 ☑
J1627	Injection, granisetron, extended-release, 0.1 mg Use this code for Sustol.	G N1
J1628	Injection, guselkumab, 1 mg Use this code for Tremfya.	K2
J1630	Injection, haloperidol, up to 5 mg Use this code for Haldol. CMS: 100-04,4,20.6.4	N N1 ☑
J1631	Injection, haloperidol decanoate, per 50 mg Use this code for Haldol Decanoate-50. CMS: 100-04,4,20.6.4	N N1 ☑
J1632	Injection, brexanolone, 1 mg Use this code for Zulresso.	K2
J1640	Injection, hemin, 1 mg Use this code for Panhematin.	K K2 ☑
J1642	Injection, heparin sodium, (heparin lock flush), per 10 units Use this code for Hep-Lock, Hep-Lock U/P, Hep-Pak, Lok-Pak. CMS: 100-04,4,20.6.4 AHA: 4Q, '05, 1-6	N N1 ☑
J1644	Injection, Heparin sodium, per 1000 units Use this code for Heparin Sodium, Liquaemin Sodium. CMS: 100-04,4,20.6.4	N N1 ☑
J1645	Injection, dalteparin sodium, per 2500 IU Use this code for Fragmin. CMS: 100-02,15,50.5; 100-04,4,20.6.4	N N1 ☑
J1650	Injection, enoxaparin sodium, 10 mg Use this code for Lovenox. CMS: 100-02,15,50.5; 100-04,4,20.6.4	N N1 ☑
J1652	Injection, fondaparinux sodium, 0.5 mg Use this code for Atrixtra. CMS: 100-02,15,50.5	N N1 ☑
J1655	Injection, tinzaparin sodium, 1000 IU Use this code for Innohep. CMS: 100-02,15,50.5; 100-04,4,20.6.4 AHA: 1Q, '02, 5	N N1 ☑
J1670	Injection, tetanus immune globulin, human, up to 250 units Use this code for HyperTET SD.	K K2 ☑
J1675	Injection, histrelin acetate, 10 mcg Use this code for Supprelin LA.	B ☑
J1700	Injection, hydrocortisone acetate, up to 25 mg Use this code for Hydrocortone Acetate. CMS: 100-04,4,20.6.4	N N1 ☑
J1710	Injection, hydrocortisone sodium phosphate, up to 50 mg Use this code for Hydrocortone Phosphate. CMS: 100-04,4,20.6.4	N N1 ☑
J1720	Injection, hydrocortisone sodium succinate, up to 100 mg Use this code for Solu-Cortef, A-Hydrocort. CMS: 100-04,4,20.6.4	N N1 ☑
J1726	Injection, hydroxyprogesterone caproate, (Makena), 10 mg	K K2

☑ Special Coverage Instructions   Noncovered by Medicare   Carrier Discretion   ☑ Quantity Alert   ● New Code   ○ Recycled/Reinstated   ▲ Revised Code

J1729	Injection, hydroxyprogesterone caproate, not otherwise specified, 10 mg	N K2
J1730	Injection, diazoxide, up to 300 mg	E ☑
J1738	Injection, meloxicam, 1 mg	K2
	Use this code for Anjeso.	
J1740	Injection, ibandronate sodium, 1 mg	K K2 ☑
	Use this code for Boniva.	
J1741	Injection, ibuprofen, 100 mg	N N1 ☑
	Use this code for Caldolor.	
J1742	Injection, ibutilide fumarate, 1 mg	K K2 ☑
	Use this code for Corvert.	
J1743	Injection, idursulfase, 1 mg	K N1 ☑
	Use this code for Elaprase.	
J1744	Injection, icatibant, 1 mg	K K2 ☑
	Use this code for Firazyr.	
	CMS: 100-02,15,50.5	
J1745	Injection, infliximab, excludes biosimilar, 10 mg	K K2 ☑
	Use this code for Remicade.	
J1746	Injection, ibalizumab-uiyk, 10 mg	K2
	Use this code for Trogarzo.	
	CMS: 100-04,4,260.1; 100-04,4,260.1.1	
J1750	Injection, iron dextran, 50 mg	K K2 ☑
	Use this code for INFeD.	
J1756	Injection, iron sucrose, 1 mg	N N1 ☑
	Use this code for Venofer.	
	CMS: 100-04,8,60.2.4; 100-04,8,60.2.4.2	
J1786	Injection, imiglucerase, 10 units	K K2 ☑
	Use this code for Cerezyme.	
J1790	Injection, droperidol, up to 5 mg	N N1 ☑
	Use this code for Inapsine.	
	CMS: 100-04,4,20.6.4	
J1800	Injection, propranolol HCl, up to 1 mg	N N1 ☑
	Use this code for Inderal.	
	CMS: 100-04,4,20.6.4	
	AHA: 4Q, '05, 1-6	
J1810	Injection, droperidol and fentanyl citrate, up to 2 ml ampule	E ☑
	AHA: 2Q, '02, 8-9	
J1815	Injection, insulin, per 5 units	N N1 ☑
	Use this code for Humalog, Humulin, Iletin, Insulin Lispo, Lantus, Levemir, NPH, Pork insulin, Regular insulin, Ultralente, Velosulin, Humulin R, Iletin II Regular Pork, Insulin Purified Pork, Relion, Lente Iletin I, Novolin R, Humulin R U-500.	
	CMS: 100-04,4,20.6.4	
	AHA: 4Q, '05, 1-6	
J1817	Insulin for administration through DME (i.e., insulin pump) per 50 units	N N1 ☑
	Use this code for Humalog, Humulin, Vesolin BR, Iletin II NPH Pork, Lispro-PFC, Novolin, Novolog, Novolog Flexpen, Novolog Mix, Relion Novolin.	
	AHA: 4Q, '05, 1-6	
J1823	Injection, inebilizumab-cdon, 1 mg	K2
	Use this code for Uplizna.	
J1826	Injection, interferon beta-1a, 30 mcg	K K2 ☑
	Use this code for AVONEX, Rebif.	
	AHA: 4Q, '14, 6; 2Q, '11, 9	
J1830	Injection interferon beta-1b, 0.25 mg (code may be used for Medicare when drug administered under the direct supervision of a physician, not for use when drug is self-administered)	K K2 ☑
	Use this code for Betaseron.	
	CMS: 100-02,15,50.5	
J1833	Injection, isavuconazonium, 1 mg	K K2 ☑
	Use this code for Cresemba.	
J1835	Injection, itraconazole, 50 mg	E ☑
	Use this code for Sporonox IV.	
	CMS: 100-04,4,20.6.4	
	AHA: 1Q, '02, 5	
J1840	Injection, kanamycin sulfate, up to 500 mg	N N1 ☑
	Use this code for Kantrex.	
	CMS: 100-04,4,20.6.4	
J1850	Injection, kanamycin sulfate, up to 75 mg	N ☑
	Use this code for Kantrex.	
	CMS: 100-04,4,20.6.4	
	AHA: 2Q, '13, 5	
J1885	Injection, ketorolac tromethamine, per 15 mg	N N1 ☑
	Use this code for Toradol.	
	CMS: 100-04,4,20.6.4	
J1890	Injection, cephalothin sodium, up to 1 g	N N1 ☑
	CMS: 100-04,4,20.6.4	
J1930	Injection, lanreotide, 1 mg	K K2 ☑
	Use this code for Somatuline.	
J1931	Injection, laronidase, 0.1 mg	K K2 ☑
	Use this code for Aldurazyme.	
	AHA: 2Q, '05, 11; 1Q, '05, 7, 9-10	
J1940	Injection, furosemide, up to 20 mg	N N1 ☑
	Use this code for Lasix.	
	CMS: 100-04,4,20.6.4	
	AHA: 4Q, '05, 1-6; 3Q, '04, 1-10	
J1943	Injection, aripiprazole lauroxil, (Aristada Initio), 1 mg	K2
J1944	Injection, aripiprazole lauroxil, (Aristada), 1 mg	K2
J1945	Injection, lepirudin, 50 mg	E ☑
	Use this code for Refludan.	
	This drug is used for patients with heparin-induced thrombocytopenia.	
J1950	Injection, leuprolide acetate (for depot suspension), per 3.75 mg	K K2 ☑
	Use this code for Lupron Depot-Pedi.	
● **J1951**	Injection, leuprolide acetate for depot suspension (Fensolvi), 0.25 mg	K2
● **J1952**	Leuprolide injectable, camcevi, 1 mg	
	Use this code for Camcevi.	
J1953	Injection, levetiracetam, 10 mg	N N1 ☑
	Use this code for Keppra.	
J1955	Injection, levocarnitine, per 1 g	B ☑
	Use this code for Carnitor.	
J1956	Injection, levofloxacin, 250 mg	N N1 ☑
	Use this code for Levaquin.	
	CMS: 100-04,4,20.6.4	
J1960	Injection, levorphanol tartrate, up to 2 mg	N N1 ☑
	Use this code for Levo-Dromoran.	
	CMS: 100-04,4,20.6.4	
J1980	Injection, hyoscyamine sulfate, up to 0.25 mg	N N1 ☑
	Use this code for Levsin.	
	CMS: 100-04,4,20.6.4	

Special Coverage Instructions   Noncovered by Medicare   Carrier Discretion   ☑ Quantity Alert   ● New Code   ○ Recycled/Reinstated   ▲ Revised Code

© 2021 Optum360, LLC   A2-Z3 ASC Pmt   CMS: IOM   AHA: Coding Clinic   ⅃ DMEPOS Paid   ⊘ SNF Excluded   J Codes — 95

J1990   **Injection, chlordiazepoxide HCl, up to 100 mg**   N N1 ☑
Use this code for Librium.
CMS: 100-04,4,20.6.4

J2001   **Injection, lidocaine HCl for intravenous infusion, 10 mg**   N N1 ☑
Use this code for Xylocaine.
CMS: 100-04,4,20.6.4

J2010   **Injection, lincomycin HCl, up to 300 mg**   N N1 ☑
Use this code for Lincocin.
CMS: 100-04,4,20.6.4

J2020   **Injection, linezolid, 200 mg**   N N1 ☑
Use this code for Zyvok.
AHA: 2Q, '02, 8-9; 1Q, '02, 5

J2060   **Injection, lorazepam, 2 mg**   N N1 ☑
Use this code for Ativan.
CMS: 100-04,4,20.6.4

J2062   **Loxapine for inhalation, 1 mg**
Use this code for Adasuve.

J2150   **Injection, mannitol, 25% in 50 ml**   N N1 ☑
Use this code for Osmitrol.
CMS: 100-04,4,20.6.4

J2170   **Injection, mecasermin, 1 mg**   N N1 ☑
Use this code for Iplex, Increlex.
CMS: 100-02,15,50.5; 100-04,4,20.6.4

J2175   **Injection, meperidine HCl, per 100 mg**   N N1 ☑
Use this code for Demerol.
CMS: 100-04,20,180; 100-04,32,411.3; 100-04,4,20.6.4

J2180   **Injection, meperidine and promethazine HCl, up to 50 mg**   N N1 ☑
Use this code for Mepergan Injection.
CMS: 100-04,4,20.6.4

J2182   **Injection, mepolizumab, 1 mg**   G K2 ☑
Use this code for Nucala.

J2185   **Injection, meropenem, 100 mg**   N N1 ☑
Use this code for Merrem.
CMS: 100-04,4,20.6.4
AHA: 2Q, '05, 11

J2186   **Injection, meropenem, vaborbactam, 10 mg/10 mg, (20 mg)**   K2
Use this code for Vabomere.
CMS: 100-04,4,260.1; 100-04,4,260.1.1

J2210   **Injection, methylergonovine maleate, up to 0.2 mg**   N N1 ☑
Use this code for Methergine.
CMS: 100-04,4,20.6.4

J2212   **Injection, methylnaltrexone, 0.1 mg**   N N1 ☑
Use this code for Relistor.
CMS: 100-02,15,50.5

J2248   **Injection, micafungin sodium, 1 mg**   N K2 ☑
Use this code for Mycamine.

J2250   **Injection, midazolam HCl, per 1 mg**   N N1 ☑
Use this code for Versed.
CMS: 100-04,4,20.6.4

J2260   **Injection, milrinone lactate, 5 mg**   N N1 ☑
Use this code for Primacor.
CMS: 100-04,20,180; 100-04,32,411.3; 100-04,4,20.6.4

J2265   **Injection, minocycline HCl, 1 mg**   K K2 ☑
Use this code for MINOCIN.

J2270   **Injection, morphine sulfate, up to 10 mg**   N N1 ☑
Use this code for Depodur, Infumorph.
CMS: 100-04,20,180; 100-04,4,20.6.4
AHA: 2Q, '13, 5; 4Q, '05, 1-6; 3Q, '04, 1-10

J2274   **Injection, morphine sulfate, preservative free for epidural or intrathecal use, 10 mg**   N N1 ☑
Use this code for DepoDur, Astromorph PF, Durarmorph PF.
CMS: 100-04,20,180
AHA: 1Q, '15, 6

J2278   **Injection, ziconotide, 1 mcg**   K K2 ☑
Use this code for Prialt.
CMS: 100-04,20,180

J2280   **Injection, moxifloxacin, 100 mg**   N N1 ☑
Use this code for Avelox.
CMS: 100-04,4,20.6.4
AHA: 2Q, '05, 11

J2300   **Injection, nalbuphine HCl, per 10 mg**   N N1 ☑
Use this code for Nubain.
CMS: 100-04,4,20.6.4

J2310   **Injection, naloxone HCl, per 1 mg**   N N1 ☑
Use this code for Narcan.

J2315   **Injection, naltrexone, depot form, 1 mg**   K K2 ☑
Use this code for Vivitrol.

J2320   **Injection, nandrolone decanoate, up to 50 mg**   K N1 ☑

J2323   **Injection, natalizumab, 1 mg**   K K2 ☑
Use this code for Tysabri.
AHA: 1Q, '08, 6

J2325   **Injection, nesiritide, 0.1 mg**   K ☑
Use this code for Natrecor.
CMS: 100-03,200.1

J2326   **Injection, nusinersen, 0.1 mg**   G K2
Use this code for Spinraza.

J2350   **Injection, ocrelizumab, 1 mg**   G K2
Use this code for Ocrevus.

J2353   **Injection, octreotide, depot form for intramuscular injection, 1 mg**   K K2 ☑
Use this code for Sandostatin LAR.

J2354   **Injection, octreotide, nondepot form for subcutaneous or intravenous injection, 25 mcg**   N N1 ☑
Use this code for Sandostatin.
CMS: 100-02,15,50.5

J2355   **Injection, oprelvekin, 5 mg**   K N1 ☑
Use this code for Neumega.
AHA: 2Q, '05, 11

J2357   **Injection, omalizumab, 5 mg**   K K2 ☑
Use this code for Xolair.
AHA: 2Q, '05, 11

J2358   **Injection, olanzapine, long-acting, 1 mg**   N K2 ☑
Use this code for ZYPREXA RELPREVV.

J2360   **Injection, orphenadrine citrate, up to 60 mg**   N N1 ☑
Use this code for Norflex.

J2370   **Injection, phenylephrine HCl, up to 1 ml**   N N1 ☑

J2400   **Injection, chloroprocaine HCl, per 30 ml**   N N1 ☑
Use this code for Nesacaine, Nesacaine-MPF.

J2405   **Injection, ondansetron HCl, per 1 mg**   N N1 ☑
Use this code for Zofran.

● **J2406**   **Injection, oritavancin (Kimyrsa), 10 mg**   K2

Special Coverage Instructions   Noncovered by Medicare   Carrier Discretion   ☑ Quantity Alert ● New Code   ○ Recycled/Reinstated   ▲ Revised Code

▲ **J2407** **Injection, oritavancin (Orbactiv), 10 mg** K K2 ☑
Use this code for Orbactiv.

J2410 **Injection, oxymorphone HCl, up to 1 mg** N N1 ☑
Use this code for Numorphan, Oxymorphone HCl.

J2425 **Injection, palifermin, 50 mcg** K K2 ☑
Use this code for Kepivance.

J2426 **Injection, paliperidone palmitate extended release, 1 mg** K K2 ☑
Use this code for INVEGA SUSTENNA.

J2430 **Injection, pamidronate disodium, per 30 mg** N N1 ☑
Use this code for Aredia.

J2440 **Injection, papaverine HCl, up to 60 mg** N N1 ☑

J2460 **Injection, oxytetracycline HCl, up to 50 mg** E ☑
Use this code for Terramycin IM.

J2469 **Injection, palonosetron HCl, 25 mcg** K N1 ☑
Use this code for Aloxi.
AHA: 2Q, '05, 11; 1Q, '05, 7, 9-10

J2501 **Injection, paricalcitol, 1 mcg** N N1 ☑
Use this code For Zemplar.

J2502 **Injection, pasireotide long acting, 1 mg** K K2 ☑
Use this code for Signifor LAR.

J2503 **Injection, pegaptanib sodium, 0.3 mg** K N1 ☑
Use this code for Macugen.

J2504 **Injection, pegademase bovine, 25 IU** K K2 ☑
Use this code for Adagen.

~~**J2505**~~ ~~**Injection, pegfilgrastim, 6 mg**~~

● **J2506** **Injection, pegfilgrastim, excludes biosimilar, 0.5 mg**
Use this code for Neulasta.

J2507 **Injection, pegloticase, 1 mg** K K2 ☑
Use this code for KRYSTEXXA.

J2510 **Injection, penicillin G procaine, aqueous, up to 600,000 units** N N1 ☑
Use this code for Wycillin, Duracillin A.S., Pfizerpen A.S., Crysticillin 300 A.S., Crysticillin 600 A.S.

J2513 **Injection, pentastarch, 10% solution, 100 ml** E ☑

J2515 **Injection, pentobarbital sodium, per 50 mg** K K2 ☑
Use this code for Nembutal Sodium Solution.

J2540 **Injection, penicillin G potassium, up to 600,000 units** N N1 ☑
Use this code for Pfizerpen.

J2543 **Injection, piperacillin sodium/tazobactam sodium, 1 g/0.125 g (1.125 g)** N N1 ☑
Use this code for Zosyn.

J2545 **Pentamidine isethionate, inhalation solution, FDA-approved final product, noncompounded, administered through DME, unit dose form, per 300 mg** B ☑
Use this code for Nebupent, Pentam 300.

J2547 **Injection, peramivir, 1 mg** K K2 ☑
Use this code for Rapivab.

J2550 **Injection, promethazine HCl, up to 50 mg** N N1 ☑
Use this code for Phenergan.

J2560 **Injection, phenobarbital sodium, up to 120 mg** N K2 ☑

J2562 **Injection, plerixafor, 1 mg** K K2 ☑
Use this code for Mozobil.

J2590 **Injection, oxytocin, up to 10 units** N N1 ☑
Use this code for Pitocin, Syntocinon.

J2597 **Injection, desmopressin acetate, per 1 mcg** K K2 ☑
Use this code for DDAVP.

J2650 **Injection, prednisolone acetate, up to 1 ml** N N1 ☑

J2670 **Injection, tolazoline HCl, up to 25 mg** N ☑

J2675 **Injection, progesterone, per 50 mg** N N1 ☑
Use this code for Gesterone, Gestrin.

J2680 **Injection, fluphenazine decanoate, up to 25 mg** N N1 ☑

J2690 **Injection, procainamide HCl, up to 1 g** N N1 ☑
Use this code for Pronestyl.

J2700 **Injection, oxacillin sodium, up to 250 mg** N N1 ☑
Use this code for Bactocill

J2704 **Injection, propofol, 10 mg** N N1 ☑
Use this code for Diprivan.
AHA: 1Q, '15, 6

J2710 **Injection, neostigmine methylsulfate, up to 0.5 mg** N N1 ☑
Use this code for Prostigmin.

J2720 **Injection, protamine sulfate, per 10 mg** N N1 ☑

J2724 **Injection, protein C concentrate, intravenous, human, 10 IU** K K2 ☑

J2725 **Injection, protirelin, per 250 mcg** E ☑
Use this code for Thyrel TRH.

J2730 **Injection, pralidoxime chloride, up to 1 g** N N1 ☑
Use this code for Protopam Chloride.

J2760 **Injection, phentolamine mesylate, up to 5 mg** K K2 ☑
Use this code for Regitine.

J2765 **Injection, metoclopramide HCl, up to 10 mg** N N1 ☑
Use this code for Reglan.

J2770 **Injection, quinupristin/dalfopristin, 500 mg (150/350)** K K2 ☑
Use this code for Synercid.

J2778 **Injection, ranibizumab, 0.1 mg** K K2 ☑
Use this code for Lucentis.
AHA: 1Q, '08, 6

J2780 **Injection, ranitidine HCl, 25 mg** N N1 ☑
Use this code for Zantac.

J2783 **Injection, rasburicase, 0.5 mg** K K2 ☑
Use this code for Elitek.
AHA: 2Q, '05, 11; 2Q, '04, 8

J2785 **Injection, regadenoson, 0.1 mg** N N1 ☑
Use this code for Lexiscan.

J2786 **Injection, reslizumab, 1 mg** G K2 ☑
Use this code for Cinqair.

J2787 **Riboflavin 5'-phosphate, ophthalmic solution, up to 3 ml**
Use this code for Photrexa Viscous.
CMS: 100-04,4,260.1; 100-04,4,260.1.1

J2788 **Injection, Rho D immune globulin, human, minidose, 50 mcg (250 IU)** N N1 ☑
Use this code for RhoGam, MiCRhoGAM.

J2790 **Injection, Rho D immune globulin, human, full dose, 300 mcg (1500 IU)** N N1 ☑
Use this code for RhoGam, HypRho SD.

J2791 **Injection, Rho D immune globulin (human), (Rhophylac), intramuscular or intravenous, 100 IU** N N1 ☑
Use this for Rhophylac.
AHA: 1Q, '08, 6

Special Coverage Instructions   Noncovered by Medicare   Carrier Discretion   ☑ Quantity Alert   ● New Code   ○ Recycled/Reinstated   ▲ Revised Code

© 2021 Optum360, LLC   A2-Z3 ASC Pmt   **CMS:** IOM   **AHA:** Coding Clinic   ᵟ DMEPOS Paid   ⊘ SNF Excluded   **J Codes — 97**

J2792 Injection, Rho D immune globulin, intravenous, human, solvent detergent, 100 IU ☒ K K2 ☑
Use this code for WINRho SDF.

J2793 Injection, rilonacept, 1 mg ☒ K ☑
Use this code for Arcalyst.
CMS: 100-02,15,50.5

J2794 Injection, risperidone (RISPERDAL CONSTA), 0.5 mg ☒ K K2 ☑
AHA: 2Q, '05, 11; 1Q, '05, 7, 9-10

J2795 Injection, ropivacaine HCl, 1 mg ☒ N N1 ☑
Use this code for Naropin.

J2796 Injection, romiplostim, 10 mcg ☒ K K2 ☑
Use this code for Nplate.

J2797 Injection, rolapitant, 0.5 mg
Use this code for Varubi.

J2798 Injection, risperidone, (Perseris), 0.5 mg ☒ K2

J2800 Injection, methocarbamol, up to 10 ml ☒ N N1 ☑
Use this code for Robaxin.

J2805 Injection, sincalide, 5 mcg ☒ N N1 ☑
Use this code for Kinevac.
AHA: 4Q, '05, 1-6

J2810 Injection, theophylline, per 40 mg ☒ N N1 ☑

J2820 Injection, sargramostim (GM-CSF), 50 mcg ☒ K K2 ☑
Use this code for Leukine.

J2840 Injection, sebelipase alfa, 1 mg ☒ G K2 ☑
Use this code for Kanuma.

J2850 Injection, secretin, synthetic, human, 1 mcg ☒ K K2 ☑

J2860 Injection, siltuximab, 10 mg ☒ K K2 ☑
Use this code for Sylvant.

J2910 Injection, aurothioglucose, up to 50 mg ☒ E ☑
Use this code for Solganal.

J2916 Injection, sodium ferric gluconate complex in sucrose injection, 12.5 mg ☒ N N1 ☑
CMS: 100-03,110.10

J2920 Injection, methylprednisolone sodium succinate, up to 40 mg ☒ N N1 ☑
Use this code for Solu-Medrol, A-methaPred.

J2930 Injection, methylprednisolone sodium succinate, up to 125 mg ☒ N N1 ☑
Use this code for Solu-Medrol, A-methaPred.

J2940 Injection, somatrem, 1 mg ☒ E ☑
Use this code for Protropin.
AHA: 2Q, '02, 8-9; 1Q, '02, 5

J2941 Injection, somatropin, 1 mg ☒ K K2 ☑
Use this code for Humatrope, Genotropin Nutropin, Biotropin, Genotropin, Genotropin Miniquick, Norditropin, Nutropin, Nutropin AQ, Saizen, Saizen Somatropin RDNA Origin, Serostim, Serostim RDNA Origin, Zorbtive.
CMS: 100-02,15,50.5
AHA: 2Q, '02, 8-9; 1Q, '02, 5

J2950 Injection, promazine HCl, up to 25 mg ☒ N N1 ☑
Use this code for Sparine, Prozine-50.

J2993 Injection, reteplase, 18.1 mg ☒ K K2 ☑
Use this code for Retavase.

J2995 Injection, streptokinase, per 250,000 IU ☒ N ☑
Use this code for Streptase.

J2997 Injection, alteplase recombinant, 1 mg ☒ K K2 ☑
Use this code for Activase, Cathflo.
AHA: 1Q, '14, 4

J3000 Injection, streptomycin, up to 1 g ☒ N N1 ☑
Use this code for Streptomycin Sulfate.

J3010 Injection, fentanyl citrate, 0.1 mg ☒ N N1 ☑
Use this code for Sublimaze.
CMS: 100-04,20,180; 100-04,32,411.3

J3030 Injection, sumatriptan succinate, 6 mg (code may be used for Medicare when drug administered under the direct supervision of a physician, not for use when drug is self-administered) ☒ N N1 ☑
Use this code for Imitrex.
CMS: 100-02,15,50.5

J3031 Injection, fremanezumab-vfrm, 1 mg (code may be used for Medicare when drug administered under the direct supervision of a physician, not for use when drug is self-administered) ☒ K2
Use this code for Ajovy.

J3032 Injection, eptinezumab-jjmr, 1 mg ☒ K2
Use this code for Vyepti.

J3060 Injection, taliglucerase alfa, 10 units ☒ K K2 ☑
Use this code for Elelyso.

J3070 Injection, pentazocine, 30 mg ☒ K N1 ☑
Use this code for Talwin.

J3090 Injection, tedizolid phosphate, 1 mg ☒ K K2 ☑
Use this code for Sivextro.

J3095 Injection, telavancin, 10 mg ☒ K K2 ☑
Use this code for VIBATIV.

J3101 Injection, tenecteplase, 1 mg ☒ K K2 ☑
Use this code for TNKase.

J3105 Injection, terbutaline sulfate, up to 1 mg ☒ N N1 ☑
For terbutaline in inhalation solution, see K0525 and K0526.

J3110 Injection, teriparatide, 10 mcg ☒ B ☑
Use this code for Forteo.
CMS: 100-02,15,50.5; 100-04,10,90.1

J3111 Injection, romosozumab-aqqg, 1 mg ☒ K2
Use this code for Evenity.
CMS: 100-04,10,90.1

J3121 Injection, testosterone enanthate, 1 mg ☒ N N1 ☑
Use this code for Delatstryl.
AHA: 1Q, '15, 6

J3145 Injection, testosterone undecanoate, 1 mg ☒ K K2 ☑
Use this code for Aveed.
AHA: 1Q, '15, 6

J3230 Injection, chlorpromazine HCl, up to 50 mg ☒ N N1 ☑
Use this code for Thorazine.

J3240 Injection, thyrotropin alpha, 0.9 mg, provided in 1.1 mg vial ☒ K K2 ☑
Use this code for Thyrogen.
AHA: 4Q, '05, 1-6; 2Q, '05, 11; 3Q, '04, 1-10

J3241 Injection, teprotumumab-trbw, 10 mg ☒ K2
Use this code for Tepezza.

J3243 Injection, tigecycline, 1 mg ☒ K K2 ☑
Use this code for Tygacil.

J3245 Injection, tildrakizumab, 1 mg ☒ K2
Use this code for Ilumya.

J3246 Injection, tirofiban HCl, 0.25 mg ☒ K K2 ☑
Use this code for Aggrastat.
AHA: 1Q, '05, 7, 9-10

J3250 Injection, trimethobenzamide HCl, up to 200 mg ☒ N N1 ☑
Use this code for Tigan, Tiject-20, Arrestin.

Special Coverage Instructions   Noncovered by Medicare   Carrier Discretion   ☑ Quantity Alert   ● New Code   ○ Recycled/Reinstated   ▲ Revised Code

Ⓐ Age Edit   Ⓜ Maternity Edit   ♀ Female Only   ♂ Male Only   Ⓐ-Ⓨ OPPS Status Indicators   © 2021 Optum360, LLC

J3260	Injection, tobramycin sulfate, up to 80 mg	N N1 ☑

Use this code for Nebcin.

J3262	Injection, tocilizumab, 1 mg	K K2 ☑

Use this code for ACTEMRA.

J3265	Injection, torsemide, 10 mg/ml	N N1 ☑

Use this code for Demadex, Torsemide.

J3280	Injection, thiethylperazine maleate, up to 10 mg	E ☑

J3285	Injection, treprostinil, 1 mg	K K2 ☑

Use this code for Remodulin.
CMS: 100-04,20,180; 100-04,32,411.3

J3300	Injection, triamcinolone acetonide, preservative free, 1 mg	K N1 ☑

Use this code for TRIVARIS, TRIESENCE.

J3301	Injection, triamcinolone acetonide, not otherwise specified, 10 mg	N N1 ☑

Use this code for Kenalog-10, Kenalog-40, Tri-Kort, Kenaject-40, Cenacort A-40, Triam-A, Trilog.
AHA: 2Q, '13, 5

J3302	Injection, triamcinolone diacetate, per 5 mg	N N1 ☑

Use this code for Aristocort, Aristocort Intralesional, Aristocort Forte, Amcort, Trilone, Cenacort Forte.

J3303	Injection, triamcinolone hexacetonide, per 5 mg	N N1 ☑

Use this code for Aristospan Intralesional, Aristospan Intra-articular.

J3304	Injection, triamcinolone acetonide, preservative-free, extended-release, microsphere formulation, 1 mg	K2

Use this code for Zilretta.

J3305	Injection, trimetrexate glucuronate, per 25 mg	E ☑

Use this code for Neutrexin.

J3310	Injection, perphenazine, up to 5 mg	N N1 ☑

Use this code for Trilafon.

J3315	Injection, triptorelin pamoate, 3.75 mg	♂ K K2 ☑

Use this code for Trelstar Depot, Trelstar Depot Plus Debioclip Kit, Trelstar LA.

J3316	Injection, triptorelin, extended-release, 3.75 mg	K2

Use this code for Triptodur.

J3320	Injection, spectinomycin dihydrochloride, up to 2 g	E ☑

Use this code for Trobicin.

J3350	Injection, urea, up to 40 g	N ☑

J3355	Injection, urofollitropin, 75 IU	E ☑

Use this code for Metrodin, Bravelle, Fertinex.
CMS: 100-02,15,50.5

J3357	Ustekinumab, for subcutaneous injection, 1 mg	K K2 ☑

Use this code for STELARA.
CMS: 100-02,15,50.5
AHA: 1Q, '17, 1-3; 4Q, '16, 10

J3358	Ustekinumab, for intravenous injection, 1 mg	G K2

Use this code for Stelara.

J3360	Injection, diazepam, up to 5 mg	N N1 ☑

Use this code for Diastat, Dizac, Valium.
CMS: 100-04,8,60.2.1
AHA: 2Q, '07, 6

J3364	Injection, urokinase, 5,000 IU vial	N N1 ☑

Use this code for Kinlytic.

J3365	Injection, IV, urokinase, 250,000 IU vial	E ☑

Use this code for Kinlytic.

J3370	Injection, vancomycin HCl, 500 mg	N N1 ☑

Use this code for Vancocin.

J3380	Injection, vedolizumab, 1 mg	K K2 ☑

Use this code for Entyvio.

J3385	Injection, velaglucerase alfa, 100 units	K K2 ☑

Use this code for VPRIV.

J3396	Injection, verteporfin, 0.1 mg	K K2 ☑

Use this code for Visudyne.
CMS: 100-03,80.2; 100-03,80.2.1; 100-03,80.3; 100-03,80.3.1; 100-04,32,300; 100-04,32,300.1; 100-04,32,300.2
AHA: 1Q, '05, 7, 9-10

J3397	Injection, vestronidase alfa-vjbk, 1 mg	N1

Use this code for Mepsevii.
CMS: 100-04,4,260.1; 100-04,4,260.1.1

J3398	Injection, voretigene neparvovec-rzyl, 1 billion vector genomes	K2

Use this code for Luxturna.

J3399	Injection, onasemnogene abeparvovec-xioi, per treatment, up to 5×10^{15} vector genomes	

Use this code for Zolgensma.

J3400	Injection, triflupromazine HCl, up to 20 mg	E ☑

J3410	Injection, hydroxyzine HCl, up to 25 mg	N N1 ☑

Use this code for Vistaril, Vistaject-25, Hyzine, Hyzine-50.

J3411	Injection, thiamine HCl, 100 mg	N N1 ☑

AHA: 2Q, '05, 11

J3415	Injection, pyridoxine HCl, 100 mg	N N1 ☑

AHA: 2Q, '05, 11

J3420	Injection, vitamin B-12 cyanocobalamin, up to 1,000 mcg	N N1 ☑

Use this code for Sytobex, Redisol, Rubramin PC, Betalin 12, Berubigen, Cobex, Cobal, Crystal B12, Cyano, Cyanocobalamin, Hydroxocobalamin, Hydroxycobal, Nutri-Twelve.

J3430	Injection, phytonadione (vitamin K), per 1 mg	N N1 ☑

Use this code for AquaMephyton, Konakion, Menadione, Phytonadione.

J3465	Injection, voriconazole, 10 mg	K N1 ☑

AHA: 2Q, '05, 11

J3470	Injection, hyaluronidase, up to 150 units	N N1 ☑

J3471	Injection, hyaluronidase, ovine, preservative free, per 1 USP unit (up to 999 USP units)	N N1 ☑

J3472	Injection, hyaluronidase, ovine, preservative free, per 1,000 USP units	N N1 ☑

J3473	Injection, hyaluronidase, recombinant, 1 USP unit	N N1 ☑

J3475	Injection, magnesium sulfate, per 500 mg	N N1 ☑

Use this code for Mag Sul, Sulfa Mag.

J3480	Injection, potassium chloride, per 2 mEq	N N1 ☑

J3485	Injection, zidovudine, 10 mg	N N1 ☑

Use this code for Retrovir, Zidovudine.

J3486	Injection, ziprasidone mesylate, 10 mg	N N1 ☑

Use this code for Geodon.
AHA: 2Q, '05, 11

J3489	Injection, zoledronic acid, 1 mg	N N1 ☑

Use this code for Reclast and Zometa.

J3490	Unclassified drugs	N N1 ☑

CMS: 100-02,15,50.5; 100-03,1,110.22; 100-03,110.22; 100-04,10,90.1; 100-04,32,280.1; 100-04,32,280.2; 100-04,32,400; 100-04,32,400.1; 100-04,32,400.2; 100-04,32,400.2.1; 100-04,32,400.2.2; 100-04,32,400.2.3; 100-04,32,400.2.4; 100-04,32,400.3; 100-04,32,400.4; 100-04,32,400.5; 100-04,4,260.1; 100-04,4,260.1.1; 100-04,8,60.2.1.1; 100-04,8,60.2.3
AHA: 1Q, '17, 8; 1Q, '17, 1-3; 3Q, '15, 7; 4Q, '14, 5; 2Q, '14, 8; 2Q, '13, 5; 1Q, '13, 9; 4Q, '12, 9; 2Q, '09, 1; 1Q, '08, 6; 4Q, '05, 1-6; 3Q, '04, 1-10

Special Coverage Instructions   Noncovered by Medicare   Carrier Discretion   ☑ Quantity Alert ● New Code ○ Recycled/Reinstated ▲ Revised Code

J3520 **Edetate disodium, per 150 mg** ☐E ☑
Use this code for Endrate, Disotate, Meritate, Chealamide, E.D.T.A. This drug is used in chelation therapy, a treatment for atherosclerosis that is not covered by Medicare.

J3530 **Nasal vaccine inhalation** ☐N ☐N1 ☑

J3535 **Drug administered through a metered dose inhaler** ☐E ☑

J3570 **Laetrile, amygdalin, vitamin B-17** ☐E ☑
The FDA has found Laetrile to have no safe or effective therapeutic purpose.

J3590 **Unclassified biologics** ☐N ☐N1 ☑
CMS: 100-02,15,50.5; 100-03,1,110.22; 100-03,110.22; 100-04,10,90.1; 100-04,32,280.1; 100-04,32,280.2; 100-04,32,400; 100-04,32,400.1; 100-04,32,400.2; 100-04,32,400.2.1; 100-04,32,400.2.2; 100-04,32,400.2.3; 100-04,32,400.2.4; 100-04,32,400.3; 100-04,32,400.4; 100-04,32,400.5
AHA: 1Q, '17, 1-3; 4Q, '16, 10; 3Q, '15, 7; 4Q, '12, 9

J3591 **Unclassified drug or biological used for ESRD on dialysis**
CMS: 100-04,4,260.1; 100-04,4,260.1.1; 100-04,8,20

J7030 **Infusion, normal saline solution, 1,000 cc** ☐N ☐N1 ☑

J7040 **Infusion, normal saline solution, sterile (500 ml=1 unit)** ☐N ☐N1 ☑

J7042 **5% dextrose/normal saline (500 ml = 1 unit)** ☐N ☐N1 ☑

J7050 **Infusion, normal saline solution, 250 cc** ☐N ☐N1 ☑

J7060 **5% dextrose/water (500 ml = 1 unit)** ☐N ☐N1 ☑

J7070 **Infusion, D-5-W, 1,000 cc** ☐N ☐N1 ☑

J7100 **Infusion, dextran 40, 500 ml** ☐N ☐N1 ☑
Use this code for Gentran, 10% LMD, Rheomacrodex.

J7110 **Infusion, dextran 75, 500 ml** ☐N ☐N1 ☑
Use this code for Gentran 75.

J7120 **Ringers lactate infusion, up to 1,000 cc** ☐N ☐N1 ☑

J7121 **5% dextrose in lactated ringers infusion, up to 1000 cc** ☐N ☐N1 ☑
AHA: 1Q, '16, 6-8

J7131 **Hypertonic saline solution, 1 ml** ☐N ☐N1 ☑

● **J7168** **Prothrombin complex concentrate (human), Kcentra, per IU of Factor IX activity** ☐K2

J7169 **Injection, coagulation Factor Xa (recombinant), inactivated-zhzo (Andexxa), 10 mg** ☐K2

J7170 **Injection, emicizumab-kxwh, 0.5 mg** ☐K2
Use this code for Hemlibra.

J7175 **Injection, Factor X, (human), 1 IU** ☐K ☐K2 ☑
Use this code for Coagadex.
AHA: 1Q, '17, 9-10

J7177 **Injection, human fibrinogen concentrate (Fibryga), 1 mg** ☐N1
CMS: 100-04,4,260.1; 100-04,4,260.1.1

J7178 **Injection, human fibrinogen concentrate, not otherwise specified, 1 mg** ☐K ☐K2 ☑
Use this code for RiaSTAP.

J7179 **Injection, von Willebrand factor (recombinant), (Vonvendi), 1 IU VWF:RCo** ☐G ☐K2 ☑
AHA: 1Q, '17, 9-10

J7180 **Injection, Factor XIII (antihemophilic factor, human), 1 IU** ☐K ☐K2 ☑
Use this code for Corifact.

J7181 **Injection, Factor XIII A-subunit, (recombinant), per IU** ☐K ☐K2 ☑
AHA: 1Q, '15, 6

J7182 **Injection, Factor VIII, (antihemophilic factor, recombinant), (NovoEight), per IU** ☐K ☐K2 ☑
AHA: 1Q, '15, 6

J7183 **Injection, von Willebrand factor complex (human), Wilate, 1 IU VWF:RCO** ☐K ☐K2 ☑

J7185 **Injection, Factor VIII (antihemophilic factor, recombinant) (Xyntha), per IU** ☐K ☐K2 ☑

J7186 **Injection, antihemophilic Factor VIII/von Willebrand factor complex (human), per Factor VIII IU** ☐K ☐K2 ☑
Use this code for Alphanate.
CMS: 100-04,17,80.4.1

J7187 **Injection, von Willebrand factor complex (Humate-P), per IU VWF:RCO** ☐K ☐K2 ☑
CMS: 100-04,17,80.4.1

J7188 **Injection, Factor VIII (antihemophilic factor, recombinant) (Obizur), per IU** ☐K ☐K2 ☑
AHA: 1Q, '16, 6-8

J7189 **Factor VIIa (antihemophilic factor, recombinant), (NovoSeven RT), 1 mcg** ☐K ☐K2 ☑
CMS: 100-04,17,80.4.1

J7190 **Factor VIII (antihemophilic factor, human) per IU** ☐K ☐K2 ☑
Use this code for Koate-DVI, Monarc-M, Monoclate-P.
CMS: 100-04,17,80.4; 100-04,17,80.4.1

J7191 **Factor VIII (antihemophilic factor (porcine)), per IU** ☐E ☑
CMS: 100-04,17,80.4; 100-04,17,80.4.1

J7192 **Factor VIII (antihemophilic factor, recombinant) per IU, not otherwise specified** ☐K ☐K2 ☑
Use this code for Advate rAHF-PFM, Antihemophilic Factor Human Method M Monoclonal Purified, Bioclate, Kogenate FS, Recombinate, Refacto.
CMS: 100-04,17,80.4; 100-04,17,80.4.1
AHA: 2Q, '13, 5

J7193 **Factor IX (antihemophilic factor, purified, nonrecombinant) per IU** ☐K ☐K2 ☑
Use this code for AlphaNine SD, Mononine.
CMS: 100-04,17,80.4; 100-04,17,80.4.1
AHA: 2Q, '02, 8-9

J7194 **Factor IX complex, per IU** ☐K ☐K2 ☑
Use this code for Konyne-80, Profilnine SD, Proplex T, Proplex T, Bebulin VH, factor IX+ complex, Profilnine SD.
CMS: 100-04,17,80.4; 100-04,17,80.4.1

J7195 **Injection, Factor IX (antihemophilic factor, recombinant) per IU, not otherwise specified** ☐K ☐K2 ☑
Use this code for Antithrombate III, Benefix, Thrombate III.
CMS: 100-04,17,80.4; 100-04,17,80.4.1
AHA: 2Q, '02, 8-9; 1Q, '02, 5

J7196 **Injection, antithrombin recombinant, 50 IU** ☐E ☐N1 ☑
Use this code for ATryn.

J7197 **Antithrombin III (human), per IU** ☐K ☐K2 ☑
Use this code for Thrombate III, ATnativ.
CMS: 100-04,17,80.4.1

J7198 **Antiinhibitor, per IU** ☐K ☐K2 ☑
Medicare jurisdiction: local contractor. Use this code for Autoplex T, Feiba VH AICC.
CMS: 100-03,110.3; 100-04,17,80.4; 100-04,17,80.4.1

J7199 **Hemophilia clotting factor, not otherwise classified** ☐B ☑
Medicare jurisdiction: local contractor.
CMS: 100-04,17,80.4; 100-04,17,80.4.1
AHA: 2Q, '13, 5

Special Coverage Instructions   Noncovered by Medicare   Carrier Discretion   ☑ Quantity Alert   ● New Code   ○ Recycled/Reinstated   ▲ Revised Code

100 — J Codes   ☐A Age Edit   ☐M Maternity Edit   ♀ Female Only   ♂ Male Only   ☐A-Y OPPS Status Indicators   © 2021 Optum360, LLC

J7200	Injection, Factor IX, (antihemophilic factor, recombinant), Rixubis, per IU K K2 ☑
	AHA: 1Q, '15, 6
J7201	Injection, Factor IX, Fc fusion protein (recombinant), Alprolix, 1 IU K K2 ☑
	AHA: 1Q, '15, 6
J7202	Injection, Factor IX, albumin fusion protein, (recombinant), Idelvion, 1 IU G K2 ☑
J7203	Injection Factor IX, (antihemophilic factor, recombinant), glycoPEGylated, (Rebinyn), 1 IU K2
J7204	Injection, Factor VIII, antihemophilic factor (recombinant) (Esperoct), glycopegylated-exei, per IU K2
J7205	Injection, Factor VIII Fc fusion protein (recombinant), per IU K K2 ☑
	Use this code for Eloctate.
J7207	Injection, Factor VIII, (antihemophilic factor, recombinant), PEGylated, 1 IU G K2 ☑
	Use this code for Adynovate.
J7208	Injection, Factor VIII, (antihemophilic factor, recombinant), PEGylated-aucl, (Jivi), 1 IU K2
J7209	Injection, Factor VIII, (antihemophilic factor, recombinant), (Nuwiq), 1 IU G K2 ☑
J7210	Injection, Factor VIII, (antihemophilic factor, recombinant), (Afstyla), 1 IU G K2
J7211	Injection, Factor VIII, (antihemophilic factor, recombinant), (Kovaltry), 1 IU K K2 ☑
J7212	Factor VIIa (antihemophilic factor, recombinant)-jncw (Sevenfact), 1 mcg K2
● **J7294**	Segesterone acetate and ethinyl estradiol 0.15 mg, 0.013 mg per 24 hours; yearly vaginal system, ea
	Use this code for Annovera vaginal ring.
● **J7295**	Ethinyl estradiol and etonogestrel 0.015 mg, 0.12 mg per 24 hours; monthly vaginal ring, ea
	Use this code for NuvaRing vaginal ring.
J7296	Levonorgestrel-releasing intrauterine contraceptive system, (Kyleena), 19.5 mg ♀ E
J7297	Levonorgestrel-releasing intrauterine contraceptive system (Liletta), 52 mg M ♀ E ☑
	AHA: 1Q, '16, 6-8
J7298	Levonorgestrel-releasing intrauterine contraceptive system (Mirena), 52 mg M ♀ E ☑
	AHA: 1Q, '16, 6-8
J7300	Intrauterine copper contraceptive E ☑
	Use this code for Paragard T380A.
J7301	Levonorgestrel-releasing intrauterine contraceptive system (Skyla), 13.5 mg M ♀ E ☑
	AHA: 4Q, '14, 6
~~**J7303**~~	~~Contraceptive supply, hormone containing vaginal ring, each~~
	To report, see ~J7294, J7294
J7304	Contraceptive supply, hormone containing patch, each E ☑
J7306	Levonorgestrel (contraceptive) implant system, including implants and supplies E ☑
J7307	Etonogestrel (contraceptive) implant system, including implant and supplies E ☑
	Use this code for Implanon and Nexplanon.

J7308	Aminolevulinic acid HCl for topical administration, 20%, single unit dosage form (354 mg) K K2 ☑
	Use this code for Levulan Kerastick.
	AHA: 2Q, '05, 11; 1Q, '02, 5
J7309	Methyl aminolevulinate (MAL) for topical administration, 16.8%, 1 g N ☑
	Use this code for Metvixia.
J7310	Ganciclovir, 4.5 mg, long-acting implant E ☑
	Use this code for Vitrasert.
J7311	Injection, fluocinolone acetonide, intravitreal implant (Retisert), 0.01 mg K K2 ☑
J7312	Injection, dexamethasone, intravitreal implant, 0.1 mg K K2 ☑
	Use this code for OZURDEX.
J7313	Injection, fluocinolone acetonide, intravitreal implant (Iluvien), 0.01 mg K K2 ☑
J7314	Injection, fluocinolone acetonide, intravitreal implant (Yutiq), 0.01 mg K2
J7315	Mitomycin, opthalmic, 0.2 mg N N1 ☑
	Use this code for Mitosol.
	AHA: 4Q, '16, 8; 2Q, '14, 8; 2Q, '13, 9
J7316	Injection, ocriplasmin, 0.125 mg K K2 ☑
	Use this code for Jetrea.
J7318	Hyaluronan or derivative, Durolane, for intra-articular injection, 1 mg K2
J7320	Hyaluronan or derivative, GenVisc 850, for intra-articular injection, 1 mg K K2 ☑
▲ **J7321**	Hyaluronan or derivative, Hyalgan, Supartz or Visco-3, for intra-articular injection, per dose K N1 ☑
	AHA: 4Q, '12, 9; 1Q, '08, 6
J7322	Hyaluronan or derivative, Hymovis, for intra-articular injection, 1 mg G K2 ☑
J7323	Hyaluronan or derivative, Euflexxa, for intra-articular injection, per dose K K2 ☑
	AHA: 4Q, '12, 9; 1Q, '08, 6
J7324	Hyaluronan or derivative, Orthovisc, for intra-articular injection, per dose K K2 ☑
	AHA: 4Q, '12, 9; 1Q, '08, 6
J7325	Hyaluronan or derivative, Synvisc or Synvisc-One, for intra-articular injection, 1 mg K K2 ☑
	AHA: 4Q, '12, 9
J7326	Hyaluronan or derivative, Gel-One, for intra-articular injection, per dose K K2 ☑
	AHA: 4Q, '12, 9
J7327	Hyaluronan or derivative, Monovisc, for intra-articular injection, per dose K K2 ☑
	AHA: 1Q, '15, 6
J7328	Hyaluronan or derivative, GELSYN-3, for intra-articular injection, 0.1 mg G K2 ☑
	AHA: 1Q, '16, 6-8
J7329	Hyaluronan or derivative, Trivisc, for intra-articular injection, 1 mg K2
	CMS: 100-04,4,260.1; 100-04,4,260.1.1
J7330	Autologous cultured chondrocytes, implant B ☑
	Medicare jurisdiction: local contractor. Use this code for Carticel.
	AHA: 4Q, '10, 1
J7331	Hyaluronan or derivative, SYNOJOYNT, for intra-articular injection, 1 mg K2

Special Coverage Instructions	Noncovered by Medicare	Carrier Discretion	☑ Quantity Alert ● New Code ○ Recycled/Reinstated ▲ Revised Code

J7332 Hyaluronan or derivative, Triluron, for intra-articular injection, 1 mg N1

~~**J7333** Hyaluronan or derivative, Visco-3, for intra-articular injection, per dose~~

J7336 Capsaicin 8% patch, per sq cm K K2 ☑
Use this code for Qutenza.
AHA: 1Q, '15, 6

J7340 Carbidopa 5 mg/levodopa 20 mg enteral suspension, 100 ml K K2 ☑
Use this code for Duopa.
AHA: 1Q, '16, 6-8

J7342 Instillation, ciprofloxacin otic suspension, 6 mg G K2 ☑
Use this code for Otipro.

J7345 Aminolevulinic acid HCl for topical administration, 10% gel, 10 mg G K2
Use this code for Ameluz.

J7351 Injection, bimatoprost, intracameral implant, 1 mcg K2
Use this code for Durysta.

J7352 Afamelanotide implant, 1 mg K2
Use this code for Scenesse.

~~**J7401** Mometasone furoate sinus implant, 10 mcg~~
To report, see ~J7402

● **J7402** Mometasone furoate sinus implant, (Sinuva), 10 mcg K2

J7500 Azathioprine, oral, 50 mg N N1 ☑
Use this code for Azasan, Imuran.
CMS: 100-04,17,80.3

J7501 Azathioprine, parenteral, 100 mg K K2 ☑
CMS: 100-04,17,80.3

J7502 Cyclosporine, oral, 100 mg N N1 ☑
Use this code for Neoral, Sandimmune, Gengraf, Sangcya.
CMS: 100-04,17,80.3

J7503 Tacrolimus, extended release, (Envarsus XR), oral, 0.25 mg G N1 ☑
AHA: 1Q, '16, 6-8

J7504 Lymphocyte immune globulin, antithymocyte globulin, equine, parenteral, 250 mg K K2 ☑
Use this code for Atgam.
CMS: 100-03,260.7; 100-04,17,80.3

J7505 Muromonab-CD3, parenteral, 5 mg K N1 ☑
Use this code for Orthoclone OKT3.
CMS: 100-04,17,80.3

J7507 Tacrolimus, immediate release, oral, 1 mg N N1 ☑
Use this code for Prograf.
CMS: 100-04,17,80.3

J7508 Tacrolimus, extended release, (Astagraf XL), oral, 0.1 mg N N1 ☑
AHA: 1Q, '16, 6-8; 1Q, '14, 6

J7509 Methylprednisolone, oral, per 4 mg N N1 ☑
Use this code for Medrol, Methylpred.
CMS: 100-04,17,80.3

J7510 Prednisolone, oral, per 5 mg N N1 ☑
Use this code for Delta-Cortef, Cotolone, Pediapred, Prednoral, Prelone.
CMS: 100-04,17,80.3

J7511 Lymphocyte immune globulin, antithymocyte globulin, rabbit, parenteral, 25 mg K K2 ☑
Use this code for Thymoglobulin.
CMS: 100-04,17,80.3
AHA: 2Q, '02, 8-9; 1Q, '02, 5

J7512 Prednisone, immediate release or delayed release, oral, 1 mg N N1 ☑
AHA: 1Q, '16, 6-8

J7513 Daclizumab, parenteral, 25 mg E ☑
Use this code for Zenapax.
CMS: 100-04,17,80.3
AHA: 2Q, '05, 11

J7515 Cyclosporine, oral, 25 mg N N1 ☑
Use this code for Neoral, Sandimmune, Gengraf, Sangcya.
CMS: 100-04,17,80.3

J7516 Cyclosporine, parenteral, 250 mg N N1 ☑
Use this code for Neoral, Sandimmune, Gengraf, Sangcya.
CMS: 100-04,17,80.3

J7517 Mycophenolate mofetil, oral, 250 mg N N1 ☑
Use this code for CellCept.
CMS: 100-04,17,80.3

J7518 Mycophenolic acid, oral, 180 mg N N1 ☑
Use this code for Myfortic Delayed Release.
CMS: 100-04,17,80.3.1
AHA: 2Q, '05, 11

J7520 Sirolimus, oral, 1 mg N N1 ☑
Use this code for Rapamune.
CMS: 100-04,17,80.3

J7525 Tacrolimus, parenteral, 5 mg K K2 ☑
Use this code for Prograf.
CMS: 100-04,17,80.3

J7527 Everolimus, oral, 0.25 mg N N1 ☑
Use this code for Zortress, Afinitor.

J7599 Immunosuppressive drug, not otherwise classified N N1 ☑
Determine if an alternative HCPCS Level II or a CPT code better describes the service being reported. This code should be used only if a more specific code is unavailable.
CMS: 100-04,17,80.3
AHA: 2Q, '13, 5

Inhalation Drugs

J7604 Acetylcysteine, inhalation solution, compounded product, administered through DME, unit dose form, per g M ☑

J7605 Arformoterol, inhalation solution, FDA-approved final product, noncompounded, administered through DME, unit dose form, 15 mcg M ☑
CMS: 100-02,15,50.5

J7606 Formoterol fumarate, inhalation solution, FDA-approved final product, noncompounded, administered through DME, unit dose form, 20 mcg M ☑
Use this code for PERFOROMIST.
CMS: 100-02,15,50.5

J7607 Levalbuterol, inhalation solution, compounded product, administered through DME, concentrated form, 0.5 mg M ☑
CMS: 100-03,200.2

J7608 Acetylcysteine, inhalation solution, FDA-approved final product, noncompounded, administered through DME, unit dose form, per g M ☑
Use this code for Acetadote, Mucomyst, Mucosil.

J7609 Albuterol, inhalation solution, compounded product, administered through DME, unit dose, 1 mg M ☑

J7610 Albuterol, inhalation solution, compounded product, administered through DME, concentrated form, 1 mg M ☑

Special Coverage Instructions   Noncovered by Medicare   Carrier Discretion   ☑ Quantity Alert ● New Code   ○ Recycled/Reinstated ▲ Revised Code

102 — J Codes   A Age Edit   M Maternity Edit   ♀ Female Only   ♂ Male Only   A-Y OPPS Status Indicators   © 2021 Optum360, LLC

J7611 **Albuterol, inhalation solution, FDA-approved final product, noncompounded, administered through DME, concentrated form, 1 mg** M ☑
Use this code for Accuneb, Proventil, Respirol, Ventolin.
AHA: 2Q, '08, 10

J7612 **Levalbuterol, inhalation solution, FDA-approved final product, noncompounded, administered through DME, concentrated form, 0.5 mg** M ☑
Use this code for Xopenex HFA.
CMS: 100-03,200.2
AHA: 2Q, '08, 10

J7613 **Albuterol, inhalation solution, FDA-approved final product, noncompounded, administered through DME, unit dose, 1 mg** M ☑
Use this code for Accuneb, Proventil, Respirol, Ventolin.
AHA: 2Q, '08, 10

J7614 **Levalbuterol, inhalation solution, FDA-approved final product, noncompounded, administered through DME, unit dose, 0.5 mg** M ☑
Use this code for Xopenex.
CMS: 100-03,200.2
AHA: 2Q, '08, 10

J7615 **Levalbuterol, inhalation solution, compounded product, administered through DME, unit dose, 0.5 mg** M ☑
CMS: 100-03,200.2

J7620 **Albuterol, up to 2.5 mg and ipratropium bromide, up to 0.5 mg, FDA-approved final product, noncompounded, administered through DME** M ☑

J7622 **Beclomethasone, inhalation solution, compounded product, administered through DME, unit dose form, per mg** M ☑
Use this code for Beclovent, Beconase.
AHA: 1Q, '02, 5

J7624 **Betamethasone, inhalation solution, compounded product, administered through DME, unit dose form, per mg** M ☑
AHA: 1Q, '02, 5

J7626 **Budesonide, inhalation solution, FDA-approved final product, noncompounded, administered through DME, unit dose form, up to 0.5 mg**
Use this code for Pulmicort, Pulmicort Flexhaler, Pulmicort Respules, Vanceril.
AHA: 1Q, '02, 5

J7627 **Budesonide, inhalation solution, compounded product, administered through DME, unit dose form, up to 0.5 mg** M ☑

J7628 **Bitolterol mesylate, inhalation solution, compounded product, administered through DME, concentrated form, per mg** M ☑

J7629 **Bitolterol mesylate, inhalation solution, compounded product, administered through DME, unit dose form, per mg** M ☑

J7631 **Cromolyn sodium, inhalation solution, FDA-approved final product, noncompounded, administered through DME, unit dose form, per 10 mg** M ☑
Use this code for Intal, Nasalcrom.

J7632 **Cromolyn sodium, inhalation solution, compounded product, administered through DME, unit dose form, per 10 mg** M ☑

J7633 **Budesonide, inhalation solution, FDA-approved final product, noncompounded, administered through DME, concentrated form, per 0.25 mg** M ☑
Use this code for Pulmicort, Pulmicort Flexhaler, Pulmicort Respules, Vanceril.

J7634 **Budesonide, inhalation solution, compounded product, administered through DME, concentrated form, per 0.25 mg** M ☑

J7635 **Atropine, inhalation solution, compounded product, administered through DME, concentrated form, per mg** M ☑

J7636 **Atropine, inhalation solution, compounded product, administered through DME, unit dose form, per mg** M ☑

J7637 **Dexamethasone, inhalation solution, compounded product, administered through DME, concentrated form, per mg** M ☑

J7638 **Dexamethasone, inhalation solution, compounded product, administered through DME, unit dose form, per mg** M ☑

J7639 **Dornase alfa, inhalation solution, FDA-approved final product, noncompounded, administered through DME, unit dose form, per mg** M ☑
Use this code for Pulmozyme.
CMS: 100-02,15,50.5

J7640 **Formoterol, inhalation solution, compounded product, administered through DME, unit dose form, 12 mcg** E ☑

J7641 **Flunisolide, inhalation solution, compounded product, administered through DME, unit dose, per mg** M ☑
Use this code for Aerobid, Flunisolide.
AHA: 1Q, '02, 5

J7642 **Glycopyrrolate, inhalation solution, compounded product, administered through DME, concentrated form, per mg** M ☑

J7643 **Glycopyrrolate, inhalation solution, compounded product, administered through DME, unit dose form, per mg** M ☑

J7644 **Ipratropium bromide, inhalation solution, FDA-approved final product, noncompounded, administered through DME, unit dose form, per mg** M ☑
Use this code for Atrovent.

J7645 **Ipratropium bromide, inhalation solution, compounded product, administered through DME, unit dose form, per mg** M ☑

J7647 **Isoetharine HCl, inhalation solution, compounded product, administered through DME, concentrated form, per mg** M ☑

J7648 **Isoetharine HCl, inhalation solution, FDA-approved final product, noncompounded, administered through DME, concentrated form, per mg** M ☑
Use this code for Beta-2.

J7649 **Isoetharine HCl, inhalation solution, FDA-approved final product, noncompounded, administered through DME, unit dose form, per mg** M ☑

J7650 **Isoetharine HCl, inhalation solution, compounded product, administered through DME, unit dose form, per mg** M ☑

J7657 **Isoproterenol HCl, inhalation solution, compounded product, administered through DME, concentrated form, per mg** M ☑

J7658 **Isoproterenol HCl, inhalation solution, FDA-approved final product, noncompounded, administered through DME, concentrated form, per mg** M ☑
Use this code for Isuprel HCl.

J7659 **Isoproterenol HCl, inhalation solution, FDA-approved final product, noncompounded, administered through DME, unit dose form, per mg** M ☑
Use this code for Isuprel HCl.

J7660 **Isoproterenol HCl, inhalation solution, compounded product, administered through DME, unit dose form, per mg** M ☑

J7665 **Mannitol, administered through an inhaler, 5 mg** N III ☑
Use this code for ARIDOL.

J7667 **Metaproterenol sulfate, inhalation solution, compounded product, concentrated form, per 10 mg** M ☑

☑ Special Coverage Instructions   Noncovered by Medicare   Carrier Discretion   ☑ Quantity Alert ● New Code   ○ Recycled/Reinstated   ▲ Revised Code

© 2021 Optum360, LLC   A2-Z3 ASC Pmt   CMS: IOM   AHA: Coding Clinic   ₺ DMEPOS Paid   ⊘ SNF Excluded   J Codes — 103

J7668 Metaproterenol sulfate, inhalation solution, FDA-approved final product, noncompounded, administered through DME, concentrated form, per 10 mg Ⓜ ☑
Use this code for Alupent.

J7669 Metaproterenol sulfate, inhalation solution, FDA-approved final product, noncompounded, administered through DME, unit dose form, per 10 mg Ⓜ ☑
Use this code for Alupent.

J7670 Metaproterenol sulfate, inhalation solution, compounded product, administered through DME, unit dose form, per 10 mg Ⓜ ☑

J7674 Methacholine chloride administered as inhalation solution through a nebulizer, per 1 mg Ⓝ Ⓜ ☑
AHA: 2Q, '05, 11

J7676 Pentamidine isethionate, inhalation solution, compounded product, administered through DME, unit dose form, per 300 mg Ⓜ ☑

J7677 Revefenacin inhalation solution, FDA-approved final product, noncompounded, administered through DME, 1 mcg
Use this code for Yupelri.

J7680 Terbutaline sulfate, inhalation solution, compounded product, administered through DME, concentrated form, per mg Ⓜ ☑
Use this code for Brethine.

J7681 Terbutaline sulfate, inhalation solution, compounded product, administered through DME, unit dose form, per mg Ⓜ ☑
Use this code for Brethine.

J7682 Tobramycin, inhalation solution, FDA-approved final product, noncompounded, unit dose form, administered through DME, per 300 mg Ⓜ ☑
Use this code for Tobi.
CMS: 100-02,15,50.5

J7683 Triamcinolone, inhalation solution, compounded product, administered through DME, concentrated form, per mg Ⓜ ☑
Use this code for Azmacort.

J7684 Triamcinolone, inhalation solution, compounded product, administered through DME, unit dose form, per mg Ⓜ ☑
Use this code for Azmacort.

J7685 Tobramycin, inhalation solution, compounded product, administered through DME, unit dose form, per 300 mg Ⓜ ☑

J7686 Treprostinil, inhalation solution, FDA-approved final product, noncompounded, administered through DME, unit dose form, 1.74 mg Ⓜ ☑
Use this code for Tyvaso.
CMS: 100-02,15,50.5

J7699 NOC drugs, inhalation solution administered through DME Ⓜ ☑
CMS: 100-02,15,50.5

J7799 NOC drugs, other than inhalation drugs, administered through DME Ⓝ Ⓝ1 ☑
CMS: 100-04,20,180; 100-04,32,411.3; 100-04,32,411.4; 100-04,32,411.5; 100-04,32,411.6
AHA: 3Q, '15, 7

J7999 Compounded drug, not otherwise classified Ⓝ Ⓝ1 ☑
CMS: 100-04,20,180; 100-04,32,411.4; 100-04,32,411.5; 100-04,32,411.6
AHA: 1Q, '17, 1-3; 4Q, '16, 8; 1Q, '16, 6-8

J8498 Antiemetic drug, rectal/suppository, not otherwise specified Ⓑ ☑
AHA: 2Q, '13, 5

J8499 Prescription drug, oral, nonchemotherapeutic, NOS Ⓔ ☑
CMS: 100-02,15,50.5
AHA: 2Q, '13, 5

J Codes Chemotherapy Drugs J8501-J9999
Oral Chemotherapy Drugs

J8501 Aprepitant, oral, 5 mg Ⓚ Ⓝ1 ☑
Use this code for Emend.
CMS: 100-02,15,50.5.4; 100-03,110.18; 100-04,17,80.2.1; 100-04,17,80.2.4
AHA: 3Q, '05, 7, 9

J8510 Busulfan, oral, 2 mg Ⓝ Ⓝ1 ☑
Use this code for Busulfex, Myleran.
CMS: 100-04,17,80.1.1

J8515 Cabergoline, oral, 0.25 mg Ⓔ ☑
Use this code for Dostinex.

J8520 Capecitabine, oral, 150 mg Ⓝ Ⓝ1 ☑
Use this code for Xeloda.
CMS: 100-04,17,80.1.1

J8521 Capecitabine, oral, 500 mg Ⓝ Ⓝ1 ☑
Use this code for Xeloda.
CMS: 100-04,17,80.1.1

J8530 Cyclophosphamide, oral, 25 mg Ⓝ Ⓝ1 ☑
Use this code for Cytoxan.
CMS: 100-04,17,80.1.1
AHA: 1Q, '02, 1-2

J8540 Dexamethasone, oral, 0.25 mg Ⓝ Ⓝ1 ☑
Use this code for Decadron.

J8560 Etoposide, oral, 50 mg Ⓚ Ⓚ2 ☑
Use this code for VePesid.
CMS: 100-04,17,80.1.1

J8562 Fludarabine phosphate, oral, 10 mg Ⓔ ☑
Use this code for Oforta.

J8565 Gefitinib, oral, 250 mg Ⓔ ☑
Use this code for Iressa.
CMS: 100-04,17,80.1.1
AHA: 4Q, '14, 6

J8597 Antiemetic drug, oral, not otherwise specified Ⓝ Ⓝ1 ☑
AHA: 2Q, '13, 5

J8600 Melphalan, oral, 2 mg Ⓝ Ⓝ1 ☑
Use this code for Alkeran.
CMS: 100-04,17,80.1.1

J8610 Methotrexate, oral, 2.5 mg Ⓝ Ⓝ1 ☑
Use this code for Trexall, RHEUMATREX.
CMS: 100-04,17,80.1.1

J8650 Nabilone, oral, 1 mg Ⓔ ☑
Use this code for Cesamet.

J8655 Netupitant 300 mg and palonosetron 0.5 mg, oral Ⓚ Ⓚ2 ☑
Use this code for Akynzeo.

J8670 Rolapitant, oral, 1 mg Ⓚ Ⓚ2 ☑
Use this code for Varubi.

J8700 Temozolomide, oral, 5 mg Ⓝ Ⓝ1 ☑
Use this code for Temodar.

J8705 Topotecan, oral, 0.25 mg Ⓚ Ⓝ1 ☑
Use this code for Hycamtin.

J8999 Prescription drug, oral, chemotherapeutic, NOS Ⓑ ☑
Determine if an alternative HCPCS Level II or a CPT code better describes the service being reported. This code should be used only if a more specific code is unavailable.
CMS: 100-04,17,80.1.1; 100-04,17,80.1.2
AHA: 2Q, '13, 5

Special Coverage Instructions   Noncovered by Medicare   Carrier Discretion   ☑ Quantity Alert ● New Code   ○ Recycled/Reinstated   ▲ Revised Code

Ⓐ Age Edit   Ⓜ Maternity Edit   ♀ Female Only   ♂ Male Only   Ⓐ-Ⓨ OPPS Status Indicators   © 2021 Optum360, LLC

Injectable Chemotherapy Drugs

These codes cover the cost of the chemotherapy drug only, not the administration.

J9000 **Injection, doxorubicin HCl, 10 mg** N N1 ☑ ⊘
Use this code for Adriamycin PFS, Adriamycin RDF, Rubex.
CMS: 100-04,20,180; 100-04,32,411.3
AHA: 4Q, '07, 5

J9015 **Injection, aldesleukin, per single use vial** K K2 ☑ ⊘
Use this code for Proleukin, IL-2, Interleukin.
AHA: 2Q, '05, 11

J9017 **Injection, arsenic trioxide, 1 mg** K K2 ☑ ⊘
Use this code for Trisenox.
AHA: 2Q, '05, 11; 2Q, '02, 8-9; 1Q, '02, 5

J9019 **Injection, asparaginase (Erwinaze), 1,000 IU** K K2 ☑

J9020 **Injection, asparaginase, not otherwise specified, 10,000 units** N ☑
Use this code for Elspar.
AHA: 2Q, '13, 5

● **J9021** **Injection, asparaginase, recombinant, (Rylaze), 0.1 mg**
Use this code for Rylaze.

J9022 **Injection, atezolizumab, 10 mg** G K2
Use this code for Tecentriq.

J9023 **Injection, avelumab, 10 mg** G K2
Use this code for Bavencio.

J9025 **Injection, azacitidine, 1 mg** K K2 ☑ ⊘
Use this code for Vidaza.

J9027 **Injection, clofarabine, 1 mg** K K2 ☑ ⊘
Use this code for Clolar.

J9030 **BCG live intravesical instillation, 1 mg** N1
Use this code for Pacis, TICE BCG.

J9032 **Injection, belinostat, 10 mg** K K2 ☑
Use this code for Beleodaq.

J9033 **Injection, bendamustine HCl (Treanda), 1 mg** K K2 ☑ ⊘

J9034 **Injection, bendamustine HCl (Bendeka), 1 mg** G K2 ☑
AHA: 1Q, '17, 9-10

J9035 **Injection, bevacizumab, 10 mg** K K2 ☑ ⊘
Use this code for Avastin.
CMS: 100-03,110.17
AHA: 3Q, '13, 9; 2Q, '13; 2Q, '05, 11

J9036 **Injection, bendamustine hydrochloride, (Belrapzo/bendamustine), 1 mg** K2

● **J9037** **Injection, belantamab mafodontin-blmf, 0.5 mg** K2
Use this code for Blenrep.

J9039 **Injection, blinatumomab, 1 mcg** K K2 ☑
Use this code for Blincyto.
CMS: 100-04,20,180; 100-04,32,411.3

J9040 **Injection, bleomycin sulfate, 15 units** N N1 ☑ ⊘
Use this code for Blenoxane.
CMS: 100-04,20,180; 100-04,32,411.3

J9041 **Injection, bortezomib (Velcade), 0.1 mg** K K2 ☑ ⊘
AHA: 2Q, '05, 11; 1Q, '05, 7, 9-10

J9042 **Injection, brentuximab vedotin, 1 mg** K K2 ☑
Use this code for Adcentris.

J9043 **Injection, cabazitaxel, 1 mg** K K2 ☑
Use this code for Jevtana.

J9044 **Injection, bortezomib, not otherwise specified, 0.1 mg** K2
CMS: 100-04,4,260.1; 100-04,4,260.1.1

J9045 **Injection, carboplatin, 50 mg** N N1 ☑ ⊘
Use this code for Paraplatin.

J9047 **Injection, carfilzomib, 1 mg** K K2 ☑
Use this code for Kyprolis.

J9050 **Injection, carmustine, 100 mg** K K2 ☑ ⊘
Use this code for BiCNU.

J9055 **Injection, cetuximab, 10 mg** K K2 ☑ ⊘
Use this code for Erbitux.
CMS: 100-03,110.17
AHA: 2Q, '05, 11

J9057 **Injection, copanlisib, 1 mg** K2
Use this code for Aliqopa.

J9060 **Injection, cisplatin, powder or solution, 10 mg** N N1 ☑ ⊘
Use this code for Plantinol AQ.
AHA: 2Q, '13, 6

● **J9061** **Injection, amivantamab-vmjw, 2 mg**
Use this code for Rybrevant.

J9065 **Injection, cladribine, per 1 mg** K K2 ☑ ⊘
Use this code for Leustatin.
CMS: 100-04,20,180; 100-04,32,411.3

J9070 **Cyclophosphamide, 100 mg** K K2 ☑ ⊘
Use this code for Endoxan-Asta.

J9098 **Injection, cytarabine liposome, 10 mg** K N1 ☑ ⊘
Use this code for Depocyt.

J9100 **Injection, cytarabine, 100 mg** N N1 ☑ ⊘
Use this code for Cytosar-U, Ara-C, Tarabin CFS.
CMS: 100-04,20,180; 100-04,32,411.3

J9118 **Injection, calaspargase pegol-mknl, 10 units**
Use this code for Asparla.

J9119 **Injection, cemiplimab-rwlc, 1 mg** K2
Use this code for Libtayo.

J9120 **Injection, dactinomycin, 0.5 mg** K K2 ☑ ⊘
Use this code for Cosmegen.

J9130 **Dacarbazine, 100 mg** N N1 ☑ ⊘
Use this code for DTIC-Dome.
AHA: 1Q, '08, 6

J9144 **Injection, daratumumab, 10 mg and hyaluronidase-fihj** K2
Use this code for Darzalex Faspro.

J9145 **Injection, daratumumab, 10 mg** G K2 ☑
Use this code for Darzalex.

J9150 **Injection, daunorubicin, 10 mg** K K2 ☑ ⊘
Use this code for Cerubidine.

J9151 **Injection, daunorubicin citrate, liposomal formulation, 10 mg** E ☑ ⊘
Use this code for Daunoxome.

J9153 **Injection, liposomal, 1 mg daunorubicin and 2.27 mg cytarabine** K2
Use this code for Vyxeos.

J9155 **Injection, degarelix, 1 mg** K K2 ☑
CMS: 100-02,15,50.5

J9160 **Injection, denileukin diftitox, 300 mcg** E ☑ ⊘
Use this code for Ontak.
AHA: 2Q, '05, 11

J9165 **Injection, diethylstilbestrol diphosphate, 250 mg** E ☑

J9171 **Injection, docetaxel, 1 mg** K N1 ☑ ⊘
Use this code for Taxotere.

J9173 **Injection, durvalumab, 10 mg** K2
Use this code for Imfinzi.

J9175 **Injection, Elliotts' B solution, 1 ml** N N1 ☑

Special Coverage Instructions   Noncovered by Medicare   Carrier Discretion   ☑ Quantity Alert ● New Code   ○ Recycled/Reinstated   ▲ Revised Code

Chemotherapy Drugs

J9176 — J9269

J9176 Injection, elotuzumab, 1 mg G K2 ☑
Use this code for Empliciti.

J9177 Injection, enfortumab vedotin-ejfv, 0.25 mg K2
Use this code for PADCEV.

J9178 Injection, epirubicin HCl, 2 mg N N1 ☑ ⊘
Use this code for Ellence.

J9179 Injection, eribulin mesylate, 0.1 mg K K2 ☑
Use this code for Halaven.

J9181 Injection, etoposide, 10 mg N N1 ☑ ⊘
Use this code for VePesid, Toposar.

J9185 Injection, fludarabine phosphate, 50 mg K N1 ☑ ⊘
Use this code for Fludara.

J9190 Injection, fluorouracil, 500 mg N N1 ☑
Use this code for Adrucil.
CMS: 100-04,20,180; 100-04,32,411.3

J9198 Injection, gemcitabine hydrochloride, (Infugem), 100 mg K2

J9200 Injection, floxuridine, 500 mg N N1 ☑ ⊘
Use this code for FUDR.
CMS: 100-04,20,180

J9201 Injection, gemcitabine HCl, not otherwise specified, 200 mg N N1 ☑ ⊘
Use this code for Gemzar.

J9202 Goserelin acetate implant, per 3.6 mg K K2 ☑
Use this code for Zoladex.

J9203 Injection, gemtuzumab ozogamicin, 0.1 mg G K2
Use this code for Mylotarg.

J9204 Injection, mogamulizumab-kpkc, 1 mg K2
Use this code for Poteligeo.

J9205 Injection, irinotecan liposome, 1 mg G K2 ☑
Use this code for Onivyde.

J9206 Injection, irinotecan, 20 mg N N1 ☑ ⊘
Use this code for Camptosar.
CMS: 100-03,110.17

J9207 Injection, ixabepilone, 1 mg K K2 ☑ ⊘
Use this code for IXEMPRA.

J9208 Injection, ifosfamide, 1 g N N1 ☑ ⊘
Use this code for IFEX, Mitoxana.

J9209 Injection, mesna, 200 mg N N1 ☑
Use this code for Mesnex.

J9210 Injection, emapalumab-lzsg, 1 mg K2
Use this code for Gamifant.

J9211 Injection, idarubicin HCl, 5 mg K N1 ☑ ⊘
Use this code for Idamycin.

J9212 Injection, interferon alfacon-1, recombinant, 1 mcg N ☑
Use this code for Infergen.

J9213 Injection, interferon, alfa-2a, recombinant, 3 million units N N1 ☑
Use this code for Roferon-A.

J9214 Injection, interferon, alfa-2b, recombinant, 1 million units K K2 ☑
Use this code for Intron A, Rebetron Kit.
CMS: 100-02,15,50.5

J9215 Injection, interferon, alfa-N3, (human leukocyte derived), 250,000 IU E ☑
Use this code for Alferon N.

J9216 Injection, interferon, gamma 1-b, 3 million units K ☑
Use this code for Actimmune.
CMS: 100-02,15,50.5
AHA: 2Q, '05, 11

J9217 Leuprolide acetate (for depot suspension), 7.5 mg K K2 ☑
Use this code for Lupron Depot, Eligard.
AHA: 3Q, '15, 3

J9218 Leuprolide acetate, per 1 mg K N1 ☑
Use this code for Lupron.
CMS: 100-02,15,50.5
AHA: 3Q, '15, 3

J9219 Leuprolide acetate implant, 65 mg E ☑
Use this code for Lupron Implant, Viadur.
AHA: 4Q, '01, 5

J9223 Injection, lurbinectedin, 0.1 mg K2
Use this code for Zepzelca.

J9225 Histrelin implant (Vantas), 50 mg K K2 ☑ ⊘

J9226 Histrelin implant (Supprelin LA), 50 mg K K2 ☑ ⊘
AHA: 1Q, '08, 6

J9227 Injection, isatuximab-irfc, 10 mg K2
Use this code for Sarclisa.

J9228 Injection, ipilimumab, 1 mg K K2 ☑
Use this code for YERVOY.

J9229 Injection, inotuzumab ozogamicin, 0.1 mg K2
Use this code for Besponsa.

J9230 Injection, mechlorethamine HCl, (nitrogen mustard), 10 mg K K2 ☑ ⊘
Use this code for Mustargen.

J9245 Injection, melphalan hydrochloride, not otherwise specified, 50 mg K K2 ☑ ⊘

J9246 Injection, melphalan (Evomela), 1 mg K2

● **J9247** Injection, melphalan flufenamide, 1 mg K2
Use this code for Pepaxto.

J9250 Methotrexate sodium, 5 mg N N1 ☑
Use this code for Folex, Folex PFS, Methotrexate LPF.

J9260 Methotrexate sodium, 50 mg N N1 ☑
Use this code for Folex, Folex PFS, Methotrexate LPF.

J9261 Injection, nelarabine, 50 mg K K2 ☑
Use this code for Arranon.

J9262 Injection, omacetaxine mepesuccinate, 0.01 mg K K2 ☑
Use this code for Synribo.
CMS: 100-02,15,50.5

J9263 Injection, oxaliplatin, 0.5 mg N N1 ☑ ⊘
Use this code for Eloxatin.
AHA: 1Q, '09, 10

J9264 Injection, paclitaxel protein-bound particles, 1 mg K K2 ☑ ⊘
Use this code for Abraxane.

J9266 Injection, pegaspargase, per single dose vial K K2 ☑ ⊘
Use this code for Oncaspar.
AHA: 2Q, '02, 8-9

J9267 Injection, paclitaxel, 1 mg N N1 ☑
Use this code for Taxol.
AHA: 1Q, '15, 6

J9268 Injection, pentostatin, 10 mg K K2 ☑ ⊘
Use this code for Nipent.

J9269 Injection, tagraxofusp-erzs, 10 mcg K2
Use this code for Elzonris.

Special Coverage Instructions Noncovered by Medicare Carrier Discretion ☑ Quantity Alert ● New Code ○ Recycled/Reinstated ▲ Revised Code

106 — J Codes A Age Edit M Maternity Edit ♀ Female Only ♂ Male Only A-Y OPPS Status Indicators © 2021 Optum360, LLC

Chemotherapy Drugs

J9270 — J9999

J9270   **Injection, plicamycin, 2.5 mg**   N K2 ☑
Use this code for Mithacin.

J9271   **Injection, pembrolizumab, 1 mg**   K K2 ☑
Use this code for Keytruda.

● **J9272**   **Injection, dostarlimab-gxly, 10 mg**
Use this code for Jemperli.

J9280   **Injection, mitomycin, 5 mg**   K K2 ☑ ⊘
Use this code for Mutamycin.
AHA: 4Q, '16, 8; 2Q, '14, 8

J9281   **Mitomycin pyelocalyceal instillation, 1 mg**   K2
Use this code for Jelmyto.

J9285   **Injection, olaratumab, 10 mg**   G K2
Use this code for Lartruvo.

J9293   **Injection, mitoxantrone HCl, per 5 mg**   K K2 ☑ ⊘
Use this code for Navantrone.

J9295   **Injection, necitumumab, 1 mg**   G K2 ☑
Use this code for Portrazza.

J9299   **Injection, nivolumab, 1 mg**   K K2 ☑
Use this code for Opdivo.

J9301   **Injection, obinutuzumab, 10 mg**   K K2 ☑
Use this code for Gazyva.
AHA: 1Q, '15, 6

J9302   **Injection, ofatumumab, 10 mg**   K K2 ☑
Use this code for Arzerra.

J9303   **Injection, panitumumab, 10 mg**   K K2 ☑ ⊘
Use this code for Vectibix.
AHA: 1Q, '08, 6

J9304   **Injection, pemetrexed (Pemfexy), 10 mg**

J9305   **Injection, pemetrexed, NOS, 10 mg**   K K2 ☑ ⊘
AHA: 2Q, '05, 11

J9306   **Injection, pertuzumab, 1 mg**   K K2 ☑
Use this code for Perjeta.

J9307   **Injection, pralatrexate, 1 mg**   K K2 ☑
Use this code for FOLOTYN.

J9308   **Injection, ramucirumab, 5 mg**   K K2 ☑
Use this code for Cyramza.

J9309   **Injection, polatuzumab vedotin-piiq, 1 mg**   K2
Use this code for Polivy.

J9311   **Injection, rituximab 10 mg and hyaluronidase**   K2
Use this code for Rituxin Hycela.

J9312   **Injection, rituximab, 10 mg**   K2
Use this code for Rituxin.

J9313   **Injection, moxetumomab pasudotox-tdfk, 0.01 mg**   K2
Use this code for Lumoxiti.

~~**J9315**   **Injection, romidepsin, 1 mg**~~
To report, see ~J9319

J9316   **Injection, pertuzumab, trastuzumab, and hyaluronidase-zzxf, per 10 mg**   K2
Use this code for PHESGO.

J9317   **Injection, sacituzumab govitecan-hziy, 2.5 mg**   K2
Use this code for Trodelvy.

● **J9318**   **Injection, romidepsin, nonlyophilized, 0.1 mg**   K2

● **J9319**   **Injection, romidepsin, lyophilized, 0.1 mg**   K2
Use this code for Istodax.

J9320   **Injection, streptozocin, 1 g**   K K2 ☑ ⊘
Use this code for Zanosar.

J9325   **Injection, talimogene laherparepvec, per 1 million plaque forming units**   G K2 ☑
Use this code for Imlygic.

J9328   **Injection, temozolomide, 1 mg**   K K2 ☑ ⊘
Use this code for Temodar.

J9330   **Injection, temsirolimus, 1 mg**   K K2 ☑ ⊘
Use this code for TORISEL.

J9340   **Injection, thiotepa, 15 mg**   K K2 ☑ ⊘
Use this code for Thioplex.

● **J9348**   **Injection, naxitamab-gqgk, 1 mg**   K2

● **J9349**   **Injection, tafasitamab-cxix, 2 mg**   K2
Use this code for Monjuvi.

J9351   **Injection, topotecan, 0.1 mg**   N N1 ☑
Use this code for Hycamtin.

J9352   **Injection, trabectedin, 0.1 mg**   G K2 ☑
Use this code for Yondelis.

● **J9353**   **Injection, margetuximab-cmkb, 5 mg**   K2

J9354   **Injection, ado-trastuzumab emtansine, 1 mg**   K K2 ☑
Use this code for Kadcyla.

J9355   **Injection, trastuzumab, excludes biosimilar, 10 mg**   K K2 ☑ ⊘
Use this code for Herceptin.

J9356   **Injection, trastuzumab, 10 mg and hyaluronidase-oysk**   K2
Use this code for Herceptin Hylecta.

J9357   **Injection, valrubicin, intravesical, 200 mg**   K K2 ☑ ⊘
Use this code for Valstar.

J9358   **Injection, fam-trastuzumab deruxtecan-nxki, 1 mg**   K2
Use this code for Enhertu.

J9360   **Injection, vinblastine sulfate, 1 mg**   N N1 ☑ ⊘
Use this code for Velban.
CMS: 100-04,20,180; 100-04,32,411.3

J9370   **Vincristine sulfate, 1 mg**   N N1 ☑ ⊘
Use this code for Oncovin, Vincasar PFS.
CMS: 100-04,20,180; 100-04,32,411.3

J9371   **Injection, vincristine sulfate liposome, 1 mg**   K K2 ☑
Use this code for Marqibo kit.
AHA: 1Q, '14, 6

J9390   **Injection, vinorelbine tartrate, 10 mg**   N N1 ☑ ⊘
Use this code for Navelbine.
AHA: 2Q, '05, 8

J9395   **Injection, fulvestrant, 25 mg**   K K2 ☑ ⊘
Use this code for Faslodex.

J9400   **Injection, ziv-aflibercept, 1 mg**   K K2 ☑
Use this code for Zaltrap.

J9600   **Injection, porfimer sodium, 75 mg**   K K2 ☑ ⊘
Use this code for Photofrin.

J9999   **Not otherwise classified, antineoplastic drugs**   N N1 ☑
Determine if an alternative HCPCS Level II or a CPT code better describes the service being reported. This code should be used only if a more specific code is unavailable.
CMS: 100-02,15,50.5; 100-04,32,400; 100-04,32,400.1; 100-04,32,400.2; 100-04,32,400.2.1; 100-04,32,400.2.2; 100-04,32,400.2.3; 100-04,32,400.2.4; 100-04,32,400.3; 100-04,32,400.4; 100-04,32,400.5; 100-04,32,411.3; 100-04,4,260.1; 100-04,4,260.1.1
AHA: 1Q, '17, 1-3; 3Q, '15, 7; 2Q, '13, 5; 1Q, '13, 9; 4Q, '12, 9; 1Q, '08, 6; 1Q, '02, 1-2

Special Coverage Instructions   Noncovered by Medicare   Carrier Discretion   ☑ Quantity Alert   ● New Code   ○ Recycled/Reinstated   ▲ Revised Code

Temporary Codes K0001-K1027

The K codes were established for use by the DME Medicare Administrative Contractors (DME MACs). The K codes are developed when the currently existing permanent national codes for supplies and certain product categories do not include the codes needed to implement a DME MAC medical review policy.

Wheelchairs and Accessories

Code	Description	Indicators
K0001	Standard wheelchair	Y ও (RR)
K0002	Standard hemi (low seat) wheelchair	Y ও (RR)
K0003	Lightweight wheelchair	Y ও (RR)
K0004	High strength, lightweight wheelchair	Y ও (RR)
K0005	Ultralightweight wheelchair	Y ও (NU, RR, UE)
K0006	Heavy-duty wheelchair	Y ও (RR)
K0007	Extra heavy-duty wheelchair	Y ও (RR)
K0008	Custom manual wheelchair/base	Y
K0009	Other manual wheelchair/base	Y ও (RR)
K0010	Standard-weight frame motorized/power wheelchair	Y ও (RR)
K0011	Standard-weight frame motorized/power wheelchair with programmable control parameters for speed adjustment, tremor dampening, acceleration control and braking CMS: 100-04,20,30.9	Y ও (RR)
K0012	Lightweight portable motorized/power wheelchair	Y ও (RR)
K0013	Custom motorized/power wheelchair base	Y
K0014	Other motorized/power wheelchair base	Y
K0015	Detachable, nonadjustable height armrest, each	Y ☑ ও (RR)
K0017	Detachable, adjustable height armrest, base, replacement only, each	Y ☑ ও (NU, RR, UE)
K0018	Detachable, adjustable height armrest, upper portion, replacement only, each	Y ☑ ও (NU, RR, UE)
K0019	Arm pad, replacement only, each	Y ☑ ও (NU, RR, UE)
K0020	Fixed, adjustable height armrest, pair	Y ☑ ও (NU, RR, UE)
K0037	High mount flip-up footrest, each	Y ☑ ও (NU, RR, UE)
K0038	Leg strap, each	Y ☑ ও (NU, RR, UE)
K0039	Leg strap, H style, each	Y ☑ ও (NU, RR, UE)
K0040	Adjustable angle footplate, each	Y ☑ ও (NU, RR, UE)
K0041	Large size footplate, each	Y ☑ ও (NU, RR, UE)
K0042	Standard size footplate, replacement only, each	Y ☑ ও (NU, RR, UE)
K0043	Footrest, lower extension tube, replacement only, each	Y ☑ ও (NU, RR, UE)
K0044	Footrest, upper hanger bracket, replacement only, each	Y ☑ ও (NU, RR, UE)
K0045	Footrest, complete assembly, replacement only, each	Y ও (NU, RR, UE)
K0046	Elevating legrest, lower extension tube, replacement only, each	Y ☑ ও (NU, RR, UE)
K0047	Elevating legrest, upper hanger bracket, replacement only, each	Y ☑ ও (NU, RR, UE)
K0050	Ratchet assembly, replacement only	Y ও (NU, RR, UE)
K0051	Cam release assembly, footrest or legrest, replacement only, each	Y ☑ ও (NU, RR, UE)
K0052	Swingaway, detachable footrests, replacement only, each	Y ☑ ও (NU, RR, UE)
K0053	Elevating footrests, articulating (telescoping), each	Y ☑ ও (NU, RR, UE)
K0056	Seat height less than 17 in or equal to or greater than 21 in for a high-strength, lightweight, or ultralightweight wheelchair	Y ☑ ও (NU, RR, UE)
K0065	Spoke protectors, each	Y ☑ ও (NU, RR, UE)
K0069	Rear wheel assembly, complete, with solid tire, spokes or molded, replacement only, each	Y ☑ ও (NU, RR, UE)
K0070	Rear wheel assembly, complete, with pneumatic tire, spokes or molded, replacement only, each	Y ☑ ও (RR)
K0071	Front caster assembly, complete, with pneumatic tire, replacement only, each	Y ☑ ও (NU, RR, UE)
K0072	Front caster assembly, complete, with semi-pneumatic tire, replacement only, each	Y ☑ ও (NU, RR, UE)
K0073	Caster pin lock, each	Y ☑ ও (NU, RR, UE)
K0077	Front caster assembly, complete, with solid tire, replacement only, each	Y ☑ ও (NU, RR, UE)
K0098	Drive belt for power wheelchair, replacement only	Y ও (NU, RR, UE)
K0105	IV hanger, each	Y ☑ ও (NU, RR, UE)
K0108	Wheelchair component or accessory, not otherwise specified	Y
K0195	Elevating legrests, pair (for use with capped rental wheelchair base)	Y ও (RR)

Equipment, Replacement, Repair, Rental

Code	Description	Indicators
K0455	Infusion pump used for uninterrupted parenteral administration of medication, (e.g., epoprostenol or treprostinol)	Y ও (RR)
K0462	Temporary replacement for patient-owned equipment being repaired, any type CMS: 100-04,20,40.1	Y
K0552	Supplies for external noninsulin drug infusion pump, syringe type cartridge, sterile, each	Y ☑ ও
K0553	Supply allowance for therapeutic continuous glucose monitor (CGM), includes all supplies and accessories, 1 month supply = 1 unit of service	Y ও (KF)
K0554	Receiver (monitor), dedicated, for use with therapeutic glucose continuous monitor system	Y ও (NU, RR, UE)
K0601	Replacement battery for external infusion pump owned by patient, silver oxide, 1.5 volt, each AHA: 2Q, '03, 7	Y ☑ ও (NU)
K0602	Replacement battery for external infusion pump owned by patient, silver oxide, 3 volt, each AHA: 2Q, '03, 7	Y ☑ ও (NU)
K0603	Replacement battery for external infusion pump owned by patient, alkaline, 1.5 volt, each AHA: 2Q, '03, 7	Y ☑ ও (NU)
K0604	Replacement battery for external infusion pump owned by patient, lithium, 3.6 volt, each AHA: 2Q, '03, 7	Y ☑ ও (NU)
K0605	Replacement battery for external infusion pump owned by patient, lithium, 4.5 volt, each AHA: 2Q, '03, 7	Y ☑ ও (NU)
K0606	Automatic external defibrillator, with integrated electrocardiogram analysis, garment type AHA: 4Q, '03, 4-5	Y (RR)

Special Coverage Instructions   Noncovered by Medicare   Carrier Discretion   ☑ Quantity Alert   ● New Code   ○ Recycled/Reinstated   ▲ Revised Code

K0607 Replacement battery for automated external defibrillator, garment type only, each   Y ☑ & (RR)
AHA: 4Q, '03, 4-5

K0608 Replacement garment for use with automated external defibrillator, each   Y ☑ & (NU, RR, UE)
AHA: 4Q, '03, 4-5

K0609 Replacement electrodes for use with automated external defibrillator, garment type only, each   Y ☑ & (KF)
AHA: 4Q, '03, 4-5

K0669 Wheelchair accessory, wheelchair seat or back cushion, does not meet specific code criteria or no written coding verification from DME PDAC   Y

K0672 Addition to lower extremity orthotic, removable soft interface, all components, replacement only, each   A ☑ &

K0730 Controlled dose inhalation drug delivery system   Y & (RR)

K0733 Power wheelchair accessory, 12 to 24 amp hour sealed lead acid battery, each (e.g., gel cell, absorbed glassmat)   Y & (NU, RR, UE)

K0738 Portable gaseous oxygen system, rental; home compressor used to fill portable oxygen cylinders; includes portable containers, regulator, flowmeter, humidifier, cannula or mask, and tubing   Y & (RR)
CMS: 100-04,20,130.6

K0739 Repair or nonroutine service for durable medical equipment other than oxygen equipment requiring the skill of a technician, labor component, per 15 minutes   Y ☑

K0740 Repair or nonroutine service for oxygen equipment requiring the skill of a technician, labor component, per 15 minutes   E ☑

K0743 Suction pump, home model, portable, for use on wounds   Y

K0744 Absorptive wound dressing for use with suction pump, home model, portable, pad size 16 sq in or less   A ☑

K0745 Absorptive wound dressing for use with suction pump, home model, portable, pad size more than 16 sq in but less than or equal to 48 sq in   A ☑

K0746 Absorptive wound dressing for use with suction pump, home model, portable, pad size greater than 48 sq in   A

Power Operated Vehicle and Accessories

K0800 Power operated vehicle, group 1 standard, patient weight capacity up to and including 300 pounds   Y & (NU, RR, UE)
CMS: 100-04,12,30.6.15.4

K0801 Power operated vehicle, group 1 heavy-duty, patient weight capacity 301 to 450 pounds   Y & (NU, RR, UE)
CMS: 100-04,12,30.6.15.4

K0802 Power operated vehicle, group 1 very heavy-duty, patient weight capacity 451 to 600 pounds   Y & (NU, RR, UE)
CMS: 100-04,12,30.6.15.4

K0806 Power operated vehicle, group 2 standard, patient weight capacity up to and including 300 pounds   Y & (NU, RR, UE)
CMS: 100-04,12,30.6.15.4

K0807 Power operated vehicle, group 2 heavy-duty, patient weight capacity 301 to 450 pounds   Y & (NU, RR, UE)
CMS: 100-04,12,30.6.15.4

K0808 Power operated vehicle, group 2 very heavy-duty, patient weight capacity 451 to 600 pounds   Y & (NU, RR, UE)
CMS: 100-04,12,30.6.15.4

K0812 Power operated vehicle, not otherwise classified   Y
CMS: 100-04,12,30.6.15.4

Power Wheelchairs

K0813 Power wheelchair, group 1 standard, portable, sling/solid seat and back, patient weight capacity up to and including 300 pounds   Y & (RR)

K0814 Power wheelchair, group 1 standard, portable, captain's chair, patient weight capacity up to and including 300 pounds   Y & (RR)

K0815 Power wheelchair, group 1 standard, sling/solid seat and back, patient weight capacity up to and including 300 pounds   Y & (RR)

K0816 Power wheelchair, group 1 standard, captain's chair, patient weight capacity up to and including 300 pounds   Y & (RR)

K0820 Power wheelchair, group 2 standard, portable, sling/solid seat/back, patient weight capacity up to and including 300 pounds   Y & (RR)

K0821 Power wheelchair, group 2 standard, portable, captain's chair, patient weight capacity up to and including 300 pounds   Y & (RR)

K0822 Power wheelchair, group 2 standard, sling/solid seat/back, patient weight capacity up to and including 300 pounds   Y & (RR)

K0823 Power wheelchair, group 2 standard, captain's chair, patient weight capacity up to and including 300 pounds   Y & (RR)

K0824 Power wheelchair, group 2 heavy-duty, sling/solid seat/back, patient weight capacity 301 to 450 pounds   Y & (RR)

K0825 Power wheelchair, group 2 heavy-duty, captain's chair, patient weight capacity 301 to 450 pounds   Y & (RR)

K0826 Power wheelchair, group 2 very heavy-duty, sling/solid seat/back, patient weight capacity 451 to 600 pounds   Y & (RR)

K0827 Power wheelchair, group 2 very heavy-duty, captain's chair, patient weight capacity 451 to 600 pounds   Y & (RR)

K0828 Power wheelchair, group 2 extra heavy-duty, sling/solid seat/back, patient weight capacity 601 pounds or more   Y & (RR)

K0829 Power wheelchair, group 2 extra heavy-duty, captain's chair, patient weight 601 pounds or more   Y & (RR)

K0830 Power wheelchair, group 2 standard, seat elevator, sling/solid seat/back, patient weight capacity up to and including 300 pounds   Y

K0831 Power wheelchair, group 2 standard, seat elevator, captain's chair, patient weight capacity up to and including 300 pounds   Y

K0835 Power wheelchair, group 2 standard, single power option, sling/solid seat/back, patient weight capacity up to and including 300 pounds   Y & (RR)

K0836 Power wheelchair, group 2 standard, single power option, captain's chair, patient weight capacity up to and including 300 pounds   Y & (RR)

K0837 Power wheelchair, group 2 heavy-duty, single power option, sling/solid seat/back, patient weight capacity 301 to 450 pounds   Y & (RR)

K0838 Power wheelchair, group 2 heavy-duty, single power option, captain's chair, patient weight capacity 301 to 450 pounds   Y & (RR)

K0839 Power wheelchair, group 2 very heavy-duty, single power option sling/solid seat/back, patient weight capacity 451 to 600 pounds   Y & (RR)

Special Coverage Instructions   Noncovered by Medicare   Carrier Discretion   ☑ Quantity Alert   ● New Code   ○ Recycled/Reinstated   ▲ Revised Code

K0840 Power wheelchair, group 2 extra heavy-duty, single power option, sling/solid seat/back, patient weight capacity 601 pounds or more ⓨ ♿ (RR)

K0841 Power wheelchair, group 2 standard, multiple power option, sling/solid seat/back, patient weight capacity up to and including 300 pounds ⓨ ♿ (RR)

K0842 Power wheelchair, group 2 standard, multiple power option, captain's chair, patient weight capacity up to and including 300 pounds ⓨ ♿ (RR)

K0843 Power wheelchair, group 2 heavy-duty, multiple power option, sling/solid seat/back, patient weight capacity 301 to 450 pounds ⓨ ♿ (RR)

K0848 Power wheelchair, group 3 standard, sling/solid seat/back, patient weight capacity up to and including 300 pounds ⓨ ♿ (RR)
CMS: 100-04,20,30.9

K0849 Power wheelchair, group 3 standard, captain's chair, patient weight capacity up to and including 300 pounds ⓨ ♿ (RR)
CMS: 100-04,20,30.9

K0850 Power wheelchair, group 3 heavy-duty, sling/solid seat/back, patient weight capacity 301 to 450 pounds ⓨ ♿ (RR)
CMS: 100-04,20,30.9

K0851 Power wheelchair, group 3 heavy-duty, captain's chair, patient weight capacity 301 to 450 pounds ⓨ ♿ (RR)
CMS: 100-04,20,30.9

K0852 Power wheelchair, group 3 very heavy-duty, sling/solid seat/back, patient weight capacity 451 to 600 pounds ⓨ ♿ (RR)
CMS: 100-04,20,30.9

K0853 Power wheelchair, group 3 very heavy-duty, captain's chair, patient weight capacity 451 to 600 pounds ⓨ ♿ (RR)
CMS: 100-04,20,30.9

K0854 Power wheelchair, group 3 extra heavy-duty, sling/solid seat/back, patient weight capacity 601 pounds or more ⓨ ♿ (RR)
CMS: 100-04,20,30.9

K0855 Power wheelchair, group 3 extra heavy-duty, captain's chair, patient weight capacity 601 pounds or more ⓨ ♿ (RR)
CMS: 100-04,20,30.9

K0856 Power wheelchair, group 3 standard, single power option, sling/solid seat/back, patient weight capacity up to and including 300 pounds ⓨ ♿ (RR)
CMS: 100-04,20,30.9

K0857 Power wheelchair, group 3 standard, single power option, captain's chair, patient weight capacity up to and including 300 pounds ⓨ ♿ (RR)
CMS: 100-04,20,30.9

K0858 Power wheelchair, group 3 heavy-duty, single power option, sling/solid seat/back, patient weight capacity 301 to 450 pounds ⓨ ♿ (RR)
CMS: 100-04,20,30.9

K0859 Power wheelchair, group 3 heavy-duty, single power option, captain's chair, patient weight capacity 301 to 450 pounds ⓨ ♿ (RR)
CMS: 100-04,20,30.9

K0860 Power wheelchair, group 3 very heavy-duty, single power option, sling/solid seat/back, patient weight capacity 451 to 600 pounds ⓨ ♿ (RR)
CMS: 100-04,20,30.9

K0861 Power wheelchair, group 3 standard, multiple power option, sling/solid seat/back, patient weight capacity up to and including 300 pounds ⓨ ♿ (RR)
CMS: 100-04,20,30.9

K0862 Power wheelchair, group 3 heavy-duty, multiple power option, sling/solid seat/back, patient weight capacity 301 to 450 pounds ⓨ ♿ (RR)
CMS: 100-04,20,30.9

K0863 Power wheelchair, group 3 very heavy-duty, multiple power option, sling/solid seat/back, patient weight capacity 451 to 600 pounds ⓨ ♿ (RR)
CMS: 100-04,20,30.9

K0864 Power wheelchair, group 3 extra heavy-duty, multiple power option, sling/solid seat/back, patient weight capacity 601 pounds or more ⓨ ♿ (RR)
CMS: 100-04,20,30.9

K0868 Power wheelchair, group 4 standard, sling/solid seat/back, patient weight capacity up to and including 300 pounds ⓨ

K0869 Power wheelchair, group 4 standard, captain's chair, patient weight capacity up to and including 300 pounds ⓨ

K0870 Power wheelchair, group 4 heavy-duty, sling/solid seat/back, patient weight capacity 301 to 450 pounds ⓨ

K0871 Power wheelchair, group 4 very heavy-duty, sling/solid seat/back, patient weight capacity 451 to 600 pounds ⓨ

K0877 Power wheelchair, group 4 standard, single power option, sling/solid seat/back, patient weight capacity up to and including 300 pounds ⓨ

K0878 Power wheelchair, group 4 standard, single power option, captain's chair, patient weight capacity up to and including 300 pounds ⓨ

K0879 Power wheelchair, group 4 heavy-duty, single power option, sling/solid seat/back, patient weight capacity 301 to 450 pounds ⓨ

K0880 Power wheelchair, group 4 very heavy-duty, single power option, sling/solid seat/back, patient weight 451 to 600 pounds ⓨ

K0884 Power wheelchair, group 4 standard, multiple power option, sling/solid seat/back, patient weight capacity up to and including 300 pounds ⓨ

K0885 Power wheelchair, group 4 standard, multiple power option, captain's chair, patient weight capacity up to and including 300 pounds ⓨ

K0886 Power wheelchair, group 4 heavy-duty, multiple power option, sling/solid seat/back, patient weight capacity 301 to 450 pounds ⓨ

K0890 Power wheelchair, group 5 pediatric, single power option, sling/solid seat/back, patient weight capacity up to and including 125 pounds ⓨ

K0891 Power wheelchair, group 5 pediatric, multiple power option, sling/solid seat/back, patient weight capacity up to and including 125 pounds ⓨ

K0898 Power wheelchair, not otherwise classified ⓨ

K0899 Power mobility device, not coded by DME PDAC or does not meet criteria ⓨ
CMS: 100-04,12,30.6.15.4

Other DME

K0900 Customized durable medical equipment, other than wheelchair ⓨ

K1001 Electronic positional obstructive sleep apnea treatment, with sensor, includes all components and accessories, any type

---

K1002 Cranial electrotherapy stimulation (CES) system, includes all supplies and accessories, any type

K1003 Whirlpool tub, walk in, portable

K1004 Low frequency ultrasonic diathermy treatment device for home use, includes all components and accessories

K1005 Disposable collection and storage bag for breast milk, any size, any type, each

K1006 Suction pump, home model, portable or stationary, electric, any type, for use with external urine management system

K1007 Bilateral hip, knee, ankle, foot (HKAFO) device, powered, includes pelvic component, single or double upright(s), knee joints any type, with or without ankle joints any type, includes all components and accessories, motors, microprocessors, sensors

K1009 Speech volume modulation system, any type, including all components and accessories

K1010 ~~Indwelling intraurethral drainage device with valve, patient inserted, replacement only, each~~

K1011 ~~Activation device for intraurethral drainage device with valve, replacement only, each~~

K1012 ~~Charger and base station for intraurethral activation device, replacement only~~

▲ **K1013** Enema tube, with or without adapter, any type, replacement only, ea

● **K1014** Addition, endoskeletal knee-shin system, 4 bar linkage or multiaxial, fluid swing and stance phase control

● **K1015** Foot, adductus positioning device, adjustable

● **K1016** Transcutaneous electrical nerve stimulator for electrical stimulation of the trigeminal nerve

● **K1017** Monthly supplies for use of device coded at K1016

● **K1018** External upper limb tremor stimulator of the peripheral nerves of the wrist

● **K1019** Monthly supplies for use of device coded at K1018

● **K1020** Noninvasive vagus nerve stimulator

● **K1021** Exsufflation belt, includes all supplies and accessories

● **K1022** Addition to lower extremity prosthesis, endoskeletal, knee disarticulation, above knee, hip disarticulation, positional rotation unit, any type

● **K1023** Distal transcutaneous electrical nerve stimulator, stimulates peripheral nerves of the upper arm

● **K1024** Nonpneumatic compression controller with sequential calibrated gradient pressure

● **K1025** Nonpneumatic sequential compression garment, full arm

● **K1026** Mechanical allergen particle barrier/inhalation filter, cream, nasal, topical

● **K1027** Oral device/appliance used to reduce upper airway collapsibility, without fixed mechanical hinge, custom fabricated, includes fitting and adjustment

Special Coverage Instructions   Noncovered by Medicare   Carrier Discretion   ☑ Quantity Alert   ● New Code   ○ Recycled/Reinstated   ▲ Revised Code

112 — K Codes   A Age Edit   M Maternity Edit   ♀ Female Only   ♂ Male Only   A-Y OPPS Status Indicators   © 2021 Optum360, LLC

Orthotic Procedures and Devices L0112-L4631

L codes include orthotic and prosthetic procedures and devices, as well as scoliosis equipment, orthopedic shoes, and prosthetic implants.

Cervical

L0112 Cranial cervical orthosis, congenital torticollis type, with or without soft interface material, adjustable range of motion joint, custom fabricated   A &

L0113 Cranial cervical orthosis, torticollis type, with or without joint, with or without soft interface material, prefabricated, includes fitting and adjustment   A &

L0120 Cervical, flexible, nonadjustable, prefabricated, off-the-shelf (foam collar)   A &

L0130 Cervical, flexible, thermoplastic collar, molded to patient   A &

L0140 Cervical, semi-rigid, adjustable (plastic collar)   A &

L0150 Cervical, semi-rigid, adjustable molded chin cup (plastic collar with mandibular/occipital piece)   A &

L0160 Cervical, semi-rigid, wire frame occipital/mandibular support, prefabricated, off-the-shelf   A &

L0170 Cervical, collar, molded to patient model   A &

L0172 Cervical, collar, semi-rigid thermoplastic foam, two piece, prefabricated, off-the-shelf   A &

L0174 Cervical, collar, semi-rigid, thermoplastic foam, two piece with thoracic extension, prefabricated, off-the-shelf   A &

Multiple Post Collar

L0180 Cervical, multiple post collar, occipital/mandibular supports, adjustable   A &

L0190 Cervical, multiple post collar, occipital/mandibular supports, adjustable cervical bars (SOMI, Guilford, Taylor types)   A &

L0200 Cervical, multiple post collar, occipital/mandibular supports, adjustable cervical bars, and thoracic extension   A &

Thoracic

L0220 Thoracic, rib belt, custom fabricated   A &

L0450 Thoracic-lumbar-sacral orthosis (TLSO), flexible, provides trunk support, upper thoracic region, produces intracavitary pressure to reduce load on the intervertebral disks with rigid stays or panel(s), includes shoulder straps and closures, prefabricated, off-the-shelf   A &

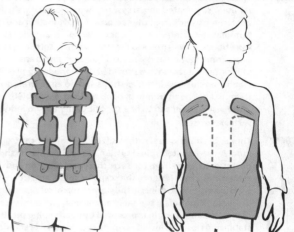

TLSO brace with adjustable straps and pads (L0450). The model at right and similar devices such as the Boston brace are molded polymer over foam and may be bivalve (front and back components)

Thoracic lumbar sacral othosis (TLSO)

L0452 Thoracic-lumbar-sacral orthosis (TLSO), flexible, provides trunk support, upper thoracic region, produces intracavitary pressure to reduce load on the intervertebral disks with rigid stays or panel(s), includes shoulder straps and closures, custom fabricated   A &

L0454 Thoracic-lumbar-sacral orthosis (TLSO), flexible, provides trunk support, extends from sacrococcygeal junction to above T-9 vertebra, restricts gross trunk motion in the sagittal plane, produces intracavitary pressure to reduce load on the intervertebral disks with rigid stays or panel(s), includes shoulder straps and closures, prefabricated item that has been trimmed, bent, molded, assembled, or otherwise customized to fit a specific patient by an individual with expertise   A &

L0455 Thoracic-lumbar-sacral orthosis (TLSO), flexible, provides trunk support, extends from sacrococcygeal junction to above T-9 vertebra, restricts gross trunk motion in the sagittal plane, produces intracavitary pressure to reduce load on the intervertebral disks with rigid stays or panel(s), includes shoulder straps and closures, prefabricated, off-the-shelf   A &

L0456 Thoracic-lumbar-sacral orthosis (TLSO), flexible, provides trunk support, thoracic region, rigid posterior panel and soft anterior apron, extends from the sacrococcygeal junction and terminates just inferior to the scapular spine, restricts gross trunk motion in the sagittal plane, produces intracavitary pressure to reduce load on the intervertebral disks, includes straps and closures, prefabricated item that has been trimmed, bent, molded, assembled, or otherwise customized to fit a specific patient by an individual with expertise   A &

L0457 Thoracic-lumbar-sacral orthosis (TLSO), flexible, provides trunk support, thoracic region, rigid posterior panel and soft anterior apron, extends from the sacrococcygeal junction and terminates just inferior to the scapular spine, restricts gross trunk motion in the sagittal plane, produces intracavitary pressure to reduce load on the intervertebral disks, includes straps and closures, prefabricated, off-the-shelf   A &

Special Coverage Instructions   Noncovered by Medicare   Carrier Discretion   ☑ Quantity Alert   ● New Code   ○ Recycled/Reinstated   ▲ Revised Code

© 2021 Optum360, LLC   A2-Z3 ASC Pmt   CMS: IOM   AHA: Coding Clinic   & DMEPOS Paid   ⊘ SNF Excluded   L Codes — 113

L0458 Thoracic-lumbar-sacral orthosis (TLSO), triplanar control, modular segmented spinal system, two rigid plastic shells, posterior extends from the sacrococcygeal junction and terminates just inferior to the scapular spine, anterior extends from the symphysis pubis to the xiphoid, soft liner, restricts gross trunk motion in the sagittal, coronal, and transverse planes, lateral strength is provided by overlapping plastic and stabilizing closures, includes straps and closures, prefabricated, includes fitting and adjustment   Ⓐ ♿

L0460 Thoracic-lumbar-sacral orthosis (TLSO), triplanar control, modular segmented spinal system, two rigid plastic shells, posterior extends from the sacrococcygeal junction and terminates just inferior to the scapular spine, anterior extends from the symphysis pubis to the sternal notch, soft liner, restricts gross trunk motion in the sagittal, coronal, and transverse planes, lateral strength is provided by overlapping plastic and stabilizing closures, includes straps and closures, prefabricated item that has been trimmed, bent, molded, assembled, or otherwise customized to fit a specific patient by an individual with expertise   Ⓐ ♿

L0462 Thoracic-lumbar-sacral orthosis (TLSO), triplanar control, modular segmented spinal system, three rigid plastic shells, posterior extends from the sacrococcygeal junction and terminates just inferior to the scapular spine, anterior extends from the symphysis pubis to the sternal notch, soft liner, restricts gross trunk motion in the sagittal, coronal, and transverse planes, lateral strength is provided by overlapping plastic and stabilizing closures, includes straps and closures, prefabricated, includes fitting and adjustment   Ⓐ ♿

L0464 Thoracic-lumbar-sacral orthosis (TLSO), triplanar control, modular segmented spinal system, four rigid plastic shells, posterior extends from sacrococcygeal junction and terminates just inferior to scapular spine, anterior extends from symphysis pubis to the sternal notch, soft liner, restricts gross trunk motion in sagittal, coronal, and transverse planes, lateral strength is provided by overlapping plastic and stabilizing closures, includes straps and closures, prefabricated, includes fitting and adjustment   Ⓐ ♿

L0466 Thoracic-lumbar-sacral orthosis (TLSO), sagittal control, rigid posterior frame and flexible soft anterior apron with straps, closures and padding, restricts gross trunk motion in sagittal plane, produces intracavitary pressure to reduce load on intervertebral disks, prefabricated item that has been trimmed, bent, molded, assembled, or otherwise customized to fit a specific patient by an individual with expertise   Ⓐ ♿

L0467 Thoracic-lumbar-sacral orthosis (TLSO), sagittal control, rigid posterior frame and flexible soft anterior apron with straps, closures and padding, restricts gross trunk motion in sagittal plane, produces intracavitary pressure to reduce load on intervertebral disks, prefabricated, off-the-shelf   Ⓐ ♿

L0468 Thoracic-lumbar-sacral orthosis (TLSO), sagittal-coronal control, rigid posterior frame and flexible soft anterior apron with straps, closures and padding, extends from sacrococcygeal junction over scapulae, lateral strength provided by pelvic, thoracic, and lateral frame pieces, restricts gross trunk motion in sagittal, and coronal planes, produces intracavitary pressure to reduce load on intervertebral disks, prefabricated item that has been trimmed, bent, molded, assembled, or otherwise customized to fit a specific patient by an individual with expertise   Ⓐ ♿

L0469 Thoracic-lumbar-sacral orthosis (TLSO), sagittal-coronal control, rigid posterior frame and flexible soft anterior apron with straps, closures and padding, extends from sacrococcygeal junction over scapulae, lateral strength provided by pelvic, thoracic, and lateral frame pieces, restricts gross trunk motion in sagittal and coronal planes, produces intracavitary pressure to reduce load on intervertebral disks, prefabricated, off-the-shelf   Ⓐ ♿

L0470 Thoracic-lumbar-sacral orthosis (TLSO), triplanar control, rigid posterior frame and flexible soft anterior apron with straps, closures and padding extends from sacrococcygeal junction to scapula, lateral strength provided by pelvic, thoracic, and lateral frame pieces, rotational strength provided by subclavicular extensions, restricts gross trunk motion in sagittal, coronal, and transverse planes, provides intracavitary pressure to reduce load on the intervertebral disks, includes fitting and shaping the frame, prefabricated, includes fitting and adjustment   Ⓐ ♿

L0472 Thoracic-lumbar-sacral orthosis (TLSO), triplanar control, hyperextension, rigid anterior and lateral frame extends from symphysis pubis to sternal notch with two anterior components (one pubic and one sternal), posterior and lateral pads with straps and closures, limits spinal flexion, restricts gross trunk motion in sagittal, coronal, and transverse planes, includes fitting and shaping the frame, prefabricated, includes fitting and adjustment   Ⓐ ♿

L0480 Thoracic-lumbar-sacral orthosis (TLSO), triplanar control, one-piece rigid plastic shell without interface liner, with multiple straps and closures, posterior extends from sacrococcygeal junction and terminates just inferior to scapular spine, anterior extends from symphysis pubis to sternal notch, anterior or posterior opening, restricts gross trunk motion in sagittal, coronal, and transverse planes, includes a carved plaster or CAD-CAM model, custom fabricated   Ⓐ ♿

L0482 Thoracic-lumbar-sacral orthosis (TLSO), triplanar control, one-piece rigid plastic shell with interface liner, multiple straps and closures, posterior extends from sacrococcygeal junction and terminates just inferior to scapular spine, anterior extends from symphysis pubis to sternal notch, anterior or posterior opening, restricts gross trunk motion in sagittal, coronal, and transverse planes, includes a carved plaster or CAD-CAM model, custom fabricated   Ⓐ ♿

L0484 Thoracic-lumbar-sacral orthosis (TLSO), triplanar control, two-piece rigid plastic shell without interface liner, with multiple straps and closures, posterior extends from sacrococcygeal junction and terminates just inferior to scapular spine, anterior extends from symphysis pubis to sternal notch, lateral strength is enhanced by overlapping plastic, restricts gross trunk motion in the sagittal, coronal, and transverse planes, includes a carved plaster or CAD-CAM model, custom fabricated   Ⓐ ♿

L0486 Thoracic-lumbar-sacral orthosis (TLSO), triplanar control, two-piece rigid plastic shell with interface liner, multiple straps and closures, posterior extends from sacrococcygeal junction and terminates just inferior to scapular spine, anterior extends from symphysis pubis to sternal notch, lateral strength is enhanced by overlapping plastic, restricts gross trunk motion in the sagittal, coronal, and transverse planes, includes a carved plaster or CAD-CAM model, custom fabricated   Ⓐ ♿

L0488 Thoracic-lumbar-sacral orthosis (TLSO), triplanar control, one-piece rigid plastic shell with interface liner, multiple straps and closures, posterior extends from sacrococcygeal junction and terminates just inferior to scapular spine, anterior extends from symphysis pubis to sternal notch, anterior or posterior opening, restricts gross trunk motion in sagittal, coronal, and transverse planes, prefabricated, includes fitting and adjustment   Ⓐ ♿

L0490 Thoracic-lumbar-sacral orthosis (TLSO), sagittal-coronal control, one-piece rigid plastic shell, with overlapping reinforced anterior, with multiple straps and closures, posterior extends from sacrococcygeal junction and terminates at or before the T-9 vertebra, anterior extends from symphysis pubis to xiphoid, anterior opening, restricts gross trunk motion in sagittal and coronal planes, prefabricated, includes fitting and adjustment   Ⓐ ♿

Special Coverage Instructions   Noncovered by Medicare   Carrier Discretion   ☑ Quantity Alert   ● New Code   ○ Recycled/Reinstated   ▲ Revised Code

114 — L Codes   Ⓐ Age Edit   Ⓜ Maternity Edit   ♀ Female Only   ♂ Male Only   Ⓐ-Ⓨ OPPS Status Indicators   © 2021 Optum360, LLC

L0491 Thoracic-lumbar-sacral orthosis (TLSO), sagittal-coronal control, modular segmented spinal system, two rigid plastic shells, posterior extends from the sacrococcygeal junction and terminates just inferior to the scapular spine, anterior extends from the symphysis pubis to the xiphoid, soft liner, restricts gross trunk motion in the sagittal and coronal planes, lateral strength is provided by overlapping plastic and stabilizing closures, includes straps and closures, prefabricated, includes fitting and adjustment Ⓐ ♿

L0492 Thoracic-lumbar-sacral orthosis (TLSO), sagittal-coronal control, modular segmented spinal system, three rigid plastic shells, posterior extends from the sacrococcygeal junction and terminates just inferior to the scapular spine, anterior extends from the symphysis pubis to the xiphoid, soft liner, restricts gross trunk motion in the sagittal and coronal planes, lateral strength is provided by overlapping plastic and stabilizing closures, includes straps and closures, prefabricated, includes fitting and adjustment Ⓐ ♿

Cervical-Thoracic-Lumbar-Sacral Orthoses

L0621 Sacroiliac orthosis, flexible, provides pelvic-sacral support, reduces motion about the sacroiliac joint, includes straps, closures, may include pendulous abdomen design, prefabricated, off-the-shelf Ⓐ ♿

L0622 Sacroiliac orthosis, flexible, provides pelvic-sacral support, reduces motion about the sacroiliac joint, includes straps, closures, may include pendulous abdomen design, custom fabricated Ⓐ ♿

L0623 Sacroiliac orthosis, provides pelvic-sacral support, with rigid or semi-rigid panels over the sacrum and abdomen, reduces motion about the sacroiliac joint, includes straps, closures, may include pendulous abdomen design, prefabricated, off-the-shelf Ⓐ ♿

L0624 Sacroiliac orthosis, provides pelvic-sacral support, with rigid or semi-rigid panels placed over the sacrum and abdomen, reduces motion about the sacroiliac joint, includes straps, closures, may include pendulous abdomen design, custom fabricated Ⓐ ♿

L0625 Lumbar orthosis, flexible, provides lumbar support, posterior extends from L-1 to below L-5 vertebra, produces intracavitary pressure to reduce load on the intervertebral discs, includes straps, closures, may include pendulous abdomen design, shoulder straps, stays, prefabricated, off-the-shelf Ⓐ ♿

L0626 Lumbar orthosis, sagittal control, with rigid posterior panel(s), posterior extends from L-1 to below L-5 vertebra, produces intracavitary pressure to reduce load on the intervertebral discs, includes straps, closures, may include padding, stays, shoulder straps, pendulous abdomen design, prefabricated item that has been trimmed, bent, molded, assembled, or otherwise customized to fit a specific patient by an individual with expertise Ⓐ ♿

L0627 Lumbar orthosis, sagittal control, with rigid anterior and posterior panels, posterior extends from L-1 to below L-5 vertebra, produces intracavitary pressure to reduce load on the intervertebral discs, includes straps, closures, may include padding, shoulder straps, pendulous abdomen design, prefabricated item that has been trimmed, bent, molded, assembled, or otherwise customized to fit a specific patient by an individual with expertise Ⓐ ♿

L0628 Lumbar-sacral orthosis (LSO), flexible, provides lumbo-sacral support, posterior extends from sacrococcygeal junction to T-9 vertebra, produces intracavitary pressure to reduce load on the intervertebral discs, includes straps, closures, may include stays, shoulder straps, pendulous abdomen design, prefabricated, off-the-shelf Ⓐ ♿

L0629 Lumbar-sacral orthosis (LSO), flexible, provides lumbo-sacral support, posterior extends from sacrococcygeal junction to T-9 vertebra, produces intracavitary pressure to reduce load on the intervertebral discs, includes straps, closures, may include stays, shoulder straps, pendulous abdomen design, custom fabricated Ⓐ ♿

L0630 Lumbar-sacral orthosis (LSO), sagittal control, with rigid posterior panel(s), posterior extends from sacrococcygeal junction to T-9 vertebra, produces intracavitary pressure to reduce load on the intervertebral discs, includes straps, closures, may include padding, stays, shoulder straps, pendulous abdomen design, prefabricated item that has been trimmed, bent, molded, assembled, or otherwise customized to fit a specific patient by an individual with expertise Ⓐ ♿

L0631 Lumbar-sacral orthosis (LSO), sagittal control, with rigid anterior and posterior panels, posterior extends from sacrococcygeal junction to T-9 vertebra, produces intracavitary pressure to reduce load on the intervertebral discs, includes straps, closures, may include padding, shoulder straps, pendulous abdomen design, prefabricated item that has been trimmed, bent, molded, assembled, or otherwise customized to fit a specific patient by an individual with expertise Ⓐ ♿

L0632 Lumbar-sacral orthosis (LSO), sagittal control, with rigid anterior and posterior panels, posterior extends from sacrococcygeal junction to T-9 vertebra, produces intracavitary pressure to reduce load on the intervertebral discs, includes straps, closures, may include padding, shoulder straps, pendulous abdomen design, custom fabricated Ⓐ ♿

L0633 Lumbar-sacral orthosis (LSO), sagittal-coronal control, with rigid posterior frame/panel(s), posterior extends from sacrococcygeal junction to T-9 vertebra, lateral strength provided by rigid lateral frame/panels, produces intracavitary pressure to reduce load on intervertebral discs, includes straps, closures, may include padding, stays, shoulder straps, pendulous abdomen design, prefabricated item that has been trimmed, bent, molded, assembled, or otherwise customized to fit a specific patient by an individual with expertise Ⓐ ♿

L0634 Lumbar-sacral orthosis (LSO), sagittal-coronal control, with rigid posterior frame/panel(s), posterior extends from sacrococcygeal junction to T-9 vertebra, lateral strength provided by rigid lateral frame/panel(s), produces intracavitary pressure to reduce load on intervertebral discs, includes straps, closures, may include padding, stays, shoulder straps, pendulous abdomen design, custom fabricated Ⓐ ♿

L0635 Lumbar-sacral orthosis (LSO), sagittal-coronal control, lumbar flexion, rigid posterior frame/panel(s), lateral articulating design to flex the lumbar spine, posterior extends from sacrococcygeal junction to T-9 vertebra, lateral strength provided by rigid lateral frame/panel(s), produces intracavitary pressure to reduce load on intervertebral discs, includes straps, closures, may include padding, anterior panel, pendulous abdomen design, prefabricated, includes fitting and adjustment Ⓐ ♿

L0636 Lumbar-sacral orthosis (LSO), sagittal-coronal control, lumbar flexion, rigid posterior frame/panels, lateral articulating design to flex the lumbar spine, posterior extends from sacrococcygeal junction to T-9 vertebra, lateral strength provided by rigid lateral frame/panels, produces intracavitary pressure to reduce load on intervertebral discs, includes straps, closures, may include padding, anterior panel, pendulous abdomen design, custom fabricated Ⓐ ♿

Special Coverage Instructions   Noncovered by Medicare   Carrier Discretion   ☑ Quantity Alert   ● New Code   ○ Recycled/Reinstated   ▲ Revised Code

© 2021 Optum360, LLC   A2-Z3 ASC Pmt   **CMS:** IOM   **AHA:** Coding Clinic   ♿ DMEPOS Paid   ⊘ SNF Excluded   **L Codes — 115**

L0637 Lumbar-sacral orthosis (LSO), sagittal-coronal control, with rigid anterior and posterior frame/panels, posterior extends from sacrococcygeal junction to T-9 vertebra, lateral strength provided by rigid lateral frame/panels, produces intracavitary pressure to reduce load on intervertebral discs, includes straps, closures, may include padding, shoulder straps, pendulous abdomen design, prefabricated item that has been trimmed, bent, molded, assembled, or otherwise customized to fit a specific patient by an individual with expertise A &

L0638 Lumbar-sacral orthosis (LSO), sagittal-coronal control, with rigid anterior and posterior frame/panels, posterior extends from sacrococcygeal junction to T-9 vertebra, lateral strength provided by rigid lateral frame/panels, produces intracavitary pressure to reduce load on intervertebral discs, includes straps, closures, may include padding, shoulder straps, pendulous abdomen design, custom fabricated A &

L0639 Lumbar-sacral orthosis (LSO), sagittal-coronal control, rigid shell(s)/panel(s), posterior extends from sacrococcygeal junction to T-9 vertebra, anterior extends from symphysis pubis to xyphoid, produces intracavitary pressure to reduce load on intervertebral discs, overall strength is provided by overlapping rigid material and stabilizing closures, includes straps, closures, may include soft interface, pendulous abdomen design, prefabricated item that has been trimmed, bent, molded, assembled, or otherwise customized to fit a specific patient by an individual with expertise A &

L0640 Lumbar-sacral orthosis (LSO), sagittal-coronal control, rigid shell(s)/panel(s), posterior extends from sacrococcygeal junction to T-9 vertebra, anterior extends from symphysis pubis to xyphoid, produces intracavitary pressure to reduce load on the intervertebral discs, overall strength is provided by overlapping rigid material and stabilizing closures, includes straps, closures, may include soft interface, pendulous abdomen design, custom fabricated A &

L0641 Lumbar orthosis, sagittal control, with rigid posterior panel(s), posterior extends from L-1 to below L-5 vertebra, produces intracavitary pressure to reduce load on the intervertebral discs, includes straps, closures, may include padding, stays, shoulder straps, pendulous abdomen design, prefabricated, off-the-shelf A &

L0642 Lumbar orthosis, sagittal control, with rigid anterior and posterior panels, posterior extends from L-1 to below L-5 vertebra, produces intracavitary pressure to reduce load on the intervertebral discs, includes straps, closures, may include padding, shoulder straps, pendulous abdomen design, prefabricated, off-the-shelf A &

L0643 Lumbar-sacral orthosis (LSO), sagittal control, with rigid posterior panel(s), posterior extends from sacrococcygeal junction to T-9 vertebra, produces intracavitary pressure to reduce load on the intervertebral discs, includes straps, closures, may include padding, stays, shoulder straps, pendulous abdomen design, prefabricated, off-the-shelf A &

L0648 Lumbar-sacral orthosis (LSO), sagittal control, with rigid anterior and posterior panels, posterior extends from sacrococcygeal junction to T-9 vertebra, produces intracavitary pressure to reduce load on the intervertebral discs, includes straps, closures, may include padding, shoulder straps, pendulous abdomen design, prefabricated, off-the-shelf A &

L0649 Lumbar-sacral orthosis (LSO), sagittal-coronal control, with rigid posterior frame/panel(s), posterior extends from sacrococcygeal junction to T-9 vertebra, lateral strength provided by rigid lateral frame/panels, produces intracavitary pressure to reduce load on intervertebral discs, includes straps, closures, may include padding, stays, shoulder straps, pendulous abdomen design, prefabricated, off-the-shelf A &

L0650 Lumbar-sacral orthosis (LSO), sagittal-coronal control, with rigid anterior and posterior frame/panel(s), posterior extends from sacrococcygeal junction to T-9 vertebra, lateral strength provided by rigid lateral frame/panel(s), produces intracavitary pressure to reduce load on intervertebral discs, includes straps, closures, may include padding, shoulder straps, pendulous abdomen design, prefabricated, off-the-shelf A &

L0651 Lumbar-sacral orthosis (LSO), sagittal-coronal control, rigid shell(s)/panel(s), posterior extends from sacrococcygeal junction to T-9 vertebra, anterior extends from symphysis pubis to xyphoid, produces intracavitary pressure to reduce load on the intervertebral discs, overall strength is provided by overlapping rigid material and stabilizing closures, includes straps, closures, may include soft interface, pendulous abdomen design, prefabricated, off-the-shelf A &

L0700 Cervical-thoracic-lumbar-sacral orthosis (CTLSO), anterior-posterior-lateral control, molded to patient model, (Minerva type) A &

L0710 Cervical-thoracic-lumbar-sacral orthosis (CTLSO), anterior-posterior-lateral control, molded to patient model, with interface material, (Minerva type) A &

Halo Procedure

L0810 Halo procedure, cervical halo incorporated into jacket vest A &

L0820 Halo procedure, cervical halo incorporated into plaster body jacket A &

L0830 Halo procedure, cervical halo incorporated into Milwaukee type orthotic A &

L0859 Addition to halo procedure, magnetic resonance image compatible systems, rings and pins, any material A &

L0861 Addition to halo procedure, replacement liner/interface material A &

Additions to Spinal Orthoses

L0970 Thoracic-lumbar-sacral orthosis (TLSO), corset front A &
L0972 Lumbar-sacral orthosis (LSO), corset front A &
L0974 Thoracic-lumbar-sacral orthosis (TLSO), full corset A &
L0976 Lumbar-sacral orthosis (LSO), full corset A &
L0978 Axillary crutch extension A &
L0980 Peroneal straps, prefabricated, off-the-shelf, pair A ☑ &
L0982 Stocking supporter grips, prefabricated, off-the-shelf, set of four (4) A ☑ &
L0984 Protective body sock, prefabricated, off-the-shelf, each A ☑ &
L0999 Addition to spinal orthosis, not otherwise specified A

Determine if an alternative HCPCS Level II or a CPT code better describes the service being reported. This code should be used only if a more specific code is unavailable.

Orthotic Devices - Scoliosis Procedures

The orthotic care of scoliosis differs from other orthotic care in that the treatment is more dynamic in nature and uses continual modification of the orthosis to the patient's changing condition. This coding structure uses the proper names - or eponyms - of the procedures because they have historic and universal acceptance in the profession. It should be recognized that variations to the basic procedures described by the founders/developers are accepted in various medical and orthotic practices throughout the country. All procedures include model of patient when indicated.

Special Coverage Instructions **Noncovered by Medicare** **Carrier Discretion** ☑ Quantity Alert ● New Code ○ Recycled/Reinstated ▲ Revised Code

116 — L Codes A Age Edit M Maternity Edit ♀ Female Only ♂ Male Only A-Y OPPS Status Indicators © 2021 Optum360, LLC

L1000 Cervical-thoracic-lumbar-sacral orthosis (CTLSO) (Milwaukee), inclusive of furnishing initial orthotic, including model Ⓐ &

A variety of configurations are available for the Milwaukee brace (L1000)

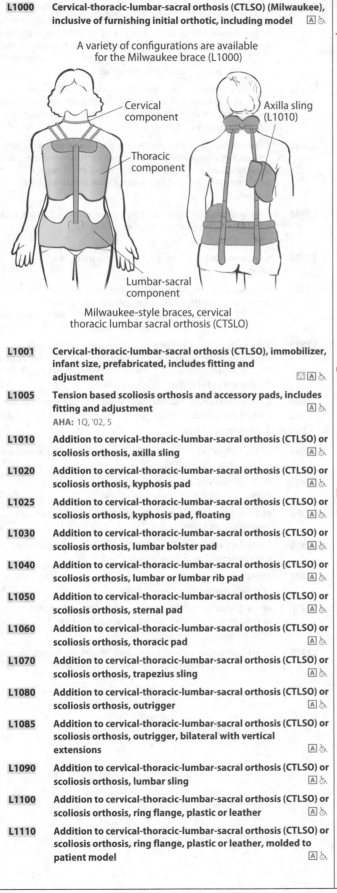

Milwaukee-style braces, cervical thoracic lumbar sacral orthosis (CTSLO)

L1001 Cervical-thoracic-lumbar-sacral orthosis (CTLSO), immobilizer, infant size, prefabricated, includes fitting and adjustment Ⓐ Ⓐ &

L1005 Tension based scoliosis orthosis and accessory pads, includes fitting and adjustment Ⓐ &
AHA: 1Q, '02, 5

L1010 Addition to cervical-thoracic-lumbar-sacral orthosis (CTLSO) or scoliosis orthosis, axilla sling Ⓐ &

L1020 Addition to cervical-thoracic-lumbar-sacral orthosis (CTLSO) or scoliosis orthosis, kyphosis pad Ⓐ &

L1025 Addition to cervical-thoracic-lumbar-sacral orthosis (CTLSO) or scoliosis orthosis, kyphosis pad, floating Ⓐ &

L1030 Addition to cervical-thoracic-lumbar-sacral orthosis (CTLSO) or scoliosis orthosis, lumbar bolster pad Ⓐ &

L1040 Addition to cervical-thoracic-lumbar-sacral orthosis (CTLSO) or scoliosis orthosis, lumbar or lumbar rib pad Ⓐ &

L1050 Addition to cervical-thoracic-lumbar-sacral orthosis (CTLSO) or scoliosis orthosis, sternal pad Ⓐ &

L1060 Addition to cervical-thoracic-lumbar-sacral orthosis (CTLSO) or scoliosis orthosis, thoracic pad Ⓐ &

L1070 Addition to cervical-thoracic-lumbar-sacral orthosis (CTLSO) or scoliosis orthosis, trapezius sling Ⓐ &

L1080 Addition to cervical-thoracic-lumbar-sacral orthosis (CTLSO) or scoliosis orthosis, outrigger Ⓐ &

L1085 Addition to cervical-thoracic-lumbar-sacral orthosis (CTLSO) or scoliosis orthosis, outrigger, bilateral with vertical extensions Ⓐ &

L1090 Addition to cervical-thoracic-lumbar-sacral orthosis (CTLSO) or scoliosis orthosis, lumbar sling Ⓐ &

L1100 Addition to cervical-thoracic-lumbar-sacral orthosis (CTLSO) or scoliosis orthosis, ring flange, plastic or leather Ⓐ &

L1110 Addition to cervical-thoracic-lumbar-sacral orthosis (CTLSO) or scoliosis orthosis, ring flange, plastic or leather, molded to patient model Ⓐ &

L1120 Addition to cervical-thoracic-lumbar-sacral orthosis (CTLSO), scoliosis orthosis, cover for upright, each Ⓐ ☑ &

Thoracic-Lumbar-Sacral Orthosis (TLSO) (Low Profile)

L1200 Thoracic-lumbar-sacral orthosis (TLSO), inclusive of furnishing initial orthosis only Ⓐ &

L1210 Addition to thoracic-lumbar-sacral orthosis (TLSO), (low profile), lateral thoracic extension Ⓐ &

L1220 Addition to thoracic-lumbar-sacral orthosis (TLSO), (low profile), anterior thoracic extension Ⓐ &

L1230 Addition to thoracic-lumbar-sacral orthosis (TLSO), (low profile), Milwaukee type superstructure Ⓐ &

L1240 Addition to thoracic-lumbar-sacral orthosis (TLSO), (low profile), lumbar derotation pad Ⓐ &

L1250 Addition to thoracic-lumbar-sacral orthosis (TLSO), (low profile), anterior ASIS pad Ⓐ &

L1260 Addition to thoracic-lumbar-sacral orthosis (TLSO), (low profile), anterior thoracic derotation pad Ⓐ &

L1270 Addition to thoracic-lumbar-sacral orthosis (TLSO), (low profile), abdominal pad Ⓐ &

L1280 Addition to thoracic-lumbar-sacral orthosis (TLSO), (low profile), rib gusset (elastic), each Ⓐ ☑ &

L1290 Addition to thoracic-lumbar-sacral orthosis (TLSO), (low profile), lateral trochanteric pad Ⓐ &

Other Scoliosis Procedures

L1300 Other scoliosis procedure, body jacket molded to patient model Ⓐ &

L1310 Other scoliosis procedure, postoperative body jacket Ⓐ &

L1499 Spinal orthosis, not otherwise specified Ⓐ
Determine if an alternative HCPCS Level II or a CPT code better describes the service being reported. This code should be used only if a more specific code is unavailable.

Hip Orthoses (HO) - Flexible

L1600 Hip orthosis (HO), abduction control of hip joints, flexible, Frejka type with cover, prefabricated item that has been trimmed, bent, molded, assembled, or otherwise customized to fit a specific patient by an individual with expertise Ⓐ &

L1610 Hip orthosis (HO), abduction control of hip joints, flexible, (Frejka cover only), prefabricated item that has been trimmed, bent, molded, assembled, or otherwise customized to fit a specific patient by an individual with expertise Ⓐ &

L1620 Hip orthosis (HO), abduction control of hip joints, flexible, (Pavlik harness), prefabricated item that has been trimmed, bent, molded, assembled, or otherwise customized to fit a specific patient by an individual with expertise Ⓐ &

L1630 Hip orthosis (HO), abduction control of hip joints, semi-flexible (Von Rosen type), custom fabricated Ⓐ &

L1640 Hip orthosis (HO), abduction control of hip joints, static, pelvic band or spreader bar, thigh cuffs, custom fabricated Ⓐ &

L1650 Hip orthosis (HO), abduction control of hip joints, static, adjustable, (Ilfled type), prefabricated, includes fitting and adjustment Ⓐ &

L1652 Hip orthosis (HO), bilateral thigh cuffs with adjustable abductor spreader bar, adult size, prefabricated, includes fitting and adjustment, any type Ⓐ &

L1660 Hip orthosis (HO), abduction control of hip joints, static, plastic, prefabricated, includes fitting and adjustment Ⓐ &

Special Coverage Instructions   Noncovered by Medicare   Carrier Discretion   ☑ Quantity Alert ● New Code   ○ Recycled/Reinstated ▲ Revised Code

© 2021 Optum360, LLC   A2–Z3 ASC Pmt   **CMS:** IOM   **AHA:** Coding Clinic   & DMEPOS Paid   ⊘ SNF Excluded   **L Codes — 117**

Orthotic Devices and Procedures

L1680 — L1920

L1680 Hip orthosis (HO), abduction control of hip joints, dynamic, pelvic control, adjustable hip motion control, thigh cuffs (Rancho hip action type), custom fabricated Ⓐ &

L1685 Hip orthosis (HO), abduction control of hip joint, postoperative hip abduction type, custom fabricated Ⓐ &

L1686 Hip orthosis (HO), abduction control of hip joint, postoperative hip abduction type, prefabricated, includes fitting and adjustment Ⓐ &

L1690 Combination, bilateral, lumbo-sacral, hip, femur orthosis providing adduction and internal rotation control, prefabricated, includes fitting and adjustment Ⓐ &

Legg Perthes

L1700 Legg Perthes orthosis, (Toronto type), custom fabricated Ⓐ &

L1710 Legg Perthes orthosis, (Newington type), custom fabricated Ⓐ &

L1720 Legg Perthes orthosis, trilateral, (Tachdijan type), custom fabricated Ⓐ &

L1730 Legg Perthes orthosis, (Scottish Rite type), custom fabricated Ⓐ &

L1755 Legg Perthes orthosis, (Patten bottom type), custom fabricated Ⓐ &

Knee Orthosis

L1810 Knee orthosis (KO), elastic with joints, prefabricated item that has been trimmed, bent, molded, assembled, or otherwise customized to fit a specific patient by an individual with expertise Ⓐ &

L1812 Knee orthosis (KO), elastic with joints, prefabricated, off-the-shelf Ⓐ &

L1820 Knee orthosis (KO), elastic with condylar pads and joints, with or without patellar control, prefabricated, includes fitting and adjustment Ⓐ &

L1830 Knee orthosis (KO), immobilizer, canvas longitudinal, prefabricated, off-the-shelf Ⓐ &

L1831 Knee orthosis (KO), locking knee joint(s), positional orthosis, prefabricated, includes fitting and adjustment Ⓐ &

L1832 Knee orthosis (KO), adjustable knee joints (unicentric or polycentric), positional orthosis, rigid support, prefabricated item that has been trimmed, bent, molded, assembled, or otherwise customized to fit a specific patient by an individual with expertise Ⓐ &

L1833 Knee orthosis (KO), adjustable knee joints (unicentric or polycentric), positional orthosis, rigid support, prefabricated, off-the shelf Ⓐ &

L1834 Knee orthosis (KO), without knee joint, rigid, custom fabricated Ⓐ &

L1836 Knee orthosis (KO), rigid, without joint(s), includes soft interface material, prefabricated, off-the-shelf Ⓐ &

L1840 Knee orthosis (KO), derotation, medial-lateral, anterior cruciate ligament, custom fabricated Ⓐ &

L1843 Knee orthosis (KO), single upright, thigh and calf, with adjustable flexion and extension joint (unicentric or polycentric), medial-lateral and rotation control, with or without varus/valgus adjustment, prefabricated item that has been trimmed, bent, molded, assembled, or otherwise customized to fit a specific patient by an individual with expertise Ⓐ &

L1844 Knee orthosis (KO), single upright, thigh and calf, with adjustable flexion and extension joint (unicentric or polycentric), medial-lateral and rotation control, with or without varus/valgus adjustment, custom fabricated Ⓐ &

L1845 Knee orthosis (KO), double upright, thigh and calf, with adjustable flexion and extension joint (unicentric or polycentric), medial-lateral and rotation control, with or without varus/valgus adjustment, prefabricated item that has been trimmed, bent, molded, assembled, or otherwise customized to fit a specific patient by an individual with expertise Ⓐ &

L1846 Knee orthosis (KO), double upright, thigh and calf, with adjustable flexion and extension joint (unicentric or polycentric), medial-lateral and rotation control, with or without varus/valgus adjustment, custom fabricated Ⓐ &

L1847 Knee orthosis (KO), double upright with adjustable joint, with inflatable air support chamber(s), prefabricated item that has been trimmed, bent, molded, assembled, or otherwise customized to fit a specific patient by an individual with expertise Ⓐ &

L1848 Knee orthosis (KO), double upright with adjustable joint, with inflatable air support chamber(s), prefabricated, off-the-shelf Ⓐ &

L1850 Knee orthosis (KO), Swedish type, prefabricated, off-the-shelf Ⓐ &

L1851 Knee orthosis (KO), single upright, thigh and calf, with adjustable flexion and extension joint (unicentric or polycentric), medial-lateral and rotation control, with or without varus/valgus adjustment, prefabricated, off-the-shelf Ⓐ &

L1852 Knee orthosis (KO), double upright, thigh and calf, with adjustable flexion and extension joint (unicentric or polycentric), medial-lateral and rotation control, with or without varus/valgus adjustment, prefabricated, off-the-shelf Ⓐ &

L1860 Knee orthosis (KO), modification of supracondylar prosthetic socket, custom fabricated (SK) Ⓐ &

Ankle-Foot Orthosis (AFO)

L1900 Ankle-foot orthosis (AFO), spring wire, dorsiflexion assist calf band, custom fabricated Ⓐ &

L1902 Ankle orthosis (AO), ankle gauntlet or similar, with or without joints, prefabricated, off-the-shelf Ⓐ &

L1904 Ankle orthosis (AO), ankle gauntlet or similar, with or without joints, custom fabricated Ⓐ &

L1906 Ankle foot orthosis (AFO), multiligamentous ankle support, prefabricated, off-the-shelf Ⓐ &

L1907 Ankle orthosis (AO), supramalleolar with straps, with or without interface/pads, custom fabricated Ⓐ &

L1910 Ankle-foot orthosis (AFO), posterior, single bar, clasp attachment to shoe counter, prefabricated, includes fitting and adjustment Ⓐ &

L1920 Ankle-foot orthosis (AFO), single upright with static or adjustable stop (Phelps or Perlstein type), custom fabricated Ⓐ &

Special Coverage Instructions   Noncovered by Medicare   Carrier Discretion   ☑ Quantity Alert ● New Code   ○ Recycled/Reinstated   ▲ Revised Code

118 — L Codes   Ⓐ Age Edit   Ⓜ Maternity Edit   ♀ Female Only   ♂ Male Only   Ⓐ-Ⓨ OPPS Status Indicators   © 2021 Optum360, LLC

L1930 Ankle-foot orthosis (AFO), plastic or other material, prefabricated, includes fitting and adjustment Ⓐ ♿

Ankle foot orthotic (AFO), plastic or other material (L1930)

Flexible carbon component

Foot component may fit inside shoe

L1932 Ankle-foot orthosis (AFO), rigid anterior tibial section, total carbon fiber or equal material, prefabricated, includes fitting and adjustment Ⓐ ♿

L1940 Ankle-foot orthosis (AFO), plastic or other material, custom fabricated Ⓐ ♿

L1945 Ankle-foot orthosis (AFO), plastic, rigid anterior tibial section (floor reaction), custom fabricated Ⓐ ♿

Rigid tibial anterior floor reaction; ankle-foot orthosis (AFO) (L1945)

Spiral; ankle foot orthosis (AFO) (L1950)

L1950 Ankle-foot orthosis (AFO), spiral, (Institute of Rehabilitative Medicine type), plastic, custom fabricated Ⓐ ♿

L1951 Ankle-foot orthosis (AFO), spiral, (Institute of rehabilitative Medicine type), plastic or other material, prefabricated, includes fitting and adjustment Ⓐ ♿

L1960 Ankle-foot orthosis (AFO), posterior solid ankle, plastic, custom fabricated Ⓐ ♿

L1970 Ankle-foot orthosis (AFO), plastic with ankle joint, custom fabricated Ⓐ ♿

L1971 Ankle-foot orthosis (AFO), plastic or other material with ankle joint, prefabricated, includes fitting and adjustment Ⓐ ♿

L1980 Ankle-foot orthosis (AFO), single upright free plantar dorsiflexion, solid stirrup, calf band/cuff (single bar 'BK' orthosis), custom fabricated Ⓐ ♿

L1990 Ankle-foot orthosis (AFO), double upright free plantar dorsiflexion, solid stirrup, calf band/cuff (double bar 'BK' orthosis), custom fabricated Ⓐ ♿

Knee-Ankle-Foot Orthosis (KAFO) - Or Any Combination

L2000 Knee-ankle-foot orthosis (KAFO), single upright, free knee, free ankle, solid stirrup, thigh and calf bands/cuffs (single bar 'AK' orthosis), custom fabricated Ⓐ ♿

L2005 Knee-ankle-foot orthosis (KAFO), any material, single or double upright, stance control, automatic lock and swing phase release, any type activation, includes ankle joint, any type, custom fabricated Ⓐ ♿

L2006 Knee ankle foot device, any material, single or double upright, swing and stance phase microprocessor control with adjustability, includes all components (e.g., sensors, batteries, charger), any type activation, with or without ankle joint(s), custom fabricated Ⓐ ♿

L2010 Knee-ankle-foot orthosis (KAFO), single upright, free ankle, solid stirrup, thigh and calf bands/cuffs (single bar 'AK' orthosis), without knee joint, custom fabricated Ⓐ ♿

L2020 Knee-ankle-foot orthosis (KAFO), double upright, free ankle, solid stirrup, thigh and calf bands/cuffs (double bar 'AK' orthosis), custom fabricated Ⓐ ♿

L2030 Knee-ankle-foot orthosis (KAFO), double upright, free ankle, solid stirrup, thigh and calf bands/cuffs, (double bar 'AK' orthosis), without knee joint, custom fabricated Ⓐ ♿

L2034 Knee-ankle-foot orthosis (KAFO), full plastic, single upright, with or without free motion knee, medial-lateral rotation control, with or without free motion ankle, custom fabricated Ⓐ ♿

L2035 Knee-ankle-foot orthosis (KAFO), full plastic, static (pediatric size), without free motion ankle, prefabricated, includes fitting and adjustment Ⓐ ♿

L2036 Knee-ankle-foot orthosis (KAFO), full plastic, double upright, with or without free motion knee, with or without free motion ankle, custom fabricated Ⓐ ♿

L2037 Knee-ankle-foot orthosis (KAFO), full plastic, single upright, with or without free motion knee, with or without free motion ankle, custom fabricated Ⓐ ♿

L2038 Knee-ankle-foot orthosis (KAFO), full plastic, with or without free motion knee, multi-axis ankle, custom fabricated Ⓐ ♿

Torsion Control: Hip-Knee-Ankle-Foot Orthosis (HKAFO)

L2040 Hip-knee-ankle-foot orthosis (HKAFO), torsion control, bilateral rotation straps, pelvic band/belt, custom fabricated Ⓐ ♿

L2050 Hip-knee-ankle-foot orthosis (HKAFO), torsion control, bilateral torsion cables, hip joint, pelvic band/belt, custom fabricated Ⓐ ♿

L2060 Hip-knee-ankle-foot orthosis (HKAFO), torsion control, bilateral torsion cables, ball bearing hip joint, pelvic band/ belt, custom fabricated Ⓐ ♿

L2070 Hip-knee-ankle-foot orthosis (HKAFO), torsion control, unilateral rotation straps, pelvic band/belt, custom fabricated Ⓐ ♿

L2080 Hip-knee-ankle-foot orthosis (HKAFO), torsion control, unilateral torsion cable, hip joint, pelvic band/belt, custom fabricated Ⓐ ♿

L2090 Hip-knee-ankle-foot orthosis (HKAFO), torsion control, unilateral torsion cable, ball bearing hip joint, pelvic band/ belt, custom fabricated Ⓐ ♿

L2106 Ankle-foot orthosis (AFO), fracture orthosis, tibial fracture cast orthosis, thermoplastic type casting material, custom fabricated Ⓐ ♿

L2108 Ankle-foot orthosis (AFO), fracture orthosis, tibial fracture cast orthosis, custom fabricated Ⓐ ♿

Special Coverage Instructions   Noncovered by Medicare   Carrier Discretion   ☑ Quantity Alert ● New Code   ○ Recycled/Reinstated   ▲ Revised Code

© 2021 Optum360, LLC   Ⓐ²-Ⓩ³ ASC Pmt   CMS: IOM   AHA: Coding Clinic   ♿ DMEPOS Paid   ⊘ SNF Excluded   L Codes — 119

Orthotic Devices and Procedures

L2112 — L2526

L2112 Ankle-foot orthosis (AFO), fracture orthosis, tibial fracture orthosis, soft, prefabricated, includes fitting and adjustment Ⓐ&

L2114 Ankle-foot orthosis (AFO), fracture orthosis, tibial fracture orthosis, semi-rigid, prefabricated, includes fitting and adjustment Ⓐ&

L2116 Ankle-foot orthosis (AFO), fracture orthosis, tibial fracture orthosis, rigid, prefabricated, includes fitting and adjustment Ⓐ&

L2126 Knee-ankle-foot orthosis (KAFO), fracture orthosis, femoral fracture cast orthosis, thermoplastic type casting material, custom fabricated Ⓐ&

L2128 Knee-ankle-foot orthosis (KAFO), fracture orthosis, femoral fracture cast orthosis, custom fabricated Ⓐ&

L2132 Knee-ankle-foot orthosis (KAFO), fracture orthosis, femoral fracture cast orthosis, soft, prefabricated, includes fitting and adjustment Ⓐ&

L2134 Knee-ankle-foot orthosis (KAFO), fracture orthosis, femoral fracture cast orthosis, semi-rigid, prefabricated, includes fitting and adjustment Ⓐ&

L2136 Knee-ankle-foot orthosis (KAFO), fracture orthosis, femoral fracture cast orthosis, rigid, prefabricated, includes fitting and adjustment Ⓐ&

Additions to Fracture Orthosis

L2180 Addition to lower extremity fracture orthosis, plastic shoe insert with ankle joints Ⓐ&

L2182 Addition to lower extremity fracture orthosis, drop lock knee joint Ⓐ&

L2184 Addition to lower extremity fracture orthosis, limited motion knee joint Ⓐ&

L2186 Addition to lower extremity fracture orthosis, adjustable motion knee joint, Lerman type Ⓐ&

L2188 Addition to lower extremity fracture orthosis, quadrilateral brim Ⓐ&

L2190 Addition to lower extremity fracture orthosis, waist belt Ⓐ&

L2192 Addition to lower extremity fracture orthosis, hip joint, pelvic band, thigh flange, and pelvic belt Ⓐ&

Additions to Lower Extremity Orthosis: Shoe-Ankle-Shin-Knee

L2200 Addition to lower extremity, limited ankle motion, each joint Ⓐ☑&

L2210 Addition to lower extremity, dorsiflexion assist (plantar flexion resist), each joint Ⓐ☑&

L2220 Addition to lower extremity, dorsiflexion and plantar flexion assist/resist, each joint Ⓐ☑&

L2230 Addition to lower extremity, split flat caliper stirrups and plate attachment Ⓐ&

L2232 Addition to lower extremity orthosisis, rocker bottom for total contact ankle-foot orthos (AFO), for custom fabricated orthosis only Ⓐ&

L2240 Addition to lower extremity, round caliper and plate attachment Ⓐ&

L2250 Addition to lower extremity, foot plate, molded to patient model, stirrup attachment Ⓐ&

L2260 Addition to lower extremity, reinforced solid stirrup (Scott-Craig type) Ⓐ&

L2265 Addition to lower extremity, long tongue stirrup Ⓐ&

L2270 Addition to lower extremity, varus/valgus correction (T) strap, padded/lined or malleolus pad Ⓐ&

L2275 Addition to lower extremity, varus/valgus correction, plastic modification, padded/lined Ⓐ&

L2280 Addition to lower extremity, molded inner boot Ⓐ&

L2300 Addition to lower extremity, abduction bar (bilateral hip involvement), jointed, adjustable Ⓐ&

L2310 Addition to lower extremity, abduction bar, straight Ⓐ&

L2320 Addition to lower extremity, nonmolded lacer, for custom fabricated orthosis only Ⓐ&

L2330 Addition to lower extremity, lacer molded to patient model, for custom fabricated orthosis only Ⓐ&

L2335 Addition to lower extremity, anterior swing band Ⓐ&

L2340 Addition to lower extremity, pretibial shell, molded to patient model Ⓐ&

L2350 Addition to lower extremity, prosthetic type, (BK) socket, molded to patient model, (used for PTB, AFO orthoses) Ⓐ&

L2360 Addition to lower extremity, extended steel shank Ⓐ&

L2370 Addition to lower extremity, Patten bottom Ⓐ&

L2375 Addition to lower extremity, torsion control, ankle joint and half solid stirrup Ⓐ&

L2380 Addition to lower extremity, torsion control, straight knee joint, each joint Ⓐ☑&

L2385 Addition to lower extremity, straight knee joint, heavy-duty, each joint Ⓐ☑&

L2387 Addition to lower extremity, polycentric knee joint, for custom fabricated knee-ankle-foot orthosis (KAFO), each joint Ⓐ☑&

L2390 Addition to lower extremity, offset knee joint, each joint Ⓐ☑&

L2395 Addition to lower extremity, offset knee joint, heavy-duty, each joint Ⓐ☑&

L2397 Addition to lower extremity orthosis, suspension sleeve Ⓐ&

Additions to Straight Knee or Offset Knee Joints

L2405 Addition to knee joint, drop lock, each Ⓐ☑&

L2415 Addition to knee lock with integrated release mechanism (bail, cable, or equal), any material, each joint Ⓐ☑&

L2425 Addition to knee joint, disc or dial lock for adjustable knee flexion, each joint Ⓐ☑&

L2430 Addition to knee joint, ratchet lock for active and progressive knee extension, each joint Ⓐ☑&

L2492 Addition to knee joint, lift loop for drop lock ring Ⓐ&

Additions: Thigh/Weight Bearing - Gluteal/Ischial Weight Bearing

L2500 Addition to lower extremity, thigh/weight bearing, gluteal/ischial weight bearing, ring Ⓐ&

L2510 Addition to lower extremity, thigh/weight bearing, quadri-lateral brim, molded to patient model Ⓐ&

L2520 Addition to lower extremity, thigh/weight bearing, quadri-lateral brim, custom fitted Ⓐ&

L2525 Addition to lower extremity, thigh/weight bearing, ischial containment/narrow M-L brim molded to patient model Ⓐ&

L2526 Addition to lower extremity, thigh/weight bearing, ischial containment/narrow M-L brim, custom fitted Ⓐ&

| L2530 | Addition to lower extremity, thigh/weight bearing, lacer, nonmolded | A & |

| L2540 | Addition to lower extremity, thigh/weight bearing, lacer, molded to patient model | A & |

| L2550 | Addition to lower extremity, thigh/weight bearing, high roll cuff | A & |

Additions: Pelvic and Thoracic Control

| L2570 | Addition to lower extremity, pelvic control, hip joint, Clevis type two-position joint, each | A ☑ & |

| L2580 | Addition to lower extremity, pelvic control, pelvic sling | A & |

| L2600 | Addition to lower extremity, pelvic control, hip joint, Clevis type, or thrust bearing, free, each | A ☑ & |

| L2610 | Addition to lower extremity, pelvic control, hip joint, Clevis or thrust bearing, lock, each | A ☑ & |

| L2620 | Addition to lower extremity, pelvic control, hip joint, heavy-duty, each | A ☑ & |

| L2622 | Addition to lower extremity, pelvic control, hip joint, adjustable flexion, each | A ☑ & |

| L2624 | Addition to lower extremity, pelvic control, hip joint, adjustable flexion, extension, abduction control, each | A ☑ & |

| L2627 | Addition to lower extremity, pelvic control, plastic, molded to patient model, reciprocating hip joint and cables | A & |

| L2628 | Addition to lower extremity, pelvic control, metal frame, reciprocating hip joint and cables | A & |

| L2630 | Addition to lower extremity, pelvic control, band and belt, unilateral | A & |

| L2640 | Addition to lower extremity, pelvic control, band and belt, bilateral | A & |

| L2650 | Addition to lower extremity, pelvic and thoracic control, gluteal pad, each | A ☑ & |

| L2660 | Addition to lower extremity, thoracic control, thoracic band | A & |

| L2670 | Addition to lower extremity, thoracic control, paraspinal uprights | A & |

| L2680 | Addition to lower extremity, thoracic control, lateral support uprights | A & |

Additions: General

| L2750 | Addition to lower extremity orthosis, plating chrome or nickel, per bar | A ☑ & |

| L2755 | Addition to lower extremity orthosis, high strength, lightweight material, all hybrid lamination/prepreg composite, per segment, for custom fabricated orthosis only | A & |

| L2760 | Addition to lower extremity orthosis, extension, per extension, per bar (for lineal adjustment for growth) | A ☑ & |

| L2768 | Orthotic side bar disconnect device, per bar | A ☑ & |
| | **AHA:** 1Q, '02, 5 | |

| L2780 | Addition to lower extremity orthosis, noncorrosive finish, per bar | A & |

| L2785 | Addition to lower extremity orthosis, drop lock retainer, each | A ☑ & |

| L2795 | Addition to lower extremity orthosis, knee control, full kneecap | A & |

| L2800 | Addition to lower extremity orthosis, knee control, knee cap, medial or lateral pull, for use with custom fabricated orthosis only | A & |

| L2810 | Addition to lower extremity orthosis, knee control, condylar pad | A & |

| L2820 | Addition to lower extremity orthosis, soft interface for molded plastic, below knee section | A & |

| L2830 | Addition to lower extremity orthosis, soft interface for molded plastic, above knee section | A & |

| L2840 | Addition to lower extremity orthosis, tibial length sock, fracture or equal, each | A ☑ & |

| L2850 | Addition to lower extremity orthosis, femoral length sock, fracture or equal, each | A ☑ & |

| L2861 | Addition to lower extremity joint, knee or ankle, concentric adjustable torsion style mechanism for custom fabricated orthotics only, each | E ☑ |

| L2999 | Lower extremity orthoses, not otherwise specified | A |
| | Determine if an alternative HCPCS Level II or a CPT code better describes the service being reported. This code should be used only if a more specific code is unavailable. | |

Orthopedic Footwear

Inserts

| L3000 | Foot insert, removable, molded to patient model, UCB type, Berkeley shell, each | A ☑ & |

| L3001 | Foot, insert, removable, molded to patient model, Spenco, each | A ☑ & |

| L3002 | Foot insert, removable, molded to patient model, Plastazote or equal, each | A ☑ & |

| L3003 | Foot insert, removable, molded to patient model, silicone gel, each | A ☑ & |

| L3010 | Foot insert, removable, molded to patient model, longitudinal arch support, each | A ☑ & |

| L3020 | Foot insert, removable, molded to patient model, longitudinal/metatarsal support, each | A ☑ & |

| L3030 | Foot insert, removable, formed to patient foot, each | A ☑ & |

| L3031 | Foot, insert/plate, removable, addition to lower extremity orthosis, high strength, lightweight material, all hybrid lamination/prepreg composite, each | A ☑ & |

Arch Support, Removable, Premolded

| L3040 | Foot, arch support, removable, premolded, longitudinal, each | A ☑ & |

| L3050 | Foot, arch support, removable, premolded, metatarsal, each | A ☑ & |

| L3060 | Foot, arch support, removable, premolded, longitudinal/metatarsal, each | A ☑ & |

Arch Support, Nonremovable, Attached to Shoe

| L3070 | Foot, arch support, nonremovable, attached to shoe, longitudinal, each | A ☑ & |

| L3080 | Foot, arch support, nonremovable, attached to shoe, metatarsal, each | A ☑ & |

| L3090 | Foot, arch support, nonremovable, attached to shoe, longitudinal/metatarsal, each | A ☑ & |

| L3100 | Hallus-valgus night dynamic splint, prefabricated, off-the-shelf | A & |

Special Coverage Instructions   Noncovered by Medicare   Carrier Discretion   ☑ Quantity Alert   ● New Code   ○ Recycled/Reinstated   ▲ Revised Code

© 2021 Optum360, LLC   A2-Z3 ASC Pmt   CMS: IOM   AHA: Coding Clinic   & DMEPOS Paid   ⊘ SNF Excluded   L Codes — 121

Abduction and Rotation Bars

| L3140 | Foot, abduction rotation bar, including shoes | Ⓐ & |

A Denis-Browne style splint is a bar that can be applied by a strap or mounted on a shoe. This type of splint generally corrects congenital conditions such as genu varus

The angle may be adjusted on a plate on the sole of the shoe

Denis-Browne splint

L3150	Foot, abduction rotation bar, without shoes	Ⓐ &
L3160	Foot, adjustable shoe-styled positioning device	Ⓐ
L3170	Foot, plastic, silicone or equal, heel stabilizer, prefabricated, off-the-shelf, each	Ⓐ ☑ &

Orthopedic Shoes and Boots

L3201	Orthopedic shoe, Oxford with supinator or pronator, infant	Ⓐ Ⓐ
L3202	Orthopedic shoe, Oxford with supinator or pronator, child	Ⓐ Ⓐ
L3203	Orthopedic shoe, Oxford with supinator or pronator, junior	Ⓐ Ⓐ
L3204	Orthopedic shoe, hightop with supinator or pronator, infant	Ⓐ Ⓐ
L3206	Orthopedic shoe, hightop with supinator or pronator, child	Ⓐ Ⓐ
L3207	Orthopedic shoe, hightop with supinator or pronator, junior	Ⓐ Ⓐ
L3208	Surgical boot, each, infant	Ⓐ Ⓐ ☑
L3209	Surgical boot, each, child	Ⓐ Ⓐ ☑
L3211	Surgical boot, each, junior	Ⓐ Ⓐ ☑
L3212	Benesch boot, pair, infant	Ⓐ Ⓐ ☑
L3213	Benesch boot, pair, child	Ⓐ Ⓐ ☑
L3214	Benesch boot, pair, junior	Ⓐ Ⓐ ☑
L3215	Orthopedic footwear, ladies shoe, Oxford, each	Ⓐ ♀ Ⓔ ☑
L3216	Orthopedic footwear, ladies shoe, depth inlay, each	Ⓐ ♀ Ⓔ ☑
L3217	Orthopedic footwear, ladies shoe, hightop, depth inlay, each	Ⓐ ♀ Ⓔ ☑
L3219	Orthopedic footwear, mens shoe, Oxford, each	Ⓐ ♂ Ⓔ ☑
L3221	Orthopedic footwear, mens shoe, depth inlay, each	Ⓐ ♂ Ⓔ ☑
L3222	Orthopedic footwear, mens shoe, hightop, depth inlay, each	Ⓐ ♂ Ⓔ ☑

L3224	Orthopedic footwear, woman's shoe, Oxford, used as an integral part of a brace (orthosis)	♀ Ⓐ &
L3225	Orthopedic footwear, man's shoe, Oxford, used as an integral part of a brace (orthosis)	♂ Ⓐ &
L3230	Orthopedic footwear, custom shoe, depth inlay, each	Ⓐ ☑
L3250	Orthopedic footwear, custom molded shoe, removable inner mold, prosthetic shoe, each	Ⓐ ☑
L3251	Foot, shoe molded to patient model, silicone shoe, each	Ⓐ ☑
L3252	Foot, shoe molded to patient model, Plastazote (or similar), custom fabricated, each	Ⓐ ☑
L3253	Foot, molded shoe, Plastazote (or similar), custom fitted, each	Ⓐ ☑
L3254	Nonstandard size or width	Ⓐ
L3255	Nonstandard size or length	Ⓐ
L3257	Orthopedic footwear, additional charge for split size	Ⓐ
L3260	Surgical boot/shoe, each	Ⓔ ☑
L3265	Plastazote sandal, each	Ⓐ ☑

Shoe Modification - Lifts

L3300	Lift, elevation, heel, tapered to metatarsals, per in	Ⓐ ☑ &
L3310	Lift, elevation, heel and sole, neoprene, per in	Ⓐ ☑ &
L3320	Lift, elevation, heel and sole, cork, per in	Ⓐ ☑
L3330	Lift, elevation, metal extension (skate)	Ⓐ &
L3332	Lift, elevation, inside shoe, tapered, up to one-half in	Ⓐ ☑ &
L3334	Lift, elevation, heel, per in	Ⓐ ☑ &

Shoe Modification - Wedges

L3340	Heel wedge, SACH	Ⓐ &
L3350	Heel wedge	Ⓐ &
L3360	Sole wedge, outside sole	Ⓐ &
L3370	Sole wedge, between sole	Ⓐ &
L3380	Clubfoot wedge	Ⓐ &
L3390	Outflare wedge	Ⓐ &
L3400	Metatarsal bar wedge, rocker	Ⓐ &
L3410	Metatarsal bar wedge, between sole	Ⓐ &
L3420	Full sole and heel wedge, between sole	Ⓐ &

Shoe Modifications - Heels

L3430	Heel, counter, plastic reinforced	Ⓐ &
L3440	Heel, counter, leather reinforced	Ⓐ &
L3450	Heel, SACH cushion type	Ⓐ &
L3455	Heel, new leather, standard	Ⓐ &
L3460	Heel, new rubber, standard	Ⓐ &
L3465	Heel, Thomas with wedge	Ⓐ &
L3470	Heel, Thomas extended to ball	Ⓐ &
L3480	Heel, pad and depression for spur	Ⓐ &
L3485	Heel, pad, removable for spur	Ⓐ

Miscellaneous Shoe Additions

| L3500 | Orthopedic shoe addition, insole, leather | Ⓐ & |
| L3510 | Orthopedic shoe addition, insole, rubber | Ⓐ & |

Special Coverage Instructions   Noncovered by Medicare   Carrier Discretion   ☑ Quantity Alert ● New Code   ○ Recycled/Reinstated   ▲ Revised Code

122 — L Codes   Ⓐ Age Edit   Ⓜ Maternity Edit   ♀ Female Only   ♂ Male Only   Ⓐ-Ⓨ OPPS Status Indicators   © 2021 Optum360, LLC

L3520	Orthopedic shoe addition, insole, felt covered with leather	A ♿
L3530	Orthopedic shoe addition, sole, half	A ♿
L3540	Orthopedic shoe addition, sole, full	A ♿
L3550	Orthopedic shoe addition, toe tap, standard	A ♿
L3560	Orthopedic shoe addition, toe tap, horseshoe	A ♿
L3570	Orthopedic shoe addition, special extension to instep (leather with eyelets)	A ♿
L3580	Orthopedic shoe addition, convert instep to Velcro closure	A ♿
L3590	Orthopedic shoe addition, convert firm shoe counter to soft counter	A ♿
L3595	Orthopedic shoe addition, March bar	A ♿

Transfer or Replacement

L3600	Transfer of an orthosis from one shoe to another, caliper plate, existing	A ♿
L3610	Transfer of an orthosis from one shoe to another, caliper plate, new	A ♿
L3620	Transfer of an orthosis from one shoe to another, solid stirrup, existing	A ♿
L3630	Transfer of an orthosis from one shoe to another, solid stirrup, new	A ♿
L3640	Transfer of an orthosis from one shoe to another, Dennis Browne splint (Riveton), both shoes	A ♿
L3649	Orthopedic shoe, modification, addition or transfer, not otherwise specified	A

Determine if an alternative HCPCS Level II or a CPT code better describes the service being reported. This code should be used only if a more specific code is unavailable.

Shoulder Orthosis (SO)

L3650	Shoulder orthosis (SO), figure of eight design abduction restrainer, prefabricated, off-the-shelf	A ♿
L3660	Shoulder orthosis (SO), figure of eight design abduction restrainer, canvas and webbing, prefabricated, off-the-shelf	A ♿
L3670	Shoulder orthosis (SO), acromio/clavicular (canvas and webbing type), prefabricated, off-the-shelf	A ♿
L3671	Shoulder orthosis (SO), shoulder joint design, without joints, may include soft interface, straps, custom fabricated, includes fitting and adjustment	A ♿
L3674	Shoulder orthosis (SO), abduction positioning (airplane design), thoracic component and support bar, with or without nontorsion joint/turnbuckle, may include soft interface, straps, custom fabricated, includes fitting and adjustment	A ♿
L3675	Shoulder orthosis (SO), vest type abduction restrainer, canvas webbing type or equal, prefabricated, off-the-shelf	A ♿
L3677	Shoulder orthosis (SO), shoulder joint design, without joints, may include soft interface, straps, prefabricated item that has been trimmed, bent, molded, assembled, or otherwise customized to fit a specific patient by an individual with expertise	A
	AHA: 1Q, '02, 5	
L3678	Shoulder orthosis (SO), shoulder joint design, without joints, may include soft interface, straps, prefabricated, off-the-shelf	A

Elbow Orthosis (EO)

L3702	Elbow orthosis (EO), without joints, may include soft interface, straps, custom fabricated, includes fitting and adjustment	A ♿
L3710	Elbow orthosis (EO), elastic with metal joints, prefabricated, off-the-shelf	A ♿
L3720	Elbow orthosis (EO), double upright with forearm/arm cuffs, free motion, custom fabricated	A ♿
L3730	Elbow orthosis (EO), double upright with forearm/arm cuffs, extension/ flexion assist, custom fabricated	A ♿
L3740	Elbow orthosis (EO), double upright with forearm/arm cuffs, adjustable position lock with active control, custom fabricated	A ♿
L3760	Elbow orthosis (EO), with adjustable position locking joint(s), prefabricated, item that has been trimmed, bent, molded, assembled, or otherwise customized to fit a specific patient by an individual with expertise	A ♿
L3761	Elbow orthosis (EO), with adjustable position locking joint(s), prefabricated, off-the-shelf	A ♿
L3762	Elbow orthosis (EO), rigid, without joints, includes soft interface material, prefabricated, off-the-shelf	A ♿
L3763	Elbow-wrist-hand orthosis (EWHO), rigid, without joints, may include soft interface, straps, custom fabricated, includes fitting and adjustment	A ♿
L3764	Elbow-wrist-hand orthosis (EWHO), includes one or more nontorsion joints, elastic bands, turnbuckles, may include soft interface, straps, custom fabricated, includes fitting and adjustment	A ♿
L3765	Elbow-wrist-hand-finger orthosis (EWHFO), rigid, without joints, may include soft interface, straps, custom fabricated, includes fitting and adjustment	A ♿
L3766	Elbow-wrist-hand-finger orthosis (EWHFO), includes one or more nontorsion joints, elastic bands, turnbuckles, may include soft interface, straps, custom fabricated, includes fitting and adjustment	A ♿

Wrist-Hand-Finger Orthosis (WHFO)

L3806	Wrist-hand-finger orthosis (WHFO), includes one or more nontorsion joint(s), turnbuckles, elastic bands/springs, may include soft interface material, straps, custom fabricated, includes fitting and adjustment	A ♿
L3807	Wrist-hand-finger orthosis (WHFO), without joint(s), prefabricated item that has been trimmed, bent, molded, assembled, or otherwise customized to fit a specific patient by an individual with expertise	A ♿
L3808	Wrist-hand-finger orthosis (WHFO), rigid without joints, may include soft interface material; straps, custom fabricated, includes fitting and adjustment	A ♿
L3809	Wrist-hand-finger orthosis (WHFO), without joint(s), prefabricated, off-the-shelf, any type	A ♿

Additions to Upper Extremity Orthosis

L3891	Addition to upper extremity joint, wrist or elbow, concentric adjustable torsion style mechanism for custom fabricated orthotics only, each	E ☑

Dynamic Flexor Hinge, Reciprocal Wrist Extension/Flexion, Finger Flexion/Extension

L3900	Wrist-hand-finger orthosis (WHFO), dynamic flexor hinge, reciprocal wrist extension/ flexion, finger flexion/extension, wrist or finger driven, custom fabricated	A ♿

Special Coverage Instructions   Noncovered by Medicare   Carrier Discretion   ☑ Quantity Alert   ● New Code   ○ Recycled/Reinstated   ▲ Revised Code

© 2021 Optum360, LLC   A2-Z3 ASC Pmt   CMS: IOM   AHA: Coding Clinic   ♿ DMEPOS Paid   ⊘ SNF Excluded   L Codes — 123

L3901 Wrist-hand-finger orthosis (WHFO), dynamic flexor hinge, reciprocal wrist extension/ flexion, finger flexion/extension, cable driven, custom fabricated Ⓐ &

External Power

L3904 Wrist-hand-finger orthosis (WHFO), external powered, electric, custom fabricated Ⓐ &

Other Upper Extremity Orthoses

L3905 Wrist-hand orthosis (WHO), includes one or more nontorsion joints, elastic bands, turnbuckles, may include soft interface, straps, custom fabricated, includes fitting and adjustment Ⓐ &

L3906 Wrist-hand orthosis (WHO), without joints, may include soft interface, straps, custom fabricated, includes fitting and adjustment Ⓐ &

L3908 Wrist-hand orthosis (WHO), wrist extension control cock-up, nonmolded, prefabricated, off-the-shelf Ⓐ &

L3912 Hand-finger orthosis (HFO), flexion glove with elastic finger control, prefabricated, off-the-shelf Ⓐ &

L3913 Hand-finger orthosis (HFO), without joints, may include soft interface, straps, custom fabricated, includes fitting and adjustment Ⓐ &

L3915 Wrist-hand orthosis (WHO), includes one or more nontorsion joint(s), elastic bands, turnbuckles, may include soft interface, straps, prefabricated item that has been trimmed, bent, molded, assembled, or otherwise customized to fit a specific patient by an individual with expertise Ⓐ &

L3916 Wrist-hand orthosis (WHO), includes one or more nontorsion joint(s), elastic bands, turnbuckles, may include soft interface, straps, prefabricated, off-the-shelf Ⓐ &

L3917 Hand orthosis (HO), metacarpal fracture orthosis, prefabricated item that has been trimmed, bent, molded, assembled, or otherwise customized to fit a specific patient by an individual with expertise Ⓐ &

L3918 Hand orthosis (HO), metacarpal fracture orthosis, prefabricated, off-the-shelf Ⓐ &

L3919 Hand orthosis (HO), without joints, may include soft interface, straps, custom fabricated, includes fitting and adjustment Ⓐ &

L3921 Hand-finger orthosis (HFO), includes one or more nontorsion joints, elastic bands, turnbuckles, may include soft interface, straps, custom fabricated, includes fitting and adjustment Ⓐ &

L3923 Hand-finger orthosis (HFO), without joints, may include soft interface, straps, prefabricated item that has been trimmed, bent, molded, assembled, or otherwise customized to fit a specific patient by an individual with expertise Ⓐ &

L3924 Hand-finger orthosis (HFO), without joints, may include soft interface, straps, prefabricated, off-the-shelf Ⓐ &

L3925 Finger orthosis (FO), proximal interphalangeal (PIP)/distal interphalangeal (DIP), nontorsion joint/spring, extension/flexion, may include soft interface material, prefabricated, off-the-shelf Ⓐ &

L3927 Finger orthosis (FO), proximal interphalangeal (PIP)/distal interphalangeal (DIP), without joint/spring, extension/flexion (e.g., static or ring type), may include soft interface material, prefabricated, off-the-shelf Ⓐ &

L3929 Hand-finger orthosis (HFO), includes one or more nontorsion joint(s), turnbuckles, elastic bands/springs, may include soft interface material, straps, prefabricated item that has been trimmed, bent, molded, assembled, or otherwise customized to fit a specific patient by an individual with expertise Ⓐ &

L3930 Hand-finger orthosis (HFO), includes one or more nontorsion joint(s), turnbuckles, elastic bands/springs, may include soft interface material, straps, prefabricated, off-the-shelf Ⓐ &

L3931 Wrist-hand-finger orthosis (WHFO), includes one or more nontorsion joint(s), turnbuckles, elastic bands/springs, may include soft interface material, straps, prefabricated, includes fitting and adjustment Ⓐ &

L3933 Finger orthosis (FO), without joints, may include soft interface, custom fabricated, includes fitting and adjustment Ⓐ &

L3935 Finger orthosis (FO), nontorsion joint, may include soft interface, custom fabricated, includes fitting and adjustment Ⓐ &

L3956 Addition of joint to upper extremity orthosis, any material; per joint Ⓐ ☑ &

Shoulder, Elbow, Wrist, Hand Orthosis

L3960 Shoulder-elbow-wrist-hand orthosis (SEWHO), abduction positioning, airplane design, prefabricated, includes fitting and adjustment Ⓐ &

L3961 Shoulder-elbow-wrist-hand orthosis (SEWHO), shoulder cap design, without joints, may include soft interface, straps, custom fabricated, includes fitting and adjustment Ⓐ &

L3962 Shoulder-elbow-wrist-hand orthosis (SEWHO), abduction positioning, Erb's palsy design, prefabricated, includes fitting and adjustment Ⓐ &

L3967 Shoulder-elbow-wrist-hand orthosis (SEWHO), abduction positioning (airplane design), thoracic component and support bar, without joints, may include soft interface, straps, custom fabricated, includes fitting and adjustment Ⓐ &

Additions to Mobile Arm Supports

L3971 Shoulder-elbow-wrist-hand orthotic (SEWHO), shoulder cap design, includes one or more nontorsion joints, elastic bands, turnbuckles, may include soft interface, straps, custom fabricated, includes fitting and adjustment Ⓐ &

L3973 Shoulder-elbow-wrist-hand orthosis (SEWHO), abduction positioning (airplane design), thoracic component and support bar, includes one or more nontorsion joints, elastic bands, turnbuckles, may include soft interface, straps, custom fabricated, includes fitting and adjustment Ⓐ &

L3975 Shoulder-elbow-wrist-hand-finger orthosis (SEWHO), shoulder cap design, without joints, may include soft interface, straps, custom fabricated, includes fitting and adjustment Ⓐ &

L3976 Shoulder-elbow-wrist-hand-finger orthosis (SEWHO), abduction positioning (airplane design), thoracic component and support bar, without joints, may include soft interface, straps, custom fabricated, includes fitting and adjustment Ⓐ &

L3977 Shoulder-elbow-wrist-hand-finger orthosis (SEWHO), shoulder cap design, includes one or more nontorsion joints, elastic bands, turnbuckles, may include soft interface, straps, custom fabricated, includes fitting and adjustment Ⓐ &

L3978 Shoulder-elbow-wrist-hand-finger orthosis (SEWHO), abduction positioning (airplane design), thoracic component and support bar, includes one or more nontorsion joints, elastic bands, turnbuckles, may include soft interface, straps, custom fabricated, includes fitting and adjustment Ⓐ &

Special Coverage Instructions   Noncovered by Medicare   Carrier Discretion   ☑ Quantity Alert ● New Code   ○ Recycled/Reinstated ▲ Revised Code

124 — L Codes   Ⓐ Age Edit   Ⓜ Maternity Edit   ♀ Female Only   ♂ Male Only   Ⓐ-Ⓨ OPPS Status Indicators   © 2021 Optum360, LLC

Fracture Orthotic

L3980 Upper extremity fracture orthosis, humeral, prefabricated, includes fitting and adjustment ☒ ♿

L3981 Upper extremity fracture orthosis, humeral, prefabricated, includes shoulder cap design, with or without joints, forearm section, may include soft interface, straps, includes fitting and adjustments ☒ ♿

L3982 Upper extremity fracture orthosis, radius/ulnar, prefabricated, includes fitting and adjustment ☒ ♿

L3984 Upper extremity fracture orthosis, wrist, prefabricated, includes fitting and adjustment ☒ ♿

L3995 Addition to upper extremity orthosis, sock, fracture or equal, each ☒ ☑ ♿

L3999 Upper limb orthosis, not otherwise specified ☒

Repairs

L4000 Replace girdle for spinal orthosis (cervical-thoracic-lumbar-sacral orthosis (CTLSO) or spinal orthosis SO) ☒ ♿

L4002 Replacement strap, any orthosis, includes all components, any length, any type ☒ ♿

L4010 Replace trilateral socket brim ☒ ♿

L4020 Replace quadrilateral socket brim, molded to patient model ☒ ♿

L4030 Replace quadrilateral socket brim, custom fitted ☒ ♿

L4040 Replace molded thigh lacer, for custom fabricated orthosis only ☒ ♿

L4045 Replace nonmolded thigh lacer, for custom fabricated orthosis only ☒ ♿

L4050 Replace molded calf lacer, for custom fabricated orthosis only ☒ ♿

L4055 Replace nonmolded calf lacer, for custom fabricated orthosis only ☒ ♿

L4060 Replace high roll cuff ☒ ♿

L4070 Replace proximal and distal upright for KAFO ☒ ♿

L4080 Replace metal bands KAFO, proximal thigh ☒ ♿

L4090 Replace metal bands KAFO-AFO, calf or distal thigh ☒ ♿

L4100 Replace leather cuff KAFO, proximal thigh ☒ ♿

L4110 Replace leather cuff KAFO-AFO, calf or distal thigh ☒ ♿

L4130 Replace pretibial shell ☒ ♿

L4205 Repair of orthotic device, labor component, per 15 minutes ☒ ☑

L4210 Repair of orthotic device, repair or replace minor parts ☒

Miscellaneous Lower Limb Supports

L4350 Ankle control orthosis, stirrup style, rigid, includes any type interface (e.g., pneumatic, gel), prefabricated, off-the-shelf ☒ ♿

L4360 Walking boot, pneumatic and/or vacuum, with or without joints, with or without interface material, prefabricated item that has been trimmed, bent, molded, or otherwise customized to fit a specific patient by an individual with expertise ☒ ♿

L4361 Walking boot, pneumatic and/or vacuum, with or without joints, with or without interface material, prefabricated, off-the-shelf ☒ ♿

L4370 Pneumatic full leg splint, prefabricated, off-the-shelf ☒ ♿

L4386 Walking boot, nonpneumatic, with or without joints, with or without interface material, prefabricated item that has been trimmed, bent, molded, assembled, or otherwise customized to fit a specific patient by an individual with expertise ☒ ♿

L4387 Walking boot, nonpneumatic, with or without joints, with or without interface material, prefabricated, off-the-shelf ☒ ♿

L4392 Replacement, soft interface material, static AFO ☒ ♿

L4394 Replace soft interface material, foot drop splint ☒ ♿

L4396 Static or dynamic ankle foot orthosis, including soft interface material, adjustable for fit, for positioning, may be used for minimal ambulation, prefabricated item that has been trimmed, bent, molded, assembled, or otherwise customized to fit a specific patient by an individual with expertise ☒ ♿

L4397 Static or dynamic ankle foot orthosis, including soft interface material, adjustable for fit, for positioning, may be used for minimal ambulation, prefabricated, off-the-shelf ☒ ♿

L4398 Foot drop splint, recumbent positioning device, prefabricated, off-the-shelf ☒ ♿

L4631 Ankle-foot orthosis (AFO), walking boot type, varus/valgus correction, rocker bottom, anterior tibial shell, soft interface, custom arch support, plastic or other material, includes straps and closures, custom fabricated ♿

Prosthetic Procedures L5000-L9900

The codes in this section are considered as "base" or "basic procedures or prosthetics" and may be modified by listing items/procedures or special materials from the "additions" sections and adding them to the base procedure.

Partial Foot

L5000 Partial foot, shoe insert with longitudinal arch, toe filler ☒ ♿

L5010 Partial foot, molded socket, ankle height, with toe filler ☒ ♿

L5020 Partial foot, molded socket, tibial tubercle height, with toe filler ☒ ♿

Ankle

L5050 Ankle, Symes, molded socket, SACH foot ☒ ⊘ ♿

L5060 Ankle, Symes, metal frame, molded leather socket, articulated ankle/foot ☒ ⊘ ♿

Below Knee

L5100 Below knee (BK), molded socket, shin, SACH foot ☒ ⊘ ♿

L5105 Below knee (BK), plastic socket, joints and thigh lacer, SACH foot ☒ ⊘ ♿

Knee Disarticulation

L5150 Knee disarticulation (or through knee), molded socket, external knee joints, shin, SACH foot ☒ ⊘ ♿

L5160 Knee disarticulation (or through knee), molded socket, bent knee configuration, external knee joints, shin, SACH foot ☒ ⊘ ♿

Above Knee

L5200 Above knee (AK), molded socket, single axis constant friction knee, shin, SACH foot ☒ ⊘ ♿

L5210 Above knee (AK), short prosthesis, no knee joint (stubbies), with foot blocks, no ankle joints, each ☒ ☑ ⊘ ♿

L5220 Above knee (AK), short prosthesis, no knee joint (stubbies), with articulated ankle/foot, dynamically aligned, each ☒ ☑ ⊘ ♿

L5230 Above knee (AK), for proximal femoral focal deficiency, constant friction knee, shin, SACH foot ☒ ⊘ ♿

Prosthetic Devices and Procedures

L5250 — L5614

Hip Disarticulation

L5250   Hip disarticulation, Canadian type; molded socket, hip joint, single axis constant friction knee, shin, SACH foot   A ⊘ ⅓

L5270   Hip disarticulation, tilt table type; molded socket, locking hip joint, single axis constant friction knee, shin, SACH foot   A ⊘ ⅓

Hemipelvectomy

L5280   Hemipelvectomy, Canadian type; molded socket, hip joint, single axis constant friction knee, shin, SACH foot   A ⊘ ⅓

L5301   Below knee (BK), molded socket, shin, SACH foot, endoskeletal system   A ⊘ ⅓
  AHA: 1Q, '02, 5

L5312   Knee disarticulation (or through knee), molded socket, single axis knee, pylon, SACH foot, endoskeletal system   A ⅓

L5321   Above knee (AK), molded socket, open end, SACH foot, endoskeletal system, single axis knee   A ⊘ ⅓
  AHA: 1Q, '02, 5

L5331   Hip disarticulation, Canadian type, molded socket, endoskeletal system, hip joint, single axis knee, SACH foot   A ⊘ ⅓
  AHA: 1Q, '02, 5

L5341   Hemipelvectomy, Canadian type, molded socket, endoskeletal system, hip joint, single axis knee, SACH foot   A ⊘ ⅓
  AHA: 1Q, '02, 5

Immediate Postsurgical or Early Fitting Procedures

L5400   Immediate postsurgical or early fitting, application of initial rigid dressing, including fitting, alignment, suspension, and one cast change, below knee (BK)   A ☑ ⅓

Above-the-knee test socket

Below-the-knee early fitting rigid dressing (L5400)

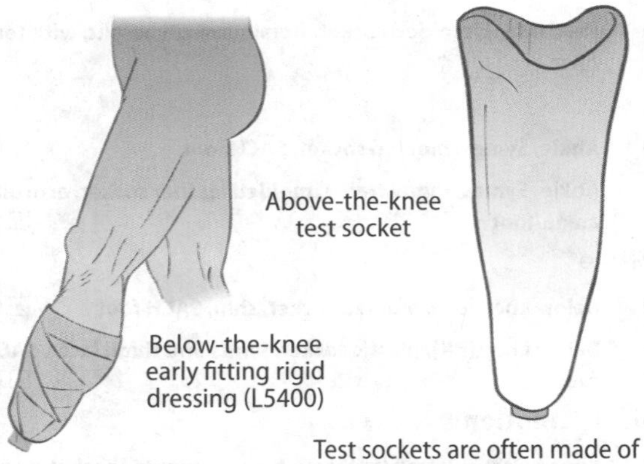

Test sockets are often made of clear plastic so the prosthetist can visualize the fit against the residual limb

L5410   Immediate postsurgical or early fitting, application of initial rigid dressing, including fitting, alignment and suspension, below knee (BK), each additional cast change and realignment   A ☑ ⅓

L5420   Immediate postsurgical or early fitting, application of initial rigid dressing, including fitting, alignment and suspension and one cast change above knee (AK) or knee disarticulation   A ☑ ⅓

L5430   Immediate postsurgical or early fitting, application of initial rigid dressing, including fitting, alignment and suspension, above knee (AK) or knee disarticulation, each additional cast change and realignment   A ☑ ⅓

L5450   Immediate postsurgical or early fitting, application of nonweight bearing rigid dressing, below knee (BK)   A ⅓

L5460   Immediate postsurgical or early fitting, application of nonweight bearing rigid dressing, above knee (AK)   A ⅓

Initial Prosthesis

L5500   Initial, below knee (BK) PTB type socket, nonalignable system, pylon, no cover, SACH foot, plaster socket, direct formed   A ⊘ ⅓

L5505   Initial, above knee (AK), knee disarticulation, ischial level socket, nonalignable system, pylon, no cover, SACH foot, plaster socket, direct formed   A ⊘ ⅓

Preparatory Prosthesis

L5510   Preparatory, below knee (BK) PTB type socket, nonalignable system, pylon, no cover, SACH foot, plaster socket, molded to model   A ⊘ ⅓

L5520   Preparatory, below knee (BK) PTB type socket, nonalignable system, pylon, no cover, SACH foot, thermoplastic or equal, direct formed   A ⊘ ⅓

L5530   Preparatory, below knee (BK) PTB type socket, nonalignable system, pylon, no cover, SACH foot, thermoplastic or equal, molded to model   A ⊘ ⅓

L5535   Preparatory, below knee (BK) PTB type socket, nonalignable system, no cover, SACH foot, prefabricated, adjustable open end socket   A ⊘ ⅓

L5540   Preparatory, below knee (BK) PTB type socket, nonalignable system, pylon, no cover, SACH foot, laminated socket, molded to model   A ⊘ ⅓

L5560   Preparatory, above knee (AK), knee disarticulation, ischial level socket, nonalignable system, pylon, no cover, SACH foot, plaster socket, molded to model   A ⊘ ⅓

L5570   Preparatory, above knee (AK), knee disarticulation, ischial level socket, nonalignable system, pylon, no cover, SACH foot, thermoplastic or equal, direct formed   A ⊘ ⅓

L5580   Preparatory, above knee (AK), knee disarticulation, ischial level socket, nonalignable system, pylon, no cover, SACH foot, thermoplastic or equal, molded to model   A ⊘ ⅓

L5585   Preparatory, above knee (AK), knee disarticulation, ischial level socket, nonalignable system, pylon, no cover, SACH foot, prefabricated adjustable open end socket   A ⊘ ⅓

L5590   Preparatory, above knee (AK), knee disarticulation, ischial level socket, nonalignable system, pylon, no cover, SACH foot, laminated socket, molded to model   A ⊘ ⅓

L5595   Preparatory, hip disarticulation/hemipelvectomy, pylon, no cover, SACH foot, thermoplastic or equal, molded to patient model   A ⊘ ⅓

L5600   Preparatory, hip disarticulation/hemipelvectomy, pylon, no cover, SACH foot, laminated socket, molded to patient model   A ⊘ ⅓

Additions

Additions: Lower Extremity

L5610   Addition to lower extremity, endoskeletal system, above knee (AK), hydracadence system   A ⊘ ⅓

L5611   Addition to lower extremity, endoskeletal system, above knee (AK), knee disarticulation, four-bar linkage, with friction swing phase control   A ⊘ ⅓

L5613   Addition to lower extremity, endoskeletal system, above knee (AK), knee disarticulation, four-bar linkage, with hydraulic swing phase control   A ⊘ ⅓

L5614   Addition to lower extremity, exoskeletal system, above knee (AK), knee disarticulation, four-bar linkage, with pneumatic swing phase control   A ⊘ ⅓

Special Coverage Instructions   Noncovered by Medicare   Carrier Discretion   ☑ Quantity Alert   ● New Code   ○ Recycled/Reinstated   ▲ Revised Code

126 — L Codes   A Age Edit   M Maternity Edit   ♀ Female Only   ♂ Male Only   A-Y OPPS Status Indicators   © 2021 Optum360, LLC

L5616 Addition to lower extremity, endoskeletal system, above knee (AK), universal multiplex system, friction swing phase control [A] ⊘ &

L5617 Addition to lower extremity, quick change self-aligning unit, above knee (AK) or below knee (BK), each [A] ☑ ⊘ &

Additions: Test Sockets

L5618 Addition to lower extremity, test socket, Symes [A] ⊘ &

L5620 Addition to lower extremity, test socket, below knee (BK) [A] ⊘ &

L5622 Addition to lower extremity, test socket, knee disarticulation [A] ⊘ &

L5624 Addition to lower extremity, test socket, above knee (AK) [A] ⊘ &

L5626 Addition to lower extremity, test socket, hip disarticulation [A] ⊘ &

L5628 Addition to lower extremity, test socket, hemipelvectomy [A] ⊘ &

L5629 Addition to lower extremity, below knee, acrylic socket [A] ⊘ &

Additions: Socket Variations

L5630 Addition to lower extremity, Symes type, expandable wall socket [A] ⊘ &

L5631 Addition to lower extremity, above knee (AK) or knee disarticulation, acrylic socket [A] ⊘ &

L5632 Addition to lower extremity, Symes type, PTB brim design socket [A] ⊘ &

L5634 Addition to lower extremity, Symes type, posterior opening (Canadian) socket [A] ⊘ &

L5636 Addition to lower extremity, Symes type, medial opening socket [A] ⊘ &

L5637 Addition to lower extremity, below knee (BK), total contact [A] ⊘ &

L5638 Addition to lower extremity, below knee (BK), leather socket [A] ⊘ &

L5639 Addition to lower extremity, below knee (BK), wood socket [A] ⊘ &

L5640 Addition to lower extremity, knee disarticulation, leather socket [A] ⊘ &

L5642 Addition to lower extremity, above knee (AK), leather socket [A] ⊘ &

L5643 Addition to lower extremity, hip disarticulation, flexible inner socket, external frame [A] ⊘ &

L5644 Addition to lower extremity, above knee (AK), wood socket [A] ⊘ &

L5645 Addition to lower extremity, below knee (BK), flexible inner socket, external frame [A] ⊘ &

L5646 Addition to lower extremity, below knee (BK), air, fluid, gel or equal, cushion socket [A] ⊘ &

L5647 Addition to lower extremity, below knee (BK), suction socket [A] ⊘ &

L5648 Addition to lower extremity, above knee (AK), air, fluid, gel or equal, cushion socket [A] ⊘ &

L5649 Addition to lower extremity, ischial containment/narrow M-L socket [A] ⊘ &

L5650 Additions to lower extremity, total contact, above knee (AK) or knee disarticulation socket [A] ⊘ &

L5651 Addition to lower extremity, above knee (AK), flexible inner socket, external frame [A] ⊘ &

L5652 Addition to lower extremity, suction suspension, above knee (AK) or knee disarticulation socket [A] ⊘ &

L5653 Addition to lower extremity, knee disarticulation, expandable wall socket [A] ⊘ &

Additions: Socket Insert and Suspension

L5654 Addition to lower extremity, socket insert, Symes, (Kemblo, Pelite, Aliplast, Plastazote or equal) [A] ⊘ &

L5655 Addition to lower extremity, socket insert, below knee (BK) (Kemblo, Pelite, Aliplast, Plastazote or equal) [A] ⊘ &

L5656 Addition to lower extremity, socket insert, knee disarticulation (Kemblo, Pelite, Aliplast, Plastazote or equal) [A] ⊘ &

L5658 Addition to lower extremity, socket insert, above knee (AK) (Kemblo, Pelite, Aliplast, Plastazote or equal) [A] ⊘ &

L5661 Addition to lower extremity, socket insert, multidurometer Symes [A] ⊘ &

L5665 Addition to lower extremity, socket insert, multidurometer, below knee (BK) [A] ⊘ &

L5666 Addition to lower extremity, below knee (BK), cuff suspension [A] ⊘ &

L5668 Addition to lower extremity, below knee (BK), molded distal cushion [A] ⊘ &

L5670 Addition to lower extremity, below knee (BK), molded supracondylar suspension (PTS or similar) [A] ⊘ &

As the suspension sleeve is donned, air is driven out through a valve

The valve is closed upon donning and a suction fit is formed around the residual limb

Residual limb

Sealing membrane

Sleeve

Open valve

Closed valve

L5671 Addition to lower extremity, below knee (BK)/above knee (AK) suspension locking mechanism (shuttle, lanyard, or equal), excludes socket insert [A] ⊘ &
  AHA: 1Q, '02, 5

L5672 Addition to lower extremity, below knee (BK), removable medial brim suspension [A] ⊘ &

L5673 Addition to lower extremity, below knee (BK)/above knee (AK), custom fabricated from existing mold or prefabricated, socket insert, silicone gel, elastomeric or equal, for use with locking mechanism [A] ⊘ &

L5676 Additions to lower extremity, below knee (BK), knee joints, single axis, pair [A] ☑ ⊘ &

Special Coverage Instructions   Noncovered by Medicare   Carrier Discretion   ☑ Quantity Alert ● New Code ○ Recycled/Reinstated ▲ Revised Code

Prosthetic Devices and Procedures

L5677 — L5824

| L5677 | Additions to lower extremity, below knee (BK), knee joints, polycentric, pair ☒☑⊘♿ |

| L5678 | Additions to lower extremity, below knee (BK), joint covers, pair ☒☑⊘♿ |

| L5679 | Addition to lower extremity, below knee (BK)/above knee (AK), custom fabricated from existing mold or prefabricated, socket insert, silicone gel, elastomeric or equal, not for use with locking mechanism ☒⊘♿ |

| L5680 | Addition to lower extremity, below knee (BK), thigh lacer, nonmolded ☒⊘♿ |

| L5681 | Addition to lower extremity, below knee (BK)/above knee (AK), custom fabricated socket insert for congenital or atypical traumatic amputee, silicone gel, elastomeric or equal, for use with or without locking mechanism, initial only (for other than initial, use code L5673 or L5679) ☒⊘♿ |

| L5682 | Addition to lower extremity, below knee (BK), thigh lacer, gluteal/ischial, molded ☒⊘♿ |

| L5683 | Addition to lower extremity, below knee (BK)/above knee (AK), custom fabricated socket insert for other than congenital or atypical traumatic amputee, silicone gel, elastomeric or equal, for use with or without locking mechanism, initial only (for other than initial, use code L5673 or L5679) ☒⊘♿ |

| L5684 | Addition to lower extremity, below knee, fork strap ☒⊘♿ |

| L5685 | Addition to lower extremity prosthesis, below knee, suspension/sealing sleeve, with or without valve, any material, each ☒⊘♿ |

| L5686 | Addition to lower extremity, below knee (BK), back check (extension control) ☒⊘♿ |

| L5688 | Addition to lower extremity, below knee (BK), waist belt, webbing ☒⊘♿ |

| L5690 | Addition to lower extremity, below knee (BK), waist belt, padded and lined ☒⊘♿ |

| L5692 | Addition to lower extremity, above knee (AK), pelvic control belt, light ☒⊘♿ |

| L5694 | Addition to lower extremity, above knee (AK), pelvic control belt, padded and lined ☒⊘♿ |

| L5695 | Addition to lower extremity, above knee (AK), pelvic control, sleeve suspension, neoprene or equal, each ☒☑⊘♿ |

| L5696 | Addition to lower extremity, above knee (AK) or knee disarticulation, pelvic joint ☒⊘♿ |

| L5697 | Addition to lower extremity, above knee (AK) or knee disarticulation, pelvic band ☒⊘♿ |

| L5698 | Addition to lower extremity, above knee (AK) or knee disarticulation, Silesian bandage ☒⊘♿ |

| L5699 | All lower extremity prostheses, shoulder harness ☒⊘♿ |

Replacements

| L5700 | Replacement, socket, below knee (BK), molded to patient model ☒⊘♿ |

| L5701 | Replacement, socket, above knee (AK)/knee disarticulation, including attachment plate, molded to patient model ☒⊘♿ |

| L5702 | Replacement, socket, hip disarticulation, including hip joint, molded to patient model ☒⊘♿ |

| L5703 | Ankle, Symes, molded to patient model, socket without solid ankle cushion heel (SACH) foot, replacement only ☒⊘♿ |

| L5704 | Custom shaped protective cover, below knee (BK) ☒⊘♿ |

| L5705 | Custom shaped protective cover, above knee (AK) ☒⊘♿ |

| L5706 | Custom shaped protective cover, knee disarticulation ☒⊘♿ |

| L5707 | Custom shaped protective cover, hip disarticulation ☒⊘♿ |

Additions: Exoskeletal Knee-Shin System

| L5710 | Addition, exoskeletal knee-shin system, single axis, manual lock ☒⊘♿ |

| L5711 | Additions exoskeletal knee-shin system, single axis, manual lock, ultra-light material ☒⊘♿ |

| L5712 | Addition, exoskeletal knee-shin system, single axis, friction swing and stance phase control (safety knee) ☒⊘♿ |

| L5714 | Addition, exoskeletal knee-shin system, single axis, variable friction swing phase control ☒⊘♿ |

| L5716 | Addition, exoskeletal knee-shin system, polycentric, mechanical stance phase lock ☒⊘♿ |

| L5718 | Addition, exoskeletal knee-shin system, polycentric, friction swing and stance phase control ☒⊘♿ |

| L5722 | Addition, exoskeletal knee-shin system, single axis, pneumatic swing, friction stance phase control ☒⊘♿ |

| L5724 | Addition, exoskeletal knee-shin system, single axis, fluid swing phase control ☒⊘♿ |

| L5726 | Addition, exoskeletal knee-shin system, single axis, external joints, fluid swing phase control ☒⊘♿ |

| L5728 | Addition, exoskeletal knee-shin system, single axis, fluid swing and stance phase control ☒⊘♿ |

| L5780 | Addition, exoskeletal knee-shin system, single axis, pneumatic/hydra pneumatic swing phase control ☒⊘♿ |

| L5781 | Addition to lower limb prosthesis, vacuum pump, residual limb volume management and moisture evacuation system ☒⊘♿ |

| L5782 | Addition to lower limb prosthesis, vacuum pump, residual limb volume management and moisture evacuation system, heavy-duty ☒⊘♿ |

Component Modification

| L5785 | Addition, exoskeletal system, below knee (BK), ultra-light material (titanium, carbon fiber or equal) ☒⊘♿ |

| L5790 | Addition, exoskeletal system, above knee (AK), ultra-light material (titanium, carbon fiber or equal) ☒⊘♿ |

| L5795 | Addition, exoskeletal system, hip disarticulation, ultra-light material (titanium, carbon fiber or equal) ☒⊘♿ |

Additions: Endoskeletal Knee-Shin System

| L5810 | Addition, endoskeletal knee-shin system, single axis, manual lock ☒⊘♿ |

| L5811 | Addition, endoskeletal knee-shin system, single axis, manual lock, ultra-light material ☒⊘♿ |

| L5812 | Addition, endoskeletal knee-shin system, single axis, friction swing and stance phase control (safety knee) ☒⊘♿ |

| L5814 | Addition, endoskeletal knee-shin system, polycentric, hydraulic swing phase control, mechanical stance phase lock ☒⊘♿ |

| L5816 | Addition, endoskeletal knee-shin system, polycentric, mechanical stance phase lock ☒⊘♿ |

| L5818 | Addition, endoskeletal knee-shin system, polycentric, friction swing and stance phase control ☒⊘♿ |

| L5822 | Addition, endoskeletal knee-shin system, single axis, pneumatic swing, friction stance phase control ☒⊘♿ |

| L5824 | Addition, endoskeletal knee-shin system, single axis, fluid swing phase control ☒⊘♿ |

Special Coverage Instructions   Noncovered by Medicare   Carrier Discretion   ☑ Quantity Alert   ● New Code   ○ Recycled/Reinstated   ▲ Revised Code

L5826 Addition, endoskeletal knee-shin system, single axis, hydraulic swing phase control, with miniature high activity frame   Ⓐ ⊘ &

L5828 Addition, endoskeletal knee-shin system, single axis, fluid swing and stance phase control   Ⓐ ⊘ &

L5830 Addition, endoskeletal knee-shin system, single axis, pneumatic/swing phase control   Ⓐ ⊘ &

L5840 Addition, endoskeletal knee-shin system, four-bar linkage or multiaxial, pneumatic swing phase control   Ⓐ ⊘ &

L5845 Addition, endoskeletal knee-shin system, stance flexion feature, adjustable   Ⓐ ⊘ &

L5848 Addition to endoskeletal knee-shin system, fluid stance extension, dampening feature, with or without adjustability   Ⓐ ⊘ &

L5850 Addition, endoskeletal system, above knee (AK) or hip disarticulation, knee extension assist   Ⓐ ⊘ &

L5855 Addition, endoskeletal system, hip disarticulation, mechanical hip extension assist   Ⓐ ⊘ &

L5856 Addition to lower extremity prosthesis, endoskeletal knee-shin system, microprocessor control feature, swing and stance phase, includes electronic sensor(s), any type   Ⓐ ⊘ &

L5857 Addition to lower extremity prosthesis, endoskeletal knee-shin system, microprocessor control feature, swing phase only, includes electronic sensor(s), any type   Ⓐ ⊘ &

L5858 Addition to lower extremity prosthesis, endoskeletal knee-shin system, microprocessor control feature, stance phase only, includes electronic sensor(s), any type   Ⓐ ⊘ &

L5859 Addition to lower extremity prosthesis, endoskeletal knee-shin system, powered and programmable flexion/extension assist control, includes any type motor(s)   Ⓐ &

L5910 Addition, endoskeletal system, below knee (BK), alignable system   Ⓐ ⊘ &

L5920 Addition, endoskeletal system, above knee (AK) or hip disarticulation, alignable system   Ⓐ ⊘ &

L5925 Addition, endoskeletal system, above knee (AK), knee disarticulation or hip disarticulation, manual lock   Ⓐ ⊘ &

L5930 Addition, endoskeletal system, high activity knee control frame   Ⓐ ⊘ &

L5940 Addition, endoskeletal system, below knee (BK), ultra-light material (titanium, carbon fiber or equal)   Ⓐ ⊘ &

L5950 Addition, endoskeletal system, above knee (AK), ultra-light material (titanium, carbon fiber or equal)   Ⓐ ⊘ &

L5960 Addition, endoskeletal system, hip disarticulation, ultra-light material (titanium, carbon fiber or equal)   Ⓐ ⊘ &

L5961 Addition, endoskeletal system, polycentric hip joint, pneumatic or hydraulic control, rotation control, with or without flexion and/or extension control   Ⓐ &

L5962 Addition, endoskeletal system, below knee (BK), flexible protective outer surface covering system   Ⓐ ⊘ &

L5964 Addition, endoskeletal system, above knee (AK), flexible protective outer surface covering system   Ⓐ ⊘ &

L5966 Addition, endoskeletal system, hip disarticulation, flexible protective outer surface covering system   Ⓐ ⊘ &

L5968 Addition to lower limb prosthesis, multiaxial ankle with swing phase active dorsiflexion feature   Ⓐ ⊘ &

L5969 Addition, endoskeletal ankle-foot or ankle system, power assist, includes any type motor(s)   Ⓐ

L5970 All lower extremity prostheses, foot, external keel, SACH foot   Ⓐ ⊘ &

L5971 All lower extremity prostheses, solid ankle cushion heel (SACH) foot, replacement only   Ⓐ ⊘ &

L5972 All lower extremity prostheses, foot, flexible keel   Ⓐ ⊘ &

L5973 Endoskeletal ankle foot system, microprocessor controlled feature, dorsiflexion and/or plantar flexion control, includes power source   Ⓐ ⊘ &

L5974 All lower extremity prostheses, foot, single axis ankle/foot   Ⓐ ⊘ &

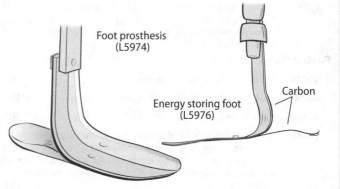

Foot prosthesis (L5974)

Energy storing foot (L5976)

Carbon

L5975 All lower extremity prostheses, combination single axis ankle and flexible keel foot   Ⓐ ⊘ &

L5976 All lower extremity prostheses, energy storing foot (Seattle Carbon Copy II or equal)   Ⓐ ⊘ &

L5978 All lower extremity prostheses, foot, multiaxial ankle/foot   Ⓐ ⊘ &

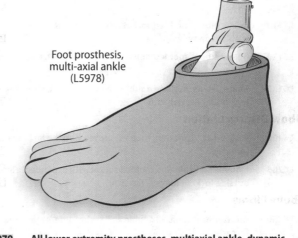

Foot prosthesis, multi-axial ankle (L5978)

L5979 All lower extremity prostheses, multiaxial ankle, dynamic response foot, one-piece system   Ⓐ ⊘ &

L5980 All lower extremity prostheses, flex-foot system   Ⓐ ⊘ &

L5981 All lower extremity prostheses, flex-walk system or equal   Ⓐ ⊘ &

L5982 All exoskeletal lower extremity prostheses, axial rotation unit   Ⓐ ⊘ &

L5984 All endoskeletal lower extremity prostheses, axial rotation unit, with or without adjustability   Ⓐ ⊘ &

Special Coverage Instructions   Noncovered by Medicare   Carrier Discretion   ☑ Quantity Alert   ● New Code   ○ Recycled/Reinstated   ▲ Revised Code

© 2021 Optum360, LLC   A2-Z3 ASC Pmt   CMS: IOM   AHA: Coding Clinic   & DMEPOS Paid   ⊘ SNF Excluded   **L Codes — 129**

Prosthetic Devices and Procedures

L5985 — L6588

L5985 All endoskeletal lower extremity prostheses, dynamic prosthetic pylon ▢Ⓐ⊘&

L5986 All lower extremity prostheses, multiaxial rotation unit (MCP or equal) Ⓐ⊘&

L5987 All lower extremity prostheses, shank foot system with vertical loading pylon Ⓐ&

L5988 Addition to lower limb prosthesis, vertical shock reducing pylon feature Ⓐ⊘&

L5990 Addition to lower extremity prosthesis, user adjustable heel height Ⓐ⊘&
AHA: 1Q, '02, 5

L5999 Lower extremity prosthesis, not otherwise specified Ⓐ
Determine if an alternative HCPCS Level II or a CPT code better describes the service being reported. This code should be used only if a more specific code is unavailable.

Partial Hand

L6000 Partial hand, thumb remaining Ⓐ&

L6010 Partial hand, little and/or ring finger remaining Ⓐ&

L6020 Partial hand, no finger remaining Ⓐ&

L6026 Transcarpal/metacarpal or partial hand disarticulation prosthesis, external power, self-suspended, inner socket with removable forearm section, electrodes and cables, two batteries, charger, myoelectric control of terminal device, excludes terminal device(s) Ⓐ&

Wrist Disarticulation

L6050 Wrist disarticulation, molded socket, flexible elbow hinges, triceps pad Ⓐ⊘&

L6055 Wrist disarticulation, molded socket with expandable interface, flexible elbow hinges, triceps pad Ⓐ⊘&

Below Elbow

L6100 Below elbow, molded socket, flexible elbow hinge, triceps pad Ⓐ⊘&

L6110 Below elbow, molded socket (Muenster or Northwestern suspension types) Ⓐ⊘&

L6120 Below elbow, molded double wall split socket, step-up hinges, half cuff Ⓐ⊘&

L6130 Below elbow, molded double wall split socket, stump activated locking hinge, half cuff Ⓐ⊘&

Elbow Disarticulation

L6200 Elbow disarticulation, molded socket, outside locking hinge, forearm Ⓐ⊘&

L6205 Elbow disarticulation, molded socket with expandable interface, outside locking hinges, forearm Ⓐ⊘&

Above Elbow

L6250 Above elbow, molded double wall socket, internal locking elbow, forearm Ⓐ⊘&

Shoulder Disarticulation

L6300 Shoulder disarticulation, molded socket, shoulder bulkhead, humeral section, internal locking elbow, forearm Ⓐ⊘&

L6310 Shoulder disarticulation, passive restoration (complete prosthesis) Ⓐ⊘&

L6320 Shoulder disarticulation, passive restoration (shoulder cap only) Ⓐ⊘&

Interscapular Thoracic

L6350 Interscapular thoracic, molded socket, shoulder bulkhead, humeral section, internal locking elbow, forearm Ⓐ⊘&

L6360 Interscapular thoracic, passive restoration (complete prosthesis) Ⓐ⊘&

L6370 Interscapular thoracic, passive restoration (shoulder cap only) Ⓐ⊘&

Immediate and Early Postsurgical Procedures

L6380 Immediate postsurgical or early fitting, application of initial rigid dressing, including fitting alignment and suspension of components, and one cast change, wrist disarticulation or below elbow Ⓐ&

L6382 Immediate postsurgical or early fitting, application of initial rigid dressing including fitting alignment and suspension of components, and one cast change, elbow disarticulation or above elbow Ⓐ▢&

L6384 Immediate postsurgical or early fitting, application of initial rigid dressing including fitting alignment and suspension of components, and one cast change, shoulder disarticulation or interscapular thoracic Ⓐ▢&

L6386 Immediate postsurgical or early fitting, each additional cast change and realignment Ⓐ▢&

L6388 Immediate postsurgical or early fitting, application of rigid dressing only Ⓐ&

Molded Socket

L6400 Below elbow, molded socket, endoskeletal system, including soft prosthetic tissue shaping Ⓐ⊘&

L6450 Elbow disarticulation, molded socket, endoskeletal system, including soft prosthetic tissue shaping Ⓐ⊘&

L6500 Above elbow, molded socket, endoskeletal system, including soft prosthetic tissue shaping Ⓐ⊘&

L6550 Shoulder disarticulation, molded socket, endoskeletal system, including soft prosthetic tissue shaping Ⓐ⊘&

L6570 Interscapular thoracic, molded socket, endoskeletal system, including soft prosthetic tissue shaping Ⓐ⊘&

Preparatory Socket

L6580 Preparatory, wrist disarticulation or below elbow, single wall plastic socket, friction wrist, flexible elbow hinges, figure of eight harness, humeral cuff, Bowden cable control, USMC or equal pylon, no cover, molded to patient model Ⓐ⊘&

L6582 Preparatory, wrist disarticulation or below elbow, single wall socket, friction wrist, flexible elbow hinges, figure of eight harness, humeral cuff, Bowden cable control, USMC or equal pylon, no cover, direct formed Ⓐ⊘&

L6584 Preparatory, elbow disarticulation or above elbow, single wall plastic socket, friction wrist, locking elbow, figure of eight harness, fair lead cable control, USMC or equal pylon, no cover, molded to patient model Ⓐ⊘&

L6586 Preparatory, elbow disarticulation or above elbow, single wall socket, friction wrist, locking elbow, figure of eight harness, fair lead cable control, USMC or equal pylon, no cover, direct formed Ⓐ⊘&

L6588 Preparatory, shoulder disarticulation or interscapular thoracic, single wall plastic socket, shoulder joint, locking elbow, friction wrist, chest strap, fair lead cable control, USMC or equal pylon, no cover, molded to patient model Ⓐ⊘&

Special Coverage Instructions   Noncovered by Medicare   Carrier Discretion   ☑ Quantity Alert ● New Code ○ Recycled/Reinstated ▲ Revised Code

130 — L Codes   Ⓐ Age Edit   Ⓜ Maternity Edit   ♀ Female Only   ♂ Male Only   Ⓐ-Ⓨ OPPS Status Indicators   © 2021 Optum360, LLC

L6590 Preparatory, shoulder disarticulation or interscapular thoracic, single wall socket, shoulder joint, locking elbow, friction wrist, chest strap, fair lead cable control, USMC or equal pylon, no cover, direct formed Ⓐ ⊘ ♿

Additions: Upper Limb

The following procedures/modifications/components may be added to other base procedures. The items in this section should reflect the additional complexity of each modification procedure, in addition to the base procedure, at the time of the original order.

L6600 Upper extremity additions, polycentric hinge, pair Ⓐ ☑ ⊘ ♿

L6605 Upper extremity additions, single pivot hinge, pair Ⓐ ☑ ⊘ ♿

L6610 Upper extremity additions, flexible metal hinge, pair Ⓐ ☑ ⊘ ♿

L6611 Addition to upper extremity prosthesis, external powered, additional switch, any type Ⓐ ⊘ ♿

L6615 Upper extremity addition, disconnect locking wrist unit Ⓐ ⊘ ♿

L6616 Upper extremity addition, additional disconnect insert for locking wrist unit, each Ⓐ ☑ ⊘ ♿

L6620 Upper extremity addition, flexion/extension wrist unit, with or without friction Ⓐ ⊘ ♿

L6621 Upper extremity prosthesis addition, flexion/extension wrist with or without friction, for use with external powered terminal device Ⓐ ⊘ ♿

L6623 Upper extremity addition, spring assisted rotational wrist unit with latch release Ⓐ ⊘ ♿

L6624 Upper extremity addition, flexion/extension and rotation wrist unit Ⓐ ⊘ ♿

L6625 Upper extremity addition, rotation wrist unit with cable lock Ⓐ ⊘ ♿

L6628 Upper extremity addition, quick disconnect hook adapter, Otto Bock or equal Ⓐ ⊘ ♿

L6629 Upper extremity addition, quick disconnect lamination collar with coupling piece, Otto Bock or equal Ⓐ ⊘ ♿

L6630 Upper extremity addition, stainless steel, any wrist Ⓐ ⊘ ♿

L6632 Upper extremity addition, latex suspension sleeve, each Ⓐ ☑ ⊘ ♿

L6635 Upper extremity addition, lift assist for elbow Ⓐ ⊘ ♿

L6637 Upper extremity addition, nudge control elbow lock Ⓐ ⊘ ♿

L6638 Upper extremity addition to prosthesis, electric locking feature, only for use with manually powered elbow Ⓐ ⊘ ♿

L6640 Upper extremity additions, shoulder abduction joint, pair Ⓐ ☑ ⊘ ♿

L6641 Upper extremity addition, excursion amplifier, pulley type Ⓐ ⊘ ♿

L6642 Upper extremity addition, excursion amplifier, lever type Ⓐ ⊘ ♿

L6645 Upper extremity addition, shoulder flexion-abduction joint, each Ⓐ ☑ ⊘ ♿

L6646 Upper extremity addition, shoulder joint, multipositional locking, flexion, adjustable abduction friction control, for use with body powered or external powered system Ⓐ ⊘ ♿

L6647 Upper extremity addition, shoulder lock mechanism, body powered actuator Ⓐ ⊘ ♿

L6648 Upper extremity addition, shoulder lock mechanism, external powered actuator Ⓐ ⊘ ♿

L6650 Upper extremity addition, shoulder universal joint, each Ⓐ ☑ ⊘ ♿

L6655 Upper extremity addition, standard control cable, extra Ⓐ ⊘ ♿

L6660 Upper extremity addition, heavy-duty control cable Ⓐ ⊘ ♿

L6665 Upper extremity addition, Teflon, or equal, cable lining Ⓐ ⊘ ♿

L6670 Upper extremity addition, hook to hand, cable adapter Ⓐ ⊘ ♿

L6672 Upper extremity addition, harness, chest or shoulder, saddle type Ⓐ ⊘ ♿

L6675 Upper extremity addition, harness, (e.g., figure of eight type), single cable design Ⓐ ⊘ ♿

L6676 Upper extremity addition, harness, (e.g., figure of eight type), dual cable design Ⓐ ⊘ ♿

L6677 Upper extremity addition, harness, triple control, simultaneous operation of terminal device and elbow Ⓐ ⊘ ♿

L6680 Upper extremity addition, test socket, wrist disarticulation or below elbow Ⓐ ⊘ ♿

L6682 Upper extremity addition, test socket, elbow disarticulation or above elbow Ⓐ ⊘ ♿

L6684 Upper extremity addition, test socket, shoulder disarticulation or interscapular thoracic Ⓐ ⊘ ♿

L6686 Upper extremity addition, suction socket Ⓐ ⊘ ♿

L6687 Upper extremity addition, frame type socket, below elbow or wrist disarticulation Ⓐ ⊘ ♿

L6688 Upper extremity addition, frame type socket, above elbow or elbow disarticulation Ⓐ ⊘ ♿

L6689 Upper extremity addition, frame type socket, shoulder disarticulation Ⓐ ⊘ ♿

L6690 Upper extremity addition, frame type socket, interscapular-thoracic Ⓐ ⊘ ♿

L6691 Upper extremity addition, removable insert, each Ⓐ ☑ ⊘ ♿

L6692 Upper extremity addition, silicone gel insert or equal, each Ⓐ ☑ ⊘ ♿

L6693 Upper extremity addition, locking elbow, forearm counterbalance Ⓐ ⊘ ♿

L6694 Addition to upper extremity prosthesis, below elbow/above elbow, custom fabricated from existing mold or prefabricated, socket insert, silicone gel, elastomeric or equal, for use with locking mechanism Ⓐ ⊘ ♿

L6695 Addition to upper extremity prosthesis, below elbow/above elbow, custom fabricated from existing mold or prefabricated, socket insert, silicone gel, elastomeric or equal, not for use with locking mechanism Ⓐ ⊘ ♿

L6696 Addition to upper extremity prosthesis, below elbow/above elbow, custom fabricated socket insert for congenital or atypical traumatic amputee, silicone gel, elastomeric or equal, for use with or without locking mechanism, initial only (for other than initial, use code L6694 or L6695) Ⓐ ⊘ ♿

L6697 Addition to upper extremity prosthesis, below elbow/above elbow, custom fabricated socket insert for other than congenital or atypical traumatic amputee, silicone gel, elastomeric or equal, for use with or without locking mechanism, initial only (for other than initial, use code L6694 or L6695) Ⓐ ⊘ ♿

L6698 Addition to upper extremity prosthesis, below elbow/above elbow, lock mechanism, excludes socket insert Ⓐ ⊘ ♿

Special Coverage Instructions | Noncovered by Medicare | Carrier Discretion | ☑ Quantity Alert | ● New Code | ○ Recycled/Reinstated | ▲ Revised Code

© 2021 Optum360, LLC | Ⓐ²-Ⓩ³ ASC Pmt | CMS: IOM | AHA: Coding Clinic | ♿ DMEPOS Paid | ⊘ SNF Excluded | L Codes — 131

Prosthetic Devices and Procedures

L6703 — L6970

Terminal Device

L6703 Terminal device, passive hand/mitt, any material, any size Ⓐ ⊘ ♿

L6704 Terminal device, sport/recreational/work attachment, any material, any size Ⓐ ⊘ ♿

L6706 Terminal device, hook, mechanical, voluntary opening, any material, any size, lined or unlined Ⓐ ⊘ ♿

L6707 Terminal device, hook, mechanical, voluntary closing, any material, any size, lined or unlined Ⓐ ⊘ ♿

L6708 Terminal device, hand, mechanical, voluntary opening, any material, any size Ⓐ ⊘ ♿

L6709 Terminal device, hand, mechanical, voluntary closing, any material, any size Ⓐ ⊘ ♿

L6711 Terminal device, hook, mechanical, voluntary opening, any material, any size, lined or unlined, pediatric Ⓐ ♿

L6712 Terminal device, hook, mechanical, voluntary closing, any material, any size, lined or unlined, pediatric Ⓐ ♿

L6713 Terminal device, hand, mechanical, voluntary opening, any material, any size, pediatric Ⓐ ♿

L6714 Terminal device, hand, mechanical, voluntary closing, any material, any size, pediatric Ⓐ ♿

L6715 Terminal device, multiple articulating digit, includes motor(s), initial issue or replacement Ⓐ ♿

L6721 Terminal device, hook or hand, heavy-duty, mechanical, voluntary opening, any material, any size, lined or unlined Ⓐ ♿

L6722 Terminal device, hook or hand, heavy-duty, mechanical, voluntary closing, any material, any size, lined or unlined Ⓐ ♿

Addition to Terminal Device

L6805 Addition to terminal device, modifier wrist unit Ⓐ ⊘ ♿

L6810 Addition to terminal device, precision pinch device Ⓐ ⊘ ♿

L6880 Electric hand, switch or myoelectric controlled, independently articulating digits, any grasp pattern or combination of grasp patterns, includes motor(s) Ⓐ ♿

L6881 Automatic grasp feature, addition to upper limb electric prosthetic terminal device Ⓐ ⊘ ♿
  AHA: 1Q, '02, 5

L6882 Microprocessor control feature, addition to upper limb prosthetic terminal device Ⓐ ⊘ ♿
  AHA: 1Q, '02, 5

Replacement Socket

L6883 Replacement socket, below elbow/wrist disarticulation, molded to patient model, for use with or without external power Ⓐ ⊘ ♿

L6884 Replacement socket, above elbow/elbow disarticulation, molded to patient model, for use with or without external power Ⓐ ⊘ ♿

L6885 Replacement socket, shoulder disarticulation/interscapular thoracic, molded to patient model, for use with or without external power Ⓐ ⊘ ♿

Hand Restoration

L6890 Addition to upper extremity prosthesis, glove for terminal device, any material, prefabricated, includes fitting and adjustment Ⓐ ♿

L6895 Addition to upper extremity prosthesis, glove for terminal device, any material, custom fabricated Ⓐ ♿

L6900 Hand restoration (casts, shading and measurements included), partial hand, with glove, thumb or one finger remaining Ⓐ ♿

L6905 Hand restoration (casts, shading and measurements included), partial hand, with glove, multiple fingers remaining Ⓐ ♿

L6910 Hand restoration (casts, shading and measurements included), partial hand, with glove, no fingers remaining Ⓐ ♿

L6915 Hand restoration (shading and measurements included), replacement glove for above Ⓐ ♿

External Power

L6920 Wrist disarticulation, external power, self-suspended inner socket, removable forearm shell, Otto Bock or equal switch, cables, two batteries and one charger, switch control of terminal device Ⓐ ⊘ ♿

L6925 Wrist disarticulation, external power, self-suspended inner socket, removable forearm shell, Otto Bock or equal electrodes, cables, two batteries and one charger, myoelectronic control of terminal device Ⓐ ⊘ ♿

L6930 Below elbow, external power, self-suspended inner socket, removable forearm shell, Otto Bock or equal switch, cables, two batteries and one charger, switch control of terminal device Ⓐ ⊘ ♿

L6935 Below elbow, external power, self-suspended inner socket, removable forearm shell, Otto Bock or equal electrodes, cables, two batteries and one charger, myoelectronic control of terminal device Ⓐ ⊘ ♿

L6940 Elbow disarticulation, external power, molded inner socket, removable humeral shell, outside locking hinges, forearm, Otto Bock or equal switch, cables, two batteries and one charger, switch control of terminal device Ⓐ ⊘ ♿

L6945 Elbow disarticulation, external power, molded inner socket, removable humeral shell, outside locking hinges, forearm, Otto Bock or equal electrodes, cables, two batteries and one charger, myoelectronic control of terminal device Ⓐ ⊘ ♿

L6950 Above elbow, external power, molded inner socket, removable humeral shell, internal locking elbow, forearm, Otto Bock or equal switch, cables, two batteries and one charger, switch control of terminal device Ⓐ ⊘ ♿

L6955 Above elbow, external power, molded inner socket, removable humeral shell, internal locking elbow, forearm, Otto Bock or equal electrodes, cables, two batteries and one charger, myoelectronic control of terminal device Ⓐ ⊘ ♿

L6960 Shoulder disarticulation, external power, molded inner socket, removable shoulder shell, shoulder bulkhead, humeral section, mechanical elbow, forearm, Otto Bock or equal switch, cables, two batteries and one charger, switch control of terminal device Ⓐ ⊘ ♿

L6965 Shoulder disarticulation, external power, molded inner socket, removable shoulder shell, shoulder bulkhead, humeral section, mechanical elbow, forearm, Otto Bock or equal electrodes, cables, two batteries and one charger, myoelectronic control of terminal device Ⓐ ⊘ ♿

L6970 Interscapular-thoracic, external power, molded inner socket, removable shoulder shell, shoulder bulkhead, humeral section, mechanical elbow, forearm, Otto Bock or equal switch, cables, two batteries and one charger, switch control of terminal device Ⓐ ⊘ ♿

Special Coverage Instructions   Noncovered by Medicare   Carrier Discretion   ☑ Quantity Alert ● New Code   ○ Recycled/Reinstated   ▲ Revised Code

132 — L Codes   Ⓐ Age Edit   Ⓜ Maternity Edit   ♀ Female Only   ♂ Male Only   Ⓐ-Ⓨ OPPS Status Indicators   © 2021 Optum360, LLC

2022 HCPCS Level II

L6975 Interscapular-thoracic, external power, molded inner socket, removable shoulder shell, shoulder bulkhead, humeral section, mechanical elbow, forearm, Otto Bock or equal electrodes, cables, two batteries and one charger, myoelectronic control of terminal device Ⓐ ⊘ ⅙

Electric Hand and Accessories

L7007 Electric hand, switch or myoelectric controlled, adult Ⓐ Ⓐ ⊘ ⅙

L7008 Electric hand, switch or myoelectric, controlled, pediatric Ⓐ Ⓐ ⊘ ⅙

L7009 Electric hook, switch or myoelectric controlled, adult Ⓐ Ⓐ ⊘ ⅙

L7040 Prehensile actuator, switch controlled Ⓐ ⊘ ⅙

L7045 Electric hook, switch or myoelectric controlled, pediatric Ⓐ ⊘ ⅙

Electronic Elbow and Accessories

L7170 Electronic elbow, Hosmer or equal, switch controlled Ⓐ ⊘ ⅙

L7180 Electronic elbow, microprocessor sequential control of elbow and terminal device Ⓐ ⊘ ⅙

L7181 Electronic elbow, microprocessor simultaneous control of elbow and terminal device Ⓐ ⊘ ⅙

L7185 Electronic elbow, adolescent, Variety Village or equal, switch controlled Ⓐ ⊘ ⅙

L7186 Electronic elbow, child, Variety Village or equal, switch controlled Ⓐ ⊘ ⅙

L7190 Electronic elbow, adolescent, Variety Village or equal, myoelectronically controlled Ⓐ ⊘ ⅙

L7191 Electronic elbow, child, Variety Village or equal, myoelectronically controlled Ⓐ ⊘ ⅙

Electronic Wrist and Accessories

L7259 Electronic wrist rotator, any type Ⓐ ⅙

Battery Components

L7360 Six volt battery, each Ⓐ ☑ ⅙

L7362 Battery charger, six volt, each Ⓐ ☑ ⊘ ⅙

L7364 Twelve volt battery, each Ⓐ ☑ ⊘ ⅙

L7366 Battery charger, 12 volt, each Ⓐ ☑ ⊘ ⅙

L7367 Lithium ion battery, rechargeable, replacement Ⓐ ⊘ ⅙

L7368 Lithium ion battery charger, replacement only Ⓐ ⊘ ⅙

Additions to Upper Extremity Prosthesis

L7400 Addition to upper extremity prosthesis, below elbow/wrist disarticulation, ultra-light material (titanium, carbon fiber or equal) Ⓐ ⊘ ⅙

L7401 Addition to upper extremity prosthesis, above elbow disarticulation, ultra-light material (titanium, carbon fiber or equal) Ⓐ ⊘ ⅙

L7402 Addition to upper extremity prosthesis, shoulder disarticulation/interscapular thoracic, ultra-light material (titanium, carbon fiber or equal) Ⓐ ⊘ ⅙

L7403 Addition to upper extremity prosthesis, below elbow/wrist disarticulation, acrylic material Ⓐ ⊘ ⅙

L7404 Addition to upper extremity prosthesis, above elbow disarticulation, acrylic material Ⓐ ⊘ ⅙

L7405 Addition to upper extremity prosthesis, shoulder disarticulation/interscapular thoracic, acrylic material Ⓐ ⊘ ⅙

L7499 Upper extremity prosthesis, not otherwise specified Ⓐ

Repairs

L7510 Repair of prosthetic device, repair or replace minor parts Ⓐ
Medicare jurisdiction: local contractor if repair of implanted prosthetic device.

L7520 Repair prosthetic device, labor component, per 15 minutes Ⓐ ☑
Medicare jurisdiction: local contractor if repair of implanted prosthetic device.

Prosthesis Supplies

L7600 Prosthetic donning sleeve, any material, each Ⓔ ☑

L7700 Gasket or seal, for use with prosthetic socket insert, any type, each Ⓐ ⅙

Male Prosthetic

L7900 Male vacuum erection system ♂ Ⓔ

L7902 Tension ring, for vacuum erection device, any type, replacement only, each ♂ Ⓔ

Breast Prosthesis

L8000 Breast prosthesis, mastectomy bra, without integrated breast prosthesis form, any size, any type ♀ Ⓐ ⅙

L8001 Breast prosthesis, mastectomy bra, with integrated breast prosthesis form, unilateral, any size, any type ♀ Ⓐ ⅙
AHA: 1Q, '02, 5

L8002 Breast prosthesis, mastectomy bra, with integrated breast prosthesis form, bilateral, any size, any type ♀ Ⓐ ⅙
AHA: 1Q, '02, 5

L8010 Breast prosthesis, mastectomy sleeve ♀ Ⓐ

L8015 External breast prosthesis garment, with mastectomy form, post mastectomy ♀ Ⓐ ⅙

L8020 Breast prosthesis, mastectomy form ♀ Ⓐ ⅙

L8030 Breast prosthesis, silicone or equal, without integral adhesive ♀ Ⓐ ⅙

L8031 Breast prosthesis, silicone or equal, with integral adhesive Ⓐ ⅙

L8032 Nipple prosthesis, prefabricated, reusable, any type, each Ⓐ ☑ ⅙

L8033 Nipple prosthesis, custom fabricated, reusable, any material, any type, each

L8035 Custom breast prosthesis, post mastectomy, molded to patient model ♀ Ⓐ ⅙

L8039 Breast prosthesis, not otherwise specified ♀ Ⓐ

Special Coverage Instructions Noncovered by Medicare Carrier Discretion ☑ Quantity Alert ● New Code ○ Recycled/Reinstated ▲ Revised Code

© 2021 Optum360, LLC Ⓐ²-Ⓩ³ ASC Pmt CMS: IOM AHA: Coding Clinic ⅙ DMEPOS Paid ⊘ SNF Excluded L Codes — 133

Prosthetic Devices and Procedures

L8040 — L8515

Face and Ear Prosthesis

L8040   Nasal prosthesis, provided by a nonphysician   Ⓐ &. (KM, KN)
CMS: 100-04,20,30.9

Nasal prosthesis (L8040)

Orbital and midfacial prosthesis (L8041-L8042)

Prosthesis ▭

Facial prosthetics are typically custom manufactured from polymers and carefully matched to the original features. The maxilla, zygoma, frontal, and nasal bones are often involved, either singly or in combination (L8040-L8044)

Frontal bone
Nasal bone
Maxilla ▬
Zygoma ▨
(L8043–L8044)

L8041   Midfacial prosthesis, provided by a nonphysician   Ⓐ &. (KM, KN)
CMS: 100-04,20,30.9

L8042   Orbital prosthesis, provided by a nonphysician   Ⓐ &. (KM, KN)
CMS: 100-04,20,30.9

L8043   Upper facial prosthesis, provided by a nonphysician   Ⓐ &. (KM, KN)
CMS: 100-04,20,30.9

L8044   Hemi-facial prosthesis, provided by a nonphysician   Ⓐ &. (KM, KN)
CMS: 100-04,20,30.9

L8045   Auricular prosthesis, provided by a nonphysician   Ⓐ &. (KM, KN)
CMS: 100-04,20,30.9

L8046   Partial facial prosthesis, provided by a nonphysician   Ⓐ &. (KM, KN)
CMS: 100-04,20,30.9

L8047   Nasal septal prosthesis, provided by a nonphysician   Ⓐ &. (KM, KN)
CMS: 100-04,20,30.9

L8048   Unspecified maxillofacial prosthesis, by report, provided by a nonphysician   Ⓐ

L8049   Repair or modification of maxillofacial prosthesis, labor component, 15 minute increments, provided by a nonphysician   Ⓐ

Trusses

L8300   Truss, single with standard pad   Ⓐ &.

L8310   Truss, double with standard pads   Ⓐ &.

L8320   Truss, addition to standard pad, water pad   Ⓐ &.

L8330   Truss, addition to standard pad, scrotal pad   ♂ Ⓐ &.

Prosthetic Socks

L8400   Prosthetic sheath, below knee, each   Ⓐ ☑ &.

L8410   Prosthetic sheath, above knee, each   Ⓐ ☑ &.

L8415   Prosthetic sheath, upper limb, each   Ⓐ ☑ &.

L8417   Prosthetic sheath/sock, including a gel cushion layer, below knee (BK) or above knee (AK), each   Ⓐ ☑ &.

L8420   Prosthetic sock, multiple ply, below knee (BK), each   Ⓐ ☑ &.

L8430   Prosthetic sock, multiple ply, above knee (AK), each   Ⓐ ☑ &.

L8435   Prosthetic sock, multiple ply, upper limb, each   Ⓐ ☑ &.

L8440   Prosthetic shrinker, below knee (BK), each   Ⓐ ☑ &.

L8460   Prosthetic shrinker, above knee (AK), each   Ⓐ ☑ &.

L8465   Prosthetic shrinker, upper limb, each   Ⓐ ☑ &.

L8470   Prosthetic sock, single ply, fitting, below knee (BK), each   Ⓐ ☑ &.

L8480   Prosthetic sock, single ply, fitting, above knee (AK), each   Ⓐ ☑ &.

L8485   Prosthetic sock, single ply, fitting, upper limb, each   Ⓐ ☑ &.

L8499   Unlisted procedure for miscellaneous prosthetic services   Ⓐ
Determine if an alternative HCPCS Level II or a CPT code better describes the service being reported. This code should be used only if a more specific code is unavailable.

Larynx and Trachea Prothetics and Accessories

L8500   Artificial larynx, any type   Ⓐ &.

L8501   Tracheostomy speaking valve   Ⓐ &.

L8505   Artificial larynx replacement battery/accessory, any type   Ⓐ
AHA: 1Q, '02, 5

L8507   Tracheo-esophageal voice prosthesis, patient inserted, any type, each   Ⓐ ☑ &.
AHA: 1Q, '02, 5

L8509   Tracheo-esophageal voice prosthesis, inserted by a licensed health care provider, any type   Ⓐ &.
AHA: 1Q, '02, 5

L8510   Voice amplifier   Ⓐ &.
AHA: 1Q, '02, 5

L8511   Insert for indwelling tracheo-esophageal prosthesis, with or without valve, replacement only, each   Ⓐ ☑ &.

L8512   Gelatin capsules or equivalent, for use with tracheo-esophageal voice prosthesis, replacement only, per 10   Ⓐ ☑ &.

L8513   Cleaning device used with tracheoesophageal voice prosthesis, pipet, brush, or equal, replacement only, each   Ⓐ ☑ &.

L8514   Tracheo-esophageal puncture dilator, replacement only, each   Ⓐ ☑ &.

L8515   Gelatin capsule, application device for use with tracheo-esophageal voice prosthesis, each   Ⓐ ☑ &.

Special Coverage Instructions   Noncovered by Medicare   Carrier Discretion   ☑ Quantity Alert   ● New Code   ○ Recycled/Reinstated   ▲ Revised Code

134 — L Codes   Ⓐ Age Edit   Ⓜ Maternity Edit   ♀ Female Only   ♂ Male Only   Ⓐ-Ⓨ OPPS Status Indicators   © 2021 Optum360, LLC

Breast Implant

L8600 **Implantable breast prosthesis, silicone or equal**   ♀ N NI &
Medicare covers implants inserted in post-mastectomy reconstruction in a breast cancer patient. Always report concurrent to the implant procedure.
CMS: 100-04,4,190

Pectoralis muscle
Rib bones
Prosthesis
Gel-type prosthesis

Bulking Agents

L8603 **Injectable bulking agent, collagen implant, urinary tract, 2.5 ml syringe, includes shipping and necessary supplies**   N NI ☑
CMS: 100-04,4,190

L8604 **Injectable bulking agent, dextranomer/hyaluronic acid copolymer implant, urinary tract, 1 ml, includes shipping and necessary supplies**   N NI ☑

L8605 **Injectable bulking agent, dextranomer/hyaluronic acid copolymer implant, anal canal, 1 ml, includes shipping and necessary supplies**   N NI &

L8606 **Injectable bulking agent, synthetic implant, urinary tract, 1 ml syringe, includes shipping and necessary supplies**   N NI ☑ &

L8607 **Injectable bulking agent for vocal cord medialization, 0.1 ml, includes shipping and necessary supplies**   N NI &

Eye and Ear Implants and Accessories

L8608 **Miscellaneous external component, supply or accessory for use with the Argus II Retinal Prosthesis System**

L8609 **Artificial cornea**   N NI &

L8610 **Ocular implant**   N NI &
CMS: 100-04,4,190

L8612 **Aqueous shunt**   N NI &
CMS: 100-04,4,190

L8613 **Ossicula implant**   N NI &
CMS: 100-04,4,190

L8614 **Cochlear device, includes all internal and external components**   N NI &
A cochlear implant is covered by Medicare when the patient has bilateral sensorineural deafness.
CMS: 100-04,14,40.8; 100-04,4,190
AHA: 3Q, '16, 10-15; 4Q, '03, 8; 3Q, '02, 4-5; 1Q, '01, 6

L8615 **Headset/headpiece for use with cochlear implant device, replacement**   A &

L8616 **Microphone for use with cochlear implant device, replacement**   A &

L8617 **Transmitting coil for use with cochlear implant device, replacement**   A &

L8618 **Transmitter cable for use with cochlear implant device or auditory osseointegrated device, replacement**   A &

L8619 **Cochlear implant, external speech processor and controller, integrated system, replacement**   A &
Medicare jurisdiction: local contractor.

L8621 **Zinc air battery for use with cochlear implant device and auditory osseointegrated sound processors, replacement, each**   A ☑ &

L8622 **Alkaline battery for use with cochlear implant device, any size, replacement, each**   A ☑ &

L8623 **Lithium ion battery for use with cochlear implant device speech processor, other than ear level, replacement, each**   A ☑ &

L8624 **Lithium ion battery for use with cochlear implant or auditory osseointegrated device speech processor, ear level, replacement, each**   A ☑ &

L8625 **External recharging system for battery for use with cochlear implant or auditory osseointegrated device, replacement only, each**   A &

L8627 **Cochlear implant, external speech processor, component, replacement**   A &

L8628 **Cochlear implant, external controller component, replacement**   A &

L8629 **Transmitting coil and cable, integrated, for use with cochlear implant device, replacement**   A &

Upper Extremity Implants

L8630 **Metacarpophalangeal joint implant**   N NI &
CMS: 100-04,4,190

Bone is cut at the MP joint (arthroplasty)

Bone may be hollowed out in both metacarpal and phalangeal sides in preparation for a prosthesis

Prosthetic joint implant

Prosthesis in place

Metacarpophalangeal prosthetic implant

L8631 **Metacarpal phalangeal joint replacement, two or more pieces, metal (e.g., stainless steel or cobalt chrome), ceramic-like material (e.g., pyrocarbon), for surgical implantation (all sizes, includes entire system)**   N NI &

Special Coverage Instructions   Noncovered by Medicare   Carrier Discretion   ☑ Quantity Alert   ● New Code   ○ Recycled/Reinstated   ▲ Revised Code

© 2021 Optum360, LLC   A2-Z3 ASC Pmt   CMS: IOM   AHA: Coding Clinic   & DMEPOS Paid   ⊘ SNF Excluded   L Codes — 135

Prosthetic Devices and Procedures

L8641 — L9900

Lower Extremity Implants

L8641   Metatarsal joint implant   N M &
CMS: 100-04,4,190

L8642   Hallux implant   N M &
CMS: 100-04,4,190

Interphalangeal Implants

L8658   Interphalangeal joint spacer, silicone or equal, each N M ☑ &
CMS: 100-04,4,190

L8659   Interphalangeal finger joint replacement, two or more pieces, metal (e.g., stainless steel or cobalt chrome), ceramic-like material (e.g., pyrocarbon) for surgical implantation, any size   N M &

Cardiovascular Implant

L8670   Vascular graft material, synthetic, implant   N M &
CMS: 100-04,4,190

Neurostimulator and Accessories

L8679   Implantable neurostimulator, pulse generator, any type   N M &

L8680   Implantable neurostimulator electrode, each   E ☑

L8681   Patient programmer (external) for use with implantable programmable neurostimulator pulse generator, replacement only   A &

L8682   Implantable neurostimulator radiofrequency receiver   N M &

L8683   Radiofrequency transmitter (external) for use with implantable neurostimulator radiofrequency receiver   A &

L8684   Radiofrequency transmitter (external) for use with implantable sacral root neurostimulator receiver for bowel and bladder management, replacement   A &

L8685   Implantable neurostimulator pulse generator, single array, rechargeable, includes extension   E

L8686   Implantable neurostimulator pulse generator, single array, nonrechargeable, includes extension   E

L8687   Implantable neurostimulator pulse generator, dual array, rechargeable, includes extension   E

L8688   Implantable neurostimulator pulse generator, dual array, nonrechargeable, includes extension   E

L8689   External recharging system for battery (internal) for use with implantable neurostimulator, replacement only   A &

Miscellaneous Prosthetics and Accessories

L8690   Auditory osseointegrated device, includes all internal and external components   N M &
CMS: 100-04,14,40.8
AHA: 3Q, '16, 10-15

L8691   Auditory osseointegrated device, external sound processor, excludes transducer/actuator, replacement only, each   A &

L8692   Auditory osseointegrated device, external sound processor, used without osseointegration, body worn, includes headband or other means of external attachment   E

L8693   Auditory osseointegrated device abutment, any length, replacement only   A &

L8694   Auditory osseointegrated device, transducer/actuator, replacement only, each   A &

L8695   External recharging system for battery (external) for use with implantable neurostimulator, replacement only   A &

L8696   Antenna (external) for use with implantable diaphragmatic/phrenic nerve stimulation device, replacement, each   A &

L8698   Miscellaneous component, supply or accessory for use with total artificial heart system

L8699   Prosthetic implant, not otherwise specified   N M
Determine if an alternative HCPCS Level II or a CPT code better describes the service being reported. This code should be used only if a more specific code is unavailable.
CMS: 100-04,4,190
AHA: 3Q, '15, 2

L8701   Powered upper extremity range of motion assist device, elbow, wrist, hand with single or double upright(s), includes microprocessor, sensors, all components and accessories, custom fabricated

L8702   Powered upper extremity range of motion assist device, elbow, wrist, hand, finger, single or double upright(s), includes microprocessor, sensors, all components and accessories, custom fabricated

L9900   Orthotic and prosthetic supply, accessory, and/or service component of another HCPCS L code   N M

▢ Special Coverage Instructions   ▢ Noncovered by Medicare   Carrier Discretion   ☑ Quantity Alert   ● New Code   ○ Recycled/Reinstated   ▲ Revised Code

136 — L Codes   A Age Edit   M Maternity Edit   ♀ Female Only   ♂ Male Only   A-Y OPPS Status Indicators   © 2021 Optum360, LLC

Medical Services M0075-M0301

Other Medical Services

M codes include office services, cellular therapy, prolotherapy, intragastric hypothermia, IV chelation therapy, and fabric wrapping of an abdominal aneurysm.

M0075 **Cellular therapy**   E

The therapeutic efficacy of injecting foreign proteins has not been established.

M0076 **Prolotherapy**   E

The therapeutic efficacy of prolotherapy and joint sclerotherapy has not been established.

M0100 **Intragastric hypothermia using gastric freezing**   E

Code with caution: This procedure is considered obsolete.

● **M0201** **COVID-19 vaccine administration inside a patient's home; reported only once per individual home, per date of service, when only COVID-19 vaccine administration is performed at the patient's home**

M0239 ~~Intravenous infusion, bamlanivimab-xxxx, includes infusion and post administration monitoring~~

● **M0240** **Intravenous infusion or subcutaneous injection, casirivimab and imdevimab, includes infusion or injection and post administration monitoring, subsequent repeat doses**

Use this code for casirivimab and imdevimab 600 mg administered as post exposure prophylaxis. Report also Q0240 for drug.

● **M0241** **Intravenous infusion or subcutaneous injection, casirivimab and imdevimab, includes infusion or injection, and post administration monitoring in the home or residence. This includes a beneficiary's home that has been made provider-based to the hospital during the covid-19 public health emergency, subsequent repeat doses**

Use this code for casirivimab and imdevimab 600 mg administered as post exposure prophylaxis. Report also Q0240 for drug.

▲ **M0243** **Intravenous infusion or subcutaneous injection, casirivimab and imdevimab, includes infusion or injection, and post administration monitoring**

Use this code for administration of Casirivimab and Imdevimab (REGN-COV2), Regeneron. Report also Q0243 for drug.

▲ **M0244** **Intravenous infusion or subcutaneous injection, casirivimab and imdevimab, includes infusion or injection and post administration monitoring in the home or residence; this includes a beneficiary's home that has been made provider-based to the hospital during the COVID-19 public health emergency**

Use this code for administration of casirivimab and imdevimab in the home setting. Report also Q0243 for drug.

● **M0245** **Intravenous infusion, bamlanivimab and etesevimab, includes infusion and post administration monitoring**

Use this code for administration of bamlanivimab (LY-CoV555) and etesevimab (LY-CoV016). Report also Q0245 for drug.

● **M0246** **Intravenous infusion, bamlanivimab and etesevimab, includes infusion and post administration monitoring in the home or residence; this includes a beneficiary's home that has been made provider-based to the hospital during the COVID-19 public health emergency**

Use this code for administration of bamlanivimab and etesevimab in the home setting. Report also Q0245 for drug.

● **M0247** **Intravenous infusion, sotrovimab, includes infusion and post administration monitoring**

● **M0248** **Intravenous infusion, sotrovimab, includes infusion and post administration monitoring in the home or residence; this includes a beneficiary's home that has been made provider-based to the hospital during the COVID-19 public health emergency**

● **M0249** **Intravenous infusion, tocilizumab, for hospitalized adults and pediatric patients (2 years of age and older) with COVID-19 who are receiving systemic corticosteroids and require supplemental oxygen, non-invasive or invasive mechanical ventilation, or extracorporeal membrane oxygenation (ECMO) only, includes infusion and post administration monitoring, first dose**

● **M0250** **Intravenous infusion, tocilizumab, for hospitalized adults and pediatric patients (2 years of age and older) with COVID-19 who are receiving systemic corticosteroids and require supplemental oxygen, non-invasive or invasive mechanical ventilation, or extracorporeal membrane oxygenation (ECMO) only, includes infusion and post administration monitoring, second dose**

Cardiovascular Services

M0300 **IV chelation therapy (chemical endarterectomy)**   E

Chelation therapy is considered experimental in the United States.
CMS: 100-03*; 100-03,20.22

M0301 **Fabric wrapping of abdominal aneurysm**   E

Code with caution: This procedure has largely been replaced with more effective treatment modalities. Submit documentation.

Quality Measures M1003-M1149

Quality Measures

M1003 **TB screening performed and results interpreted within 12 months prior to initiation of first-time biologic disease modifying antirheumatic drug therapy**

M1004 **Documentation of medical reason for not screening for TB or interpreting results (i.e., patient positive for TB and documentation of past treatment; patient who has recently completed a course of anti-TB therapy)**

M1005 **TB screening not performed or results not interpreted, reason not given**

M1006 **Disease activity not assessed, reason not given**

M1007 **>=50% of total number of a patient's outpatient RA encounters assessed**

M1008 **<50% of total number of a patient's outpatient RA encounters assessed**

M1009 **Discharge/discontinuation of the episode of care documented in the medical record**

M1010 **Discharge/discontinuation of the episode of care documented in the medical record**

M1011 **Discharge/discontinuation of the episode of care documented in the medical record**

M1012 **Discharge/discontinuation of the episode of care documented in the medical record**

M1013 **Discharge/discontinuation of the episode of care documented in the medical record**

M1014 **Discharge/discontinuation of the episode of care documented in the medical record**

M1016 **Female patients unable to bear children**

M1017 **Patient admitted to palliative care services**

M1018 **Patients with an active diagnosis or history of cancer (except basal cell and squamous cell skin carcinoma), patients who are heavy tobacco smokers, lung cancer screening patients**

M1019 **Adolescent patients 12 to 17 years of age with major depression or dysthymia who reached remission at 12 months as demonstrated by a 12 month (+/-60 days) PHQ-9 or PHQ-9M score of less than 5**

Special Coverage Instructions   Noncovered by Medicare   Carrier Discretion   ☑ Quantity Alert   ● New Code   ○ Recycled/Reinstated   ▲ Revised Code

© 2021 Optum360, LLC   A2-Z3 ASC Pmt   **CMS:** IOM   **AHA:** Coding Clinic   ⅄ DMEPOS Paid   ⊘ SNF Excluded   **M Codes — 137**

Quality Measures

M1020 — M1089

M1020 Adolescent patients 12 to 17 years of age with major depression or dysthymia who did not reach remission at 12 months as demonstrated by a 12 month (+/-60 days) PHQ-9 or PHQ-9M score of less than 5. Either PHQ-9 or PHQ-9M score was not assessed or is greater than or equal to 5

M1021 Patient had only urgent care visits during the performance period

M1022 Patients who were in hospice at any time during the performance period

M1025 Patients who were in hospice at any time during the performance period

M1026 Patients who were in hospice at any time during the performance period

M1027 Imaging of the head (CT or MRI) was obtained

M1028 Documentation of patients with primary headache diagnosis and imaging other than CT or MRI obtained

M1029 Imaging of the head (CT or MRI) was not obtained, reason not given

M1031 Patients with no clinical indications for imaging of the head

M1032 Adults currently taking pharmacotherapy for OUD

M1034 Adults who have at least 180 days of continuous pharmacotherapy with a medication prescribed for OUD without a gap of more than seven days

M1035 Adults who are deliberately phased out of medication assisted treatment (MAT) prior to 180 days of continuous treatment

M1036 Adults who have not had at least 180 days of continuous pharmacotherapy with a medication prescribed for OUD without a gap of more than seven days

M1037 Patients with a diagnosis of lumbar spine region cancer at the time of the procedure

M1038 Patients with a diagnosis of lumbar spine region fracture at the time of the procedure

M1039 Patients with a diagnosis of lumbar spine region infection at the time of the procedure

M1040 Patients with a diagnosis of lumbar idiopathic or congenital scoliosis

M1041 Patient had cancer, acute fracture or infection related to the lumbar spine or patient had neuromuscular, idiopathic or congenital lumbar scoliosis

M1043 Functional status was not measured by the Oswestry Disability Index (ODI version 2.1a) at 1 year (9 to 15 months) postoperatively

M1045 Functional status measured by the Oxford Knee Score (OKS) at one year (9 to 15 months) postoperatively was greater than or equal to 37 or knee injury and osteoarthritis outcome score joint replacement (KOOS, JR.) was greater than or equal to 71

M1046 Functional status measured by the Oxford Knee Score (OKS) at one year (9 to 15 months) postoperatively was less than 37 or the knee injury and osteoarthritis outcome score joint replacement (KOOS, JR.) was less than 71 postoperatively

M1049 Functional status was not measured by the Oswestry Disability Index (ODI version 2.1a) at 3 months (6 to 20 weeks) postoperatively

M1051 Patient had cancer, acute fracture or infection related to the lumbar spine or patient had neuromuscular, idiopathic or congenital lumbar scoliosis

M1052 Leg pain was not measured by the visual analog scale (VAS) at 1 year (9 to 15 months) postoperatively

M1054 Patient had only urgent care visits during the performance period

M1055 Aspirin or another antiplatelet therapy used

M1056 Prescribed anticoagulant medication during the performance period, history of GI bleeding, history of intracranial bleeding, bleeding disorder and specific provider documented reasons: allergy to aspirin or antiplatelets, use of nonsteroidal antiinflammatory agents, drug-drug interaction, uncontrolled hypertension > 180/110 mm Hg or gastroesophageal reflux disease

M1057 Aspirin or another antiplatelet therapy not used, reason not given

M1058 Patient was a permanent nursing home resident at any time during the performance period

M1059 Patient was in hospice or receiving palliative care at any time during the performance period

M1060 Patient died prior to the end of the performance period

M1067 Hospice services for patient provided any time during the measurement period

M1068 Adults who are not ambulatory

M1069 Patient screened for future fall risk

M1070 Patient not screened for future fall risk, reason not given

M1071 Patient had any additional spine procedures performed on the same date as the lumbar discectomy/laminotomy

● **M1072** Radiation therapy for anal cancer under the Radiation Oncology model, 90-day episode, professional component

● **M1073** Radiation therapy for anal cancer under the Radiation Oncology model, 90-day episode, technical component

● **M1074** Radiation therapy for bladder cancer under the Radiation Oncology model, 90-day episode, professional component

● **M1075** Radiation therapy for bladder cancer under the Radiation Oncology model, 90-day episode, technical component

● **M1076** Radiation therapy for bone metastases under the Radiation Oncology model, 90-day episode, professional component

● **M1077** Radiation therapy for bone metastases under the Radiation Oncology model, 90-day episode, technical component

● **M1078** Radiation therapy for brain metastases under the Radiation Oncology model, 90-day episode, professional component

● **M1079** Radiation therapy for brain metastases under the Radiation Oncology model, 90-day episode, technical component

● **M1080** Radiation therapy for breast cancer under the Radiation Oncology model, 90-day episode, professional component

● **M1081** Radiation therapy for breast cancer under the Radiation Oncology model, 90-day episode, technical component

● **M1082** Radiation therapy for cervical cancer under the Radiation Oncology model, 90-day episode, professional component

● **M1083** Radiation therapy for cervical cancer under the Radiation Oncology model, 90-day episode, technical component

● **M1084** Radiation therapy for CNS tumors under the Radiation Oncology model, 90-day episode, professional component

● **M1085** Radiation therapy for CNS tumors under the Radiation Oncology model, 90-day episode, technical component

● **M1086** Radiation therapy for colorectal cancer under the Radiation Oncology model, 90-day episode, professional component

● **M1087** Radiation therapy for colorectal cancer under the Radiation Oncology model, 90-day episode, technical component

● **M1088** Radiation therapy for head and neck cancer under the Radiation Oncology model, 90-day episode, professional component

● **M1089** Radiation therapy for head and neck cancer under the Radiation Oncology model, 90-day episode, technical component

---

Special Coverage Instructions   Noncovered by Medicare   Carrier Discretion   ☑ Quantity Alert   ● New Code   ○ Recycled/Reinstated   ▲ Revised Code

   Ⓐ Age Edit   Ⓜ Maternity Edit   ♀ Female Only   ♂ Male Only   Ⓐ-Ⓨ OPPS Status Indicators   © 2021 Optum360, LLC

● **M1094** Radiation therapy for lung cancer under the Radiation Oncology model, 90-day episode, professional component

● **M1095** Radiation therapy for lung cancer under the Radiation Oncology model, 90-day episode, technical component

● **M1096** Radiation therapy for lymphoma under the Radiation Oncology model, 90-day episode, professional component

● **M1097** Radiation therapy for lymphoma under the Radiation Oncology model, 90-day episode, technical component

● **M1098** Radiation therapy for pancreatic cancer under the Radiation Oncology model, 90-day episode, professional component

● **M1099** Radiation therapy for pancreatic cancer under the Radiation Oncology model, 90-day episode, technical component

● **M1100** Radiation therapy for prostate cancer under the Radiation Oncology model, 90-day episode, professional component

● **M1101** Radiation therapy for prostate cancer under the Radiation Oncology model, 90-day episode, technical component

● **M1102** Radiation therapy for upper GI cancer under the Radiation Oncology model, 90-day episode, professional component

● **M1103** Radiation therapy for upper GI cancer under the Radiation Oncology model, 90-day episode, technical component

● **M1104** Radiation therapy for uterine cancer under the Radiation Oncology model, 90-day episode, professional component

● **M1105** Radiation therapy for uterine cancer under the Radiation Oncology model, 90-day episode, technical component

M1106 The start of an episode of care documented in the medical record

M1107 Documentation stating patient has a diagnosis of a degenerative neurological condition such as ALS, MS, or Parkinson's diagnosed at any time before or during the episode of care

M1108 Ongoing care not clinically indicated because the patient needed a home program only, referral to another provider or facility, or consultation only, as documented in the medical record

M1109 Ongoing care not medically possible because the patient was discharged early due to specific medical events, documented in the medical record, such as the patient became hospitalized or scheduled for surgery

M1110 Ongoing care not possible because the patient self-discharged early (e.g., financial or insurance reasons, transportation problems, or reason unknown)

M1111 The start of an episode of care documented in the medical record

M1112 Documentation stating patient has a diagnosis of a degenerative neurological condition such as ALS, MS, or Parkinson's diagnosed at any time before or during the episode of care

M1113 Ongoing care not clinically indicated because the patient needed a home program only, referral to another provider or facility, or consultation only, as documented in the medical record

M1114 Ongoing care not medically possible because the patient was discharged early due to specific medical events, documented in the medical record, such as the patient became hospitalized or scheduled for surgery

M1115 Ongoing care not possible because the patient self-discharged early (e.g., financial or insurance reasons, transportation problems, or reason unknown)

M1116 The start of an episode of care documented in the medical record

M1117 Documentation stating patient has a diagnosis of a degenerative neurological condition such as ALS, MS, or Parkinson's diagnosed at any time before or during the episode of care

M1118 Ongoing care not clinically indicated because the patient needed a home program only, referral to another provider or facility, or consultation only, as documented in the medical record

M1119 Ongoing care not medically possible because the patient was discharged early due to specific medical events, documented in the medical record, such as the patient became hospitalized or scheduled for surgery

M1120 Ongoing care not possible because the patient self-discharged early (e.g., financial or insurance reasons, transportation problems, or reason unknown)

M1121 The start of an episode of care documented in the medical record

M1122 Documentation stating patient has a diagnosis of a degenerative neurological condition such as ALS, MS, or Parkinson's diagnosed at any time before or during the episode of care

M1123 Ongoing care not clinically indicated because the patient needed a home program only, referral to another provider or facility, or consultation only, as documented in the medical record

M1124 Ongoing care not medically possible because the patient was discharged early due to specific medical events, documented in the medical record, such as the patient became hospitalized or scheduled for surgery

M1125 Ongoing care not possible because the patient self-discharged early (e.g., financial or insurance reasons, transportation problems, or reason unknown)

M1126 The start of an episode of care documented in the medical record

M1127 Documentation stating patient has a diagnosis of a degenerative neurological condition such as ALS, MS, or Parkinson's diagnosed at any time before or during the episode of care

M1128 Ongoing care not clinically indicated because the patient needed a home program only, referral to another provider or facility, or consultation only, as documented in the medical record

M1129 Ongoing care not medically possible because the patient was discharged early due to specific medical events, documented in the medical record, such as the patient became hospitalized or scheduled for surgery

M1130 Ongoing care not possible because the patient self-discharged early (e.g., financial or insurance reasons, transportation problems, or reason unknown)

M1131 Documentation stating patient has a diagnosis of a degenerative neurological condition such as ALS, MS, or Parkinson's diagnosed at any time before or during the episode of care

M1132 Ongoing care not clinically indicated because the patient needed a home program only, referral to another provider or facility, or consultation only, as documented in the medical record

M1133 Ongoing care not medically possible because the patient was discharged early due to specific medical events, documented in the medical record, such as the patient became hospitalized or scheduled for surgery

M1134 Ongoing care not possible because the patient self-discharged early (e.g., financial or insurance reasons, transportation problems, or reason unknown)

M1135 The start of an episode of care documented in the medical record

M1141 Functional status was not measured by the Oxford Knee Score (OKS) or the knee injury and osteoarthritis outcome score joint replacement (KOOS, JR.) at one year (9 to 15 months) postoperatively

M1142 Emergent cases

M1143 Initiated episode of rehabilitation therapy, medical, or chiropractic care for neck impairment

Special Coverage Instructions   Noncovered by Medicare   Carrier Discretion   ☑ Quantity Alert ● New Code ○ Recycled/Reinstated ▲ Revised Code

© 2021 Optum360, LLC   A2–Z3 ASC Pmt   **CMS:** IOM   **AHA:** Coding Clinic   & DMEPOS Paid   ⊘ SNF Excluded   **M Codes — 139**

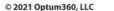

Quality Measures

M1145 — M1149

M1145 Most favored nation (MFN) model drug add-on amount, per dose, (do not bill with line items that have the JW modifier)

M1146 Ongoing care not clinically indicated because the patient needed a home program only, referral to another provider or facility, or consultation only, as documented in the medical record

M1147 Ongoing care not medically possible because the patient was discharged early due to specific medical events, documented in the medical record, such as the patient became hospitalized or scheduled for surgery

M1148 Ongoing care not possible because the patient self-discharged early (e.g., financial or insurance reasons, transportation problems, or reason unknown)

M1149 Patient unable to complete the neck FS PROM at initial evaluation and/or discharge due to blindness, illiteracy, severe mental incapacity or language incompatibility, and an adequate proxy is not available

Special Coverage Instructions   Noncovered by Medicare   Carrier Discretion   ☑ Quantity Alert ● New Code   ○ Recycled/Reinstated ▲ Revised Code

140 — M Codes   Ⓐ Age Edit   Ⓜ Maternity Edit   ♀ Female Only   ♂ Male Only   Ⓐ-Ⓨ OPPS Status Indicators   © 2021 Optum360, LLC

Pathology and Laboratory Services P2028-P9615

P codes include chemistry, toxicology, and microbiology tests, screening Papanicolaou procedures, and various blood products.

Chemistry and Toxicology Tests

P2028   **Cephalin floculation, blood**   Ⓐ
Code with caution: This test is considered obsolete. Submit documentation.

P2029   **Congo red, blood**   Ⓐ
Code with caution: This test is considered obsolete. Submit documentation.

P2031   **Hair analysis (excluding arsenic)**   Ⓔ

P2033   **Thymol turbidity, blood**   Ⓐ
Code with caution: This test is considered obsolete. Submit documentation.

P2038   **Mucoprotein, blood (seromucoid) (medical necessity procedure)**   Ⓐ
Code with caution: This test is considered obsolete. Submit documentation.

Pathology Screening Tests

P3000   **Screening Papanicolaou smear, cervical or vaginal, up to three smears, by technician under physician supervision**   Ⓐ ♀Ⓐ
One Pap test is covered by Medicare every two years, unless the physician suspects cervical abnormalities and shortens the interval. See also G0123-G0124.
CMS: 100-02,15,280.4; 100-03,210.2.1; 100-04,18,30.2.1; 100-04,18,30.5; 100-04,18,30.6

P3001   **Screening Papanicolaou smear, cervical or vaginal, up to three smears, requiring interpretation by physician**   Ⓐ ♀Ⓑ ⊘
One Pap test is covered by Medicare every two years, unless the physician suspects cervical abnormalities and shortens the interval. See also G0123-G0124.
CMS: 100-02,15,280.4; 100-03,210.2.1; 100-04,18,30.2.1; 100-04,18,30.5; 100-04,18,30.6

Microbiology Tests

P7001   **Culture, bacterial, urine; quantitative, sensitivity study**   Ⓔ

Miscellaneous

P9010   **Blood (whole), for transfusion, per unit**   Ⓡ ☑
CMS: 100-01,3,20.5; 100-01,3,20.5.2; 100-01,3,20.5.3; 100-02,1,10; 100-04,3,40.2.2
AHA: 3Q, '04, 11-13

P9011   **Blood, split unit**   Ⓡ ☑
CMS: 100-01,3,20.5; 100-01,3,20.5.2; 100-01,3,20.5.3; 100-02,1,10; 100-04,3,40.2.2; 100-04,4,231.4
AHA: 2Q, '05, 1-3; 3Q, '04, 11-13

P9012   **Cryoprecipitate, each unit**   Ⓡ ☑
CMS: 100-02,1,10; 100-04,3,40.2.2
AHA: 3Q, '04, 11-13

P9016   **Red blood cells, leukocytes reduced, each unit**   Ⓡ ☑
CMS: 100-02,1,10; 100-04,3,40.2.2
AHA: 4Q, '04, 2; 3Q, '04, 11-13

P9017   **Fresh frozen plasma (single donor), frozen within 8 hours of collection, each unit**   Ⓡ ☑
CMS: 100-02,1,10; 100-04,3,40.2.2
AHA: 3Q, '04, 11-13

P9019   **Platelets, each unit**   Ⓡ ☑
CMS: 100-02,1,10; 100-04,3,40.2.2
AHA: 3Q, '04, 11-13

P9020   **Platelet rich plasma, each unit**   Ⓡ ☑
CMS: 100-04,3,40.2.2
AHA: 3Q, '04, 11-13

P9021   **Red blood cells, each unit**   Ⓡ ☑
CMS: 100-01,3,20.5; 100-01,3,20.5.2; 100-01,3,20.5.3; 100-02,1,10; 100-04,3,40.2.2
AHA: 4Q, '04, 2; 3Q, '04, 11-13

P9022   **Red blood cells, washed, each unit**   Ⓡ ☑
CMS: 100-01,3,20.5; 100-01,3,20.5.2; 100-01,3,20.5.3; 100-02,1,10; 100-04,3,40.2.2
AHA: 3Q, '04, 11-13

P9023   **Plasma, pooled multiple donor, solvent/detergent treated, frozen, each unit**   Ⓡ ☑
CMS: 100-02,1,10; 100-04,3,40.2.2
AHA: 3Q, '04, 11-13

● **P9025**   **Plasma, cryoprecipitate reduced, pathogen reduced, each unit**

● **P9026**   **Cryoprecipitated fibrinogen complex, pathogen reduced, each unit**

P9031   **Platelets, leukocytes reduced, each unit**   Ⓡ ☑
CMS: 100-02,1,10; 100-04,3,40.2.2
AHA: 3Q, '04, 11-13

P9032   **Platelets, irradiated, each unit**   Ⓡ ☑
CMS: 100-02,1,10; 100-04,3,40.2.2
AHA: 2Q, '05, 1-3; 3Q, '04, 11-13

P9033   **Platelets, leukocytes reduced, irradiated, each unit**   Ⓡ ☑
CMS: 100-02,1,10; 100-04,3,40.2.2
AHA: 2Q, '05, 1-3; 3Q, '04, 11-13

P9034   **Platelets, pheresis, each unit**   Ⓡ ☑
CMS: 100-02,1,10; 100-04,3,40.2.2
AHA: 3Q, '04, 11-13

P9035   **Platelets, pheresis, leukocytes reduced, each unit**   Ⓡ ☑
CMS: 100-02,1,10; 100-04,3,40.2.2
AHA: 3Q, '04, 11-13

P9036   **Platelets, pheresis, irradiated, each unit**   Ⓡ ☑
CMS: 100-02,1,10; 100-04,3,40.2.2
AHA: 2Q, '05, 1-3; 3Q, '04, 11-13

P9037   **Platelets, pheresis, leukocytes reduced, irradiated, each unit**   Ⓡ ☑
CMS: 100-02,1,10; 100-04,3,40.2.2
AHA: 2Q, '05, 1-3; 3Q, '04, 11-13

P9038   **Red blood cells, irradiated, each unit**   Ⓡ ☑
CMS: 100-01,3,20.5; 100-01,3,20.5.2; 100-01,3,20.5.3; 100-02,1,10; 100-04,3,40.2.2
AHA: 2Q, '05, 1-3; 3Q, '04, 11-13

P9039   **Red blood cells, deglycerolized, each unit**   Ⓡ ☑
CMS: 100-02,1,10; 100-04,3,40.2.2
AHA: 3Q, '04, 11-13

P9040   **Red blood cells, leukocytes reduced, irradiated, each unit**   Ⓡ ☑
CMS: 100-02,1,10; 100-04,3,40.2.2
AHA: 2Q, '05, 1-3; 3Q, '04, 11-13

P9041   **Infusion, albumin (human), 5%, 50 ml**   Ⓚ K2 ☑
CMS: 100-02,1,10; 100-04,3,40.2.2
AHA: 3Q, '04, 11-13

P9043   **Infusion, plasma protein fraction (human), 5%, 50 ml**   Ⓡ ☑
CMS: 100-02,1,10; 100-04,3,40.2.2
AHA: 3Q, '04, 11-13

P9044   **Plasma, cryoprecipitate reduced, each unit**   Ⓡ ☑
CMS: 100-02,1,10; 100-04,3,40.2.2
AHA: 3Q, '04, 11-13

Special Coverage Instructions   Noncovered by Medicare   Carrier Discretion   ☑ Quantity Alert   ● New Code   ○ Recycled/Reinstated   ▲ Revised Code

© 2021 Optum360, LLC   A2-Z3 ASC Pmt   **CMS:** IOM   **AHA:** Coding Clinic   ⅅ DMEPOS Paid   ⊘ SNF Excluded   **P Codes — 141**

Pathology and Laboratory Services

P9045 — P9615

P9045   Infusion, albumin (human), 5%, 250 ml   K K2 ☑
CMS: 100-02,1,10; 100-04,3,40.2.2
AHA: 3Q, '04, 11-13; 1Q, '02, 5

P9046   Infusion, albumin (human), 25%, 20 ml   K K2 ☑
CMS: 100-02,1,10; 100-04,3,40.2.2
AHA: 3Q, '04, 11-13; 1Q, '02, 5

P9047   Infusion, albumin (human), 25%, 50 ml   K K2 ☑
CMS: 100-02,1,10; 100-04,3,40.2.2
AHA: 3Q, '04, 11-13; 1Q, '02, 5

P9048   Infusion, plasma protein fraction (human), 5%, 250 ml   R ☑
CMS: 100-02,1,10; 100-04,3,40.2.2
AHA: 3Q, '04, 11-13; 1Q, '02, 5

P9050   Granulocytes, pheresis, each unit   E ☑
CMS: 100-02,1,10; 100-03,110.5; 100-04,3,40.2.2
AHA: 3Q, '04, 11-13; 1Q, '02, 5

P9051   Whole blood or red blood cells, leukocytes reduced, CMV-negative, each unit   R ☑
CMS: 100-02,1,10; 100-04,3,40.2.2
AHA: 3Q, '04, 11-13

P9052   Platelets, HLA-matched leukocytes reduced, apheresis/pheresis, each unit   R ☑
CMS: 100-02,1,10; 100-04,3,40.2.2
AHA: 3Q, '04, 11-13

P9053   Platelets, pheresis, leukocytes reduced, CMV-negative, irradiated, each unit   R ☑
CMS: 100-02,1,10; 100-04,3,40.2.2
AHA: 2Q, '05, 1-3; 3Q, '04, 11-13

P9054   Whole blood or red blood cells, leukocytes reduced, frozen, deglycerol, washed, each unit   R ☑
CMS: 100-02,1,10; 100-04,3,40.2.2
AHA: 3Q, '04, 11-13

P9055   Platelets, leukocytes reduced, CMV-negative, apheresis/pheresis, each unit   R ☑
CMS: 100-02,1,10; 100-04,3,40.2.2
AHA: 3Q, '04, 11-13

P9056   Whole blood, leukocytes reduced, irradiated, each unit   R ☑
CMS: 100-02,1,10; 100-04,3,40.2.2
AHA: 2Q, '05, 1-3; 3Q, '04, 11-13

P9057   Red blood cells, frozen/deglycerolized/washed, leukocytes reduced, irradiated, each unit   R ☑
CMS: 100-02,1,10; 100-04,3,40.2.2
AHA: 2Q, '05, 1-3; 3Q, '04, 11-13

P9058   Red blood cells, leukocytes reduced, CMV-negative, irradiated, each unit   R ☑
CMS: 100-02,1,10; 100-04,3,40.2.2
AHA: 2Q, '05, 1-3; 3Q, '04, 11-13

P9059   Fresh frozen plasma between 8-24 hours of collection, each unit   R ☑
CMS: 100-02,1,10; 100-04,3,40.2.2
AHA: 3Q, '04, 11-13

P9060   Fresh frozen plasma, donor retested, each unit   R ☑
CMS: 100-02,1,10; 100-04,3,40.2.2
AHA: 3Q, '04, 11-13

P9070   Plasma, pooled multiple donor, pathogen reduced, frozen, each unit   R
AHA: 1Q, '16, 7

P9071   Plasma (single donor), pathogen reduced, frozen, each unit   R
AHA: 1Q, '16, 7

P9073   Platelets, pheresis, pathogen-reduced, each unit   R

P9099   Blood component or product not otherwise classified

P9100   Pathogen(s) test for platelets   S

P9603   Travel allowance, one way in connection with medically necessary laboratory specimen collection drawn from homebound or nursing homebound patient; prorated miles actually travelled   A ☑
CMS: 100-04,16,60; 100-04,16,60.2

P9604   Travel allowance, one way in connection with medically necessary laboratory specimen collection drawn from homebound or nursing homebound patient; prorated trip charge   A ☑
CMS: 100-04,16,60; 100-04,16,60.2

P9612   Catheterization for collection of specimen, single patient, all places of service   A
CMS: 100-04,16,60
AHA: 2Q, '09, 1; 3Q, '07, 5

P9615   Catheterization for collection of specimen(s) (multiple patients)   N
CMS: 100-04,16,60; 100-04,16,60.1.4

Special Coverage Instructions   Noncovered by Medicare   Carrier Discretion   ☑ Quantity Alert   ● New Code   ○ Recycled/Reinstated   ▲ Revised Code

Q Codes (Temporary) Q0035-Q9992

Temporary Q codes are used to pay health care providers for supplies, drugs, and biologicals to which no permanent code has been assigned.

Q0035   **Cardiokymography**   Q1

Covered only in conjunction with electrocardiographic stress testing in male patients with atypical angina or nonischemic chest pain, or female patients with angina.

Q0081   **Infusion therapy, using other than chemotherapeutic drugs, per visit**   B ☑

AHA: 1Q, '05, 7, 9-10; 4Q, '04, 6; 2Q, '04, 11; 1Q, '04, 4-5; 4Q, '02, 6-7; 2Q, '02, 8-9; 2Q, '02; 1Q, '02, 7

Q0083   **Chemotherapy administration by other than infusion technique only (e.g., subcutaneous, intramuscular, push), per visit**   B ☑

AHA: 1Q, '05, 7, 9-10; 4Q, '04, 6; 1Q, '04, 4-5; 1Q, '02, 7; 1Q, '02, 1-2

Q0084   **Chemotherapy administration by infusion technique only, per visit**   B ☑

AHA: 1Q, '05, 7, 9-10; 4Q, '04, 6; 2Q, '04, 11; 1Q, '04, 4-5; 1Q, '02, 7; 1Q, '02, 1-2

Q0085   **Chemotherapy administration by both infusion technique and other technique(s) (e.g. subcutaneous, intramuscular, push), per visit**   B ☑

AHA: 4Q, '04, 6; 1Q, '04, 4-5; 1Q, '02, 7; 1Q, '02, 1-2

Q0091   **Screening Papanicolaou smear; obtaining, preparing and conveyance of cervical or vaginal smear to laboratory**   A ♀ S ⊘

One pap test is covered by Medicare every two years for low risk patients and every one year for high risk patients. Q0091 can be reported with an E/M code when a separately identifiable E/M service is provided.

CMS: 100-02,13,220; 100-02,13,220.1; 100-02,13,220.3; 100-02,15,280.4; 100-03,210.2.1; 100-04,18,30.2.1; 100-04,18,30.5; 100-04,18,30.6; 1004-04,13,220.1

AHA: 4Q, '08, 3; 4Q, '02, 8

Q0092   **Set-up portable x-ray equipment**   N

CMS: 100-04,13,90.4

Q0111   **Wet mounts, including preparations of vaginal, cervical or skin specimens**   A

Q0112   **All potassium hydroxide (KOH) preparations**   A

Q0113   **Pinworm examinations**   A

Q0114   **Fern test**   ♀ A

Q0115   **Postcoital direct, qualitative examinations of vaginal or cervical mucous**   A ♀

Q0138   **Injection, ferumoxytol, for treatment of iron deficiency anemia, 1 mg (non-ESRD use)**   K K2 ☑

Use this code for Feraheme.

Q0139   **Injection, ferumoxytol, for treatment of iron deficiency anemia, 1 mg (for ESRD on dialysis)**   K K2 ☑

Use this code for Feraheme.

Q0144   **Azithromycin dihydrate, oral, capsules/powder, 1 g**   E ☑

Use this code for Zithromax, Zithromax Z-PAK.

Q0161   **Chlorpromazine HCl, 5 mg, oral, FDA-approved prescription antiemetic, for use as a complete therapeutic substitute for an IV antiemetic at the time of chemotherapy treatment, not to exceed a 48-hour dosage regimen**   N N1 ☑

CMS: 100-02,15,50.5.4; 100-03,110.18; 100-04,17,80.2.1

AHA: 1Q, '14, 7

Q0162   **Ondansetron 1 mg, oral, FDA-approved prescription antiemetic, for use as a complete therapeutic substitute for an IV antiemetic at the time of chemotherapy treatment, not to exceed a 48-hour dosage regimen**   N N1 ☑

Use this code for Zofran, Zuplenz.

CMS: 100-02,15,50.5.4; 100-03,110.18; 100-04,17,80.2.1

Q0163   **Diphenhydramine HCl, 50 mg, oral, FDA-approved prescription antiemetic, for use as a complete therapeutic substitute for an IV antiemetic at time of chemotherapy treatment not to exceed a 48-hour dosage regimen**   N N1 ☑

See also J1200. Medicare covers at the time of chemotherapy if regimen doesn't exceed 48 hours. Submit on the same claim as the chemotherapy. Use this code for Truxadryl.

CMS: 100-02,15,50.5.4; 100-03,110.18; 100-04,17,80.2.1

AHA: 2Q, '12, 9; 1Q, '08, 1; 1Q, '02, 1-2

Q0164   **Prochlorperazine maleate, 5 mg, oral, FDA-approved prescription antiemetic, for use as a complete therapeutic substitute for an IV antiemetic at the time of chemotherapy treatment, not to exceed a 48-hour dosage regimen**   N N1 ☑

Medicare covers at the time of chemotherapy if regimen doesn't exceed 48 hours. Submit on the same claim as the chemotherapy. Use this code for Compazine.

CMS: 100-02,15,50.5.4; 100-03,110.18; 100-04,17,80.2.1

AHA: 1Q, '08, 1

Q0166   **Granisetron HCl, 1 mg, oral, FDA-approved prescription antiemetic, for use as a complete therapeutic substitute for an IV antiemetic at the time of chemotherapy treatment, not to exceed a 24-hour dosage regimen**   N N1 ☑

Medicare covers at the time of chemotherapy if regimen doesn't exceed 48 hours. Submit on the same claim as the chemotherapy. Use this code for Kytril.

CMS: 100-02,15,50.5.4; 100-03,110.18; 100-04,17,80.2.1

AHA: 1Q, '08, 1

Q0167   **Dronabinol, 2.5 mg, oral, FDA-approved prescription antiemetic, for use as a complete therapeutic substitute for an IV antiemetic at the time of chemotherapy treatment, not to exceed a 48-hour dosage regimen**   N N1 ☑

Medicare covers at the time of chemotherapy if regimen doesn't exceed 48 hours. Submit on the same claim as the chemotherapy. Use this code for Marinol.

CMS: 100-02,15,50.5.4; 100-03,110.18; 100-04,17,80.2.1

AHA: 1Q, '08, 1

Q0169   **Promethazine HCl, 12.5 mg, oral, FDA-approved prescription antiemetic, for use as a complete therapeutic substitute for an IV antiemetic at the time of chemotherapy treatment, not to exceed a 48-hour dosage regimen**   N N1 ☑

Medicare covers at the time of chemotherapy if regimen doesn't exceed 48 hours. Submit on the same claim as the chemotherapy. Use this code for Phenergan, Amergan.

CMS: 100-02,15,50.5.4; 100-03,110.18; 100-04,17,80.2.1

AHA: 1Q, '08, 1

Q0173   **Trimethobenzamide HCl, 250 mg, oral, FDA-approved prescription antiemetic, for use as a complete therapeutic substitute for an IV antiemetic at the time of chemotherapy treatment, not to exceed a 48-hour dosage regimen**   N N1 ☑

Medicare covers at the time of chemotherapy if regimen doesn't exceed 48 hours. Submit on the same claim as the chemotherapy. Use this code for Tebamide, T-Gen, Ticon, Tigan, Triban, Thimazide.

CMS: 100-02,15,50.5.4; 100-03,110.18; 100-04,17,80.2.1

AHA: 1Q, '08, 1

Q0174   **Thiethylperazine maleate, 10 mg, oral, FDA-approved prescription antiemetic, for use as a complete therapeutic substitute for an IV antiemetic at the time of chemotherapy treatment, not to exceed a 48-hour dosage regimen**   E ☑

Medicare covers at the time of chemotherapy if regimen doesn't exceed 48 hours. Submit on the same claim as the chemotherapy.

CMS: 100-02,15,50.5.4; 100-03,110.18; 100-04,17,80.2.1

AHA: 1Q, '08, 1

Special Coverage Instructions   Noncovered by Medicare   Carrier Discretion   ☑ Quantity Alert   ● New Code   ○ Recycled/Reinstated   ▲ Revised Code

© 2021 Optum360, LLC   A2 – Z3 ASC Pmt   CMS: IOM   AHA: Coding Clinic   ⅊ DMEPOS Paid   ⊘ SNF Excluded   Q Codes (Temporary) — 143

Q Codes (Temporary)

Q0175 — Q0494

Q0175 **Perphenazine, 4 mg, oral, FDA-approved prescription antiemetic, for use as a complete therapeutic substitute for an IV antiemetic at the time of chemotherapy treatment, not to exceed a 48-hour dosage regimen** N N1 ☑

Medicare covers at the time of chemotherapy if regimen doesn't exceed 48 hours. Submit on the same claim as the chemotherapy. Use this code for Trilifon.

CMS: 100-02,15,50.5.4; 100-03,110.18; 100-04,17,80.2.1
AHA: 1Q, '08, 1

Q0177 **Hydroxyzine pamoate, 25 mg, oral, FDA-approved prescription antiemetic, for use as a complete therapeutic substitute for an IV antiemetic at the time of chemotherapy treatment, not to exceed a 48-hour dosage regimen** N N1 ☑

Medicare covers at the time of chemotherapy if regimen doesn't exceed 48 hours. Submit on the same claim as the chemotherapy. Use this code for Vistaril.

CMS: 100-02,15,50.5.4; 100-03,110.18; 100-04,17,80.2.1
AHA: 1Q, '08, 1

Q0180 **Dolasetron mesylate, 100 mg, oral, FDA-approved prescription antiemetic, for use as a complete therapeutic substitute for an IV antiemetic at the time of chemotherapy treatment, not to exceed a 24-hour dosage regimen** N N1 ☑

Medicare covers at the time of chemotherapy if regimen doesn't exceed 24 hours. Submit on the same claim as the chemotherapy. Use this code for Anzemet.

CMS: 100-02,15,50.5.4; 100-03,110.18; 100-04,17,80.2.1
AHA: 1Q, '08, 1

Q0181 **Unspecified oral dosage form, FDA-approved prescription antiemetic, for use as a complete therapeutic substitute for an IV antiemetic at the time of chemotherapy treatment, not to exceed a 48-hour dosage regimen** N N1 ☑

Medicare covers at the time of chemotherapy if regimen doesn't exceed 48-hours. Submit on the same claim as the chemotherapy.

CMS: 100-02,15,50.5.4; 100-03,110.18; 100-04,17,80.2.1
AHA: 2Q, '12, 9; 1Q, '08, 1

Q0239 ~~Injection, bamlanivimab-xxxx, 700 mg~~

● **Q0240** **Injection, casirivimab and imdevimab, 600 mg** L1

Use this code for casirivimab and imdevimab 600 mg administered as post exposure prophylaxis. Report also M0240 or M0241 for administration.

Q0243 **Injection, casirivimab and imdevimab, 2400 mg**

Use this code for Casirivimab and Imdevimab (REGN-COV2), Regeneron.

● **Q0244** **Injection, casirivimab and imdevimab, 1200 mg** L1

● **Q0245** **Injection, bamlanivimab and etesevimab, 2100 mg** L1

Use this code for Eli Lilly's bamlanivimab (LY-CoV555) 700 mg and etesevimab (LY-CoV016) 1400 mg, administered together.

● **Q0247** **Injection, sotrovimab, 500 mg** L1

● **Q0249** **Injection, tocilizumab, for hospitalized adults and pediatric patients (2 years of age and older) with COVID-19 who are receiving systemic corticosteroids and require supplemental oxygen, non-invasive or invasive mechanical ventilation, or extracorporeal membrane oxygenation (ECMO) only, 1 mg** L1

Q0477 **Power module patient cable for use with electric or electric/pneumatic ventricular assist device, replacement only** A ♿

Q0478 **Power adapter for use with electric or electric/pneumatic ventricular assist device, vehicle type** A ♿

Q0479 **Power module for use with electric or electric/pneumatic ventricular assist device, replacement only** A ♿

Q0480 **Driver for use with pneumatic ventricular assist device, replacement only** A ♿

CMS: 100-04,32,320.3.4
AHA: 3Q, '05, 1-2

Q0481 **Microprocessor control unit for use with electric ventricular assist device, replacement only** A ♿

CMS: 100-04,32,320.3.4
AHA: 3Q, '05, 1-2

Q0482 **Microprocessor control unit for use with electric/pneumatic combination ventricular assist device, replacement only** A ♿

CMS: 100-04,32,320.3.4
AHA: 3Q, '05, 1-2

Q0483 **Monitor/display module for use with electric ventricular assist device, replacement only** A ♿

CMS: 100-04,32,320.3.4
AHA: 3Q, '05, 1-2

Q0484 **Monitor/display module for use with electric or electric/pneumatic ventricular assist device, replacement only** A ♿

CMS: 100-04,32,320.3.4
AHA: 3Q, '05, 1-2

Q0485 **Monitor control cable for use with electric ventricular assist device, replacement only** A ♿

CMS: 100-04,32,320.3.4
AHA: 3Q, '05, 1-2

Q0486 **Monitor control cable for use with electric/pneumatic ventricular assist device, replacement only** A ♿

CMS: 100-04,32,320.3.4
AHA: 3Q, '05, 1-2

Q0487 **Leads (pneumatic/electrical) for use with any type electric/pneumatic ventricular assist device, replacement only** A ♿

CMS: 100-04,32,320.3.4
AHA: 3Q, '05, 1-2

Q0488 **Power pack base for use with electric ventricular assist device, replacement only** A

CMS: 100-04,32,320.3.4
AHA: 3Q, '05, 1-2

Q0489 **Power pack base for use with electric/pneumatic ventricular assist device, replacement only** A ♿

CMS: 100-04,32,320.3.4
AHA: 3Q, '05, 1-2

Q0490 **Emergency power source for use with electric ventricular assist device, replacement only** A ♿

CMS: 100-04,32,320.3.4
AHA: 3Q, '05, 1-2

Q0491 **Emergency power source for use with electric/pneumatic ventricular assist device, replacement only** A ♿

CMS: 100-04,32,320.3.4
AHA: 3Q, '05, 1-2

Q0492 **Emergency power supply cable for use with electric ventricular assist device, replacement only** A ♿

CMS: 100-04,32,320.3.4
AHA: 3Q, '05, 1-2

Q0493 **Emergency power supply cable for use with electric/pneumatic ventricular assist device, replacement only** A ♿

CMS: 100-04,32,320.3.4
AHA: 3Q, '05, 1-2

Q0494 **Emergency hand pump for use with electric or electric/pneumatic ventricular assist device, replacement only** A ♿

CMS: 100-04,32,320.3.4
AHA: 3Q, '05, 1-2

Special Coverage Instructions   Noncovered by Medicare   Carrier Discretion   ☑ Quantity Alert   ● New Code   ○ Recycled/Reinstated   ▲ Revised Code

144 — Q Codes (Temporary)   A Age Edit   M Maternity Edit   ♀ Female Only   ♂ Male Only   A-Y OPPS Status Indicators   © 2021 Optum360, LLC

Q0495	**Battery/power pack charger for use with electric or electric/pneumatic ventricular assist device, replacement only** [A] [&]
	CMS: 100-04,32,320.3.4
	AHA: 3Q, '05, 1-2
Q0496	**Battery, other than lithium-ion, for use with electric or electric/pneumatic ventricular assist device, replacement only** [A] [&]
	CMS: 100-04,32,320.3.4
	AHA: 3Q, '05, 1-2
Q0497	**Battery clips for use with electric or electric/pneumatic ventricular assist device, replacement only** [A] [&]
	CMS: 100-04,32,320.3.4
	AHA: 3Q, '05, 1-2
Q0498	**Holster for use with electric or electric/pneumatic ventricular assist device, replacement only** [A] [&]
	CMS: 100-04,32,320.3.4
	AHA: 3Q, '05, 1-2
Q0499	**Belt/vest/bag for use to carry external peripheral components of any type ventricular assist device, replacement only** [A] [&]
	CMS: 100-04,32,320.3.4
	AHA: 3Q, '05, 1-2
Q0500	**Filters for use with electric or electric/pneumatic ventricular assist device, replacement only** [A] [✓] [&]
	The base unit for this code is for each filter.
	CMS: 100-04,32,320.3.4
	AHA: 3Q, '05, 1-2
Q0501	**Shower cover for use with electric or electric/pneumatic ventricular assist device, replacement only** [A] [&]
	CMS: 100-04,32,320.3.4
	AHA: 3Q, '05, 1-2
Q0502	**Mobility cart for pneumatic ventricular assist device, replacement only** [A] [&]
	CMS: 100-04,32,320.3.4
	AHA: 3Q, '05, 1-2
Q0503	**Battery for pneumatic ventricular assist device, replacement only, each** [A] [✓] [&]
	CMS: 100-04,32,320.3.4
	AHA: 3Q, '05, 1-2
Q0504	**Power adapter for pneumatic ventricular assist device, replacement only, vehicle type** [A] [&]
	CMS: 100-04,32,320.3.4
	AHA: 3Q, '05, 1-2
Q0506	**Battery, lithium-ion, for use with electric or electric/pneumatic ventricular assist device, replacement only** [A] [&]
	CMS: 100-04,32,320.3.4
Q0507	**Miscellaneous supply or accessory for use with an external ventricular assist device** [A]
	CMS: 100-04,32,320.3.4
Q0508	**Miscellaneous supply or accessory for use with an implanted ventricular assist device** [A]
	CMS: 100-04,32,320.3.4
Q0509	**Miscellaneous supply or accessory for use with any implanted ventricular assist device for which payment was not made under Medicare Part A** [A]
	CMS: 100-04,32,320.3.4
Q0510	**Pharmacy supply fee for initial immunosuppressive drug(s), first month following transplant** [B] [✓]
Q0511	**Pharmacy supply fee for oral anticancer, oral antiemetic, or immunosuppressive drug(s); for the first prescription in a 30-day period** [B] [✓]

Q0512	**Pharmacy supply fee for oral anticancer, oral antiemetic, or immunosuppressive drug(s); for a subsequent prescription in a 30-day period** [B] [✓]
Q0513	**Pharmacy dispensing fee for inhalation drug(s); per 30 days** [B] [✓]
Q0514	**Pharmacy dispensing fee for inhalation drug(s); per 90 days** [B] [✓]
Q0515	**Injection, sermorelin acetate, 1 mcg** [E] [✓]
Q1004	**New technology, intraocular lens, category 4 as defined in Federal Register notice** [E]
Q1005	**New technology, intraocular lens, category 5 as defined in Federal Register notice** [E]
Q2004	**Irrigation solution for treatment of bladder calculi, for example renacidin, per 500 ml** [N] [N1] [✓]
Q2009	**Injection, fosphenytoin, 50 mg phenytoin equivalent** [K] [N1] [✓]
	Use this code for Cerebyx.
Q2017	**Injection, teniposide, 50 mg** [K] [K2] [✓]
	Use this code for Vumon.
Q2026	**Injection, Radiesse, 0.1 ml** [E] [K2] [✓]
	CMS: 100-03,250.5; 100-04,32,260.1; 100-04,32,260.2.1; 100-04,32,260.2.2
Q2028	**Injection, sculptra, 0.5 mg** [E] [K2] [✓]
	CMS: 100-04,32,260.2.2
	AHA: 1Q, '14, 7
Q2034	**Influenza virus vaccine, split virus, for intramuscular use (Agriflu)** [L] [L1] [✓]
	CMS: 100-04,18,10.1.2
	AHA: 3Q, '12, 10
Q2035	**Influenza virus vaccine, split virus, when administered to individuals 3 years of age and older, for intramuscular use (AFLURIA)** [A] [L] [L1] [✓]
	CMS: 100-02,15,50.4.4.2; 100-04,18,10.1.2
Q2036	**Influenza virus vaccine, split virus, when administered to individuals 3 years of age and older, for intramuscular use (FLULAVAL)** [A] [L] [L1] [✓]
	CMS: 100-02,15,50.4.4.2; 100-04,18,10.1.2
Q2037	**Influenza virus vaccine, split virus, when administered to individuals 3 years of age and older, for intramuscular use (FLUVIRIN)** [A] [L] [L1] [✓]
	CMS: 100-02,15,50.4.4.2; 100-04,18,10.1.2
Q2038	**Influenza virus vaccine, split virus, when administered to individuals 3 years of age and older, for intramuscular use (Fluzone)** [A] [L] [L1] [✓]
	CMS: 100-02,15,50.4.4.2; 100-04,18,10.1.2
Q2039	**Influenza virus vaccine, not otherwise specified** [A] [L] [L1] [✓]
	CMS: 100-02,15,50.4.4.2; 100-04,18,10.1.2
Q2041	**Axicabtagene ciloleucel, up to 200 million autologous anti-CD19 CAR positive T cells, including leukapheresis and dose preparation procedures, per therapeutic dose** [G]
	Use this code for Yescarta.
	CMS: 100-04,32,400; 100-04,32,400.1; 100-04,32,400.2; 100-04,32,400.2.1; 100-04,32,400.2.2; 100-04,32,400.2.3; 100-04,32,400.2.4; 100-04,32,400.3; 100-04,32,400.4; 100-04,32,400.5; 100-04,32,66.2
Q2042	**Tisagenlecleucel, up to 600 million CAR-positive viable T cells, including leukapheresis and dose preparation procedures, per therapeutic dose**
	Use this code for Kymriah.
	CMS: 100-04,32,400; 100-04,32,400.1; 100-04,32,400.2; 100-04,32,400.2.1; 100-04,32,400.2.2; 100-04,32,400.2.3; 100-04,32,400.2.4; 100-04,32,400.3; 100-04,32,400.4; 100-04,32,400.5; 100-04,32,66.2

Special Coverage Instructions   Noncovered by Medicare   Carrier Discretion   ☑ Quantity Alert   ● New Code   ○ Recycled/Reinstated   ▲ Revised Code

© 2021 Optum360, LLC   [A2]–[Z3] ASC Pmt   CMS: IOM   AHA: Coding Clinic   & DMEPOS Paid   ⊘ SNF Excluded   Q Codes (Temporary) — 145

Q Codes (Temporary)

Q2043 — Q4019

Q2043 Sipuleucel-T, minimum of 50 million autologous CD54+ cells activated with PAP-GM-CSF, including leukapheresis and all other preparatory procedures, per infusion ♂ K K2 ☑
Use this code for PROVENGE.
CMS: 100-03,1,110.22; 100-03,110.22; 100-04,32,280.1; 100-04,32,280.2; 100-04,32,280.4; 100-04,32,280.5
AHA: 2Q, '12, 7; 3Q, '11, 9

Q2049 Injection, doxorubicin HCl, liposomal, imported Lipodox, 10 mg K K2 ☑
AHA: 3Q, '12, 10

Q2050 Injection, doxorubicin HCl, liposomal, not otherwise specified, 10 mg K K2 ☑ ◯
AHA: 4Q, '13, 8-10; 3Q, '13, 10

Q2052 Services, supplies and accessories used in the home under the Medicare intravenous immune globulin (IVIG) demonstration E ☑
AHA: 2Q, '14, 8

● **Q2053** Brexucabtagene autoleucel, up to 200 million autologous anti-CD19 CAR positive viable T cells, including leukapheresis and dose preparation procedures, per therapeutic dose
Use this code for Tecartus.
CMS: 100-04,32,400; 100-04,32,400.1; 100-04,32,400.2; 100-04,32,400.2.1; 100-04,32,400.2.2; 100-04,32,400.2.3; 100-04,32,400.2.4; 100-04,32,400.3; 100-04,32,400.4; 100-04,32,400.5

● **Q2054** Lisocabtagene maraleucel, up to 110 million autologous anti-CD19 CAR-positive viable T cells, including leukapheresis and dose preparation procedures, per therapeutic dose
Use this code for Breyanzi.

● **Q2055** Idecabtagene vicleucel, up to 460 million autologous B-cell maturation antigen (BCMA) directed CAR-positive T cells, including leukapheresis and dose preparation procedures, per therapeutic dose
Use this code for Abecma.

Q3001 Radioelements for brachytherapy, any type, each B ☑ ◯

Q3014 Telehealth originating site facility fee A ◯
CMS: 100-04,12,190.5; 100-04,12,190.6; 100-04,39,30.5

Q3027 Injection, interferon beta-1a, 1 mcg for intramuscular use K K2 ☑
Use this code for Avonex.
CMS: 100-02,15,50.5
AHA: 1Q, '14, 7

Q3028 Injection, interferon beta-1a, 1 mcg for subcutaneous use E ☑
Use this code for Rebif.
CMS: 100-02,15,50.5

Q3031 Collagen skin test N N1

Q4001 Casting supplies, body cast adult, with or without head, plaster A B ♿
CMS: 100-04,20,170
AHA: 2Q, '02, 1-3

Q4002 Cast supplies, body cast adult, with or without head, fiberglass A B ♿
CMS: 100-04,20,170
AHA: 2Q, '02, 1-3

Q4003 Cast supplies, shoulder cast, adult (11 years +), plaster A B ♿
CMS: 100-04,20,170
AHA: 2Q, '02, 1-3

Q4004 Cast supplies, shoulder cast, adult (11 years +), fiberglass A B ♿
CMS: 100-04,20,170
AHA: 2Q, '02, 1-3

Q4005 Cast supplies, long arm cast, adult (11 years +), plaster A B ♿
CMS: 100-04,20,170
AHA: 2Q, '02, 1-3

Q4006 Cast supplies, long arm cast, adult (11 years +), fiberglass A B ♿
CMS: 100-04,20,170
AHA: 2Q, '02, 1-3

Q4007 Cast supplies, long arm cast, pediatric (0-10 years), plaster A B ♿
CMS: 100-04,20,170
AHA: 2Q, '02, 1-3

Q4008 Cast supplies, long arm cast, pediatric (0-10 years), fiberglass A B ♿
CMS: 100-04,20,170
AHA: 2Q, '02, 1-3

Q4009 Cast supplies, short arm cast, adult (11 years +), plaster A B ♿
CMS: 100-04,20,170
AHA: 2Q, '02, 1-3

Q4010 Cast supplies, short arm cast, adult (11 years +), fiberglass A B ♿
CMS: 100-04,20,170
AHA: 2Q, '02, 1-3

Q4011 Cast supplies, short arm cast, pediatric (0-10 years), plaster A B ♿
CMS: 100-04,20,170
AHA: 2Q, '02, 1-3

Q4012 Cast supplies, short arm cast, pediatric (0-10 years), fiberglass A B ♿
CMS: 100-04,20,170
AHA: 2Q, '02, 1-3

Q4013 Cast supplies, gauntlet cast (includes lower forearm and hand), adult (11 years +), plaster A B ♿
CMS: 100-04,20,170
AHA: 2Q, '02, 1-3

Q4014 Cast supplies, gauntlet cast (includes lower forearm and hand), adult (11 years +), fiberglass A B ♿
CMS: 100-04,20,170
AHA: 2Q, '02, 1-3

Q4015 Cast supplies, gauntlet cast (includes lower forearm and hand), pediatric (0-10 years), plaster A B ♿
CMS: 100-04,20,170
AHA: 2Q, '02, 1-3

Q4016 Cast supplies, gauntlet cast (includes lower forearm and hand), pediatric (0-10 years), fiberglass A B ♿
CMS: 100-04,20,170
AHA: 2Q, '02, 1-3

Q4017 Cast supplies, long arm splint, adult (11 years +), plaster A B ♿
CMS: 100-04,20,170
AHA: 2Q, '02, 1-3

Q4018 Cast supplies, long arm splint, adult (11 years +), fiberglass A B ♿
CMS: 100-04,20,170
AHA: 2Q, '02, 1-3

Q4019 Cast supplies, long arm splint, pediatric (0-10 years), plaster A B ♿
CMS: 100-04,20,170
AHA: 2Q, '02, 1-3

■ Special Coverage Instructions   ■ Noncovered by Medicare   ■ Carrier Discretion   ☑ Quantity Alert   ● New Code   ◯ Recycled/Reinstated   ▲ Revised Code

146 — Q Codes (Temporary)   A Age Edit   M Maternity Edit   ♀ Female Only   ♂ Male Only   A-Y OPPS Status Indicators   © 2021 Optum360, LLC

Q Codes (Temporary)

Q4020 — Q4049

Q4020   Cast supplies, long arm splint, pediatric (0-10 years), fiberglass   A B &
CMS: 100-04,20,170
AHA: 2Q, '02, 1-3

Q4021   Cast supplies, short arm splint, adult (11 years +), plaster   A B &
CMS: 100-04,20,170
AHA: 2Q, '02, 1-3

Q4022   Cast supplies, short arm splint, adult (11 years +), fiberglass   A B &
CMS: 100-04,20,170
AHA: 2Q, '02, 1-3

Q4023   Cast supplies, short arm splint, pediatric (0-10 years), plaster   A B &
CMS: 100-04,20,170
AHA: 2Q, '02, 1-3

Q4024   Cast supplies, short arm splint, pediatric (0-10 years), fiberglass   A B &
CMS: 100-04,20,170
AHA: 2Q, '02, 1-3

Q4025   Cast supplies, hip spica (one or both legs), adult (11 years +), plaster   A B &
CMS: 100-04,20,170
AHA: 2Q, '02, 1-3

Q4026   Cast supplies, hip spica (one or both legs), adult (11 years +), fiberglass   A B &
CMS: 100-04,20,170
AHA: 2Q, '02, 1-3

Q4027   Cast supplies, hip spica (one or both legs), pediatric (0-10 years), plaster   A B &
CMS: 100-04,20,170
AHA: 2Q, '02, 1-3

Q4028   Cast supplies, hip spica (one or both legs), pediatric (0-10 years), fiberglass   A B &
CMS: 100-04,20,170
AHA: 2Q, '02, 1-3

Q4029   Cast supplies, long leg cast, adult (11 years +), plaster   A B &
CMS: 100-04,20,170
AHA: 2Q, '02, 1-3

Q4030   Cast supplies, long leg cast, adult (11 years +), fiberglass   A B &
CMS: 100-04,20,170
AHA: 2Q, '02, 1-3

Q4031   Cast supplies, long leg cast, pediatric (0-10 years), plaster   A B &
CMS: 100-04,20,170
AHA: 2Q, '02, 1-3

Q4032   Cast supplies, long leg cast, pediatric (0-10 years), fiberglass   A B &
CMS: 100-04,20,170
AHA: 2Q, '02, 1-3

Q4033   Cast supplies, long leg cylinder cast, adult (11 years +), plaster   A B &
CMS: 100-04,20,170
AHA: 2Q, '02, 1-3

Q4034   Cast supplies, long leg cylinder cast, adult (11 years +), fiberglass   A B &
CMS: 100-04,20,170
AHA: 2Q, '02, 1-3

Q4035   Cast supplies, long leg cylinder cast, pediatric (0-10 years), plaster   A B &
CMS: 100-04,20,170
AHA: 2Q, '02, 1-3

Q4036   Cast supplies, long leg cylinder cast, pediatric (0-10 years), fiberglass   A B &
CMS: 100-04,20,170
AHA: 2Q, '02, 1-3

Q4037   Cast supplies, short leg cast, adult (11 years +), plaster   A B &
CMS: 100-04,20,170
AHA: 2Q, '02, 1-3

Q4038   Cast supplies, short leg cast, adult (11 years +), fiberglass   A B &
CMS: 100-04,20,170
AHA: 2Q, '02, 1-3

Q4039   Cast supplies, short leg cast, pediatric (0-10 years), plaster   A B &
CMS: 100-04,20,170
AHA: 2Q, '02, 1-3

Q4040   Cast supplies, short leg cast, pediatric (0-10 years), fiberglass   A B &
CMS: 100-04,20,170
AHA: 2Q, '02, 1-3

Q4041   Cast supplies, long leg splint, adult (11 years +), plaster   A B &
CMS: 100-04,20,170
AHA: 2Q, '02, 1-3

Q4042   Cast supplies, long leg splint, adult (11 years +), fiberglass   A B &
CMS: 100-04,20,170
AHA: 2Q, '02, 1-3

Q4043   Cast supplies, long leg splint, pediatric (0-10 years), plaster   A B &
CMS: 100-04,20,170
AHA: 2Q, '02, 1-3

Q4044   Cast supplies, long leg splint, pediatric (0-10 years), fiberglass   A B &
CMS: 100-04,20,170
AHA: 2Q, '02, 1-3

Q4045   Cast supplies, short leg splint, adult (11 years +), plaster   A B &
CMS: 100-04,20,170
AHA: 2Q, '02, 1-3

Q4046   Cast supplies, short leg splint, adult (11 years +), fiberglass   A B &
CMS: 100-04,20,170
AHA: 2Q, '02, 1-3

Q4047   Cast supplies, short leg splint, pediatric (0-10 years), plaster   A B &
CMS: 100-04,20,170
AHA: 2Q, '02, 1-3

Q4048   Cast supplies, short leg splint, pediatric (0-10 years), fiberglass   A B &
CMS: 100-04,20,170
AHA: 2Q, '02, 1-3

Q4049   Finger splint, static   B &
CMS: 100-04,20,170
AHA: 2Q, '07, 10; 2Q, '02, 1-3

Special Coverage Instructions   Noncovered by Medicare   Carrier Discretion   ☑ Quantity Alert   ● New Code   ○ Recycled/Reinstated   ▲ Revised Code

Q4050 **Cast supplies, for unlisted types and materials of casts** B
CMS: 100-04,20,170
AHA: 2Q, '02, 1-3

Q4051 **Splint supplies, miscellaneous (includes thermoplastics, strapping, fasteners, padding and other supplies)** B
CMS: 100-04,20,170
AHA: 2Q, '02, 1-3

Q4074 **Iloprost, inhalation solution, FDA-approved final product, noncompounded, administered through DME, unit dose form, up to 20 mcg** Y ☑
CMS: 100-02,15,50.5

Q4081 **Injection, epoetin alfa, 100 units (for ESRD on dialysis)** N ☑
CMS: 100-04,8,60.4; 100-04,8,60.4.1; 100-04,8,60.4.2; 100-04,8,60.4.4; 100-04,8,60.4.4.1; 100-04,8,60.4.4.2; 100-04,8,60.4.5.1

Q4082 **Drug or biological, not otherwise classified, Part B drug competitive acquisition program (CAP)** B ☑

Q4100 **Skin substitute, not otherwise specified** N N1 ☑
CMS: 100-04,4,260.1; 100-04,4,260.1.1
AHA: 2Q, '12, 7; 2Q, '10, 2, 3

Q4101 **Apligraf, per sq cm** N N1 ☑
CMS: 100-04,4,260.1; 100-04,4,260.1.1
AHA: 2Q, '12, 7; 2Q, '10, 2, 3

Q4102 **Oasis wound matrix, per sq cm** N N1 ☑
CMS: 100-04,4,260.1; 100-04,4,260.1.1
AHA: 3Q, '12, 8; 2Q, '12, 7; 2Q, '10, 2, 3

Q4103 **Oasis burn matrix, per sq cm** N N1 ☑
CMS: 100-04,4,260.1; 100-04,4,260.1.1
AHA: 2Q, '12, 7; 2Q, '10, 2, 3

Q4104 **Integra bilayer matrix wound dressing (BMWD), per sq cm** N N1 ☑
CMS: 100-04,4,260.1; 100-04,4,260.1.1
AHA: 3Q, '14, 4; 2Q, '12, 7; 2Q, '10, 8; 2Q, '10, 2, 3

Q4105 **Integra dermal regeneration template (DRT) or Integra Omnigraft dermal regeneration matrix, per sq cm** N N1 ☑
CMS: 100-04,4,260.1; 100-04,4,260.1.1
AHA: 2Q, '12, 7; 2Q, '10, 8; 2Q, '10, 2, 3

Q4106 **Dermagraft, per sq cm** N N1 ☑
CMS: 100-04,4,260.1; 100-04,4,260.1.1
AHA: 2Q, '12, 7; 2Q, '10, 2, 3

Q4107 **GRAFTJACKET, per sq cm** N N1 ☑
CMS: 100-04,4,260.1; 100-04,4,260.1.1
AHA: 2Q, '12, 7; 2Q, '10, 2, 3

Q4108 **Integra matrix, per sq cm** N N1 ☑
CMS: 100-04,4,260.1; 100-04,4,260.1.1
AHA: 2Q, '12, 7; 2Q, '10, 8; 2Q, '10, 2, 3

Q4110 **PriMatrix, per sq cm** N N1 ☑
CMS: 100-04,4,260.1; 100-04,4,260.1.1
AHA: 2Q, '12, 7; 2Q, '10, 2, 3

Q4111 **GammaGraft, per sq cm** N N1 ☑
CMS: 100-04,4,260.1; 100-04,4,260.1.1
AHA: 2Q, '12, 7; 2Q, '10, 2, 3

Q4112 **Cymetra, injectable, 1 cc** N N1 ☑
AHA: 2Q, '12, 7; 2Q, '10, 2, 3

Q4113 **GRAFTJACKET XPRESS, injectable, 1 cc** N N1 ☑
AHA: 2Q, '12, 7; 2Q, '10, 2, 3

Q4114 **Integra flowable wound matrix, injectable, 1 cc** N N1 ☑
AHA: 2Q, '12, 7; 2Q, '10, 8; 2Q, '10, 2, 3

Q4115 **AlloSkin, per sq cm** N N1 ☑
CMS: 100-04,4,260.1; 100-04,4,260.1.1
AHA: 2Q, '12, 7; 2Q, '10, 2, 3

Q4116 **AlloDerm, per sq cm** N N1 ☑
CMS: 100-04,4,260.1; 100-04,4,260.1.1
AHA: 2Q, '12, 7; 2Q, '10, 2, 3

Q4117 **HYALOMATRIX, per sq cm** N N1 ☑
CMS: 100-04,4,260.1; 100-04,4,260.1.1

Q4118 **MatriStem micromatrix, 1 mg** N N1 ☑
AHA: 4Q, '13, 1-2; 2Q, '12, 7

Q4121 **TheraSkin, per sq cm** N N1 ☑
CMS: 100-04,4,260.1; 100-04,4,260.1.1
AHA: 2Q, '12, 7

Q4122 **DermACELL, DermACELL AWM or DermACELL AWM Porous, per sq cm** N N1 ☑
CMS: 100-04,4,260.1; 100-04,4,260.1.1
AHA: 2Q, '12, 7

Q4123 **AlloSkin RT, per sq cm** N N1 ☑
CMS: 100-04,4,260.1; 100-04,4,260.1.1

Q4124 **OASIS ultra tri-layer wound matrix, per sq cm** N N1 ☑
CMS: 100-04,4,260.1; 100-04,4,260.1.1
AHA: 2Q, '12, 7

Q4125 **ArthroFlex, per sq cm** N N1 ☑

Q4126 **MemoDerm, DermaSpan, TranZgraft or InteguPly, per sq cm** N N1 ☑
CMS: 100-04,4,260.1; 100-04,4,260.1.1

Q4127 **Talymed, per sq cm** N N1 ☑
CMS: 100-04,4,260.1; 100-04,4,260.1.1
AHA: 2Q, '13, 9

Q4128 **FlexHD, AllopatchHD, or Matrix HD, per sq cm** N N1 ☑
CMS: 100-04,4,260.1; 100-04,4,260.1.1

Q4130 **Strattice TM, per sq cm** N N1 ☑
AHA: 2Q, '12, 7

Q4132 **Grafix Core and GrafixPL Core, per sq cm** N N1 ☑
CMS: 100-04,4,260.1; 100-04,4,260.1.1

Q4133 **Grafix PRIME, GrafixPL PRIME, Stravix and StravixPL, per sq cm** N N1 ☑
CMS: 100-04,4,260.1; 100-04,4,260.1.1

Q4134 **HMatrix, per sq cm** N N1 ☑
CMS: 100-04,4,260.1; 100-04,4,260.1.1

Q4135 **Mediskin, per sq cm** N N1 ☑
CMS: 100-04,4,260.1; 100-04,4,260.1.1

Q4136 **E-Z Derm, per sq cm** N N1 ☑
CMS: 100-04,4,260.1; 100-04,4,260.1.1

Q4137 **AmnioExcel, AmnioExcel Plus or BioDExcel, per sq cm** N N1 ☑
CMS: 100-04,4,260.1; 100-04,4,260.1.1
AHA: 1Q, '14, 6

Q4138 **BioDFence DryFlex, per sq cm** N N1 ☑
CMS: 100-04,4,260.1; 100-04,4,260.1.1
AHA: 1Q, '14, 6

Q4139 **AmnioMatrix or BioDMatrix, injectable, 1 cc** N N1 ☑
AHA: 1Q, '14, 6

Q4140 **BioDFence, per sq cm** N N1 ☑
CMS: 100-04,4,260.1; 100-04,4,260.1.1
AHA: 1Q, '14, 6

Special Coverage Instructions   Noncovered by Medicare   Carrier Discretion   ☑ Quantity Alert ● New Code   ○ Recycled/Reinstated ▲ Revised Code

148 — Q Codes (Temporary)   A Age Edit   M Maternity Edit   ♀ Female Only   ♂ Male Only   A-Y OPPS Status Indicators   © 2021 Optum360, LLC

Q4141   **AlloSkin AC, per sq cm**   N N1 ☑
CMS: 100-04,4,260.1; 100-04,4,260.1.1
AHA: 1Q, '14, 6

Q4142   **XCM biologic tissue matrix, per sq cm**   N N1 ☑
AHA: 1Q, '14, 6

Q4143   **Repriza, per sq cm**   N N1 ☑
CMS: 100-04,4,260.1; 100-04,4,260.1.1
AHA: 1Q, '14, 6

Q4145   **EpiFix, injectable, 1 mg**   N N1 ☑
AHA: 1Q, '14, 6

Q4146   **Tensix, per sq cm**   N N1 ☑
CMS: 100-04,4,260.1; 100-04,4,260.1.1
AHA: 1Q, '14, 6

Q4147   **Architect, Architect PX, or Architect FX, extracellular matrix, per sq cm**   N N1 ☑
CMS: 100-04,4,260.1; 100-04,4,260.1.1
AHA: 1Q, '14, 6

Q4148   **Neox Cord 1K, Neox Cord RT, or Clarix Cord 1K, per sq cm**   N N1 ☑
CMS: 100-04,4,260.1; 100-04,4,260.1.1
AHA: 1Q, '14, 6

Q4149   **Excellagen, 0.1 cc**   N N1 ☑
AHA: 1Q, '14, 6

Q4150   **AlloWrap DS or dry, per sq cm**   N N1 ☑
CMS: 100-04,4,260.1; 100-04,4,260.1.1

Q4151   **AmnioBand or Guardian, per sq cm**   N N1 ☑
CMS: 100-04,4,260.1; 100-04,4,260.1.1

Q4152   **DermaPure, per sq cm**   N N1 ☑
CMS: 100-04,4,260.1; 100-04,4,260.1.1

Q4153   **Dermavest and Plurivest, per sq cm**   N N1 ☑
CMS: 100-04,4,260.1; 100-04,4,260.1.1
AHA: 1Q, '16, 6-8

Q4154   **Biovance, per sq cm**   N N1 ☑
CMS: 100-04,4,260.1; 100-04,4,260.1.1

Q4155   **Neox Flo or Clarix Flo 1 mg**   N N1 ☑

Q4156   **Neox 100 or Clarix 100, per sq cm**   N N1 ☑
CMS: 100-04,4,260.1; 100-04,4,260.1.1

Q4157   **Revitalon, per sq cm**   N N1 ☑
CMS: 100-04,4,260.1; 100-04,4,260.1.1

Q4158   **Kerecis Omega3, per sq cm**   N N1 ☑
CMS: 100-04,4,260.1; 100-04,4,260.1.1

Q4159   **Affinity, per sq cm**   N N1 ☑
CMS: 100-04,4,260.1; 100-04,4,260.1.1

Q4160   **Nushield, per sq cm**   N N1 ☑
CMS: 100-04,4,260.1; 100-04,4,260.1.1

Q4161   **bio-ConneKt wound matrix, per sq cm**   N N1 ☑
CMS: 100-04,4,260.1; 100-04,4,260.1.1
AHA: 1Q, '16, 6-8

Q4162   **WoundEx Flow, BioSkin Flow, 0.5 cc**   N N1 ☑
AHA: 1Q, '16, 6-8

Q4163   **WoundEx, BioSkin, per sq cm**   N N1 ☑
CMS: 100-04,4,260.1; 100-04,4,260.1.1
AHA: 1Q, '16, 6-8

Q4164   **Helicoll, per sq cm**   N N1 ☑
CMS: 100-04,4,260.1; 100-04,4,260.1.1
AHA: 1Q, '16, 6-8

Q4165   **Keramatrix or Kerasorb, per sq cm**   N N1 ☑
CMS: 100-04,4,260.1; 100-04,4,260.1.1
AHA: 1Q, '16, 6-8

Q4166   **Cytal, per sq cm**   N N1 ☑
CMS: 100-04,4,260.1; 100-04,4,260.1.1
AHA: 1Q, '17, 9-10

Q4167   **Truskin, per sq cm**   N N1 ☑
CMS: 100-04,4,260.1; 100-04,4,260.1.1
AHA: 1Q, '17, 9-10

Q4168   **AmnioBand, 1 mg**   N N1 ☑
AHA: 1Q, '17, 9-10

Q4169   **Artacent wound, per sq cm**   N N1 ☑
CMS: 100-04,4,260.1; 100-04,4,260.1.1
AHA: 1Q, '17, 9-10

Q4170   **Cygnus, per sq cm**   N N1 ☑
CMS: 100-04,4,260.1; 100-04,4,260.1.1
AHA: 1Q, '17, 9-10

Q4171   **Interfyl, 1 mg**   N N1 ☑
AHA: 1Q, '17, 9-10

Q4173   **PalinGen or PalinGen XPlus, per sq cm**   N N1 ☑
CMS: 100-04,4,260.1; 100-04,4,260.1.1
AHA: 1Q, '17, 9-10

Q4174   **PalinGen or ProMatrX, 0.36 mg per 0.25 cc**   N N1 ☑
AHA: 1Q, '17, 9-10

Q4175   **Miroderm, per sq cm**   N N1 ☑
CMS: 100-04,4,260.1; 100-04,4,260.1.1
AHA: 1Q, '17, 9-10

Q4176   **Neopatch or therion, per square centimeter**   N N1
CMS: 100-04,4,260.1; 100-04,4,260.1.1

Q4177   **FlowerAmnioFlo, 0.1 cc**   N N1

Q4178   **FlowerAmnioPatch, per sq cm**   N N1
CMS: 100-04,4,260.1; 100-04,4,260.1.1

Q4179   **FlowerDerm, per sq cm**   N N1
CMS: 100-04,4,260.1; 100-04,4,260.1.1

Q4180   **Revita, per sq cm**   N N1
CMS: 100-04,4,260.1; 100-04,4,260.1.1

Q4181   **Amnio Wound, per sq cm**   N N1
CMS: 100-04,4,260.1; 100-04,4,260.1.1

Q4182   **Transcyte, per sq cm**   N N1
CMS: 100-04,4,260.1; 100-04,4,260.1.1

Q4183   **Surgigraft, per sq cm**   N1
CMS: 100-04,4,260.1; 100-04,4,260.1.1

Q4184   **Cellesta or Cellesta Duo, per sq cm**   N1
CMS: 100-04,4,260.1; 100-04,4,260.1.1

Q4185   **Cellesta Flowable Amnion (25 mg per cc); per 0.5 cc**   N1
CMS: 100-04,4,260.1; 100-04,4,260.1.1

Q4186   **Epifix, per sq cm**   N1
CMS: 100-04,4,260.1; 100-04,4,260.1.1

Q4187   **Epicord, per sq cm**   N1
CMS: 100-04,4,260.1; 100-04,4,260.1.1

Q4188   **AmnioArmor, per sq cm**   N1
CMS: 100-04,4,260.1; 100-04,4,260.1.1

Q4189   **Artacent AC, 1 mg**   N1
CMS: 100-04,4,260.1; 100-04,4,260.1.1

Q4190   **Artacent AC, per sq cm**   N1
CMS: 100-04,4,260.1; 100-04,4,260.1.1

Special Coverage Instructions   Noncovered by Medicare   Carrier Discretion   ☑ Quantity Alert   ● New Code   ○ Recycled/Reinstated   ▲ Revised Code

Code	Description	Indicator
Q4191	Restorigin, per sq cm CMS: 100-04,4,260.1; 100-04,4,260.1.1	N1
Q4192	Restorigin, 1 cc CMS: 100-04,4,260.1; 100-04,4,260.1.1	N1
Q4193	Coll-e-Derm, per sq cm CMS: 100-04,4,260.1; 100-04,4,260.1.1	N1
Q4194	Novachor, per sq cm CMS: 100-04,4,260.1; 100-04,4,260.1.1	N1
Q4195	PuraPly, per sq cm CMS: 100-04,4,260.1; 100-04,4,260.1.1	N1
Q4196	PuraPly AM, per sq cm CMS: 100-04,4,260.1; 100-04,4,260.1.1	N1
Q4197	PuraPly XT, per sq cm CMS: 100-04,4,260.1; 100-04,4,260.1.1	N1
Q4198	Genesis Amniotic Membrane, per sq cm CMS: 100-04,4,260.1; 100-04,4,260.1.1	N1
● Q4199	Cygnus matrix, per sq cm	
Q4200	SkinTE, per sq cm CMS: 100-04,4,260.1; 100-04,4,260.1.1	N1
Q4201	Matrion, per sq cm CMS: 100-04,4,260.1; 100-04,4,260.1.1	N1
Q4202	Keroxx (2.5 g/cc), 1 cc CMS: 100-04,4,260.1; 100-04,4,260.1.1	N1
Q4203	Derma-Gide, per sq cm CMS: 100-04,4,260.1; 100-04,4,260.1.1	N1
Q4204	XWRAP, per sq cm CMS: 100-04,4,260.1; 100-04,4,260.1.1	N1
Q4205	Membrane Graft or Membrane Wrap, per sq cm	N1
Q4206	Fluid Flow or Fluid GF, 1 cc	N1
Q4208	Novafix, per sq cm	N1
Q4209	SurGraft, per sq cm	N1
Q4210	Axolotl Graft or Axolotl DualGraft, per sq cm	N1
Q4211	Amnion Bio or AxoBioMembrane, per sq cm	N1
Q4212	AlloGen, per cc	
Q4213	Ascent, 0.5 mg	
Q4214	Cellesta Cord, per sq cm	N1
Q4215	Axolotl Ambient or Axolotl Cryo, 0.1 mg	
Q4216	Artacent Cord, per sq cm	N1
Q4217	WoundFix, BioWound, WoundFix Plus, BioWound Plus, WoundFix Xplus or BioWound Xplus, per sq cm	N1
Q4218	SurgiCORD, per sq cm	N1
Q4219	SurgiGRAFT-DUAL, per sq cm	N1
Q4220	BellaCell HD or Surederm, per sq cm	N1
Q4221	Amnio Wrap2, per sq cm	N1
Q4222	ProgenaMatrix, per sq cm	N1
Q4226	MyOwn Skin, includes harvesting and preparation procedures, per sq cm	N1
Q4227	AmnioCore™, per sq cm	N1
Q4228	BioNextPATCH, per sq cm	
Q4229	Cogenex Amniotic Membrane, per sq cm	N1
Q4230	Cogenex Flowable Amnion, per 0.5 cc	N1

Code	Description	Indicator
Q4231	Corplex P, per cc	N1
Q4232	Corplex, per sq cm	N1
Q4233	SurFactor or NuDyn, per 0.5 cc	N1
Q4234	XCellerate, per sq cm	N1
Q4235	AMNIOREPAIR or AltiPly, per sq cm	N1
Q4236	carePATCH, per sq cm	
Q4237	Cryo-Cord, per sq cm	N1
Q4238	Derm-Maxx, per sq cm	N1
Q4239	Amnio-Maxx or Amnio-Maxx Lite, per sq cm	N1
Q4240	CoreCyte, for topical use only, per 0.5 cc	N1
Q4241	PolyCyte, for topical use only, per 0.5 cc	N1
Q4242	AmnioCyte Plus, per 0.5 cc	N1
Q4244	Procenta, per 200 mg	N1
Q4245	AmnioText, per cc	N1
Q4246	CoreText or ProText, per cc	N1
Q4247	Amniotext patch, per sq cm	N1
Q4248	Dermacyte Amniotic Membrane Allograft, per sq cm	N1
Q4249	AMNIPLY, for topical use only, per sq cm	N1
Q4250	AmnioAmp-MP, per sq cm	N1
● Q4251	Vim, per sq cm	N1
● Q4252	Vendaje, per sq cm	N1
● Q4253	Zenith Amniotic Membrane, per sq cm	N1
Q4254	Novafix DL, per sq cm	N1
Q4255	REGUaRD, for topical use only, per sq cm	N1
Q5001	Hospice or home health care provided in patient's home/residence CMS: 100-01,3,30.3; 100-04,10,40.2; 100-04,11,10; 100-04,11,130.1; 100-04,11,30.3	B
Q5002	Hospice or home health care provided in assisted living facility CMS: 100-01,3,30.3; 100-04,10,40.2; 100-04,11,10; 100-04,11,130.1; 100-04,11,30.3	B
Q5003	Hospice care provided in nursing long-term care facility (LTC) or nonskilled nursing facility (NF) CMS: 100-01,3,30.3; 100-04,11,10; 100-04,11,130.1; 100-04,11,30.3	B
Q5004	Hospice care provided in skilled nursing facility (SNF) CMS: 100-01,3,30.3; 100-04,11,10; 100-04,11,130.1; 100-04,11,30.3	B
Q5005	Hospice care provided in inpatient hospital CMS: 100-01,3,30.3; 100-04,11,10; 100-04,11,130.1; 100-04,11,30.3	B
Q5006	Hospice care provided in inpatient hospice facility CMS: 100-01,3,30.3; 100-04,11,10; 100-04,11,130.1; 100-04,11,30.3	B
Q5007	Hospice care provided in long-term care facility CMS: 100-01,3,30.3; 100-04,11,10; 100-04,11,130.1; 100-04,11,30.3	B
Q5008	Hospice care provided in inpatient psychiatric facility CMS: 100-01,3,30.3; 100-04,11,10; 100-04,11,130.1; 100-04,11,30.3	B
Q5009	Hospice or home health care provided in place not otherwise specified (NOS) CMS: 100-01,3,30.3; 100-04,10,40.2; 100-04,11,10; 100-04,11,130.1; 100-04,11,30.3	B
Q5010	Hospice home care provided in a hospice facility CMS: 100-01,3,30.3; 100-04,11,10; 100-04,11,130.1; 100-04,11,30.3	B

Special Coverage Instructions   Noncovered by Medicare   Carrier Discretion   ☑ Quantity Alert   ● New Code   ○ Recycled/Reinstated   ▲ Revised Code

Q5101 Injection, filgrastim-sndz, biosimilar, (Zarxio), 1 mcg `G` `K2`
AHA: 2Q, '16, 6-7; 4Q, '15, 4; 3Q, '15, 7

Q5103 Injection, infliximab-dyyb, biosimilar, (Inflectra), 10 mg `G` `K2`

Q5104 Injection, infliximab-abda, biosimilar, (Renflexis), 10 mg `G` `K2`

Q5105 Injection, epoetin alfa-epbx, biosimilar, (Retacrit) (for ESRD on dialysis), 100 units `N1`
CMS: 100-04,8,60.4.2

Q5106 Injection, epoetin alfa-epbx, biosimilar, (Retacrit) (for non-ESRD use), 1000 units `K2`

Q5107 Injection, bevacizumab-awwb, biosimilar, (Mvasi), 10 mg `K2`
CMS: 100-04,4,260.1; 100-04,4,260.1.1

Q5108 Injection, pegfilgrastim-jmdb, biosimilar, (Fulphila), 0.5 mg `K2`
CMS: 100-04,4,260.1; 100-04,4,260.1.1

Q5109 Injection, infliximab-qbtx, biosimilar, (Ixifi), 10 mg `K2`
CMS: 100-04,4,260.1; 100-04,4,260.1.1

Q5110 Injection, filgrastim-aafi, biosimilar, (Nivestym), 1 mcg `K2`
CMS: 100-04,4,260.1; 100-04,4,260.1.1

Q5111 Injection, pegfilgrastim-cbqv, biosimilar, (Udenyca), 0.5 mg `K2`
CMS: 100-04,4,260.1; 100-04,4,260.1.1

Q5112 Injection, trastuzumab-dttb, biosimilar, (Ontruzant), 10 mg `K2`

Q5113 Injection, trastuzumab-pkrb, biosimilar, (Herzuma), 10 mg `K2`

Q5114 Injection, Trastuzumab-dkst, biosimilar, (Ogivri), 10 mg `K2`

Q5115 Injection, rituximab-abbs, biosimilar, (Truxima), 10 mg `K2`

Q5116 Injection, trastuzumab-qyyp, biosimilar, (Trazimera), 10 mg `K2`

Q5117 Injection, trastuzumab-anns, biosimilar, (Kanjinti), 10 mg `K2`

Q5118 Injection, bevacizumab-bvzr, biosimilar, (Zirabev), 10 mg `K2`

Q5119 Injection, rituximab-pvvr, biosimilar, (RUXIENCE), 10 mg `K2`

Q5120 Injection, pegfilgrastim-bmez, biosimilar, (ZIEXTENZO), 0.5 mg `K2`

Q5121 Injection, infliximab-axxq, biosimilar, (AVSOLA), 10 mg `K2`

Q5122 Injection, pegfilgrastim-apgf, biosimilar, (Nyvepria), 0.5 mg `K2`

● **Q5123** Injection, rituximab-arrx, biosimilar, (Riabni), 10 mg `K2`

Q9001 Assessment by Department of Veterans Affairs Chaplain Services

Q9002 Counseling, individual, by Department of Veterans Affairs Chaplain Services

Q9003 Counseling, group, by Department of Veterans Affairs Chaplain Services

● **Q9004** Department of Veterans Affairs Whole Health Partner Services

Q9950 Injection, sulfur hexafluoride lipid microspheres, per ml `N` `N1`
Use this code for Lumason.
CMS: 100-03,1,220.2
AHA: 4Q, '16, 9

Q9951 Low osmolar contrast material, 400 or greater mg/ml iodine concentration, per ml `N` `N1` ☑
CMS: 100-03,1,220.2
AHA: 3Q, '12, 8

Q9953 Injection, iron-based magnetic resonance contrast agent, per ml `N` `N1` ☑
CMS: 100-03,1,220.2
AHA: 3Q, '12, 8

Q9954 Oral magnetic resonance contrast agent, per 100 ml `N` `N1` ☑
CMS: 100-03,1,220.2
AHA: 3Q, '12, 8

Q9955 Injection, perflexane lipid microspheres, per ml `N` `N1` ☑
AHA: 3Q, '12, 8

Q9956 Injection, octafluoropropane microspheres, per ml `N` `N1` ☑
Use this code for Optison.
AHA: 3Q, '12, 8

Q9957 Injection, perflutren lipid microspheres, per ml `N` `N1` ☑
Use this code for Definity.
AHA: 3Q, '12, 8

Q9958 High osmolar contrast material, up to 149 mg/ml iodine concentration, per ml `N` `N1` ☑
CMS: 100-03,1,220.2
AHA: 3Q, '12, 8; 4Q, '11, 6; 1Q, '07, 6; 3Q, '05, 7, 9

Q9959 High osmolar contrast material, 150-199 mg/ml iodine concentration, per ml `N` `N1` ☑
CMS: 100-03,1,220.2
AHA: 3Q, '12, 8; 4Q, '11, 6; 3Q, '05, 7, 9

Q9960 High osmolar contrast material, 200-249 mg/ml iodine concentration, per ml `N` `N1` ☑
CMS: 100-03,1,220.2
AHA: 3Q, '12, 8; 4Q, '11, 6; 1Q, '07, 6; 3Q, '05, 7, 9

Q9961 High osmolar contrast material, 250-299 mg/ml iodine concentration, per ml `N` `N1` ☑
CMS: 100-03,1,220.2
AHA: 3Q, '12, 8; 4Q, '11, 6; 3Q, '05, 7, 9

Q9962 High osmolar contrast material, 300-349 mg/ml iodine concentration, per ml `N` `N1` ☑
CMS: 100-03,1,220.2
AHA: 3Q, '12, 8; 4Q, '11, 6; 3Q, '05, 7, 9

Q9963 High osmolar contrast material, 350-399 mg/ml iodine concentration, per ml `N` `N1` ☑
CMS: 100-03,1,220.2
AHA: 3Q, '12, 8; 4Q, '11, 6; 3Q, '05, 7, 9

Q9964 High osmolar contrast material, 400 or greater mg/ml iodine concentration, per ml `N` `N1` ☑
CMS: 100-03,1,220.2
AHA: 3Q, '12, 8; 4Q, '11, 6; 3Q, '05, 7, 9

Q9965 Low osmolar contrast material, 100-199 mg/ml iodine concentration, per ml `N` `N1` ☑
Use this code for Omnipaque 140, Omnipaque 180, Optiray 160, Optiray 140, ULTRAVIST 150.
CMS: 100-03,1,220.2
AHA: 3Q, '12, 8; 4Q, '11, 6; 1Q, '08, 6

Q9966 Low osmolar contrast material, 200-299 mg/ml iodine concentration, per ml `N` `N1` ☑
Use this code for Omnipaque 240, Optiray 240, ULTRAVIST 240.
CMS: 100-03,1,220.2
AHA: 3Q, '12, 8; 4Q, '11, 6; 1Q, '08, 6

Q9967 Low osmolar contrast material, 300-399 mg/ml iodine concentration, per ml `N` `N1` ☑
Use this code for Omnipaque 300, Omnipaque 350, Optiray, Optiray 300, Optiray 320, Oxilan 300, Oxilan 350, ULTRAVIST 300, ULTRAVIST 370.
CMS: 100-03,1,220.2
AHA: 3Q, '12, 8; 4Q, '11, 6; 1Q, '08, 6

Q Codes (Temporary)

Q9968 — Q9992

Q9968 Injection, nonradioactive, noncontrast, visualization adjunct (e.g., methylene blue, isosulfan blue), 1 mg K K2 ☑

Q9969 Tc-99m from nonhighly enriched uranium source, full cost recovery add-on, per study dose K ☑

Q9982 Flutemetamol F18, diagnostic, per study dose, up to 5 mCi G N1
Use this code for Vizamyl.

Q9983 Florbetaben F18, diagnostic, per study dose, up to 8.1 mCi G N1
Use this code for Neuraceq.

Q9991 Injection, buprenorphine extended-release (Sublocade), less than or equal to 100 mg K2

Q9992 Injection, buprenorphine extended-release (Sublocade), greater than 100 mg K2

Special Coverage Instructions   Noncovered by Medicare   Carrier Discretion   ☑ Quantity Alert ● New Code ○ Recycled/Reinstated ▲ Revised Code

152 — Q Codes (Temporary)   A Age Edit   M Maternity Edit   ♀ Female Only   ♂ Male Only   A-Y OPPS Status Indicators   © 2021 Optum360, LLC

Diagnostic Radiology Services R0070-R0076

R codes are used for the transportation of portable x-ray and/or EKG equipment.

R0070   **Transportation of portable x-ray equipment and personnel to home or nursing home, per trip to facility or location, one patient seen**   B ☑

Only a single, reasonable transportation charge is allowed for each trip the portable x-ray supplier makes to a location. When more than one patient is x-rayed at the same location, prorate the single allowable transport charge among all patients.
CMS: 100-04,13,90.3

R0075   **Transportation of portable x-ray equipment and personnel to home or nursing home, per trip to facility or location, more than one patient seen**   B ☑

Only a single, reasonable transportation charge is allowed for each trip the portable x-ray supplier makes to a location. When more than one patient is x-rayed at the same location, prorate the single allowable transport charge among all patients.
CMS: 100-04,13,90.3

R0076   **Transportation of portable EKG to facility or location, per patient**   B ☑

Only a single, reasonable transportation charge is allowed for each trip the portable EKG supplier makes to a location. When more than one patient is tested at the same location, prorate the single allowable transport charge among all patients.
CMS: 100-04,13,90.3; 100-04,6,20.3

Special Coverage Instructions   Noncovered by Medicare   Carrier Discretion   ☑ Quantity Alert   ● New Code   ○ Recycled/Reinstated   ▲ Revised Code

© 2021 Optum360, LLC   A2-Z3 ASC Pmt   **CMS:** IOM   **AHA:** Coding Clinic   ⅄ DMEPOS Paid   ⊘ SNF Excluded   **R Codes — 153**

Temporary National Codes (Non-Medicare) S0012-S9999

The S codes are used by the Blue Cross/Blue Shield Association (BCBSA) and the Health Insurance Association of America (HIAA) to report drugs, services, and supplies for which there are no national codes but for which codes are needed by the private sector to implement policies, programs, or claims processing. They are for the purpose of meeting the particular needs of the private sector. These codes are also used by the Medicaid program, but they are not payable by Medicare.

S0012 **Butorphanol tartrate, nasal spray, 25 mg** ☑
Use this code for Stadol NS.

S0013 **Esketamine, nasal spray, 1 mg** ☑
Use this code for Spravato.

S0014 **Tacrine HCl, 10 mg** ☑
Use this code for Cognex.

S0017 **Injection, aminocaproic acid, 5 g** ☑
Use this code for Amicar.

S0020 **Injection, bupivicaine HCl, 30 ml** ☑
Use this code for Marcaine, Sensorcaine.

S0021 **Injection, cefoperazone sodium, 1 g** ☑
Use this code for Cefobid.

S0023 **Injection, cimetidine HCl, 300 mg** ☑
Use this code for Tagamet HCl.

S0028 **Injection, famotidine, 20 mg** ☑
Use this code for Pepcid.

S0030 **Injection, metronidazole, 500 mg** ☑
Use this code for Flagyl IV RTU.

S0032 **Injection, nafcillin sodium, 2 g** ☑
Use this code for Nallpen, Unipen.

S0034 **Injection, ofloxacin, 400 mg** ☑
Use this code for Floxin IV.

S0039 **Injection, sulfamethoxazole and trimethoprim, 10 ml** ☑
Use this code for Bactrim IV, Septra IV, SMZ-TMP, Sulfutrim.

S0040 **Injection, ticarcillin disodium and clavulanate potassium, 3.1 g** ☑
Use this code for Timentin.

S0073 **Injection, aztreonam, 500 mg** ☑
Use this code for Azactam.

S0074 **Injection, cefotetan disodium, 500 mg** ☑
Use this code for Cefotan.

S0077 **Injection, clindamycin phosphate, 300 mg** ☑
Use this code for Cleocin Phosphate.

S0078 **Injection, fosphenytoin sodium, 750 mg** ☑
Use this code for Cerebryx.

S0080 **Injection, pentamidine isethionate, 300 mg** ☑
Use this code for NebuPent, Pentam 300, Pentacarinat. See also code J2545.

S0081 **Injection, piperacillin sodium, 500 mg** ☑
Use this code for Pipracil.

S0088 **Imatinib, 100 mg** ☑
Use this code for Gleevec.

S0090 **Sildenafil citrate, 25 mg** Ⓐ ☑
Use this code for Viagra.

S0091 **Granisetron HCl, 1 mg (for circumstances falling under the Medicare statute, use Q0166)** ☑
Use this code for Kytril.

S0092 **Injection, hydromorphone HCl, 250 mg (loading dose for infusion pump)** ☑
Use this code for Dilaudid, Hydromophone. See also J1170.

S0093 **Injection, morphine sulfate, 500 mg (loading dose for infusion pump)** ☑
Use this code for Duramorph, MS Contin, Morphine Sulfate. See also J2270, J2271, J2275.

S0104 **Zidovudine, oral, 100 mg** ☑
See also J3485 for Retrovir.

S0106 **Bupropion HCl sustained release tablet, 150 mg, per bottle of 60 tablets** ☑
Use this code for Wellbutrin SR tablets.

S0108 **Mercaptopurine, oral, 50 mg** ☑
Use this code for Purinethol oral.

S0109 **Methadone, oral, 5 mg** ☑
Use this code for Dolophine.

S0117 **Tretinoin, topical, 5 g** ☑

S0119 **Ondansetron, oral, 4 mg (for circumstances falling under the Medicare statute, use HCPCS Q code)** ☑
Use this code for Zofran, Zuplenz.

S0122 **Injection, menotropins, 75 IU** ☑
Use this code for Humegon, Pergonal, Repronex.
CMS: 100-02,15,50.5

S0126 **Injection, follitropin alfa, 75 IU** ☑
Use this code for Gonal-F.
CMS: 100-02,15,50.5

S0128 **Injection, follitropin beta, 75 IU** ♀☑
Use this code for Follistim.
CMS: 100-02,15,50.5

S0132 **Injection, ganirelix acetate, 250 mcg** ♀☑
Use this code for Antagon.
CMS: 100-02,15,50.5

S0136 **Clozapine, 25 mg** ☑
Use this code for Clozaril.

S0137 **Didanosine (ddI), 25 mg** ☑
Use this code for Videx.

S0138 **Finasteride, 5 mg** ♂☑
Use this code for Propecia (oral), Proscar (oral).

S0139 **Minoxidil, 10 mg** ☑

S0140 **Saquinavir, 200 mg** ☑
Use this code for Fortovase (oral), Invirase (oral).

S0142 **Colistimethate sodium, inhalation solution administered through DME, concentrated form, per mg** ☑

S0145 **Injection, PEGylated interferon alfa-2A, 180 mcg per ml** ☑
Use this code for Pegasys.
CMS: 100-02,15,50.5

S0148 **Injection, PEGylated interferon alfa-2B, 10 mcg** ☑
CMS: 100-02,15,50.5

S0155 **Sterile dilutant for epoprostenol, 50 ml** ☑
Use this code for Flolan.

S0156 **Exemestane, 25 mg** ☑
Use this code for Aromasin.

S0157 **Becaplermin gel 0.01%, 0.5 gm** ☑
Use this code for Regraex Gel.

S0160 **Dextroamphetamine sulfate, 5 mg** ☑

S0164 **Injection, pantoprazole sodium, 40 mg** ☑
Use this code for Protonix IV.

S0166 **Injection, olanzapine, 2.5 mg** ☑
Use this code for Zyprexa.

Special Coverage Instructions Noncovered by Medicare Carrier Discretion ☑ Quantity Alert ● New Code ○ Recycled/Reinstated ▲ Revised Code

S0169 **Calcitrol, 0.25 mcg** ☑
Use this code for Calcijex.

S0170 **Anastrozole, oral, 1 mg** ☑
Use this code for Arimidex.

S0171 **Injection, bumetanide, 0.5 mg** ☑
Use this code for Bumex.

S0172 **Chlorambucil, oral, 2 mg** ☑
Use this code for Leukeran.

S0174 **Dolasetron mesylate, oral 50 mg (for circumstances falling under the Medicare statute, use Q0180)** ☑
Use this code for Anzemet.

S0175 **Flutamide, oral, 125 mg** ☑
Use this code for Eulexin.

S0176 **Hydroxyurea, oral, 500 mg** ☑
Use this code for Droxia, Hydrea, Mylocel.

S0177 **Levamisole HCl, oral, 50 mg** ☑
Use this code for Ergamisol.

S0178 **Lomustine, oral, 10 mg** ☑
Use this code for Ceenu.

S0179 **Megestrol acetate, oral, 20 mg** ☑
Use this code for Megace.

S0182 **Procarbazine HCl, oral, 50 mg** ☑
Use this code for Matulane.

S0183 **Prochlorperazine maleate, oral, 5 mg (for circumstances falling under the Medicare statute, use Q0164)** ☑
Use this code for Compazine.

S0187 **Tamoxifen citrate, oral, 10 mg** ☑
Use this code for Nolvadex.

S0189 **Testosterone pellet, 75 mg** ☑

S0190 **Mifepristone, oral, 200 mg** ♀☑
Use this code for Mifoprex 200 mg oral.

S0191 **Misoprostol, oral, 200 mcg** ☑

S0194 **Dialysis/stress vitamin supplement, oral, 100 capsules** ☑

S0197 **Prenatal vitamins, 30-day supply** ♀☑

S0199 **Medically induced abortion by oral ingestion of medication including all associated services and supplies (e.g., patient counseling, office visits, confirmation of pregnancy by HCG, ultrasound to confirm duration of pregnancy, ultrasound to confirm completion of abortion) except drugs** ♀

S0201 **Partial hospitalization services, less than 24 hours, per diem**

S0207 **Paramedic intercept, nonhospital-based ALS service (nonvoluntary), nontransport**

S0208 **Paramedic intercept, hospital-based ALS service (nonvoluntary), nontransport**

S0209 **Wheelchair van, mileage, per mile** ☑

S0215 **Nonemergency transportation; mileage, per mile** ☑
See also codes A0021-A0999 for transportation.

S0220 **Medical conference by a physician with interdisciplinary team of health professionals or representatives of community agencies to coordinate activities of patient care (patient is present); approximately 30 minutes** ☑

S0221 **Medical conference by a physician with interdisciplinary team of health professionals or representatives of community agencies to coordinate activities of patient care (patient is present); approximately 60 minutes** ☑

S0250 **Comprehensive geriatric assessment and treatment planning performed by assessment team** Ⓐ

S0255 **Hospice referral visit (advising patient and family of care options) performed by nurse, social worker, or other designated staff**
CMS: 100-04,11,10

S0257 **Counseling and discussion regarding advance directives or end of life care planning and decisions, with patient and/or surrogate (list separately in addition to code for appropriate evaluation and management service)**

S0260 **History and physical (outpatient or office) related to surgical procedure (list separately in addition to code for appropriate evaluation and management service)**

S0265 **Genetic counseling, under physician supervision, each 15 minutes** ☑

S0270 **Physician management of patient home care, standard monthly case rate (per 30 days)** ☑

S0271 **Physician management of patient home care, hospice monthly case rate (per 30 days)** ☑

S0272 **Physician management of patient home care, episodic care monthly case rate (per 30 days)** ☑

S0273 **Physician visit at member's home, outside of a capitation arrangement**

S0274 **Nurse practitioner visit at member's home, outside of a capitation arrangement**

S0280 **Medical home program, comprehensive care coordination and planning, initial plan**

S0281 **Medical home program, comprehensive care coordination and planning, maintenance of plan**

S0285 **Colonoscopy consultation performed prior to a screening colonoscopy procedure**

S0302 **Completed early periodic screening diagnosis and treatment (EPSDT) service (list in addition to code for appropriate evaluation and management service)**

S0310 **Hospitalist services (list separately in addition to code for appropriate evaluation and management service)**

S0311 **Comprehensive management and care coordination for advanced illness, per calendar month**

S0315 **Disease management program; initial assessment and initiation of the program**

S0316 **Disease management program, follow-up/reassessment**

S0317 **Disease management program; per diem** ☑

S0320 **Telephone calls by a registered nurse to a disease management program member for monitoring purposes; per month**

S0340 **Lifestyle modification program for management of coronary artery disease, including all supportive services; first quarter/stage**

S0341 **Lifestyle modification program for management of coronary artery disease, including all supportive services; second or third quarter/stage**

S0342 **Lifestyle modification program for management of coronary artery disease, including all supportive services; fourth quarter/stage**

S0353 **Treatment planning and care coordination management for cancer initial treatment**

S0354 **Treatment planning and care coordination management for cancer established patient with a change of regimen**

S0390 **Routine foot care; removal and/or trimming of corns, calluses and/or nails and preventive maintenance in specific medical conditions (e.g., diabetes), per visit**

Special Coverage Instructions　　Noncovered by Medicare　　Carrier Discretion　　☑ Quantity Alert　● New Code　○ Recycled/Reinstated　▲ Revised Code

156 — S Codes　　Ⓐ Age Edit　Ⓜ Maternity Edit　♀ Female Only　♂ Male Only　Ⓐ-Ⓨ OPPS Status Indicators　　© 2021 Optum360, LLC

S0395	Impression casting of a foot performed by a practitioner other than the manufacturer of the orthotic	
S0400	Global fee for extracorporeal shock wave lithotripsy treatment of kidney stone(s)	
S0500	Disposable contact lens, per lens	☑
S0504	Single vision prescription lens (safety, athletic, or sunglass), per lens	☑
S0506	Bifocal vision prescription lens (safety, athletic, or sunglass), per lens	☑
S0508	Trifocal vision prescription lens (safety, athletic, or sunglass), per lens	☑
S0510	Nonprescription lens (safety, athletic, or sunglass), per lens	☑
S0512	Daily wear specialty contact lens, per lens	☑
S0514	Color contact lens, per lens	☑
S0515	Scleral lens, liquid bandage device, per lens	
S0516	Safety eyeglass frames	
S0518	Sunglasses frames	
S0580	Polycarbonate lens (list this code in addition to the basic code for the lens)	
S0581	Nonstandard lens (list this code in addition to the basic code for the lens)	
S0590	Integral lens service, miscellaneous services reported separately	
S0592	Comprehensive contact lens evaluation	
S0595	Dispensing new spectacle lenses for patient supplied frame	
S0596	Phakic intraocular lens for correction of refractive error	☑
S0601	Screening proctoscopy	♂
S0610	Annual gynecological examination, new patient	A ♀
S0612	Annual gynecological examination, established patient	A ♀
S0613	Annual gynecological examination; clinical breast examination without pelvic evaluation	♀
S0618	Audiometry for hearing aid evaluation to determine the level and degree of hearing loss	
S0620	Routine ophthalmological examination including refraction; new patient	
S0621	Routine ophthalmological examination including refraction; established patient	
S0622	Physical exam for college, new or established patient (list separately in addition to appropriate evaluation and management code)	
S0630	Removal of sutures; by a physician other than the physician who originally closed the wound	
S0800	Laser in situ keratomileusis (LASIK)	
S0810	Photorefractive keratectomy (PRK)	
S0812	Phototherapeutic keratectomy (PTK)	
S1001	Deluxe item, patient aware (list in addition to code for basic item) CMS: 100-02,15,110	
S1002	Customized item (list in addition to code for basic item)	
S1015	IV tubing extension set	
S1016	Non-PVC (polyvinyl chloride) intravenous administration set, for use with drugs that are not stable in PVC, e.g., Paclitaxel	
S1030	Continuous noninvasive glucose monitoring device, purchase (for physician interpretation of data, use CPT code)	
S1031	Continuous noninvasive glucose monitoring device, rental, including sensor, sensor replacement, and download to monitor (for physician interpretation of data, use CPT code)	
S1034	Artificial pancreas device system (e.g., low glucose suspend [LGS] feature) including continuous glucose monitor, blood glucose device, insulin pump and computer algorithm that communicates with all of the devices	
S1035	Sensor; invasive (e.g., subcutaneous), disposable, for use with artificial pancreas device system	
S1036	Transmitter; external, for use with artificial pancreas device system	
S1037	Receiver (monitor); external, for use with artificial pancreas device system	
S1040	Cranial remolding orthotic, pediatric, rigid, with soft interface material, custom fabricated, includes fitting and adjustment(s)	
● S1091	Stent, noncoronary, temporary, with delivery system (Propel)	
S2053	Transplantation of small intestine and liver allografts	
S2054	Transplantation of multivisceral organs	
S2055	Harvesting of donor multivisceral organs, with preparation and maintenance of allografts; from cadaver donor	
S2060	Lobar lung transplantation	
S2061	Donor lobectomy (lung) for transplantation, living donor	
S2065	Simultaneous pancreas kidney transplantation	
S2066	Breast reconstruction with gluteal artery perforator (GAP) flap, including harvesting of the flap, microvascular transfer, closure of donor site and shaping the flap into a breast, unilateral	
S2067	Breast reconstruction of a single breast with "stacked" deep inferior epigastric perforator (DIEP) flap(s) and/or gluteal artery perforator (GAP) flap(s), including harvesting of the flap(s), microvascular transfer, closure of donor site(s) and shaping the flap into a breast, unilateral	
S2068	Breast reconstruction with deep inferior epigastric perforator (DIEP) flap or superficial inferior epigastric artery (SIEA) flap, including harvesting of the flap, microvascular transfer, closure of donor site and shaping the flap into a breast, unilateral	
S2070	Cystourethroscopy, with ureteroscopy and/or pyeloscopy; with endoscopic laser treatment of ureteral calculi (includes ureteral catheterization)	
S2079	Laparoscopic esophagomyotomy (Heller type)	
S2080	Laser-assisted uvulopalatoplasty (LAUP)	
S2083	Adjustment of gastric band diameter via subcutaneous port by injection or aspiration of saline	
S2095	Transcatheter occlusion or embolization for tumor destruction, percutaneous, any method, using yttrium-90 microspheres	
S2102	Islet cell tissue transplant from pancreas; allogeneic	
S2103	Adrenal tissue transplant to brain	
S2107	Adoptive immunotherapy i.e. development of specific antitumor reactivity (e.g., tumor-infiltrating lymphocyte therapy) per course of treatment	
S2112	Arthroscopy, knee, surgical for harvesting of cartilage (chondrocyte cells)	
S2115	Osteotomy, periacetabular, with internal fixation	
S2117	Arthroereisis, subtalar	
S2118	Metal-on-metal total hip resurfacing, including acetabular and femoral components	
S2120	Low density lipoprotein (LDL) apheresis using heparin-induced extracorporeal LDL precipitation	

Special Coverage Instructions   Noncovered by Medicare   Carrier Discretion   ☑ Quantity Alert   ● New Code   ○ Recycled/Reinstated   ▲ Revised Code

© 2021 Optum360, LLC   A2-Z3 ASC Pmt   CMS: IOM   AHA: Coding Clinic   ⅄ DMEPOS Paid   ⊘ SNF Excluded   S Codes — 157

S2140 Cord blood harvesting for transplantation, allogeneic

S2142 Cord blood-derived stem-cell transplantation, allogeneic

S2150 Bone marrow or blood-derived stem cells (peripheral or umbilical), allogeneic or autologous, harvesting, transplantation, and related complications; including: pheresis and cell preparation/storage; marrow ablative therapy; drugs, supplies, hospitalization with outpatient follow-up; medical/surgical, diagnostic, emergency, and rehabilitative services; and the number of days of pre- and posttransplant care in the global definition

S2152 Solid organ(s), complete or segmental, single organ or combination of organs; deceased or living donor(s), procurement, transplantation, and related complications; including: drugs; supplies; hospitalization with outpatient follow-up; medical/surgical, diagnostic, emergency, and rehabilitative services, and the number of days of pre- and posttransplant care in the global definition

S2202 Echosclerotherapy

S2205 Minimally invasive direct coronary artery bypass surgery involving mini-thoracotomy or mini-sternotomy surgery, performed under direct vision; using arterial graft(s), single coronary arterial graft

S2206 Minimally invasive direct coronary artery bypass surgery involving mini-thoracotomy or mini-sternotomy surgery, performed under direct vision; using arterial graft(s), two coronary arterial grafts

S2207 Minimally invasive direct coronary artery bypass surgery involving mini-thoracotomy or mini-sternotomy surgery, performed under direct vision; using venous graft only, single coronary venous graft

S2208 Minimally invasive direct coronary artery bypass surgery involving mini-thoracotomy or mini-sternotomy surgery, performed under direct vision; using single arterial and venous graft(s), single venous graft

S2209 Minimally invasive direct coronary artery bypass surgery involving mini-thoracotomy or mini-sternotomy surgery, performed under direct vision; using two arterial grafts and single venous graft

S2225 Myringotomy, laser-assisted

S2230 Implantation of magnetic component of semi-implantable hearing device on ossicles in middle ear

S2235 Implantation of auditory brain stem implant

S2260 Induced abortion, 17 to 24 weeks Ⓜ ♀

S2265 Induced abortion, 25 to 28 weeks Ⓜ ♀

S2266 Induced abortion, 29 to 31 weeks Ⓜ ♀

S2267 Induced abortion, 32 weeks or greater Ⓜ ♀

S2300 Arthroscopy, shoulder, surgical; with thermally-induced capsulorrhaphy

S2325 Hip core decompression

S2340 Chemodenervation of abductor muscle(s) of vocal cord

S2341 Chemodenervation of adductor muscle(s) of vocal cord

S2342 Nasal endoscopy for postoperative debridement following functional endoscopic sinus surgery, nasal and/or sinus cavity(s), unilateral or bilateral

S2348 Decompression procedure, percutaneous, of nucleus pulposus of intervertebral disc, using radiofrequency energy, single or multiple levels, lumbar

S2350 Diskectomy, anterior, with decompression of spinal cord and/or nerve root(s), including osteophytectomy; lumbar, single interspace

S2351 Diskectomy, anterior, with decompression of spinal cord and/or nerve root(s), including osteophytectomy; lumbar, each additional interspace (list separately in addition to code for primary procedure)

S2400 Repair, congenital diaphragmatic hernia in the fetus using temporary tracheal occlusion, procedure performed in utero Ⓜ ♀

S2401 Repair, urinary tract obstruction in the fetus, procedure performed in utero Ⓜ ♀

S2402 Repair, congenital cystic adenomatoid malformation in the fetus, procedure performed in utero Ⓜ ♀

S2403 Repair, extralobar pulmonary sequestration in the fetus, procedure performed in utero Ⓜ ♀

S2404 Repair, myelomeningocele in the fetus, procedure performed in utero Ⓜ ♀

S2405 Repair of sacrococcygeal teratoma in the fetus, procedure performed in utero Ⓜ ♀

S2409 Repair, congenital malformation of fetus, procedure performed in utero, not otherwise classified Ⓜ ♀

S2411 Fetoscopic laser therapy for treatment of twin-to-twin transfusion syndrome Ⓜ ♀

S2900 Surgical techniques requiring use of robotic surgical system (list separately in addition to code for primary procedure)
AHA: 2Q, '10, 6

S3000 Diabetic indicator; retinal eye exam, dilated, bilateral

S3005 Performance measurement, evaluation of patient self assessment, depression

S3600 STAT laboratory request (situations other than S3601)

S3601 Emergency STAT laboratory charge for patient who is homebound or residing in a nursing facility

S3620 Newborn metabolic screening panel, includes test kit, postage and the laboratory tests specified by the state for inclusion in this panel (e.g., galactose; hemoglobin, electrophoresis; hydroxyprogesterone, 17-d; phenylalanine (PKU); and thyroxine, total) Ⓐ

S3630 Eosinophil count, blood, direct

S3645 HIV-1 antibody testing of oral mucosal transudate

S3650 Saliva test, hormone level; during menopause Ⓐ ♀

S3652 Saliva test, hormone level; to assess preterm labor risk Ⓜ ♀

S3655 Antisperm antibodies test (immunobead) Ⓜ ♀

S3708 Gastrointestinal fat absorption study

S3722 Dose optimization by area under the curve (AUC) analysis, for infusional 5-fluorouracil

S3800 Genetic testing for amyotrophic lateral sclerosis (ALS)

S3840 DNA analysis for germline mutations of the RET proto-oncogene for susceptibility to multiple endocrine neoplasia type 2

S3841 Genetic testing for retinoblastoma

S3842 Genetic testing for Von Hippel-Lindau disease

S3844 DNA analysis of the connexin 26 gene (GJB2) for susceptibility to congenital, profound deafness

S3845 Genetic testing for alpha-thalassemia

S3846 Genetic testing for hemoglobin E beta-thalassemia

S3849 Genetic testing for Niemann-Pick disease

S3850 Genetic testing for sickle cell anemia

S3852 DNA analysis for APOE epsilon 4 allele for susceptibility to Alzheimer's disease

Special Coverage Instructions   Noncovered by Medicare   Carrier Discretion   ☑ Quantity Alert ● New Code   ○ Recycled/Reinstated ▲ Revised Code

158 — S Codes   Ⓐ Age Edit   Ⓜ Maternity Edit   ♀ Female Only   ♂ Male Only   Ⓐ-Ⓨ OPPS Status Indicators   © 2021 Optum360, LLC

S3853	Genetic testing for myotonic muscular dystrophy	
S3854	Gene expression profiling panel for use in the management of breast cancer treatment	
	AHA: 2Q, '16, 5	
S3861	Genetic testing, sodium channel, voltage-gated, type V, alpha subunit (SCN5A) and variants for suspected Brugada Syndrome	
S3865	Comprehensive gene sequence analysis for hypertrophic cardiomyopathy	
S3866	Genetic analysis for a specific gene mutation for hypertrophic cardiomyopathy (HCM) in an individual with a known HCM mutation in the family	
S3870	Comparative genomic hybridization (CGH) microarray testing for developmental delay, autism spectrum disorder and/or intellectual disability	
S3900	Surface electromyography (EMG)	
S3902	Ballistocardiogram	
S3904	Masters two step	
S4005	Interim labor facility global (labor occurring but not resulting in delivery)	M ♀
S4011	In vitro fertilization; including but not limited to identification and incubation of mature oocytes, fertilization with sperm, incubation of embryo(s), and subsequent visualization for determination of development	M ♀
S4013	Complete cycle, gamete intrafallopian transfer (GIFT), case rate	M ♀
S4014	Complete cycle, zygote intrafallopian transfer (ZIFT), case rate	M ♀
S4015	Complete in vitro fertilization cycle, not otherwise specified, case rate	M ♀
S4016	Frozen in vitro fertilization cycle, case rate	M ♀
S4017	Incomplete cycle, treatment cancelled prior to stimulation, case rate	M ♀
S4018	Frozen embryo transfer procedure cancelled before transfer, case rate	M ♀
S4020	In vitro fertilization procedure cancelled before aspiration, case rate	M ♀
S4021	In vitro fertilization procedure cancelled after aspiration, case rate	M ♀
S4022	Assisted oocyte fertilization, case rate	M ♀
S4023	Donor egg cycle, incomplete, case rate	M ♀
S4025	Donor services for in vitro fertilization (sperm or embryo), case rate	A ♀
S4026	Procurement of donor sperm from sperm bank	♂
S4027	Storage of previously frozen embryos	M ♀
S4028	Microsurgical epididymal sperm aspiration (MESA)	A ♂
S4030	Sperm procurement and cryopreservation services; initial visit	A ♂
S4031	Sperm procurement and cryopreservation services; subsequent visit	A ♂
S4035	Stimulated intrauterine insemination (IUI), case rate	M ♀
S4037	Cryopreserved embryo transfer, case rate	M ♀
S4040	Monitoring and storage of cryopreserved embryos, per 30 days	M ♀
S4042	Management of ovulation induction (interpretation of diagnostic tests and studies, nonface-to-face medical management of the patient), per cycle	
S4981	Insertion of levonorgestrel-releasing intrauterine system	♀
S4989	Contraceptive intrauterine device (e.g., Progestacert IUD), including implants and supplies	M ♀
S4990	Nicotine patches, legend	☑
S4991	Nicotine patches, nonlegend	☑
S4993	Contraceptive pills for birth control	M ♀☑
S4995	Smoking cessation gum	☑
S5000	Prescription drug, generic	☑
S5001	Prescription drug, brand name	☑
S5010	5% dextrose and 0.45% normal saline, 1000 ml	☑
S5012	5% dextrose with potassium chloride, 1000 ml	☑
S5013	5% dextrose/0.45% normal saline with potassium chloride and magnesium sulfate, 1000 ml	☑
S5014	5% dextrose/0.45% normal saline with potassium chloride and magnesium sulfate, 1500 ml	☑
S5035	Home infusion therapy, routine service of infusion device (e.g., pump maintenance)	
S5036	Home infusion therapy, repair of infusion device (e.g., pump repair)	
S5100	Day care services, adult; per 15 minutes	A☑
S5101	Day care services, adult; per half day	A☑
S5102	Day care services, adult; per diem	A☑
S5105	Day care services, center-based; services not included in program fee, per diem	☑
S5108	Home care training to home care client, per 15 minutes	☑
S5109	Home care training to home care client, per session	☑
S5110	Home care training, family; per 15 minutes	☑
S5111	Home care training, family; per session	
S5115	Home care training, nonfamily; per 15 minutes	☑
S5116	Home care training, nonfamily; per session	☑
S5120	Chore services; per 15 minutes	☑
S5121	Chore services; per diem	☑
S5125	Attendant care services; per 15 minutes	☑
S5126	Attendant care services; per diem	☑
S5130	Homemaker service, NOS; per 15 minutes	☑
S5131	Homemaker service, NOS; per diem	☑
S5135	Companion care, adult (e.g., IADL/ADL); per 15 minutes	A☑
S5136	Companion care, adult (e.g., IADL/ADL); per diem	A☑
S5140	Foster care, adult; per diem	A☑
S5141	Foster care, adult; per month	A☑
S5145	Foster care, therapeutic, child; per diem	A☑
S5146	Foster care, therapeutic, child; per month	A☑
S5150	Unskilled respite care, not hospice; per 15 minutes	☑
S5151	Unskilled respite care, not hospice; per diem	☑
S5160	Emergency response system; installation and testing	
S5161	Emergency response system; service fee, per month (excludes installation and testing)	☑

Special Coverage Instructions   Noncovered by Medicare   Carrier Discretion   ☑ Quantity Alert   ● New Code   ○ Recycled/Reinstated   ▲ Revised Code

© 2021 Optum360, LLC   A2-Z3 ASC Pmt   CMS: IOM   AHA: Coding Clinic   DMEPOS Paid   ⊘ SNF Excluded   S Codes — 159

S5162	Emergency response system; purchase only	
S5165	Home modifications; per service	
S5170	Home delivered meals, including preparation; per meal	
S5175	Laundry service, external, professional; per order	
S5180	Home health respiratory therapy, initial evaluation	
S5181	Home health respiratory therapy, NOS, per diem	
S5185	Medication reminder service, nonface-to-face; per month	☑
S5190	Wellness assessment, performed by nonphysician	
S5199	Personal care item, NOS, each	
S5497	Home infusion therapy, catheter care/maintenance, not otherwise classified; includes administrative services, professional pharmacy services, care coordination, and all necessary supplies and equipment (drugs and nursing visits coded separately), per diem	☑
S5498	Home infusion therapy, catheter care/maintenance, simple (single lumen), includes administrative services, professional pharmacy services, care coordination and all necessary supplies and equipment, (drugs and nursing visits coded separately), per diem	☑
S5501	Home infusion therapy, catheter care/maintenance, complex (more than one lumen), includes administrative services, professional pharmacy services, care coordination, and all necessary supplies and equipment (drugs and nursing visits coded separately), per diem	☑
S5502	Home infusion therapy, catheter care/maintenance, implanted access device, includes administrative services, professional pharmacy services, care coordination and all necessary supplies and equipment (drugs and nursing visits coded separately), per diem (use this code for interim maintenance of vascular access not currently in use)	☑
S5517	Home infusion therapy, all supplies necessary for restoration of catheter patency or declotting	
S5518	Home infusion therapy, all supplies necessary for catheter repair	
S5520	Home infusion therapy, all supplies (including catheter) necessary for a peripherally inserted central venous catheter (PICC) line insertion	
S5521	Home infusion therapy, all supplies (including catheter) necessary for a midline catheter insertion	
S5522	Home infusion therapy, insertion of peripherally inserted central venous catheter (PICC), nursing services only (no supplies or catheter included)	
S5523	Home infusion therapy, insertion of midline venous catheter, nursing services only (no supplies or catheter included)	
S5550	Insulin, rapid onset, 5 units	☑
S5551	Insulin, most rapid onset (Lispro or Aspart); 5 units	☑
S5552	Insulin, intermediate acting (NPH or LENTE); 5 units	☑
S5553	Insulin, long acting; 5 units CMS: 100-02,15,50.5	☑
S5560	Insulin delivery device, reusable pen; 1.5 ml size	☑
S5561	Insulin delivery device, reusable pen; 3 ml size	☑
S5565	Insulin cartridge for use in insulin delivery device other than pump; 150 units	☑
S5566	Insulin cartridge for use in insulin delivery device other than pump; 300 units	☑
S5570	Insulin delivery device, disposable pen (including insulin); 1.5 ml size CMS: 100-02,15,50.5	☑
S5571	Insulin delivery device, disposable pen (including insulin); 3 ml size CMS: 100-02,15,50.5	☑
S8030	Scleral application of tantalum ring(s) for localization of lesions for proton beam therapy	
S8035	Magnetic source imaging	
S8037	Magnetic resonance cholangiopancreatography (MRCP)	
S8040	Topographic brain mapping	
S8042	Magnetic resonance imaging (MRI), low-field	
S8055	Ultrasound guidance for multifetal pregnancy reduction(s), technical component (only to be used when the physician doing the reduction procedure does not perform the ultrasound, guidance is included in the CPT code for multifetal pregnancy reduction (59866)	Ⓜ ♀
S8080	Scintimammography (radioimmunoscintigraphy of the breast), unilateral, including supply of radiopharmaceutical	
S8085	Fluorine-18 fluorodeoxyglucose (F-18 FDG) imaging using dual-head coincidence detection system (nondedicated PET scan)	
S8092	Electron beam computed tomography (also known as ultrafast CT, cine CT)	
S8096	Portable peak flow meter	
S8097	Asthma kit (including but not limited to portable peak expiratory flow meter, instructional video, brochure, and/or spacer)	☑
S8100	Holding chamber or spacer for use with an inhaler or nebulizer; without mask	
S8101	Holding chamber or spacer for use with an inhaler or nebulizer; with mask	
S8110	Peak expiratory flow rate (physician services)	
S8120	Oxygen contents, gaseous, 1 unit equals 1 cubic foot	☑
S8121	Oxygen contents, liquid, 1 unit equals 1 pound	☑
S8130	Interferential current stimulator, 2 channel	
S8131	Interferential current stimulator, 4 channel	
S8185	Flutter device	
S8186	Swivel adaptor	
S8189	Tracheostomy supply, not otherwise classified	
S8210	Mucus trap	
S8265	Haberman feeder for cleft lip/palate	
S8270	Enuresis alarm, using auditory buzzer and/or vibration device	
S8301	Infection control supplies, not otherwise specified	
S8415	Supplies for home delivery of infant	Ⓜ ♀
S8420	Gradient pressure aid (sleeve and glove combination), custom made	
S8421	Gradient pressure aid (sleeve and glove combination), ready made	
S8422	Gradient pressure aid (sleeve), custom made, medium weight	
S8423	Gradient pressure aid (sleeve), custom made, heavy weight	
S8424	Gradient pressure aid (sleeve), ready made	
S8425	Gradient pressure aid (glove), custom made, medium weight	
S8426	Gradient pressure aid (glove), custom made, heavy weight	
S8427	Gradient pressure aid (glove), ready made	

Special Coverage Instructions   Noncovered by Medicare   Carrier Discretion   ☑ Quantity Alert ● New Code ○ Recycled/Reinstated ▲ Revised Code

160 — S Codes   Ⓐ Age Edit   Ⓜ Maternity Edit   ♀ Female Only   ♂ Male Only   Ⓐ-Ⓨ OPPS Status Indicators   © 2021 Optum360, LLC

S8428	Gradient pressure aid (gauntlet), ready made	
S8429	Gradient pressure exterior wrap	
S8430	Padding for compression bandage, roll	☑
S8431	Compression bandage, roll	☑
S8450	Splint, prefabricated, digit (specify digit by use of modifier)	☑

Various types of digit splints (S8450)

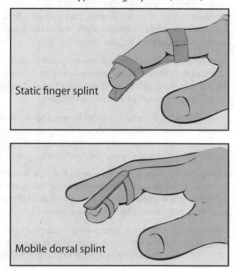

Static finger splint

Mobile dorsal splint

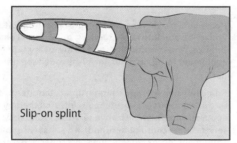

Slip-on splint

S8451	Splint, prefabricated, wrist or ankle	☑
S8452	Splint, prefabricated, elbow	☑
S8460	Camisole, postmastectomy	
S8490	Insulin syringes (100 syringes, any size)	☑
S8930	Electrical stimulation of auricular acupuncture points; each 15 minutes of personal one-on-one contact with patient	☑
S8940	Equestrian/hippotherapy, per session	
S8948	Application of a modality (requiring constant provider attendance) to one or more areas; low-level laser; each 15 minutes	☑
S8950	Complex lymphedema therapy, each 15 minutes	☑
S8990	Physical or manipulative therapy performed for maintenance rather than restoration	
S8999	Resuscitation bag (for use by patient on artificial respiration during power failure or other catastrophic event)	
S9001	Home uterine monitor with or without associated nursing services	Ⓜ ♀
S9007	Ultrafiltration monitor	
S9024	Paranasal sinus ultrasound	
S9025	Omnicardiogram/cardiointegram	

S9034	Extracorporeal shockwave lithotripsy for gall stones (if performed with ERCP, use 43265)	
S9055	Procuren or other growth factor preparation to promote wound healing	
S9056	Coma stimulation per diem	☑
S9061	Home administration of aerosolized drug therapy (e.g., Pentamidine); administrative services, professional pharmacy services, care coordination, all necessary supplies and equipment (drugs and nursing visits coded separately), per diem	☑
S9083	Global fee urgent care centers	
S9088	Services provided in an urgent care center (list in addition to code for service)	
S9090	Vertebral axial decompression, per session	☑
S9097	Home visit for wound care	
S9098	Home visit, phototherapy services (e.g., Bili-lite), including equipment rental, nursing services, blood draw, supplies, and other services, per diem	☑
S9110	Telemonitoring of patient in their home, including all necessary equipment; computer system, connections, and software; maintenance; patient education and support; per month	
S9117	Back school, per visit	☑
S9122	Home health aide or certified nurse assistant, providing care in the home; per hour	☑
S9123	Nursing care, in the home; by registered nurse, per hour (use for general nursing care only, not to be used when CPT codes 99500-99602 can be used)	☑
S9124	Nursing care, in the home; by licensed practical nurse, per hour	☑
S9125	Respite care, in the home, per diem	☑
S9126	Hospice care, in the home, per diem **CMS:** 100-04,11,10	☑
S9127	Social work visit, in the home, per diem	☑
S9128	Speech therapy, in the home, per diem	☑
S9129	Occupational therapy, in the home, per diem	☑
S9131	Physical therapy; in the home, per diem	☑
S9140	Diabetic management program, follow-up visit to non-MD provider	☑
S9141	Diabetic management program, follow-up visit to MD provider	☑
S9145	Insulin pump initiation, instruction in initial use of pump (pump not included)	
S9150	Evaluation by ocularist	
S9152	Speech therapy, re-evaluation	
S9208	Home management of preterm labor, including administrative services, professional pharmacy services, care coordination, and all necessary supplies or equipment (drugs and nursing visits coded separately), per diem (do not use this code with any home infusion per diem code)	Ⓜ ♀ ☑
S9209	Home management of preterm premature rupture of membranes (PPROM), including administrative services, professional pharmacy services, care coordination, and all necessary supplies or equipment (drugs and nursing visits coded separately), per diem (do not use this code with any home infusion per diem code)	Ⓜ ♀ ☑

S9211 Home management of gestational hypertension, includes administrative services, professional pharmacy services, care coordination and all necessary supplies and equipment (drugs and nursing visits coded separately); per diem (do not use this code with any home infusion per diem code) Ⓜ ♀ ☑

S9212 Home management of postpartum hypertension, includes administrative services, professional pharmacy services, care coordination, and all necessary supplies and equipment (drugs and nursing visits coded separately), per diem (do not use this code with any home infusion per diem code) ♀ ☑

S9213 Home management of preeclampsia, includes administrative services, professional pharmacy services, care coordination, and all necessary supplies and equipment (drugs and nursing services coded separately); per diem (do not use this code with any home infusion per diem code) Ⓜ ♀ ☑

S9214 Home management of gestational diabetes, includes administrative services, professional pharmacy services, care coordination, and all necessary supplies and equipment (drugs and nursing visits coded separately); per diem (do not use this code with any home infusion per diem code) Ⓜ ♀ ☑

S9325 Home infusion therapy, pain management infusion; administrative services, professional pharmacy services, care coordination, and all necessary supplies and equipment, (drugs and nursing visits coded separately), per diem (do not use this code with S9326, S9327 or S9328) ☑

S9326 Home infusion therapy, continuous (24 hours or more) pain management infusion; administrative services, professional pharmacy services, care coordination and all necessary supplies and equipment (drugs and nursing visits coded separately), per diem ☑

S9327 Home infusion therapy, intermittent (less than 24 hours) pain management infusion; administrative services, professional pharmacy services, care coordination, and all necessary supplies and equipment (drugs and nursing visits coded separately), per diem ☑

S9328 Home infusion therapy, implanted pump pain management infusion; administrative services, professional pharmacy services, care coordination, and all necessary supplies and equipment (drugs and nursing visits coded separately), per diem ☑

S9329 Home infusion therapy, chemotherapy infusion; administrative services, professional pharmacy services, care coordination, and all necessary supplies and equipment (drugs and nursing visits coded separately), per diem (do not use this code with S9330 or S9331) ☑

S9330 Home infusion therapy, continuous (24 hours or more) chemotherapy infusion; administrative services, professional pharmacy services, care coordination, and all necessary supplies and equipment (drugs and nursing visits coded separately), per diem ☑

S9331 Home infusion therapy, intermittent (less than 24 hours) chemotherapy infusion; administrative services, professional pharmacy services, care coordination, and all necessary supplies and equipment (drugs and nursing visits coded separately), per diem ☑

S9335 Home therapy, hemodialysis; administrative services, professional pharmacy services, care coordination, and all necessary supplies and equipment (drugs and nursing services coded separately), per diem ☑

S9336 Home infusion therapy, continuous anticoagulant infusion therapy (e.g., Heparin), administrative services, professional pharmacy services, care coordination and all necessary supplies and equipment (drugs and nursing visits coded separately), per diem ☑

S9338 Home infusion therapy, immunotherapy, administrative services, professional pharmacy services, care coordination, and all necessary supplies and equipment (drugs and nursing visits coded separately), per diem ☑

S9339 Home therapy; peritoneal dialysis, administrative services, professional pharmacy services, care coordination and all necessary supplies and equipment (drugs and nursing visits coded separately), per diem ☑

S9340 Home therapy; enteral nutrition; administrative services, professional pharmacy services, care coordination, and all necessary supplies and equipment (enteral formula and nursing visits coded separately), per diem ☑

S9341 Home therapy; enteral nutrition via gravity; administrative services, professional pharmacy services, care coordination, and all necessary supplies and equipment (enteral formula and nursing visits coded separately), per diem ☑

S9342 Home therapy; enteral nutrition via pump; administrative services, professional pharmacy services, care coordination, and all necessary supplies and equipment (enteral formula and nursing visits coded separately), per diem ☑

S9343 Home therapy; enteral nutrition via bolus; administrative services, professional pharmacy services, care coordination, and all necessary supplies and equipment (enteral formula and nursing visits coded separately), per diem ☑

S9345 Home infusion therapy, antihemophilic agent infusion therapy (e.g., Factor VIII); administrative services, professional pharmacy services, care coordination, and all necessary supplies and equipment (drugs and nursing visits coded separately), per diem ☑

S9346 Home infusion therapy, alpha-1-proteinase inhibitor (e.g., Prolastin); administrative services, professional pharmacy services, care coordination, and all necessary supplies and equipment (drugs and nursing visits coded separately), per diem ☑

S9347 Home infusion therapy, uninterrupted, long-term, controlled rate intravenous or subcutaneous infusion therapy (e.g., epoprostenol); administrative services, professional pharmacy services, care coordination, and all necessary supplies and equipment (drugs and nursing visits coded separately), per diem ☑

S9348 Home infusion therapy, sympathomimetic/inotropic agent infusion therapy (e.g., Dobutamine); administrative services, professional pharmacy services, care coordination, all necessary supplies and equipment (drugs and nursing visits coded separately), per diem ☑

S9349 Home infusion therapy, tocolytic infusion therapy; administrative services, professional pharmacy services, care coordination, and all necessary supplies and equipment (drugs and nursing visits coded separately), per diem Ⓜ ♀ ☑

S9351 Home infusion therapy, continuous or intermittent antiemetic infusion therapy; administrative services, professional pharmacy services, care coordination, and all necessary supplies and equipment (drugs and visits coded separately), per diem ☑

S9353 Home infusion therapy, continuous insulin infusion therapy; administrative services, professional pharmacy services, care coordination, and all necessary supplies and equipment (drugs and nursing visits coded separately), per diem ☑

S9355 Home infusion therapy, chelation therapy; administrative services, professional pharmacy services, care coordination, and all necessary supplies and equipment (drugs and nursing visits coded separately), per diem ☑

Special Coverage Instructions   Noncovered by Medicare   Carrier Discretion   ☑ Quantity Alert   ● New Code   ○ Recycled/Reinstated   ▲ Revised Code

   Ⓐ Age Edit   Ⓜ Maternity Edit   ♀ Female Only   ♂ Male Only   Ⓐ-Ⓨ OPPS Status Indicators   © 2021 Optum360, LLC

S9357 Home infusion therapy, enzyme replacement intravenous therapy; (e.g., Imiglucerase); administrative services, professional pharmacy services, care coordination, and all necessary supplies and equipment (drugs and nursing visits coded separately), per diem ☑

S9359 Home infusion therapy, antitumor necrosis factor intravenous therapy; (e.g., Infliximab); administrative services, professional pharmacy services, care coordination, and all necessary supplies and equipment (drugs and nursing visits coded separately), per diem ☑

S9361 Home infusion therapy, diuretic intravenous therapy; administrative services, professional pharmacy services, care coordination, and all necessary supplies and equipment (drugs and nursing visits coded separately), per diem ☑

S9363 Home infusion therapy, antispasmotic therapy; administrative services, professional pharmacy services, care coordination, and all necessary supplies and equipment (drugs and nursing visits coded separately), per diem ☑

S9364 Home infusion therapy, total parenteral nutrition (TPN); administrative services, professional pharmacy services, care coordination, and all necessary supplies and equipment including standard TPN formula (lipids, specialty amino acid formulas, drugs other than in standard formula and nursing visits coded separately), per diem (do not use with home infusion codes S9365-S9368 using daily volume scales) ☑

S9365 Home infusion therapy, total parenteral nutrition (TPN); one liter per day, administrative services, professional pharmacy services, care coordination, and all necessary supplies and equipment including standard TPN formula (lipids, specialty amino acid formulas, drugs other than in standard formula and nursing visits coded separately), per diem ☑

S9366 Home infusion therapy, total parenteral nutrition (TPN); more than one liter but no more than two liters per day, administrative services, professional pharmacy services, care coordination, and all necessary supplies and equipment including standard TPN formula (lipids, specialty amino acid formulas, drugs other than in standard formula and nursing visits coded separately), per diem ☑

S9367 Home infusion therapy, total parenteral nutrition (TPN); more than two liters but no more than three liters per day, administrative services, professional pharmacy services, care coordination, and all necessary supplies and equipment including standard TPN formula (lipids, specialty amino acid formulas, drugs other than in standard formula and nursing visits coded separately), per diem ☑

S9368 Home infusion therapy, total parenteral nutrition (TPN); more than three liters per day, administrative services, professional pharmacy services, care coordination, and all necessary supplies and equipment including standard TPN formula (lipids, specialty amino acid formulas, drugs other than in standard formula and nursing visits coded separately), per diem ☑

S9370 Home therapy, intermittent antiemetic injection therapy; administrative services, professional pharmacy services, care coordination, and all necessary supplies and equipment (drugs and nursing visits coded separately), per diem ☑

S9372 Home therapy; intermittent anticoagulant injection therapy (e.g., Heparin); administrative services, professional pharmacy services, care coordination, and all necessary supplies and equipment (drugs and nursing visits coded separately), per diem (do not use this code for flushing of infusion devices with Heparin to maintain patency) ☑

S9373 Home infusion therapy, hydration therapy; administrative services, professional pharmacy services, care coordination, and all necessary supplies and equipment (drugs and nursing visits coded separately), per diem (do not use with hydration therapy codes S9374-S9377 using daily volume scales) ☑

S9374 Home infusion therapy, hydration therapy; 1 liter per day, administrative services, professional pharmacy services, care coordination, and all necessary supplies and equipment (drugs and nursing visits coded separately), per diem ☑

S9375 Home infusion therapy, hydration therapy; more than 1 liter but no more than 2 liters per day, administrative services, professional pharmacy services, care coordination, and all necessary supplies and equipment (drugs and nursing visits coded separately), per diem ☑

S9376 Home infusion therapy, hydration therapy; more than 2 liters but no more than 3 liters per day, administrative services, professional pharmacy services, care coordination, and all necessary supplies and equipment (drugs and nursing visits coded separately), per diem ☑

S9377 Home infusion therapy, hydration therapy; more than 3 liters per day, administrative services, professional pharmacy services, care coordination, and all necessary supplies (drugs and nursing visits coded separately), per diem ☑

S9379 Home infusion therapy, infusion therapy, not otherwise classified; administrative services, professional pharmacy services, care coordination, and all necessary supplies and equipment (drugs and nursing visits coded separately), per diem ☑

S9381 Delivery or service to high risk areas requiring escort or extra protection, per visit

S9401 Anticoagulation clinic, inclusive of all services except laboratory tests, per session

S9430 Pharmacy compounding and dispensing services

● **S9432** Medical foods for noninborn errors of metabolism

S9433 Medical food nutritionally complete, administered orally, providing 100% of nutritional intake

S9434 Modified solid food supplements for inborn errors of metabolism

S9435 Medical foods for inborn errors of metabolism

S9436 Childbirth preparation/Lamaze classes, nonphysician provider, per session Ⓜ ♀☑

S9437 Childbirth refresher classes, nonphysician provider, per session Ⓜ ♀

S9438 Cesarean birth classes, nonphysician provider, per session Ⓜ ♀☑

S9439 VBAC (vaginal birth after cesarean) classes, nonphysician provider, per session Ⓜ ♀☑

S9441 Asthma education, nonphysician provider, per session ☑

S9442 Birthing classes, nonphysician provider, per session Ⓜ ♀☑

S9443 Lactation classes, nonphysician provider, per session Ⓜ ♀☑

S9444 Parenting classes, nonphysician provider, per session ☑

S9445 Patient education, not otherwise classified, nonphysician provider, individual, per session ☑

S9446 Patient education, not otherwise classified, nonphysician provider, group, per session ☑

S9447 Infant safety (including CPR) classes, nonphysician provider, per session ☑

Temporary National Codes (Non-Medicare)

S9449 — S9975

S9449 Weight management classes, nonphysician provider, per session ☑

S9451 Exercise classes, nonphysician provider, per session

S9452 Nutrition classes, nonphysician provider, per session

S9453 Smoking cessation classes, nonphysician provider, per session

S9454 Stress management classes, nonphysician provider, per session

S9455 Diabetic management program, group session

S9460 Diabetic management program, nurse visit

S9465 Diabetic management program, dietitian visit

S9470 Nutritional counseling, dietitian visit

S9472 Cardiac rehabilitation program, nonphysician provider, per diem

S9473 Pulmonary rehabilitation program, nonphysician provider, per diem

S9474 Enterostomal therapy by a registered nurse certified in enterostomal therapy, per diem

S9475 Ambulatory setting substance abuse treatment or detoxification services, per diem

S9476 Vestibular rehabilitation program, nonphysician provider, per diem

S9480 Intensive outpatient psychiatric services, per diem

S9482 Family stabilization services, per 15 minutes ☑

S9484 Crisis intervention mental health services, per hour ☑

S9485 Crisis intervention mental health services, per diem

S9490 Home infusion therapy, corticosteroid infusion; administrative services, professional pharmacy services, care coordination, and all necessary supplies and equipment (drugs and nursing visits coded separately), per diem ☑

S9494 Home infusion therapy, antibiotic, antiviral, or antifungal therapy; administrative services, professional pharmacy services, care coordination, and all necessary supplies and equipment (drugs and nursing visits coded separately), per diem (do not use this code with home infusion codes for hourly dosing schedules S9497-S9504) ☑

S9497 Home infusion therapy, antibiotic, antiviral, or antifungal therapy; once every 3 hours; administrative services, professional pharmacy services, care coordination, and all necessary supplies and equipment (drugs and nursing visits coded separately), per diem ☑

S9500 Home infusion therapy, antibiotic, antiviral, or antifungal therapy; once every 24 hours; administrative services, professional pharmacy services, care coordination, and all necessary supplies and equipment (drugs and nursing visits coded separately), per diem ☑

S9501 Home infusion therapy, antibiotic, antiviral, or antifungal therapy; once every 12 hours; administrative services, professional pharmacy services, care coordination, and all necessary supplies and equipment (drugs and nursing visits coded separately), per diem ☑

S9502 Home infusion therapy, antibiotic, antiviral, or antifungal therapy; once every 8 hours, administrative services, professional pharmacy services, care coordination, and all necessary supplies and equipment (drugs and nursing visits coded separately), per diem ☑

S9503 Home infusion therapy, antibiotic, antiviral, or antifungal; once every 6 hours; administrative services, professional pharmacy services, care coordination, and all necessary supplies and equipment (drugs and nursing visits coded separately), per diem ☑

S9504 Home infusion therapy, antibiotic, antiviral, or antifungal; once every 4 hours; administrative services, professional pharmacy services, care coordination, and all necessary supplies and equipment (drugs and nursing visits coded separately), per diem ☑

S9529 Routine venipuncture for collection of specimen(s), single homebound, nursing home, or skilled nursing facility patient ☑

S9537 Home therapy; hematopoietic hormone injection therapy (e.g., erythropoietin, G-CSF, GM-CSF); administrative services, professional pharmacy services, care coordination, and all necessary supplies and equipment (drugs and nursing visits coded separately), per diem ☑

S9538 Home transfusion of blood product(s); administrative services, professional pharmacy services, care coordination and all necessary supplies and equipment (blood products, drugs, and nursing visits coded separately), per diem ☑

S9542 Home injectable therapy, not otherwise classified, including administrative services, professional pharmacy services, care coordination, and all necessary supplies and equipment (drugs and nursing visits coded separately), per diem ☑

S9558 Home injectable therapy; growth hormone, including administrative services, professional pharmacy services, care coordination, and all necessary supplies and equipment (drugs and nursing visits coded separately), per diem ☑

S9559 Home injectable therapy, interferon, including administrative services, professional pharmacy services, care coordination, and all necessary supplies and equipment (drugs and nursing visits coded separately), per diem ☑

S9560 Home injectable therapy; hormonal therapy (e.g., leuprolide, goserelin), including administrative services, professional pharmacy services, care coordination, and all necessary supplies and equipment (drugs and nursing visits coded separately), per diem ☑

S9562 Home injectable therapy, palivizumab, including administrative services, professional pharmacy services, care coordination, and all necessary supplies and equipment (drugs and nursing visits coded separately), per diem ☑

S9590 Home therapy, irrigation therapy (e.g., sterile irrigation of an organ or anatomical cavity); including administrative services, professional pharmacy services, care coordination, and all necessary supplies and equipment (drugs and nursing visits coded separately), per diem ☑

S9810 Home therapy; professional pharmacy services for provision of infusion, specialty drug administration, and/or disease state management, not otherwise classified, per hour (do not use this code with any per diem code) ☑

S9900 Services by a Journal-listed Christian Science practitioner for the purpose of healing, per diem

S9901 Services by a Journal-listed Christian Science nurse, per hour

S9960 Ambulance service, conventional air services, nonemergency transport, one way (fixed wing)

S9961 Ambulance service, conventional air service, nonemergency transport, one way (rotary wing)

S9970 Health club membership, annual

S9975 Transplant related lodging, meals and transportation, per diem

Special Coverage Instructions   Noncovered by Medicare   Carrier Discretion   ☑ Quantity Alert ● New Code   ○ Recycled/Reinstated ▲ Revised Code

164 — S Codes   Ⓐ Age Edit   Ⓜ Maternity Edit   ♀ Female Only   ♂ Male Only   Ⓐ-Ⓨ OPPS Status Indicators   © 2021 Optum360, LLC

S9976	Lodging, per diem, not otherwise classified
S9977	Meals, per diem, not otherwise specified
S9981	Medical records copying fee, administrative
S9982	Medical records copying fee, per page ☑
S9986	Not medically necessary service (patient is aware that service not medically necessary)
S9988	Services provided as part of a Phase I clinical trial
S9989	Services provided outside of the United States of America (list in addition to code(s) for services(s))
S9990	Services provided as part of a Phase II clinical trial
S9991	Services provided as part of a Phase III clinical trial
S9992	Transportation costs to and from trial location and local transportation costs (e.g., fares for taxicab or bus) for clinical trial participant and one caregiver/companion
S9994	Lodging costs (e.g., hotel charges) for clinical trial participant and one caregiver/companion
S9996	Meals for clinical trial participant and one caregiver/companion
S9999	Sales tax

Special Coverage Instructions Noncovered by Medicare Carrier Discretion ☑ Quantity Alert ● New Code ○ Recycled/Reinstated ▲ Revised Code

© 2021 Optum360, LLC A2-Z6 ASC Pmt **CMS:** IOM **AHA:** Coding Clinic ♿ DMEPOS Paid ⊘ SNF Excluded **S Codes — 165**

National T Codes Established for State Medicaid Agencies T1000-T5999

The T codes are designed for use by Medicaid state agencies to establish codes for items for which there are no permanent national codes but for which codes are necessary to administer the Medicaid program (T codes are not accepted by Medicare but can be used by private insurers). This range of codes describes nursing and home health-related services, substance abuse treatment, and certain training-related procedures.

T1000 Private duty/independent nursing service(s), licensed, up to 15 minutes ☑

T1001 Nursing assessment/evaluation

T1002 RN services, up to 15 minutes ☑

T1003 LPN/LVN services, up to 15 minutes ☑

T1004 Services of a qualified nursing aide, up to 15 minutes ☑

T1005 Respite care services, up to 15 minutes ☑

T1006 Alcohol and/or substance abuse services, family/couple counseling

T1007 Alcohol and/or substance abuse services, treatment plan development and/or modification

T1009 Child sitting services for children of the individual receiving alcohol and/or substance abuse services

T1010 Meals for individuals receiving alcohol and/or substance abuse services (when meals not included in the program)

T1012 Alcohol and/or substance abuse services, skills development

T1013 Sign language or oral interpretive services, per 15 minutes ☑

T1014 Telehealth transmission, per minute, professional services bill separately

T1015 Clinic visit/encounter, all-inclusive
AHA: 1Q, '02, 5

T1016 Case management, each 15 minutes ☑

T1017 Targeted case management, each 15 minutes ☑

T1018 School-based individualized education program (IEP) services, bundled

T1019 Personal care services, per 15 minutes, not for an inpatient or resident of a hospital, nursing facility, ICF/MR or IMD, part of the individualized plan of treatment (code may not be used to identify services provided by home health aide or certified nurse assistant) ☑

T1020 Personal care services, per diem, not for an inpatient or resident of a hospital, nursing facility, ICF/MR or IMD, part of the individualized plan of treatment (code may not be used to identify services provided by home health aide or certified nurse assistant)

T1021 Home health aide or certified nurse assistant, per visit

T1022 Contracted home health agency services, all services provided under contract, per day

T1023 Screening to determine the appropriateness of consideration of an individual for participation in a specified program, project or treatment protocol, per encounter

T1024 Evaluation and treatment by an integrated, specialty team contracted to provide coordinated care to multiple or severely handicapped children, per encounter Ⓐ

T1025 Intensive, extended multidisciplinary services provided in a clinic setting to children with complex medical, physical, mental and psychosocial impairments, per diem Ⓐ

T1026 Intensive, extended multidisciplinary services provided in a clinic setting to children with complex medical, physical, medical and psychosocial impairments, per hour Ⓐ

T1027 Family training and counseling for child development, per 15 minutes ☑

T1028 Assessment of home, physical and family environment, to determine suitability to meet patient's medical needs

T1029 Comprehensive environmental lead investigation, not including laboratory analysis, per dwelling

T1030 Nursing care, in the home, by registered nurse, per diem ☑

T1031 Nursing care, in the home, by licensed practical nurse, per diem ☑

T1040 Medicaid certified community behavioral health clinic services, per diem

T1041 Medicaid certified community behavioral health clinic services, per month

T1502 Administration of oral, intramuscular and/or subcutaneous medication by health care agency/professional, per visit ☑

T1503 Administration of medication, other than oral and/or injectable, by a health care agency/professional, per visit ☑

T1505 Electronic medication compliance management device, includes all components and accessories, not otherwise classified

T1999 Miscellaneous therapeutic items and supplies, retail purchases, not otherwise classified; identify product in "remarks"

T2001 Nonemergency transportation; patient attendant/escort

T2002 Nonemergency transportation; per diem ☑

T2003 Nonemergency transportation; encounter/trip

T2004 Nonemergency transport; commercial carrier, multipass

T2005 Nonemergency transportation; stretcher van

T2007 Transportation waiting time, air ambulance and nonemergency vehicle, one-half (1/2) hour increments ☑

T2010 Preadmission screening and resident review (PASRR) Level I identification screening, per screen ☑

T2011 Preadmission screening and resident review (PASRR) Level II evaluation, per evaluation

T2012 Habilitation, educational; waiver, per diem ☑

T2013 Habilitation, educational, waiver; per hour ☑

T2014 Habilitation, prevocational, waiver; per diem ☑

T2015 Habilitation, prevocational, waiver; per hour ☑

T2016 Habilitation, residential, waiver; per diem ☑

T2017 Habilitation, residential, waiver; 15 minutes ☑

T2018 Habilitation, supported employment, waiver; per diem ☑

T2019 Habilitation, supported employment, waiver; per 15 minutes ☑

T2020 Day habilitation, waiver; per diem ☑

T2021 Day habilitation, waiver; per 15 minutes ☑

T2022 Case management, per month ☑

T2023 Targeted case management; per month ☑

T2024 Service assessment/plan of care development, waiver

T2025 Waiver services; not otherwise specified (NOS)

T2026 Specialized childcare, waiver; per diem ☑

T2027 Specialized childcare, waiver; per 15 minutes ☑

T2028 Specialized supply, not otherwise specified, waiver

T2029 Specialized medical equipment, not otherwise specified, waiver

---

Special Coverage Instructions   Noncovered by Medicare   Carrier Discretion   ☑ Quantity Alert   ● New Code   ○ Recycled/Reinstated   ▲ Revised Code

National T Codes

T2030 — T5999

T2030	Assisted living, waiver; per month	☑
T2031	Assisted living; waiver, per diem	☑
T2032	Residential care, not otherwise specified (NOS), waiver; per month	☑
T2033	Residential care, not otherwise specified (NOS), waiver; per diem	☑
T2034	Crisis intervention, waiver; per diem	☑
T2035	Utility services to support medical equipment and assistive technology/devices, waiver	
T2036	Therapeutic camping, overnight, waiver; each session	☑
T2037	Therapeutic camping, day, waiver; each session	☑
T2038	Community transition, waiver; per service	☑
T2039	Vehicle modifications, waiver; per service	☑
T2040	Financial management, self-directed, waiver; per 15 minutes	☑
T2041	Supports brokerage, self-directed, waiver; per 15 minutes	☑
T2042	Hospice routine home care; per diem CMS: 100-04,11,10	☑
T2043	Hospice continuous home care; per hour CMS: 100-04,11,10	☑
T2044	Hospice inpatient respite care; per diem CMS: 100-04,11,10	☑
T2045	Hospice general inpatient care; per diem CMS: 100-04,11,10	☑
T2046	Hospice long-term care, room and board only; per diem CMS: 100-04,11,10	☑
T2047	Habilitation, prevocational, waiver; per 15 minutes	
T2048	Behavioral health; long-term care residential (nonacute care in a residential treatment program where stay is typically longer than 30 days), with room and board, per diem	☑
T2049	Nonemergency transportation; stretcher van, mileage; per mile	☑
T2101	Human breast milk processing, storage and distribution only	♀
T4521	Adult sized disposable incontinence product, brief/diaper, small, each	☑
T4522	Adult sized disposable incontinence product, brief/diaper, medium, each	☑
T4523	Adult sized disposable incontinence product, brief/diaper, large, each	☑
T4524	Adult sized disposable incontinence product, brief/diaper, extra large, each	☑
T4525	Adult sized disposable incontinence product, protective underwear/pull-on, small size, each	☑
T4526	Adult sized disposable incontinence product, protective underwear/pull-on, medium size, each	☑
T4527	Adult sized disposable incontinence product, protective underwear/pull-on, large size, each	☑
T4528	Adult sized disposable incontinence product, protective underwear/pull-on, extra large size, each	☑
T4529	Pediatric sized disposable incontinence product, brief/diaper, small/medium size, each	☑
T4530	Pediatric sized disposable incontinence product, brief/diaper, large size, each	☑
T4531	Pediatric sized disposable incontinence product, protective underwear/pull-on, small/medium size, each	☑
T4532	Pediatric sized disposable incontinence product, protective underwear/pull-on, large size, each	☑
T4533	Youth sized disposable incontinence product, brief/diaper, each	☑
T4534	Youth sized disposable incontinence product, protective underwear/pull-on, each	☑
T4535	Disposable liner/shield/guard/pad/undergarment, for incontinence, each	☑
T4536	Incontinence product, protective underwear/pull-on, reusable, any size, each	☑
T4537	Incontinence product, protective underpad, reusable, bed size, each	☑
T4538	Diaper service, reusable diaper, each diaper	☑
T4539	Incontinence product, diaper/brief, reusable, any size, each	☑
T4540	Incontinence product, protective underpad, reusable, chair size, each	☑
T4541	Incontinence product, disposable underpad, large, each	☑
T4542	Incontinence product, disposable underpad, small size, each	☑
T4543	Adult sized disposable incontinence product, protective brief/diaper, above extra large, each	☑
T4544	Adult sized disposable incontinence product, protective underwear/pull-on, above extra large, each	
T4545	Incontinence product, disposable, penile wrap, each	
T5001	Positioning seat for persons with special orthopedic needs	
T5999	Supply, not otherwise specified	

Special Coverage Instructions   Noncovered by Medicare   Carrier Discretion   ☑ Quantity Alert ● New Code   ○ Recycled/Reinstated   ▲ Revised Code

168 — T Codes   A Age Edit   M Maternity Edit   ♀ Female Only   ♂ Male Only   A-Y OPPS Status Indicators   © 2021 Optum360, LLC

Coronavirus Services U0001-U0005

U0001 **CDC 2019 Novel Coronavirus (2019-nCoV) Real-Time RT-PCR Diagnostic Panel**
Use this code for CDC created tests.

U0002 **2019-nCoV Coronavirus, SARS-CoV-2/2019-nCoV (COVID-19), any technique, multiple types or subtypes (includes all targets), non-CDC**
Use this code for non-CDC created tests.

U0003 **Infectious agent detection by nucleic acid (DNA or RNA); Severe Acute Respiratory Syndrome Coronavirus 2 (SARS-CoV-2) (Coronavirus disease [COVID-19]), amplified probe technique, making use of high throughput technologies as described by CMS-2020-01-R**
Use this code for testing performed with high throughput technologies.

U0004 **2019-nCoV Coronavirus, SARS-CoV-2/2019-nCoV (COVID-19), any technique, multiple types or subtypes (includes all targets), non-CDC, making use of high throughput technologies as described by CMS-2020-01-R**
Use this code for testing performed with high throughput technologies.

U0005 **Infectious agent detection by nucleic acid (DNA or RNA); Severe Acute Respiratory Syndrome Coronavirus 2 (SARS-CoV-2) (Coronavirus disease [COVID-19]), amplified probe technique, CDC or non-CDC, making use of high throughput technologies, completed within 2 calendar days from date of specimen collection (list separately in addition to either HCPCS code U0003 or U0004) as described by CMS-2020-01-R2**

Special Coverage Instructions   Noncovered by Medicare   Carrier Discretion   ☑ Quantity Alert ● New Code   ○ Recycled/Reinstated   ▲ Revised Code

© 2021 Optum360, LLC   A2-Z3 ASC Pmt   CMS: IOM   AHA: Coding Clinic   ♿ DMEPOS Paid   ⊘ SNF Excluded   U Codes — 169

Vision Services

Vision Services V2020-V2799

These V codes include vision-related supplies, including spectacles, lenses, contact lenses, prostheses, intraocular lenses, and miscellaneous lenses.

Frames

V2020   Frames, purchases   Ⓐ ⚥

V2025   Deluxe frame   Ⓔ
CMS: 100-04,1,30.3.5

Single Vision, Glass, or Plastic

V2100   Sphere, single vision, plano to plus or minus 4.00, per lens   Ⓐ ☑ ♿

Monofocal spectacles (V2100–V2114)

Trifocal spectacles (V2300–V2314)

Low vision aids mounted to spectacles (V2610)

Telescopic or other compound lens fitted on spectacles as a low vision aid (V2615)

V2101   Sphere, single vision, plus or minus 4.12 to plus or minus 7.00d, per lens   Ⓐ ☑ ♿

V2102   Sphere, single vision, plus or minus 7.12 to plus or minus 20.00d, per lens   Ⓐ ☑ ♿

V2103   Spherocylinder, single vision, plano to plus or minus 4.00d sphere, 0.12 to 2.00d cylinder, per lens   Ⓐ ☑ ♿

V2104   Spherocylinder, single vision, plano to plus or minus 4.00d sphere, 2.12 to 4.00d cylinder, per lens   Ⓐ ☑ ♿

V2105   Spherocylinder, single vision, plano to plus or minus 4.00d sphere, 4.25 to 6.00d cylinder, per lens   Ⓐ ☑ ♿

V2106   Spherocylinder, single vision, plano to plus or minus 4.00d sphere, over 6.00d cylinder, per lens   Ⓐ ☑ ♿

V2107   Spherocylinder, single vision, plus or minus 4.25 to plus or minus 7.00 sphere, 0.12 to 2.00d cylinder, per lens   Ⓐ ☑ ♿

V2108   Spherocylinder, single vision, plus or minus 4.25d to plus or minus 7.00d sphere, 2.12 to 4.00d cylinder, per lens   Ⓐ ☑ ♿

V2109   Spherocylinder, single vision, plus or minus 4.25 to plus or minus 7.00d sphere, 4.25 to 6.00d cylinder, per lens   Ⓐ ☑ ♿

V2110   Spherocylinder, single vision, plus or minus 4.25 to 7.00d sphere, over 6.00d cylinder, per lens   Ⓐ ☑ ♿

V2111   Spherocylinder, single vision, plus or minus 7.25 to plus or minus 12.00d sphere, 0.25 to 2.25d cylinder, per lens   Ⓐ ☑ ♿

V2112   Spherocylinder, single vision, plus or minus 7.25 to plus or minus 12.00d sphere, 2.25d to 4.00d cylinder, per lens   Ⓐ ☑ ♿

V2113   Spherocylinder, single vision, plus or minus 7.25 to plus or minus 12.00d sphere, 4.25 to 6.00d cylinder, per lens   Ⓐ ☑ ♿

V2114   Spherocylinder, single vision, sphere over plus or minus 12.00d, per lens   Ⓐ ☑ ♿

V2115   Lenticular (myodisc), per lens, single vision   Ⓐ ☑ ♿

V2118   Aniseikonic lens, single vision   Ⓐ ♿

V2121   Lenticular lens, per lens, single   Ⓐ ☑ ♿

V2199   Not otherwise classified, single vision lens   Ⓐ

Bifocal, Glass, or Plastic

V2200   Sphere, bifocal, plano to plus or minus 4.00d, per lens   Ⓐ ☑ ♿

V2201   Sphere, bifocal, plus or minus 4.12 to plus or minus 7.00d, per lens   Ⓐ ☑ ♿

V2202   Sphere, bifocal, plus or minus 7.12 to plus or minus 20.00d, per lens   Ⓐ ☑ ♿

V2203   Spherocylinder, bifocal, plano to plus or minus 4.00d sphere, 0.12 to 2.00d cylinder, per lens   Ⓐ ☑ ♿

V2204   Spherocylinder, bifocal, plano to plus or minus 4.00d sphere, 2.12 to 4.00d cylinder, per lens   Ⓐ ☑ ♿

V2205   Spherocylinder, bifocal, plano to plus or minus 4.00d sphere, 4.25 to 6.00d cylinder, per lens   Ⓐ ☑ ♿

V2206   Spherocylinder, bifocal, plano to plus or minus 4.00d sphere, over 6.00d cylinder, per lens   Ⓐ ☑ ♿

V2207   Spherocylinder, bifocal, plus or minus 4.25 to plus or minus 7.00d sphere, 0.12 to 2.00d cylinder, per lens   Ⓐ ☑ ♿

V2208   Spherocylinder, bifocal, plus or minus 4.25 to plus or minus 7.00d sphere, 2.12 to 4.00d cylinder, per lens   Ⓐ ☑ ♿

V2209   Spherocylinder, bifocal, plus or minus 4.25 to plus or minus 7.00d sphere, 4.25 to 6.00d cylinder, per lens   Ⓐ ☑ ♿

V2210   Spherocylinder, bifocal, plus or minus 4.25 to plus or minus 7.00d sphere, over 6.00d cylinder, per lens   Ⓐ ☑ ♿

V2211   Spherocylinder, bifocal, plus or minus 7.25 to plus or minus 12.00d sphere, 0.25 to 2.25d cylinder, per lens   Ⓐ ☑ ♿

V2212   Spherocylinder, bifocal, plus or minus 7.25 to plus or minus 12.00d sphere, 2.25 to 4.00d cylinder, per lens   Ⓐ ☑ ♿

V2213   Spherocylinder, bifocal, plus or minus 7.25 to plus or minus 12.00d sphere, 4.25 to 6.00d cylinder, per lens   Ⓐ ☑ ♿

V2214   Spherocylinder, bifocal, sphere over plus or minus 12.00d, per lens   Ⓐ ☑ ♿

V2215   Lenticular (myodisc), per lens, bifocal   Ⓐ ☑ ♿

V2218   Aniseikonic, per lens, bifocal   Ⓐ ☑ ♿

V2219   Bifocal seg width over 28mm   Ⓐ ☑ ♿

V2220   Bifocal add over 3.25d   Ⓐ ☑ ♿

V2221   Lenticular lens, per lens, bifocal   Ⓐ ♿

V2299   Specialty bifocal (by report)   Ⓐ
Pertinent documentation to evaluate medical appropriateness should be included when this code is reported.

Trifocal, Glass, or Plastic

V2300   Sphere, trifocal, plano to plus or minus 4.00d, per lens   Ⓐ ☑ ♿

V2301   Sphere, trifocal, plus or minus 4.12 to plus or minus 7.00d per lens   Ⓐ ☑ ♿

V2302   Sphere, trifocal, plus or minus 7.12 to plus or minus 20.00, per lens   Ⓐ ☑ ♿

V2303   Spherocylinder, trifocal, plano to plus or minus 4.00d sphere, 0.12 to 2.00d cylinder, per lens   Ⓐ ☑ ♿

V2304   Spherocylinder, trifocal, plano to plus or minus 4.00d sphere, 2.25 to 4.00d cylinder, per lens   Ⓐ ☑ ♿

V2305   Spherocylinder, trifocal, plano to plus or minus 4.00d sphere, 4.25 to 6.00 cylinder, per lens   Ⓐ ☑ ♿

V2020 — V2305

Special Coverage Instructions   Noncovered by Medicare   Carrier Discretion   ☑ Quantity Alert   ● New Code   ○ Recycled/Reinstated   ▲ Revised Code

170 — V Codes   Ⓐ Age Edit   Ⓜ Maternity Edit   ♀ Female Only   ♂ Male Only   Ⓐ-Ⓨ OPPS Status Indicators   © 2021 Optum360, LLC

V2306   Spherocylinder, trifocal, plano to plus or minus 4.00d sphere, over 6.00d cylinder, per lens   Ⓐ ☑ &

V2307   Spherocylinder, trifocal, plus or minus 4.25 to plus or minus 7.00d sphere, 0.12 to 2.00d cylinder, per lens   Ⓐ ☑ &

V2308   Spherocylinder, trifocal, plus or minus 4.25 to plus or minus 7.00d sphere, 2.12 to 4.00d cylinder, per lens   Ⓐ ☑ &

V2309   Spherocylinder, trifocal, plus or minus 4.25 to plus or minus 7.00d sphere, 4.25 to 6.00d cylinder, per lens   Ⓐ ☑ &

V2310   Spherocylinder, trifocal, plus or minus 4.25 to plus or minus 7.00d sphere, over 6.00d cylinder, per lens   Ⓐ ☑ &

V2311   Spherocylinder, trifocal, plus or minus 7.25 to plus or minus 12.00d sphere, 0.25 to 2.25d cylinder, per lens   Ⓐ ☑ &

V2312   Spherocylinder, trifocal, plus or minus 7.25 to plus or minus 12.00d sphere, 2.25 to 4.00d cylinder, per lens   Ⓐ ☑ &

V2313   Spherocylinder, trifocal, plus or minus 7.25 to plus or minus 12.00d sphere, 4.25 to 6.00d cylinder, per lens   Ⓐ ☑ &

V2314   Spherocylinder, trifocal, sphere over plus or minus 12.00d, per lens   Ⓐ ☑ &

V2315   Lenticular, (myodisc), per lens, trifocal   Ⓐ ☑ &

V2318   Aniseikonic lens, trifocal   Ⓐ &

V2319   Trifocal seg width over 28 mm   Ⓐ ☑ &

V2320   Trifocal add over 3.25d   Ⓐ ☑ &

V2321   Lenticular lens, per lens, trifocal   Ⓐ &

V2399   Specialty trifocal (by report)   Ⓐ
Pertinent documentation to evaluate medical appropriateness should be included when this code is reported.

Variable Asphericity Lens, Glass, or Plastic

V2410   Variable asphericity lens, single vision, full field, glass or plastic, per lens   Ⓐ ☑ &

V2430   Variable asphericity lens, bifocal, full field, glass or plastic, per lens   Ⓐ ☑ &

V2499   Variable sphericity lens, other type   Ⓐ

Contact Lens

V2500   Contact lens, PMMA, spherical, per lens   Ⓐ ☑ &

V2501   Contact lens, PMMA, toric or prism ballast, per lens   Ⓐ ☑ &

V2502   Contact lens PMMA, bifocal, per lens   Ⓐ ☑ &

V2503   Contact lens, PMMA, color vision deficiency, per lens   Ⓐ ☑ &

V2510   Contact lens, gas permeable, spherical, per lens   Ⓐ ☑ &

V2511   Contact lens, gas permeable, toric, prism ballast, per lens   Ⓐ ☑ &

V2512   Contact lens, gas permeable, bifocal, per lens   Ⓐ ☑ &

V2513   Contact lens, gas permeable, extended wear, per lens   Ⓐ ☑ &

V2520   Contact lens, hydrophilic, spherical, per lens   Ⓐ ☑ &
Hydrophilic contact lenses are covered by Medicare only for aphakic patients. Local contractor if incident to physician services.

V2521   Contact lens, hydrophilic, toric, or prism ballast, per lens   Ⓐ ☑ &
Hydrophilic contact lenses are covered by Medicare only for aphakic patients. Local contractor if incident to physician services.

V2522   Contact lens, hydrophilic, bifocal, per lens   Ⓐ ☑ &
Hydrophilic contact lenses are covered by Medicare only for aphakic patients. Local contractor if incident to physician services.

V2523   Contact lens, hydrophilic, extended wear, per lens   Ⓐ ☑ &
Hydrophilic contact lenses are covered by Medicare only for aphakic patients.

V2524   Contact lens, hydrophilic, spherical, photochromic additive, per lens

V2530   Contact lens, scleral, gas impermeable, per lens (for contact lens modification, see 92325)   Ⓐ ☑ &

V2531   Contact lens, scleral, gas permeable, per lens (for contact lens modification, see 92325)   Ⓐ ☑ &

V2599   Contact lens, other type   Ⓐ
Local contractor if incident to physician services.

Vision Aids

V2600   Hand held low vision aids and other nonspectacle mounted aids   Ⓐ

V2610   Single lens spectacle mounted low vision aids   Ⓐ

V2615   Telescopic and other compound lens system, including distance vision telescopic, near vision telescopes and compound microscopic lens system   Ⓐ

Prosthetic Eye

V2623   Prosthetic eye, plastic, custom   Ⓐ &

Implant

Peg

One type of eye implant

Reverse angle

Previously placed prosthetic receptacle

Implant

Peg

Peg hole drilled into prosthetic

Side view

V2624   Polishing/resurfacing of ocular prosthesis   Ⓐ &

V2625   Enlargement of ocular prosthesis   Ⓐ &

V2626   Reduction of ocular prosthesis   Ⓐ &

V2627   Scleral cover shell   Ⓐ &
A scleral shell covers the cornea and the anterior sclera. Medicare covers a scleral shell when it is prescribed as an artificial support to a shrunken and sightless eye or as a barrier in the treatment of severe dry eye.

V2628   Fabrication and fitting of ocular conformer   Ⓐ &

V2629   Prosthetic eye, other type   Ⓐ

Intraocular Lenses

V2630   Anterior chamber intraocular lens   Ⓝ Ⓜ &
The IOL must be FDA-approved for reimbursement. Medicare payment for an IOL is included in the payment for ASC facility services. Medicare jurisdiction: local contractor.

Special Coverage Instructions   Noncovered by Medicare   Carrier Discretion   ☑ Quantity Alert   ● New Code   ○ Recycled/Reinstated   ▲ Revised Code

© 2021 Optum360, LLC   Ⓐ²-Ⓩ³ ASC Pmt   CMS: IOM   AHA: Coding Clinic   & DMEPOS Paid   ⊘ SNF Excluded   V Codes — 171

Vision Services

V2631 — V2799

V2631 Iris supported intraocular lens [N] [N1]
The IOL must be FDA-approved for reimbursement. Medicare payment for an IOL is included in the payment for ASC facility services. Medicare jurisdiction: local contractor.

V2632 Posterior chamber intraocular lens [N] [N1]
The IOL must be FDA-approved for reimbursement. Medicare payment for an IOL is included in the payment for ASC facility services. Medicare jurisdiction: local contractor.
CMS: 100-04,32,120.2

Miscellaneous

V2700	Balance lens, per lens	[A] ☑ ♿
V2702	Deluxe lens feature	[E]
V2710	Slab off prism, glass or plastic, per lens	[A] ☑ ♿
V2715	Prism, per lens	[A] ☑ ♿
V2718	Press-on lens, Fresnel prism, per lens	[A] ☑ ♿
V2730	Special base curve, glass or plastic, per lens	[A] ☑ ♿
V2744	Tint, photochromatic, per lens	[A] ☑ ♿
V2745	Addition to lens; tint, any color, solid, gradient or equal, excludes photochromatic, any lens material, per lens	[A] ☑ ♿
V2750	Antireflective coating, per lens	[A] ☑ ♿
V2755	U-V lens, per lens	[A] ☑ ♿
V2756	Eye glass case	[E]
V2760	Scratch resistant coating, per lens	[E] ☑ ♿
V2761	Mirror coating, any type, solid, gradient or equal, any lens material, per lens	[B] ☑
V2762	Polarization, any lens material, per lens	[E] ☑ ♿
V2770	Occluder lens, per lens	[A] ☑ ♿
V2780	Oversize lens, per lens	[A] ☑ ♿
V2781	Progressive lens, per lens	[B] ☑
V2782	Lens, index 1.54 to 1.65 plastic or 1.60 to 1.79 glass, excludes polycarbonate, per lens	[A] ☑ ♿
V2783	Lens, index greater than or equal to 1.66 plastic or greater than or equal to 1.80 glass, excludes polycarbonate, per lens	[A] ☑ ♿
V2784	Lens, polycarbonate or equal, any index, per lens	[A] ☑ ♿

V2785 Processing, preserving and transporting corneal tissue [F] [F4]
Medicare jurisdiction: local contractor.
CMS: 100-04,4,200.1

V2786 Specialty occupational multifocal lens, per lens [E] ☑ ♿

V2787 Astigmatism correcting function of intraocular lens [E]
CMS: 100-04,32,120.1; 100-04,32,120.2

V2788 Presbyopia correcting function of intraocular lens [E]
CMS: 100-04,32,120.1; 100-04,32,120.2

V2790 Amniotic membrane for surgical reconstruction, per procedure [N] [N1]
Medicare jurisdiction: local contractor.
CMS: 100-04,4,200.4

V2797 Vision supply, accessory and/or service component of another HCPCS vision code [E]

V2799 Vision item or service, miscellaneous [A]
Determine if an alternative HCPCS Level II or a CPT code better describes the service being reported. This code should be used only if a more specific code is unavailable.

Hearing Services V5008-V5364

This range of codes describes hearing tests and related supplies and equipment, speech-language pathology screenings, and repair of augmentative communicative system.

Hearing Services

V5008	Hearing screening	[E]
V5010	Assessment for hearing aid	[E]
V5011	Fitting/orientation/checking of hearing aid	[E]
V5014	Repair/modification of a hearing aid	[E]
V5020	Conformity evaluation	[E]

Monaural Hearing Aid

V5030	Hearing aid, monaural, body worn, air conduction	[E]
V5040	Hearing aid, monaural, body worn, bone conduction	[E]
V5050	Hearing aid, monaural, in the ear	[E]
V5060	Hearing aid, monaural, behind the ear	[E]

Other Hearing Services

V5070	Glasses, air conduction	[E]
V5080	Glasses, bone conduction	[E]
V5090	Dispensing fee, unspecified hearing aid	[E]
V5095	Semi-implantable middle ear hearing prosthesis	[E]
V5100	Hearing aid, bilateral, body worn	[E]
V5110	Dispensing fee, bilateral	[E]

Hearing Aids, Services, and Accessories

V5120	Binaural, body	[E]
V5130	Binaural, in the ear	[E]
V5140	Binaural, behind the ear	[E]
V5150	Binaural, glasses	[E]
V5160	Dispensing fee, binaural	[E]
V5171	Hearing aid, contralateral routing device, monaural, in the ear (ITE)	
V5172	Hearing aid, contralateral routing device, monaural, in the canal (ITC)	
V5181	Hearing aid, contralateral routing device, monaural, behind the ear (BTE)	
V5190	Hearing aid, contralateral routing, monaural, glasses	[E]
V5200	Dispensing fee, contralateral, monaural	[E]
V5211	Hearing aid, contralateral routing system, binaural, ITE/ITE	
V5212	Hearing aid, contralateral routing system, binaural, ITE/ITC	
V5213	Hearing aid, contralateral routing system, binaural, ITE/BTE	
V5214	Hearing aid, contralateral routing system, binaural, ITC/ITC	
V5215	Hearing aid, contralateral routing system, binaural, ITC/BTE	
V5221	Hearing aid, contralateral routing system, binaural, BTE/BTE	
V5230	Hearing aid, contralateral routing system, binaural, glasses	[E]
V5240	Dispensing fee, contralateral routing system, binaural	[E]

V5241 Dispensing fee, monaural hearing aid, any type [E]
AHA: 1Q, '02, 5

V5242 Hearing aid, analog, monaural, CIC (completely in the ear canal) [E]
AHA: 1Q, '02, 5

☑ Special Coverage Instructions   [M] Noncovered by Medicare   Carrier Discretion   ☑ Quantity Alert   ● New Code   ○ Recycled/Reinstated   ▲ Revised Code

172 — V Codes   [A] Age Edit   [M] Maternity Edit   ♀ Female Only   ♂ Male Only   [A]-[Y] OPPS Status Indicators   © 2021 Optum360, LLC

V5243	Hearing aid, analog, monaural, ITC (in the canal) AHA: 1Q, '02, 5	E
V5244	Hearing aid, digitally programmable analog, monaural, CIC AHA: 1Q, '02, 5	E
V5245	Hearing aid, digitally programmable, analog, monaural, ITC AHA: 1Q, '02, 5	E
V5246	Hearing aid, digitally programmable analog, monaural, ITE (in the ear) AHA: 1Q, '02, 5	E
V5247	Hearing aid, digitally programmable analog, monaural, BTE (behind the ear) AHA: 1Q, '02, 5	E
V5248	Hearing aid, analog, binaural, CIC AHA: 1Q, '02, 5	E
V5249	Hearing aid, analog, binaural, ITC AHA: 1Q, '02, 5	E
V5250	Hearing aid, digitally programmable analog, binaural, CIC AHA: 1Q, '02, 5	E
V5251	Hearing aid, digitally programmable analog, binaural, ITC AHA: 1Q, '02, 5	E
V5252	Hearing aid, digitally programmable, binaural, ITE AHA: 1Q, '02, 5	E
V5253	Hearing aid, digitally programmable, binaural, BTE AHA: 1Q, '02, 5	E
V5254	Hearing aid, digital, monaural, CIC AHA: 1Q, '02, 5	E
V5255	Hearing aid, digital, monaural, ITC AHA: 1Q, '02, 5	E
V5256	Hearing aid, digital, monaural, ITE AHA: 1Q, '02, 5	E
V5257	Hearing aid, digital, monaural, BTE AHA: 1Q, '02, 5	E
V5258	Hearing aid, digital, binaural, CIC AHA: 1Q, '02, 5	E
V5259	Hearing aid, digital, binaural, ITC AHA: 1Q, '02, 5	E
V5260	Hearing aid, digital, binaural, ITE AHA: 1Q, '02, 5	E
V5261	Hearing aid, digital, binaural, BTE AHA: 1Q, '02, 5	E
V5262	Hearing aid, disposable, any type, monaural AHA: 1Q, '02, 5	E
V5263	Hearing aid, disposable, any type, binaural AHA: 1Q, '02, 5	E
V5264	Ear mold/insert, not disposable, any type AHA: 1Q, '02, 5	E
V5265	Ear mold/insert, disposable, any type AHA: 1Q, '02, 5	E
V5266	Battery for use in hearing device AHA: 1Q, '02, 5	E
V5267	Hearing aid or assistive listening device/supplies/accessories, not otherwise specified AHA: 1Q, '02, 5	E

Assistive Listening Device

V5268	Assistive listening device, telephone amplifier, any type AHA: 1Q, '02, 5	E
V5269	Assistive listening device, alerting, any type AHA: 1Q, '02, 5	E
V5270	Assistive listening device, television amplifier, any type AHA: 1Q, '02, 5	E
V5271	Assistive listening device, television caption decoder AHA: 1Q, '02, 5	E
V5272	Assistive listening device, TDD AHA: 1Q, '02, 5	E
V5273	Assistive listening device, for use with cochlear implant AHA: 1Q, '02, 5	E
V5274	Assistive listening device, not otherwise specified AHA: 1Q, '02, 5	E

Miscellaneous Hearing Services

V5275	Ear impression, each AHA: 1Q, '02, 5	E ☑
V5281	Assistive listening device, personal FM/DM system, monaural (1 receiver, transmitter, microphone), any type	E
V5282	Assistive listening device, personal FM/DM system, binaural (2 receivers, transmitter, microphone), any type	E
V5283	Assistive listening device, personal FM/DM neck, loop induction receiver	E
V5284	Assistive listening device, personal FM/DM, ear level receiver	E
V5285	Assistive listening device, personal FM/DM, direct audio input receiver	E
V5286	Assistive listening device, personal blue tooth FM/DM receiver	E
V5287	Assistive listening device, personal FM/DM receiver, not otherwise specified	E
V5288	Assistive listening device, personal FM/DM transmitter assistive listening device	E
V5289	Assistive listening device, personal FM/DM adapter/boot coupling device for receiver, any type	E
V5290	Assistive listening device, transmitter microphone, any type	E
V5298	Hearing aid, not otherwise classified	E
V5299	Hearing service, miscellaneous Determine if an alternative HCPCS Level II or a CPT code better describes the service being reported. This code should be used only if a more specific code is unavailable.	B ⊘

Speech-Language Pathology Services

V5336	Repair/modification of augmentative communicative system or device (excludes adaptive hearing aid) Medicare jurisdiction: DME regional contractor.	E
V5362	Speech screening	E
V5363	Language screening	E
V5364	Dysphagia screening	E

Special Coverage Instructions   Noncovered by Medicare   Carrier Discretion   ☑ Quantity Alert   ● New Code   ○ Recycled/Reinstated   ▲ Revised Code

© 2021 Optum360, LLC   A2 – Z3 ASC Pmt   CMS: IOM   AHA: Coding Clinic   DMEPOS Paid   ⊘ SNF Excluded   **V Codes — 173**

Appendix 1 — Table of Drugs and Biologicals

INTRODUCTION AND DIRECTIONS

The HCPCS 2022 Table of Drugs and Biologicals is designed to quickly and easily direct the user to drug names and their corresponding codes. Both generic and brand or trade names are alphabetically listed in the "Drug Name" column of the table. The associated A, C, J, K, Q, or S code is given only for the generic name of the drug. While every effort is made to make the table comprehensive, it is not all-inclusive.

The "Unit Per" column lists the stated amount for the referenced generic drug as provided by CMS. "Up to" listings are inclusive of all quantities up to and including the listed amount. All other listings are for the amount of the drug as listed. The editors recognize that the availability of some drugs in the quantities listed is dependent on many variables beyond the control of the clinical ordering clerk. The availability in your area of regularly used drugs in the most cost-effective quantities should be relayed to your third-party payers.

The "Route of Administration" column addresses the most common methods of delivering the referenced generic drug as described in current pharmaceutical literature. The official definitions for Level II drug codes generally describe administration other than by oral method. Therefore, with a handful of exceptions, oral-delivered options for most drugs are omitted from the Route of Administration column.

Intravenous administration includes all methods, such as gravity infusion, injections, and timed pushes. When several routes of administration are listed, the first listing is simply the first, or most common, method as described in current reference literature. The "VAR" posting denotes various routes of administration and is used for drugs that are commonly administered into joints, cavities, tissues, or topical applications, in addition to other parenteral administrations. Listings posted with "OTH" alert the user to other administration methods, such as suppositories or catheter injections.

Please be reminded that the Table of Drugs and Biologicals, as well as all HCPCS Level II national definitions and listings, constitutes a post-treatment medical reference for billing purposes only. Although the editors have exercised all normal precautions to ensure the accuracy of the table and related material, the use of any of this information to select medical treatment is entirely inappropriate. Do not code directly from the table. Refer to the tabular section for complete information.

See Appendix 3 for abbreviations.

Drug Name	Unit Per	Route	Code
10% LMD	500 ML	IV	J7100
4-FACTOR PROTHROMBIN COMPLEX CONCENTRATE	1 IU	IV	C9132
5% DEXTROSE AND .45% NORMAL SALINE	1000 ML	IV	S5010
5% DEXTROSE IN LACTATED RINGERS	1000 CC	IV	J7121
5% DEXTROSE WITH POTASSIUM CHLORIDE	1000 ML	IV	S5012
5% DEXTROSE/.45% NS WITH KCL AND MAG SULFATE	1000ML	IV	S5013
5% DEXTROSE/.45% NS WITH KCL AND MAG SULFATE	1500 ML	IV	S5014
5% DEXTROSE/NORMAL SALINE	5%	VAR	J7042
5% DEXTROSE/WATER	500 ML	IV	J7060
A-HYDROCORT	100 MG	IV, IM, SC	J1720
A-METHAPRED	40 MG	IM, IV	J2920
A-METHAPRED	125 MG	IM, IV	J2930
ABATACEPT	10 MG	IV	J0129
ABCIXIMAB	10 MG	IV	J0130

Drug Name	Unit Per	Route	Code
ABECMA	UP TO 460 MILLION CELLSM	IV	C9081
ABECMA	UP TO 460 MILLION CELLS	IV	Q2055
ABELCET	10 MG	IV	J0287
ABILIFY	0.25 MG	IM	J0400
ABILIFY MAINTENA KIT	1 MG	IM	J0401
ABLAVAR	1 ML	IV	A9583
ABOBOTULINUMTOXINA	5 UNITS	IM	J0586
ABRAXANE	1 MG	IV	J9264
ACCELULAR PERICARDIAL TISSUE MATRIX NONHUMAN	SQ CM	OTH	C9354
ACCUNEB NONCOMPOUNDED, CONCENTRATED	1 MG	INH	J7611
ACCUNEB NONCOMPOUNDED, UNIT DOSE	1 MG	INH	J7613
ACETADOTE	1 G	INH	J7608
ACETADOTE	100 MG	IV	J0132
ACETAMINOPHEN	10 MG	IV	J0131
ACETAZOLAMIDE SODIUM	500 MG	IM, IV	J1120
ACETYLCYSTEINE COMPOUNDED	PER G	INH	J7604
ACETYLCYSTEINE NONCOMPOUNDED	1 G	INH	J7608
ACTEMRA	1 MG	IV	J3262
ACTEMRA	1 MG	IV	Q0249
ACTHREL	1 MCG	IV	J0795
ACTIMMUNE	3 MU	SC	J9216
ACTIVASE	1 MG	IV	J2997
ACUTECT	STUDY DOSE UP TO 20 MCI	IV	A9504
ACYCLOVIR	5 MG	IV	J0133
ADAGEN	25 IU	IM	J2504
ADAKVEO	5 MG	IV	J0791
ADALIMUMAB	20 MG	SC	J0135
ADASUVE	1 MG	INH	J2062
ADCETRIS	1 MG	IV	J9042
ADENOCARD	1 MG	IV	J0153
ADENOSINE	1 MG	IV	J0153
ADENSOSCAN	1 MG	IV	J0153
ADO-TRASTUZUMAB EMTANSINE	1 MG	IV	J9354
ADRENALIN	0.1 MG	IM, IV, SC	J0171
ADRENOCORT	1 MG	IM, IV, OTH	J1100
ADRIAMYCIN	10 MG	IV	J9000
ADRUCIL	500 MG	IV	J9190
ADUCANUMAB-AVWA	2 MG	IV	J0172
ADUHELM	2 MG	IV	J0172
ADYNOVATE	1 IU	IV	J7207
AEROBID	1 MG	INH	J7641

Drug Name	Unit Per	Route	Code
AFAMELANOTIDE IMPLANT	1 MG	OTH	J7352
AFFINITY	SQ CM	OTH	Q4159
AFINITOR	0.25 MG	ORAL	J7527
AFLIBERCEPT	1 MG	OTH	J0178
AFLURIA	EA	IM	Q2035
AFSTYLA	1 I.U.	IV	J7210
AGALSIDASE BETA	1 MG	IV	J0180
AGGRASTAT	12.5 MG	IM, IV	J3246
AGRIFLU	UNKNOWN	IM	Q2034
AJOVY	1 MG	SC	J3031
AKYNZEO	300 MG/0.5 MG	ORAL	J8655
AKYNZEO	235 MG/0.25 MG	IV	J1454
ALATROFLOXACIN MESYLATE	100 MG	IV	J0200
ALBUTEROL AND IPRATROPIUM BROMIDE NONCOMPOUNDED	2.5MG/0.5 MG	INH	J7620
ALBUTEROL COMPOUNDED, CONCENTRATED	1 MG	INH	J7610
ALBUTEROL COMPOUNDED, UNIT DOSE	1 MG	INH	J7609
ALBUTEROL NONCOMPOUNDED, UNIT DOSE	1 MG	INH	J7613
ALBUTEROL, NONCOMPOUNDED, CONCENTRATED FORM	1 MG	INH	J7611
ALDESLEUKIN	1 VIAL	IV	J9015
ALDURAZYME	0.1 MG	IV	J1931
ALEFACEPT	0.5 MG	IV, IM	J0215
ALEMTUZUMAB	1 MG	IV	J0202
ALFERON N	250,000 IU	IM	J9215
ALGLUCERASE	10 U	IV	J0205
ALGLUCOSIDASE ALFA (LUMIZYME)	10 MG	IV	J0221
ALIQOPA	1 MG	IV	J9057
ALKERAN	2 MG	ORAL	J8600
ALLODERM	SQ CM	OTH	Q4116
ALLOGEN	1 CC	OTH	Q4212
ALLOGRAFT, CYMETRA	1 CC	INJ	Q4112
ALLOGRAFT, GRAFTJACKET EXPRESS	1 CC	INJ	Q4113
ALLOPATCHHD	SQ CM	OTH	Q4128
ALLOSKIN	SQ CM	OTH	Q4115
ALLOSKIN AC	SQ CM	OTH	Q4141
ALLOSKIN RT	SQ CM	OTH	Q4123
ALLOWRAP DS OR DRY	SQ CM	OTH	Q4150
ALOXI	25 MCG	IV	J2469
ALPHA 1-PROTENIASE INHIBITOR (HUMAN) (GLASSIA)	10 MG	IV	J0257
ALPHANATE	PER FACTOR VIII IU	IV	J7186
ALPHANINE SD	1 IU	IV	J7193
ALPROLIX	IU	IV	J7201
ALPROSTADIL	1.25 MCG	IV	J0270
ALPROSTADIL	EA	OTH	J0275
ALTEPLASE RECOMBINANT	1 MG	IV	J2997
ALTIPLY	SQ CM	OTH	Q4235

Drug Name	Unit Per	Route	Code
ALUPENT, NONCOMPOUNDED, CONCENTRATED	10 MG	INH	J7668
ALUPENT, NONCOMPOUNDED, UNIT DOSE	10 MG	INH	J7669
AMANTADINE HCL (DEMONSTRATION PROJECT)	100 MG	ORAL	G9017
AMANTADINE HYDROCHLORIDE (BRAND NAME) (DEMONSTRTION PROJECT)	100 MG	ORAL	G9033
AMANTADINE HYDROCHLORIDE (GENERIC)	100 MG	ORAL	G9017
AMBISOME	10 MG	IV	J0289
AMCORT	5 MG	IM	J3302
AMELUZ	10 MG	OTH	J7345
AMERGAN	12.5 MG	ORAL	Q0169
AMEVIVE	0.5 MG	IV, IM	J0215
AMICAR	5 G	IV	S0017
AMIFOSTINE	500 MG	IV	J0207
AMIKACIN SULFATE	100 MG	IM, IV	J0278
AMINOCAPRIOC ACID	5 G	IV	S0017
AMINOLEVULINIC ACID HCL	354 MG	OTH	J7308
AMINOLEVULINIC ACID HCL	10 MG	OTH	J7345
AMINOPHYLLINE	250 MG	IV	J0280
AMIODARONE HCL	30 MG	IV	J0282
AMITRIPTYLINE HCL	20 MG	IM	J1320
~~AMIVANTAMAB-VMJW~~	~~10 MG~~	~~IV~~	~~C9083~~
AMIVANTAMAB-VMJW	2 MG	IV	J9061
AMMONIA N-13	STUDY DOSE UP TO 40 MCI	IV	A9526
AMNIO-MAXX	SQ CM	OTH	Q4239
AMNIO-MAXX LITE	SQ CM	OTH	Q4239
AMNIOAMP-MP	SQ CM	OTH	Q4250
AMNIOARMOR	SQ CM	OTH	Q4188
AMNIOBAND	SQ CM	OTH	Q4151
AMNIOBAND	1 MG	OTH	Q4168
AMNIOCORE	SQ CM	OTH	Q4227
AMNIOCYTE PLUS	0.5 CC	OTH	Q4242
AMNIOEXCEL	SQ CM	OTH	Q4137
AMNIOEXCEL PLUS	SQ CM	OTH	Q4137
AMNIOMATRIX	1 CC	OTH	Q4139
AMNION BIO	SQ CM	OTH	Q4211
AMNIOREPAIR	SQ CM	OTH	Q4235
AMNIOTEXT	1 CC	OTH	Q4245
AMNIOTEXT PATCH	SQ CM	OTH	Q4247
AMNIOWOUND	SQ CM	OTH	Q4181
AMNIOWRAP2	SQ CM	OTH	Q4221
AMNIPLY	SQ CM	OTH	Q4249
AMOBARBITAL	125 MG	IM, IV	J0300
~~AMONDYS 45~~	~~10 MG~~	~~IV~~	~~C9075~~
AMONDYS 45	10 MG	IV	J1426
AMPHOCIN	50 MG	IV	J0285
AMPHOTEC	10 MG	IV	J0287
AMPHOTERICIN B	50 MG	IV	J0285
AMPHOTERICIN B CHOLESTERYL SULFATE COMPLEX	10 MG	IV	J0288
AMPHOTERICIN B LIPID COMPLEX	10 MG	IV	J0287

Drug Name	Unit Per	Route	Code
AMPHOTERICIN B LIPOSOME	10 MG	IV	J0289
AMPICILLIN SODIUM	500 MG	IM, IV	J0290
AMPICILLIN SODIUM/SULBACTAM SODIUM	1.5 G	IM, IV	J0295
AMYGDALIN	VAR	INJ	J3570
AMYTAL	125 MG	IM, IV	J0300
AMYVID	UP TO 10 MILLICUIRES	IV	A9586
AN-DTPA DIAGNOSTIC	STUDY DOSE UP TO 25 MCI	IV	A9539
AN-DTPA THERAPEUTIC	STUDY DOSE UP TO 25 MCI	INH	A9567
ANASCORP	UP TO 120 MG	IV	J0716
ANASTROZOLE	1 MG	ORAL	S0170
ANAVIP	120 MG	IV	J0841
ANCEF	500 MG	IM, IV	J0690
ANDEXXA	10 MG	IV	J7169
ANECTINE	20 MG	IM, IV	J0330
ANGIOMAX	1 MG	IV	J0583
ANIDULAFUNGIN	1 MG	IV	J0348
ANIFROLUMAB-FNIA	1 MG	IV	C9086
ANISTREPLASE	30 U	IV	J0350
ANJESO	1 MG	IV	J1738
ANNOVERA VAGINAL RING	0.15 MG/0.013 MG	OTH	J7294
ANTAGON	250 MCG	SC	S0132
ANTI-INHIBITOR	1 IU	IV	J7198
ANTI-THYMOCYTE GLOBULIN,EQUINE	250 MG	OTH	J7504
ANTIEMETIC DRUG NOS	VAR	ORAL	J8597
ANTIHEMOPHILIC FACTOR PORCINE	1 IU	IV	J7191
ANTIHEMOPHILIC FACTOR VIII, XYNTHA, RECOMBINANT	1 IU	IV	J7185
ANTIHEMOPHILIC FACTOR VIII/VON WILLEBRAND FACTOR COMPLEX, HUMAN	PER FACTOR VIII IU	IV	J7186
ANTITHROMBIN RECOMBINANT	50 IU	IV	J7196
ANTIZOL	15 MG	IV	J1451
ANZEMET	10 MG	IV	J1260
ANZEMET	50 MG	ORAL	S0174
ANZEMET	100 MG	ORAL	Q0180
APIS	SQ CM	OTH	A2010
APLIGRAF	SQ CM	OTH	Q4101
APOKYN	1 MG	SC	J0364
APOMORPHINE HYDROCHLORIDE	1 MG	SC	J0364
APREPITANT	1 MG	IV	J0185
APREPITANT	5 MG	ORAL	J8501
APROTININ	10,000 KIU	IV	J0365
AQUAMEPHYTON	1 MG	IM, SC, IV	J3430
ARA-C	100 MG	SC, IV	J9100
ARALEN	UP TO 250 MG	IM, IV	J0390
ARAMINE	10 MG	IV, IM, SC	J0380
ARANESP, ESRD USE	1 MCG	SC, IV	J0882
ARANESP, NON-ESRD USE	1 MCG	SC, IV	J0881
ARBUTAMINE HCL	1 MG	IV	J0395
ARCALYST	1 MG	SC	J2793

Drug Name	Unit Per	Route	Code
ARCHITECT EXTRACELLULAR MATRIX	SQ CM	OTH	Q4147
AREDIA	30 MG	IV	J2430
ARFORMOTEROL	15 MCG	INH	J7605
ARGATROBAN	1 MG	IV	J0883
ARGATROBAN	1 MG	IV	J0884
ARIDOL	5 MG	INH	J7665
ARIMIDEX	1 MG	ORAL	S0170
ARIPIPRAZOLE	0.25 MG	IM	J0400
ARIPIPRAZOLE LAUROXIL	1 MG	IM	J1943
ARIPIPRAZOLE LAUROXIL	1 MG	IM	J1944
ARIPIPRAZOLE, EXTENDED RELEASE	1 MG	IM	J0401
ARISTADA	1 MG	IM	J1944
ARISTADA INITIO	1 MG	IM	J1943
ARISTOCORT	5 MG	IM	J3302
ARISTOCORTE FORTE	5 MG	IM	J3302
ARISTOCORTE INTRALESIONAL	5 MG	OTH	J3302
ARISTOSPAN	5 MG	VAR	J3303
ARIXTRA	0.5 MG	SC	J1652
AROMASIN	25 MG	ORAL	S0156
ARRANON	50 MG	IV	J9261
ARRESTIN	200 MG	IM	J3250
ARSENIC TRIOXIDE	1 MG	IV	J9017
ARTACENT AC	1 MG	OTH	Q4189
ARTACENT AC	SQ CM	OTH	Q4190
ARTACENT CORD	SQ CM	OTH	Q4216
ARTACENT WOUND	SQ CM	OTH	Q4169
ARTHROFLEX	SQ CM	OTH	Q4125
ARTISS FIBRIN SEALANT	2 ML	OTH	C9250
ARZERRA	10 MG	IV	J9302
ASCENIV	500 MG	IV	C9072
ASCENIV	500 MG	IV	J1554
ASCENT	0.5 MG	OTH	Q4213
ASPARAGINASE	1,000 IU	IM,IV,SC	J9019
ASPARAGINASE, RECOMBINANT	0.1 MG	IM	J9021
ASPARLAS	10 UNITS	IV	J9118
ASTAGRAF XL	0.1 MG	ORAL	J7508
ASTRAMORPH PF	10 MG	OTH	J2274
ATEZOLIZUMAB	10 MG	INF	J9022
ATGAM	250 MG	OTH	J7504
ATIVAN	2 MG	IM, IV	J2060
ATOPICLAIR	ANY SIZE	OTH	A6250
ATROPEN	0.01 MG	IM	J0461
ATROPINE SULFATE	0.01 MG	IM, IV, SC	J0461
ATROPINE, COMPOUNDED, CONCENTRATED	I MG	INH	J7635
ATROPINE, COMPOUNDED, UNIT DOSE	1 MG	INH	J7636
ATROVENT, NONCOMPOUNDED, UNIT DOSE	1 MG	INH	J7644
ATRYN	50 IU	IV	J7196
AUROTHIOGLUCOSE	50 MG	IM	J2910
AUTOPLEX T	1 IU	IV	J7198
AVALGLUCOSIDASE ALFA-NGPT	4 MG	IV	C9085

Drug Name	Unit Per	Route	Code
AVASTIN	0.25 MG	IV	C9257
AVASTIN	10 MG	IV	J9035
AVEED	1 MG	IM	J3145
AVELOX	100 MG	IV	J2280
AVELUMAB	10 MG	INF	J9023
AVONEX	30 MCG	IM	J1826
AVONEX	1 MCG	IM	Q3027
AVSOLA	10 MG	IV	Q5121
AVYCAZ	0.5 G/0.125 G	IV	J0714
AXICABTAGENE CILOLEUCEL	UP TO 200 MILLION CELLS	IV	Q2041
AXOBIOMEMBRANE	SQ CM	OTH	Q4211
AXOLOTL AMBIENT, AXOLOTL CRYO	0.1 MG	OTH	Q4215
AXOLOTL GRAFT, AXOLOTL DUALGRAFT	SQ CM	OTH	Q4210
AXUMIN	1 MCI	IV	A9588
AZACITIDINE	1 MG	SC	J9025
AZACTAM	500 MG	IV	S0073
AZASAN	50 MG	ORAL	J7500
AZATHIOPRINE	50 MG	ORAL	J7500
AZATHIOPRINE	100 MG	OTH	J7501
AZEDRA	1 MCI	IV	A9590
AZITHROMYCIN	1 G	ORAL	Q0144
AZITHROMYCIN	500 MG	IV	J0456
AZMACORT	PER MG	INH	J7684
AZMACORT CONCENTRATED	PER MG	INH	J7683
AZTREONAM	500 MG	IV, IM	S0073
BACLOFEN	50 MCG	IT	J0476
BACLOFEN	10 MG	IT	J0475
BACTOCILL	250 MG	IM, IV	J2700
BACTRIM IV	10 ML	IV	S0039
BAL	100 MG	IM	J0470
BAMLANIVIMAB AND ETESEVIMAB	2100 MG	IV	Q0245
BAMLANIVIMAB-XXXX	700 MG	IV	Q0239
BASILIXIMAB	20 MG	IV	J0480
BAVENCIO	10 MG	INF	J9023
BAXDELA	1 MG	ORAL, IV	C9462
BCG LIVE INTRAVESICAL	1 MG	OTH	J9030
BEBULIN VH	1 IU	IV	J7194
BECAPLERMIN GEL 0.01%	0.5 G	OTH	S0157
BECLOMETHASONE COMPOUNDED	1 MG	INH	J7622
BECLOVENT COMPOUNDED	1 MG	INH	J7622
BECONASE COMPOUNDED	1 MG	INH	J7622
BELANTAMAB MAFODONTIN-BLMF	0.5 MG	IV	C9069
BELANTAMAB MAFODONTIN-BLMF	0.5 MG	IV	J9037
BELATACEPT	1 MG	IV	J0485
BELEODAQ	10 MG	IV	J9032
BELIMUMAB	10 MG	IV	J0490
BELINOSTAT	10 MG	IV	J9032
BELLACELL HD	SQ CM	OTH	Q4220
BELRAPZO	1 MG	IV	J9036

Drug Name	Unit Per	Route	Code
BENA-D 10	50 MG	IV, IM	J1200
BENA-D 50	50 MG	IV, IM	J1200
BENADRYL	50 MG	IV, IM	J1200
BENAHIST 10	50 MG	IV, IM	J1200
BENAHIST 50	50 MG	IV, IM	J1200
BENDAMUSTINE HCL	1 MG	IV	J9033
BENDAMUSTINE HCL	1 MG	IV	J9034
BENDAMUSTINE HYDROCHLORIDE	1 MG	IV	J9036
BENDEKA	1 MG	IV	J9034
BENLYSTA	10 MG	IV	J0490
BENOJECT-10	50 MG	IV, IM	J1200
BENOJECT-50	50 MG	IV, IM	J1200
BENRALIZUMAB	1 MG	SC	J0517
BENTYL	20 MG	IM	J0500
BENZTROPINE MESYLATE	1 MG	IM, IV	J0515
BEOVU	1 MG	INJ	J0179
BERINERT	10 U	IV	J0597
BERUBIGEN	1,000 MCG	SC, IM	J3420
BESPONSA	0.1 MG	IV	J9229
BETA-2	1 MG	INH	J7648
BETALIN 12	1,000 MCG	SC, IM	J3420
BETAMETHASONE ACETATE AND BETAMETHASONE SODIUM PHOSPHATE	3 MG, OF EACH	IM	J0702
BETAMETHASONE COMPOUNDED, UNIT DOSE	1 MG	INH	J7624
BETASERON	0.25 MG	SC	J1830
BETHANECHOL CHLORIDE, MYOTONACHOL OR URECHOLINE	5 MG	SC	J0520
BEVACIZUMAB	10 MG	IV	J9035
BEVACIZUMAB	0.25 MG	IV	C9257
BEVACIZUMAB-AWWB, BIOSIMILAR	10 MG	IV	Q5107
BEVACIZUMAB-BVZR, BIOSIMILAR	10 MG	IV	Q5118
BEZLOTOXUMAB	10 MG	INF	J0565
BICILLIN CR	100,000 UNITS	IM	J0558
BICILLIN CR 900/300	100,000 UNITS	IM	J0558
BICILLIN CR TUBEX	100,000 UNITS	IM	J0558
BICILLIN LA	100,000 U	IM	J0561
BICNU	100 MG	IV	J9050
BIMATOPROST, INTRACAMERAL IMPLANT	1 MCG	OTH	J7351
BIO-CONNEKT	SQ CM	OTH	Q4161
BIO-CONNEKT WOUND MATRIX	SQ CM	OTH	A2003
BIODEXCEL	SQ CM	OTH	Q4137
BIODFENCE	SQ CM	OTH	Q4140
BIODFENCE DRYFLEX	SQ CM	OTH	Q4138
BIODMATRIX	1 CC	OTH	Q4139
BIONEXTPATCH	SQ CM	OTH	Q4228
BIOSKIN	SQ CM	OTH	Q4163
BIOSKIN FLOW	SQ CM	OTH	Q4162
BIOTROPIN	1 MG	SC	J2941
BIOVANCE	SQ CM	OTH	Q4154

Drug Name	Unit Per	Route	Code	Drug Name	Unit Per	Route	Code
BIOWOUND, BIOWOUND PLUS, BIOWOUND XPLUS	SQ CM	OTH	Q4217	BUPIVACAINE, COLLAGEN-MATRIX IMPLANT	1 MG	OTH	C9089
BIPERIDEN LACTATE	5 MG	IM, IV	J0190	BUPRENEX	0.1 MG	IM, IV	J0592
BITOLTEROL MESYLATE, COMPOUNDED CONCENTRATED	PER MG	INH	J7628	BUPRENORPHIN/NALOXONE	UP TO 3 MG	ORAL	J0572
BITOLTEROL MESYLATE, COMPOUNDED UNIT DOSE	PER MG	INH	J7629	BUPRENORPHIN/NALOXONE	> 10 MG	ORAL	J0575
BIVALIRUDIN	1 MG	IV	J0583	BUPRENORPHINE EXTENDED-RELEASE	> 100 MG	SC	Q9992
BIVIGAM	500 MG	IV	J1556	BUPRENORPHINE EXTENDED-RELEASE	≤ 100 MG	SC	Q9991
BLENOXANE	15 U	IM, IV, SC	J9040	BUPRENORPHINE HCL	0.1 MG	IM, IV	J0592
BLENREP	0.5 MG	IV	C9069	BUPRENORPHINE IMPLANT	74.2 MG	OTH	J0570
BLENREP	0.5 MG	IV	J9037	BUPRENORPHINE ORAL	1 MG	ORAL	J0571
BLEOMYCIN LYOPHILLIZED	15 U	IM, IV, SC	J9040	BUPRENORPHINE/NALOXONE	3.1 TO 6 MG	ORAL	J0573
BLEOMYCIN SULFATE	15 U	IM, IV, SC	J9040	BUPRENORPHINE/NALOXONE	6.1 TO 10 MG	ORAL	J0574
BLINATUMOMAB	1 MCG	IV	J9039	BUPROPION HCL	150 MG	ORAL	S0106
BLINCYTO	1 MCG	IV	J9039	BUROSUMAB-TWZA	1 MG	SC	J0584
BONIVA	1 MG	IV	J1740	BUSULFAN	1 MG	IV	J0594
BORTEZOMIB	0.1 MG	IV, SC	J9041	BUSULFAN	2 MG	ORAL	J8510
BOTOX	1 UNIT	IM, OTH	J0585	BUSULFEX	2 MG	ORAL	J8510
BOTOX COSMETIC	1 UNIT	IM, OTH	J0585	BUTORPHANOL TARTRATE	2 MG	IM, IV	J0595
BOTULINUM TOXIN TYPE A	1 UNIT	IM, OTH	J0585	BUTORPHANOL TARTRATE	25 MG	OTH	S0012
BOTULINUM TOXIN TYPE B	100 U	OTH	J0587	C-1 ESTERASE INHIBITOR (HUMAN)	10 UNITS	SC	J0599
BRAVELLE	75 IU	SC, IM	J3355	C1 ESTERASE INHIBITOR (HUMAN) (BERINERT)	10 UNITS	IV	J0597
BRENTUXIMAB VENDOTIN	1 MG	IV	J9042	C1 ESTERASE INHIBITOR (HUMAN) (CINRYZE)	10 UNITS	IV	J0598
BRETHINE	PER MG	INH	J7681	C1 ESTERASE INHIBITOR (RECOMBINANT)	10 UNITS	IV	J0596
BRETHINE CONCENTRATED	PER MG	INH	J7680	CABAZITAXEL	1 MG	IV	J9043
BREXANOLONE	1 MG	IV	J1632	CABENUVA	2 MG/3 MG	IM	C9077
BREXUCABTAGENE AUTOLEUCEL	UP TO 200 MILLION CELLS	IV	C9073	CABENUVA	2 MG/3 MG	IM	J0741
BREXUCABTAGENE AUTOLEUCEL	UP TO 200 MILLION CELLS	IV	Q2053	CABERGOLINE	0.25 MG	ORAL	J8515
BREYANZI	UP TO 110 MILLION CELLS	IV	C9076	CABLIVI	1 MG	IV, SC	C9047
BREYANZI	UP TO 110 MILLION CELLS	IV	Q2054	CABOTEGRAVIR AND RILPIVIRINE	2 MG/3 MG	IM	C9077
BRICANYL	PER MG	INH	J7681	CABOTEGRAVIR AND RILPIVIRINE	2 MG/3 MG	IM	J0741
BRICANYL CONCENTRATED	PER MG	INH	J7680	CAFCIT	5 MG	IV	J0706
BRINEURA	1 MG	OTH	J0567	CAFFEINE CITRATE	5 MG	IV	J0706
BROLUCIZUMAB-DBLL	1 MG	INJ	J0179	CALASPARGASE PEGOL-MKNL	10 UNITS	IV	J9118
BROM-A-COT	10 MG	IM, SC, IV	J0945	CALCIJEX	0.25 MCG	INJ	S0169
BROMPHENIRAMINE MALEATE	10 MG	IM, SC, IV	J0945	CALCIJEX	0.1 MCG	IM	J0636
BUDESONIDE COMPOUNDED, CONCETRATED	0.25 MG	INH	J7634	CALCIMAR	UP TO 400 U	SC, IM	J0630
BUDESONIDE, COMPOUNDED, UNIT DOSE	0.5 MG	INH	J7627	CALCITONIN SALMON	400 U	SC, IM	J0630
BUDESONIDE, NONCOMPOUNDED, CONCENTRATED	0.25 MG	INH	J7633	CALCITRIOL	0.1 MCG	IM	J0636
				CALCITROL	0.25 MCG	IM	S0169
BUDESONIDE, NONCOMPOUNDED, UNIT DOSE	0.5 MG	INH	J7626	CALCIUM DISODIUM VERSENATE	1,000 MG	IV, SC, IM	J0600
BUMETANIDE	0.5 MG	IM, IV	S0171	CALCIUM GLUCONATE	10 ML	IV	J0610
BUNAVAIL	2.1 MG	ORAL	J0572	CALCIUM GLYCEROPHOSPHATE AND CALCIUM LACTATE	10 ML	IM, SC	J0620
BUNAVAIL	6.3 MG	ORAL	J0574	CALDOLOR	100 MG	IV	J1741
BUNAVAIL	4.2 MG	ORAL	J0573	CAMCEVI	1 MG	SC	J1952
BUPIVACAINE AND MELOXICAM	1 MG/0.03 MG	OTH	C9088	CAMPTOSAR	20 MG	IV	J9206
BUPIVACAINE HCL	30 ML	VAR	S0020	CANAKINUMAB	1 MG	SC	J0638
BUPIVACAINE LIPOSOME	1 MG	VAR	C9290	CANCIDAS	5 MG	IV	J0637
				CAPECITABINE	150 MG	ORAL	J8520
				CAPLACIZUMAB-YHDP	1 MG	IV, SC	C9047

Drug Name	Unit Per	Route	Code
CAPROMAB PENDETIDE	STUDY DOSE UP TO 10 MCI	IV	A9507
CAPSAICIN 8% PATCH	1 SQ CM	OTH	J7336
CARBIDOPA/LEVODOPA	5 MG/20 MG	ORAL	J7340
CARBOCAINE	10 ML	VAR	J0670
CARBOPLATIN	50 MG	IV	J9045
CARDIOGEN 82	STUDY DOSE UP TO 60 MCI	IV	A9555
CARDIOLITE	STUDY DOSE	IV	A9500
CAREPATCH	SQ CM	OTH	Q4236
CARFILZOMIB	1 MG	IV	J9047
CARMUSTINE	100 MG	IV	J9050
CARNITOR	1 G	IV	J1955
CARTICEL		OTH	J7330
CASIMERSEN	10 MG	IV	C9075
CASIMERSEN	10 MG	IV	J1426
CASIRIVIMAB AND IMDEVIMAB	2400 MG	IV	Q0243
CASIRIVIMAB AND IMDEVIMAB	600 MG	IV	Q0240
CASIRIVIMAB AND IMDEVIMAB	1200 MG	IV	Q0244
CASPOFUNGIN ACETATE	5 MG	IV	J0637
CATAPRES	1 MG	OTH	J0735
CATHFLO	1 MG	IV	J2997
CAVERJECT	1.25 MCG	VAR	J0270
CEA SCAN	STUDY DOSE UP TO 45 MCI	IV	A9568
CEENU	10 MG	ORAL	S0178
CEFAZOLIN SODIUM	500 MG	IM, IV	J0690
CEFEPIME HCL	500 MG	IV	J0692
CEFIDEROCOL	5 MG	IV	J0693
CEFIDEROCOL	10 MG	IV	J0699
CEFIZOX	500 MG	IV, IM	J0715
CEFOBID	1 G	IV	S0021
CEFOPERAZONE SODIUM	1 G	IV	S0021
CEFOTAN	500 MG	IM, IV	S0074
CEFOTAXIME SODIUM	1 GM	IV, IM	J0698
CEFOTETAN DISODIUM	500 MG	IM. IV	S0074
CEFOXITIN SODIUM	1 GM	IV, IM	J0694
CEFTAROLINE FOSAMIL	10 MG	IV	J0712
CEFTAZIDIME	500 MG	IM, IV	J0713
CEFTAZIDIME AND AVIBACTAM	0.5 G/0.125 G	IV	J0714
CEFTIZOXIME SODIUM	500 MG	IV, IM	J0715
CEFTOLOZANE AND TAZOBACTAM	50 MG/25 MG	IV	J0695
CEFTRIAXONE SODIUM	250 MG	IV, IM	J0696
CEFUROXIME	750 MG	IM, IV	J0697
CEFUROXIME SODIUM STERILE	750 MG	IM, IV	J0697
CELESTONE SOLUSPAN	3 MG	IM	J0702
CELLCEPT	250 MG	ORAL	J7517
CELLESTA CORD	SQ CM	OTH	Q4214
CELLESTA FLOWABLE AMNION	0.5 CC	OTH	Q4185
CELLESTA OR CELLESTA DUO	SQ CM	OTH	Q4184
CEMIPLIMAB-RWLC	1 MG	IV	J9119
CENACORT FORTE	5 MG	IM	J3302
CENTRUROIDES (SCORPION) IMMUNE F(AB)2 (EQUINE)	UP TO 120 MG	IV	J0716

Drug Name	Unit Per	Route	Code
CEPHALOTHIN SODIUM	UP TO 1 G	INJ	J1890
CEPHAPIRIN SODIUM	1 G	IV	J0710
CEPTAZ	500 MG	IM, IV	J0713
CEREBRYX	50 MG	IM, IV	Q2009
CEREBRYX	750 MG	IM, IV	S0078
CEREDASE	10 U	IV	J0205
CERETEC	STUDY DOSE UP TO 25 MCI	IV	A9521
CEREZYME	10 U	IV	J1786
CERIANNA	1 MCI	IV	A9591
CERLIPONASE ALFA	1 MG	OTH	J0567
CERTOLIZUMAB PEGOL	1 MG	SC	J0717
CERUBIDINE	10 MG	IV	J9150
CESAMET	1 MG	ORAL	J8650
CETIRIZINE HCL	0.5 MG	IV	J1201
CETUXIMAB	10 MG	IV	J9055
CHEALAMIDE	150 MG	IV	J3520
CHLORAMBUCIL	2 MG	ORAL	S0172
CHLORAMPHENICOL SODIUM SUCCINATE	1 G	IV	J0720
CHLORDIAZEPOXIDE HCL	100 MG	IM, IV	J1990
CHLOROMYCETIN	1 G	IV	J0720
CHLOROPROCAINE HCL	30 ML	VAR	J2400
CHLOROQUINE HCL	UP TO 250 MG	IM, IV	J0390
CHLOROTHIAZIDE SODIUM	500 MG	IV	J1205
CHLORPROMAZINE HCL	5 MG	ORAL	Q0161
CHLORPROMAZINE HCL	50 MG	IM, IV	J3230
CHOLETEC	STUDY DOSE UP TO 15 MCI	IV	A9537
CHOLINE C 11, DIAGNOSTIC, PER STUDY DOSE	UP TO 20 MCI	IV	A9515
CHOREX	1000 USP	IM	J0725
CHORIONIC GONADOTROPIN	1,000 USP U	IM	J0725
CHROMIC PHOSPHATE P32 (THERAPEUTIC)	1 MCI	IV	A9564
CHROMITOPE SODIUM	STUDY DOSE UP TO 250 UCI	IV	A9553
CHROMIUM CR-51 SODIUM IOTHALAMATE, DIAGNOSTIC	STUDY DOSE UP TO 250 UCI	IV	A9553
CIDOFOVIR	375 MG	IV	J0740
CILASTATIN SODIUM	250 MG	IV, IM	J0743
CIMETIDINE HCL	300 MG	IM, IV	S0023
CIMZIA	1 MG	SC	J0717
CINACALCET	1 MG	ORAL	J0604
CINQUAIR	1 MG	IV	J2786
CINRZYE	10 UNITS	IV	J0598
CINVANTI	1 MG	IV	J0185
CIPRO	200 MG	IV	J0744
CIPROFLOXACIN FOR INTRAVENOUS INFUSION	200 MG	IV	J0744
CIPROFLOXACIN OTIC SUSPENSION	6 MG	OTIC	J7342
CIS-MDP	STUDY DOSE UP TO 30 MCI	IV	A9503
CIS-PYRO	STUDY DOSE UP TO 25 MCI	IV	A9538
CISPLATIN	10 MG	IV	J9060

Drug Name	Unit Per	Route	Code
CLADRIBINE	1 MG	IV	J9065
CLAFORAN	1 GM	IV, IM	J0698
CLARIX 100	SQ MC	OTH	Q4156
CLARIX CORD 1K	SQ CM	OTH	Q4148
CLARIXFLO	1 MG	OTH	Q4155
CLEOCIN PHOSPHATE	300 MG	IV	S0077
CLEVIDIPINE BUTYRATE	1 MG	IV	C9248
CLEVIPREX	1 MG	IV	C9248
CLINDAMYCIN PHOSPHATE	300 MG	IV	S0077
CLOFARABINE	1 MG	IV	J9027
CLOLAR	1 MG	IV	J9027
CLONIDINE HCL	1 MG	OTH	J0735
CLOZAPINE	25 MG	ORAL	S0136
CLOZARIL	25 MG	ORAL	S0136
COAGADEX	1 IU	IV	J7175
COAGULATION FACTOR XA (RECOMBINANT), INACTIVATED-ZHZO	10 MG	IV	J7169
COBAL	1,000 MCG	IM, SC	J3420
COBALT CO-57 CYNOCOBALAMIN, DIAGNOSTIC	STUDY DOSE UP TO 1 UCI	ORAL	A9559
COBATOPE 57	STUDY DOSE UP TO 1 UCI	ORAL	A9559
COBEX	1,000 MCG	SC, IM	J3420
COCAINE HYDROCHLORIDE NASAL SOLUTION	1 MG	OTH	C9046
CODEINE PHOSPHATE	30 MG	IM, IV, SC	J0745
COGENEX AMNIOTIC MEMBRANE	SQ CM	OTH	Q4229
COGENEX FLOWABLE AMNION	0.5 CC	OTH	Q4230
COGENTIN	1 MG	IM, IV	J0515
COGNEX	10 MG	ORAL	S0014
COLCHICINE	1 MG	IV	J0760
COLHIST	10 MG	IM, SC, IV	J0945
COLISTIMETHATE SODIUM	1 MG	INH	S0142
COLISTIMETHATE SODIUM	150 MG	IM, IV	J0770
COLL-E-DERM	SQ CM	OTH	Q4193
COLLAGEN BASED WOUND FILLER DRY FOAM	1 GM	OTH	A6010
COLLAGEN BASED WOUND FILLER, GEL/PASTE	1 GM	OTH	A6011
COLLAGEN MATRIX NERVE WRAP	0.5 CM	OTH	C9361
COLLAGEN NERVE CUFF	0.5 CM LENGTH	OTH	C9355
COLLAGEN WOUND DRESSING	SQ CM	OTH	Q4164
COLLAGENASE, CLOSTRIDIUM HISTOLYTICUM	0.01 MG	OTH	J0775
COLY-MYCIN M	150 MG	IM, IV	J0770
COMPAZINE	10 MG	IM, IV	J0780
COMPAZINE	5 MG	ORAL	S0183
COMPAZINE	5 MG	ORAL	Q0164
CONIVAPTAN HYDROCHLORIDE	1 MG	INJ	C9488
CONTRACEPTIVE SUPPLY, HORMONE CONTAINING PATCH	EACH	OTH	J7304
CONTRAST FOR ECHOCARDIOGRAM	STUDY	IV	A9700
COPANLISIB	1 MG	IV	J9057
COPAXONE	20 MG	SC	J1595

Drug Name	Unit Per	Route	Code
COPPER CU-64, DOTATATE, DIAGNOSTIC	1 MCI	IV	C9068
COPPER CU-64, DOTATATE, DIAGNOSTIC	1 MCI	IV	A9592
COPPER T MODEL TCU380A IUD COPPER WIRE/COPPER COLLAR	EA	OTH	J7300
CORDARONE	30 MG	IV	J0282
CORECYTE	0.5 CC	OTH	Q4240
CORETEXT	1 CC	OTH	Q4246
CORIFACT	1 IU	IV	J7180
CORPLEX	SQ CM	OTH	Q4232
CORPLEX P	1 CC	OTH	Q4231
CORTASTAT	1 MG	IM, IV, OTH	J1100
CORTASTAT LA	1 MG	IM	J1094
CORTICORELIN OVINE TRIFLUTATE	1 MCG	IV	J0795
CORTICOTROPIN	40 U	IV, IM, SC	J0800
CORTIMED	80 MG	IM	J1040
CORTROSYN	0.25 MG	IM, IV	J0834
CORVERT	1 MG	IV	J1742
COSELA	1 MG	IV	C9078
COSELA	1 MG	IV	J1448
COSMEGEN	0.5 MG	IV	J9120
COSYNTROPIN	0.25 MG	IM, IV	J0834
COTOLONE	5 MG	ORAL	J7510
CRESEMBA	1 MG	IV	J1833
CRIZANLIZUMAB-TMCA	5 MG	IV	J0791
CROFAB	UP TO 1 GM	IV	J0840
CROMOLYN SODIUM COMPOUNDED	PER 10 MG	INH	J7632
CROMOLYN SODIUM NONCOMPOUNDED	10 MG	INH	J7631
CROTALIDAE IMMUNE F(AB')2 (EQUINE)	120 MG	IV	J0841
CROTALIDAE POLYVALENT IMMUNE FAB (OVINE)	UP TO 1 GM	IV	J0840
CRYO-CORD	SQ CM	OTH	Q4237
CRYSTAL B12	1,000 MCG	IM, SC	J3420
CRYSTICILLIN 300 A.S.	600,000 UNITS	IM, IV	J2510
CRYSTICILLIN 600 A.S.	600,000 UNITS	IM, IV	J2510
CRYSVITA	1 MG	SC	J0584
CUBICIN	1 MG	IV	J0878
CUVITRU	100 MG	SC	J1555
CYANO	1,000 MCG	IM, SC	J3420
CYANOCOBALAMIN	1,000 MCG	IM, SC	J3420
CYANOCOBALAMIN COBALT 57/58	STUDY DOSE UP TO 1 UCI	IV	A9546
CYANOCOBALAMIN COBALT CO-57	STUDY DOSE UP TO 1 UCI	ORAL	A9559
CYCLOPHOSPHAMIDE	25 MG	ORAL	J8530
CYCLOPHOSPHAMIDE	10 MG	IV	C9087
CYCLOPHOSPHAMIDE	100 MG	IV	J9070
CYCLOSPORINE	25 MG	ORAL	J7515
CYCLOSPORINE	100 MG	ORAL	J7502
CYCLOSPORINE	250 MG	IV	J7516
CYGNUS	SQ CM	OTH	Q4170
CYGNUS MATRIX	SQ CM	OTH	Q4199

Drug Name	Unit Per	Route	Code
CYMETRA	1 CC	INJ	Q4112
CYRAMZA	5 MG	IV	J9308
CYSVIEW	STUDY DOSE	OTH	A9589
CYTAL	SQ CM	OTH	Q4166
CYTARABINE	100 MG	SC, IV	J9100
CYTARABINE LIPOSOME	10 MG	IT	J9098
CYTOGAM	VIAL	IV	J0850
CYTOMEGALOVIRUS IMMUNE GLOB	VIAL	IV	J0850
CYTOSAR-U	100 MG	SC, IV	J9100
CYTOTEC	200 MCG	ORAL	S0191
CYTOVENE	500 MG	IV	J1570
CYTOXAN	25 MG	ORAL	J8530
CYTOXAN	100 MG	IV	J9070
D.H.E. 45	1 MG	IM, IV	J1110
DACARBAZINE	100 MG	IV	J9130
DACLIZUMAB	25 MG	OTH	J7513
DACOGEN	1 MG	IV	J0894
DACTINOMYCIN	0.5 MG	IV	J9120
DALALONE	1 MG	IM, IV, OTH	J1100
DALALONE LA	1 MG	IM	J1094
DALBAVANCIN	5 MG	IV	J0875
DALTEPARIN SODIUM	2,500 IU	SC	J1645
DALVANCE	5 MG	IV	J0875
DANYELZA	1 MG	IV	J9348
DAPTOMYCIN	1 MG	IV	J0878
DARATUMUMAB	10 MG	IV	J9145
DARATUMUMAB AND HYALURONIDASE-FIHJ	10 MG	SC	J9144
DARBEPOETIN ALFA, ESRD USE	1 MCG	SC, IV	J0882
DARBEPOETIN ALFA, NON-ESRD USE	1 MCG	SC, IV	J0881
DARZALEX	10 MG	IV	J9145
DARZALEX FASPRO	10 MG	SC	J9144
DATSCAN	STUDY DOSE	IV	A9584
DAUNORUBICIN	10 MG	IV	J9150
DAUNORUBICIN CITRATE, LIPOOSOMAL FORMULATION	10 MG	IV	J9151
DAUNOXOME	10 MG	IV	J9151
DDAVP	1 MCG	IV, SC	J2597
DECADRON	0.25 MG	ORAL	J8540
DECAJECT	1 MG	IM, IV, OTH	J1100
DECITABINE	1 MG	IV	J0894
DECOLONE-50	50 MG	IM	J2320
DEFEROXAMINE MESYLATE	500 MG	IM, SC, IV	J0895
DEGARELIX	1 MG	SC	J9155
DELAFLOXACIN	1 MG	ORAL, IV	C9462
DELATESTRYL	1 MG	IM	J3121
DELESTROGEN	10 MG	IM	J1380
DELTA-CORTEF	5 MG	ORAL	J7510
DEMADEX	10 MG	IV	J3265
DEMEROL	100 MG	IM, IV, SC	J2175
DENILEUKIN DIFTITOX	300 MCG	IV	J9160
DENOSUMAB	1 MG	SC	J0897
DEOXYCHOLIC ACID	1 MG	SC	J0591

Drug Name	Unit Per	Route	Code
DEPGYNOGEN	UP TO 5 MG	IM	J1000
DEPHENACEN-50	50 MG	IM, IV	J1200
DEPMEDALONE	40 MG	IM	J1030
DEPMEDALONE	80 MG	IM	J1040
DEPO-ESTRADIOL CYPIONATE	UP TO 5 MG	IM	J1000
DEPO-MEDROL	40 MG	IM, OTH	J1030
DEPO-MEDROL	80 MG	IM, OTH	J1040
DEPO-MEDROL	20 MG	IM, OTH	J1020
DEPO-TESTOSTERONE	1 MG	IM	J1071
DEPOCYT	10 MG	IT	J9098
DEPOGEN	UP TO 5 MG	IM	J1000
DERM-MAXX	SQ CM	OTH	Q4238
DERMA-GIDE	SQ CM	OTH	Q4203
DERMACELL, DERMACELL AWM OR DERMACELL AWM POROUS	SQ CM	OTH	Q4122
DERMACYTE AMNIOTIC MEMBRANE ALLOGRAFT	SQ CM	OTH	Q4248
DERMAGRAFT	SQ CM	OTH	Q4106
DERMAL SUBSTITUTE, NATIVE, NONDENATURED COLLAGEN, FETAL	0.5 SQ CM	OTH	C9358
DERMAL SUBSTITUTE, NATIVE, NONDENATURED COLLAGEN, NEONATAL	0.5 SQ CM	OTH	C9360
DERMAPURE	SQ CM	OTH	Q4152
DERMAVEST AND PLURIVEST	SQ CM	OTH	Q4153
DESFERAL	500 MG	IM, SC, IV	J0895
DESMOPRESSIN ACETATE	1 MCG	IV, SC	J2597
~~DETECTNET~~	~~1 MCI~~	~~IV~~	~~C9068~~
DETECTNET	1 MCI	IV	A9592
DEXAMETHASONE	0.25 MG	ORAL	J8540
DEXAMETHASONE 9%	1 MCG	OTH	J1095
DEXAMETHASONE ACETATE	1 MG	IM	J1094
DEXAMETHASONE ACETATE ANHYDROUS	1 MG	IM	J1094
DEXAMETHASONE INTRAVITREAL IMPLANT	0.1 MG	OTH	J7312
DEXAMETHASONE SODIUM PHOSPHATE	1 MG	IM, IV, OTH	J1100
DEXAMETHASONE, COMPOUNDED, CONCENTRATED	1 MG	INH	J7637
DEXAMETHASONE, COMPOUNDED, UNIT DOSE	1 MG	INH	J7638
DEXAMETHASONE, LACRIMAL OPHTHALMIC INSERT	0.1 MG	OTH	J1096
DEXASONE	1 MG	IM, IV, OTH	J1100
DEXEDRINE	5 MG	ORAL	S0160
DEXIM	1 MG	IM, IV, OTH	J1100
DEXONE	0.25 MG	ORAL	J8540
DEXONE	1 MG	IM, IV, OTH	J1100
DEXONE LA	1 MG	IM	J1094
DEXRAZOXANE HCL	250 MG	IV	J1190
DEXTENZA	0.1 MG	OTH	J1096
DEXTRAN 40	500 ML	IV	J7100
DEXTROAMPHETAMINE SULFATE	5 MG	ORAL	S0160
DEXTROSE	500 ML	IV	J7060

Drug Name	Unit Per	Route	Code
DEXTROSE, STERILE WATER, AND/OR DEXTROSE DILUENT/FLUSH	10 ML	VAR	A4216
DEXTROSE/SODIUM CHLORIDE	5%	VAR	J7042
DEXTROSE/THEOPHYLLINE	40 MG	IV	J2810
DEXTROSTAT	5 MG	ORAL	S0160
DEXYCU	1 MCG	OTH	J1095
DI-SPAZ	UP TO 20 MG	IM	J0500
DIALYSIS/STRESS VITAMINS	100 CAPS	ORAL	S0194
DIAMOX	500 MG	IM, IV	J1120
DIASTAT	5 MG	IV, IM	J3360
DIAZEPAM	5 MG	IV, IM	J3360
DIAZOXIDE	300 MG	IV	J1730
DIBENT	UP TO 20 MG	IM	J0500
DICLOFENAC SODIUM	0.5 MG	OTH	J1130
DICYCLOMINE HCL	20 MG	IM	J0500
DIDANOSINE (DDI)	25 MG	ORAL	S0137
DIDRONEL	300 MG	IV	J1436
DIETHYLSTILBESTROL DIPHOSPHATE	250 MG	INJ	J9165
DIFLUCAN	200 MG	IV	J1450
DIGIBIND	VIAL	IV	J1162
DIGIFAB	VIAL	IV	J1162
DIGOXIN	0.5 MG	IM, IV	J1160
DIGOXIN IMMUNE FAB	VIAL	IV	J1162
DIHYDROERGOTAMINE MESYLATE	1 MG	IM, IV	J1110
DILANTIN	50 MG	IM, IV	J1165
DILAUDID	250 MG	OTH	S0092
DILAUDID	4 MG	SC, IM, IV	J1170
DIMENHYDRINATE	50 MG	IM, IV	J1240
DIMERCAPROL	100 MG	IM	J0470
DIMINE	50 MG	IV, IM	J1200
DINATE	50 MG	IM, IV	J1240
DIOVAL	10 MG	IM	J1380
DIOVAL 40	10 MG	IM	J1380
DIOVAL XX	10 MG	IM	J1380
DIPHENHYDRAMINE HCL	50 MG	ORAL	Q0163
DIPHENHYDRAMINE HCL	50 MG	IV, IM	J1200
DIPRIVAN	10 MG	IV	J2704
DIPYRIDAMOLE	10 MG	IV	J1245
DISOTATE	150 MG	IV	J3520
DIURIL	500 MG	IV	J1205
DIURIL SODIUM	500 MG	IV	J1205
DIZAC	5 MG	IV, IM	J3360
DMSO, DIMETHYL SULFOXIDE	50%, 50 ML	OTH	J1212
DOBUTAMINE HCL	250 MG	IV	J1250
DOBUTREX	250 MG	IV	J1250
DOCETAXEL	1 MG	IV	J9171
DOLASETRON MESYLATE	100 MG	ORAL	Q0180
DOLASETRON MESYLATE	10 MG	IV	J1260
DOLASETRON MESYLATE	50 MG	ORAL	S0174
DOLOPHINE	5 MG	ORAL	S0109
DOLOPHINE HCL	10 MG	IM, SC	J1230
DOMMANATE	50 MG	IM, IV	J1240

Drug Name	Unit Per	Route	Code
DOPAMINE HCL	40 MG	IV	J1265
DORIBAX	10 MG	IV	J1267
DORIPENEM	10 MG	IV	J1267
DORNASE ALPHA, NONCOMPOUNDED, UNIT DOSE	1 MG	INH	J7639
~~DOSTARLIMAB-GXLY~~	~~100 MG~~	~~IV~~	~~C9082~~
DOSTARLIMAB-GXLY	10 MG	IV	J9272
DOSTINEX	0.25 MG	ORAL	J8515
DOTAREM	0.1 ML	IV	A9575
DOXERCALCIFEROL	1 MG	IV	J1270
DOXORUBICIN HCL	10 MG	IV	J9000
DOXORUBICIN HYDROCHLORIDE, LIPOSOMAL, IMPORTED LIPODOX	10 MG	IV	Q2049
DRAMAMINE	50 MG	IM, IV	J1240
DRAMANATE	50 MG	IM, IV	J1240
DRAMILIN	50 MG	IM, IV	J1240
DRAMOCEN	50 MG	IM, IV	J1240
DRAMOJECT	50 MG	IM, IV	J1240
DRAXIMAGE MDP-10	STUDY DOSE UP TO 30 MCI	IV	A9503
DRAXIMAGE MDP-25	STUDY DOSE UP TO 30 MCI	IV	A9503
DRONABINAL	2.5 MG	ORAL	Q0167
DROPERIDOL	5 MG	IM, IV	J1790
DROPERIDOL AND FENTANYL CITRATE	2 ML	IM, IV	J1810
DROXIA	500 MG	ORAL	S0176
DTIC-DOME	100 MG	IV	J9130
DTPA	STUDY DOSE UP TO 25 MCI	IV	A9539
DTPA	STUDY DOSE UP TO 25 MCI	INH	A9567
DUOPA	5 MG/20 MG	ORAL	J7340
DURACILLIN A.S.	600,000 UNITS	IM, IV	J2510
DURACLON	1 MG	OTH	J0735
DURAGEN-10	10 MG	IM	J1380
DURAGEN-20	10 MG	IM	J1380
DURAGEN-40	10 MG	IM	J1380
DURAMORPH	500 MG	OTH	S0093
DURAMORPH PF	10 MG	OTH	J2274
DURO CORT	80 MG	IM	J1040
DUROLANE	1 MG	INJ	J7318
DURVALUMAB	10 MG	IV	J9173
DURYSTA	1 MCG	OTH	J7351
DYLOJECT	0.5 MG	OTH	J1130
DYMENATE	50 MG	IM, IV	J1240
DYPHYLLINE	500 MG	IM	J1180
DYSPORT	5 UNITS	IM	J0586
E.D.T.A.	150 MG	IV	J3520
ECALLANTIDE	1 MG	SC	J1290
ECHOCARDIOGRAM IMAGE ENHANCER OCTAFLUOROPROPANE	1 ML	IV	Q9956
ECHOCARDIOGRAM IMAGE ENHANCER PERFLEXANE	1 ML	IV	Q9955
ECULIZUMAB	10 MG	IV	J1300
EDARAVONE	1 MG	IV	J1301

Drug Name	Unit Per	Route	Code	Drug Name	Unit Per	Route	Code
EDETATE CALCIUM DISODIUM	1,000 MG	IV, SC, IM	J0600	ERGONOVINE MALEATE	0.2 MG	IM, IV	J1330
EDETATE DISODIUM	150 MG	IV	J3520	ERIBULIN MESYLATE	0.1 MG	IV	J9179
EDEX	1.25 MCG	VAR	J0270	ERTAPENEM SODIUM	500 MG	IM, IV	J1335
ELAPRASE	1 MG	IV	J1743	ERYTHROCIN LACTOBIONATE	500 MG	IV	J1364
ELAVIL	20 MG	IM	J1320	ESKETAMINE, NASAL SPRAY	1 MG	OTH	S0013
ELELYSO	10 U	IV	J3060	ESPEROCT	1 IU	IV	J7204
ELIGARD	7.5 MG	SC	J9217	ESTONE AQUEOUS	1 MG	IM, IV	J1435
ELITEK	0.5 MG	IM	J2783	ESTRA-L 20	10 MG	IM	J1380
ELLENCE	2 MG	IV	J9178	ESTRA-L 40	10 MG	IM	J1380
ELLIOTTS B SOLUTION	1 ML	IV, IT	J9175	ESTRADIOL CYPIONATE	UP TO 5 MG	IM	J1000
ELOCTATE	IU	IV	J7205	ESTRADIOL L.A.	10 MG	IM	J1380
ELOSULFASE ALFA	1 MG	IV	J1322	ESTRADIOL L.A. 20	10 MG	IM	J1380
ELOTUZUMAB	1 MG	IV	J9176	ESTRADIOL L.A. 40	10 MG	IM	J1380
ELOXATIN	0.5 MG	IV	J9263	ESTRADIOL VALERATE	10 MG	IM	J1380
ELSPAR	1,000 IU	IM,IV, SC	J9019	ESTRAGYN	1 MG	IV, IM	J1435
ELZONRIS	10 MCG	IV	J9269	ESTRO-A	1 MG	IV, IM	J1435
EMAPALUMAB-LZSG	1 MG	IV	J9210	ESTROGEN CONJUGATED	25 MG	IV, IM	J1410
EMEND	5 MG	ORAL	J8501	ESTRONE	1 MG	IV, IM	J1435
EMEND	1 MG	IV	J1453	ESTRONOL	1 MG	IM, IV	J1435
EMICIZUMAB-KXWH	0.5 MG	SC	J7170	ETANERCEPT	25 MG	IM, IV	J1438
EMINASE	30 U	IV	J0350	ETELCALCETIDE	0.1 MG	IV	J0606
EMPLICITI	1 MG	IV	J9176	ETEPLIRSEN	10 MG	INF	J1428
ENBREL	25 MG	IM, IV	J1438	ETHAMOLIN	100 MG	IV	J1430
ENDOXAN-ASTA	100 MG	IV	J9070	ETHANOLAMINE OLEATE	100 MG	IV	J1430
ENDRATE	150 MG	IV	J3520	ETHINYL ESTRADIOL AND ETONOGESTREL VAGINAL RING	0.015 MG/0.12 MG	OTH	J7295
ENFORTUMAB VEDOTIN-EJFV	0.25 MG	IV	J9177	ETHYOL	500 MG	IV	J0207
ENFUVIRTIDE	1 MG	SC	J1324	ETIDRONATE DISODIUM	300 MG	IV	J1436
ENHERTU	1 MG	IV	J9358	ETONOGESTREL	IMPLANT	OTH	J7307
ENOXAPARIN SODIUM	10 MG	SC	J1650	ETOPOSIDE	50 MG	ORAL	J8560
ENTYVIO	1 MG	IV	J3380	ETOPOSIDE	10 MG	IV	J9181
ENVARSUS XR	0.25 MG	ORAL	J7503	EUFLEXXA	PER DOSE	INJ	J7323
EOVIST	1 ML	IV	A9581	EULEXIN	125 MG	ORAL	S0175
EPICORD	SQ CM	OTH	Q4187	EVENITY	1 MG	SC	J3111
EPIFIX	SQ CM	OTH	Q4186	EVEROLIMUS	0.25 MG	ORAL	J7527
EPIFIX, INJECTABLE	1 MG	OTH	Q4145	~~EVINACUMAB-DGNB~~	~~5 MG~~	~~IV~~	~~C9079~~
EPINEPHRINE	0.1 MG	IM, IV, SC	J0171	EVINACUMAB-DGNB	5 MG	IV	J1305
EPIRUBICIN HCL	2 MG	IV	J9178	~~EVKEEZA~~	~~5 MG~~	~~IV~~	~~C9079~~
EPOETIN ALFA FOR ESRD DIALYSIS	100 U	INJ	Q4081	EVKEEZA	5 MG	IV	J1305
EPOETIN ALFA, BIOSIMILAR	100 UNITS	INJ, IV	Q5105	EVOMELA	1 MG	IV	J9246
EPOETIN ALFA, BIOSIMILAR	1000 UNITS	INJ, IV	Q5106	EXAMETAZIME LABELED AUTOLOGOUS WHITE BLOOD CELLS, TECHNETIUM TC-99M	STUDY DOSE	IV	A9569
EPOETIN ALFA, NON-ESRD USE	1,000 U	SC, IV	J0885	EXCELLAGEN	0.1 CC	OTH	Q4149
EPOETIN BETA FOR ESRD ON DIALYSIS	1 MCG	IV	J0887	EXMESTANE	25 MG	ORAL	S0156
EPOETIN BETA FOR NON-ESRD	1 MCG	IV, SC	J0888	EXONDYS 51	10 MG	INF	J1428
EPOGEN/NON-ESRD	1,000 U	SC, IV	J0885	EXPAREL	1 MG	VAR	C9290
EPOPROSTENOL	0.5 MG	IV	J1325	EZ-DERM	SQ CM	OTH	Q4136
EPOPROSTENOL STERILE DILUTANT	50 ML	IV	S0155	FABRAZYME	1 MG	IV	J0180
EPTIFIBATIDE	5 MG	IM, IV	J1327	FACTOR IX (ANTIHEMOPHILIC FACTOR, RECOMBINANT), RIXIBUS, PER I.U.	IU	IV	J7200
EPTINEZUMAB-JJMR	1 MG	IV	J3032				
ERAVACYCLINE	1 MG	IV	J0122	FACTOR IX NON-RECOMBINANT	1 IU	IV	J7193
ERAXIS	1 MG	IV	J0348	FACTOR IX+ COMPLEX	1 IU	IV	J7194
ERBITUX	10 MG	IV	J9055				
ERGAMISOL	50 MG	ORAL	S0177				

Drug Name	Unit Per	Route	Code
FACTOR IX, (ANTIHEMOPHILIC FACTOR, RECOMBINANT), GLYCOPEGYLATED	1 IU	IV	J7203
FACTOR IX, ALBUMIN FUSION PROTEIN, (RECOMBINANT)	1 IU	IV	J7202
FACTOR IX, FC FUSION PROTEIN (ANTIHEMOPHILIC FACTOR, RECOMBINANT), ALPROLIX	IU	IV	J7201
FACTOR VIIA (ANTIHEMOPHILIC FACTOR, RECOMBINANT)-JNCW	1 MCG	IV	J7212
FACTOR VIIA RECOMBINANT	1 MCG	IV	J7189
FACTOR VIII (ANTIHEMOPHILIC FACTOR, RECOMBINANT)	1 IU	IV	J7209
FACTOR VIII (ANTIHEMOPHILIC FACTOR, RECOMBINANT)	IU	IV	J7188
FACTOR VIII (ANTIHEMOPHILIC FACTOR, RECOMBINANT) (NOVOEIGHT), PER IU	IU	IV	J7182
FACTOR VIII (ANTIHEMOPHILIC FACTOR, RECOMBINANT) PEGYLATED	1 IU	IV	J7207
FACTOR VIII FC FUSION (RECOMBINANT)	IU	IV	J7205
FACTOR VIII PORCINE	1 IU	IV	J7191
FACTOR VIII, (ANTIHEMOPHILIC FACTOR, RECOMBINANT) (AFSTYLA)	1 I.U.	IV	J7210
FACTOR VIII, (ANTIHEMOPHILIC FACTOR, RECOMBINANT) (KOVALTRY)	1 I.U.	IV	J7211
FACTOR VIII, (ANTIHEMOPHILIC FACTOR, RECOMBINANT), PEGYLATED-AUCL	1 IU	IV	J7208
FACTOR VIII, ANTIHEMOPHILIC FACTOR (RECOMBINANT), GLYCOPEGYLATED-EXEI	1 IU	IV	J7204
FACTOR VIII, HUMAN	1 IU	IV	J7190
FACTOR X (HUMAN)	1 IU	IV	J7175
FACTOR XIII (ANTIHEMOPHILIC FACTOR, HUMAN)	1 IU	IV	J7180
FACTOR XIII A-SUBUNIT (RECOMBINANT)	10 IU	IV	J7181
FACTREL	100 MCG	SC, IV	J1620
FAM-TRASTUZUMAB DERUXTECAN-NXKI	1 MG	IV	J9358
FAMOTIDINE	20 MG	IV	S0028
FASENRA	1 MG	SC	J0517
FASLODEX	25 MG	IM	J9395
FDG	STUDY DOSE UP TO 45 MCI	IV	A9552
FEIBA-VH AICC	1 IU	IV	J7198
FENSOLVI	0.25 MG	SC	J1951
FENTANYL CITRATE	0.1 MG	IM, IV	J3010
FERAHEME (FOR ESRD)	1 MG	IV	Q0139
FERAHEME (NON-ESRD)	1 MG	IV	Q0138
FERIDEX IV	1 ML	IV	Q9953
FERRIC CARBOXYMALTOSE	1 MG	IV	J1439
FERRIC DERISOMALTOSE	10 MG	IV	J1437
FERRIC PYROPHOSPHATE CITRATE POWDER	0.1 MG	IV	J1444

Drug Name	Unit Per	Route	Code
FERRIC PYROPHOSPHATE CITRATE SOLUTION	0.1 MG	IV	J1443
FERRIC PYROPHOSPHATE CITRATE SOLUTION	0.1 MG	IV	J1445
FERRLECIT	12.5 MG	IV	J2916
FERTINEX	75 IU	SC	J3355
FERUMOXYTOL (FOR ESRD)	1 MG	IV	Q0139
FERUMOXYTOL (NON-ESRD)	1 MG	IV	Q0138
FETROJA	5 MG	IV	J0693
FETROJA	10 MG	IV	J0699
FIBRIN SEALANT (HUMAN)	2 ML	OTH	C9250
FIBRYGA	1 MG	IV	J7177
FILGRASTIM	1 MCG	SC, IV	J1442
FILGRASTIM-AAFI, BIOSIMILAR	1 MCG	INJ	Q5110
FILGRASTIM-SNDZ, BIOSIMILAR	1 MCG	IV, SC	Q5101
FINASTERIDE	5 MG	ORAL	S0138
FIRAZYR	1 MG	SC	J1744
FIRMAGON	1 MG	SC	J9155
FISH OIL TRIGLYCERIDES	10 G	IV	B4187
FLAGYL	500 MG	IV	S0030
FLEBOGAMMA	500 MG	IV	J1572
FLEXHD	SQ CM	OTH	Q4128
FLEXON	60 MG	IV, IM	J2360
FLOLAN	0.5 MG	IV	J1325
FLORBETABEN F18, DIAGNOSTIC	STUDY DOSE UP TO 8.1 MCI	IV	Q9983
FLOWERAMNIOFLO	SQ CM	OTH	Q4177
FLOWERAMNIOPATCH	SQ CM	OTH	Q4178
FLOWERDERM	SQ CM	OTH	Q4179
FLOXIN IV	400 MG	IV	S0034
FLOXURIDINE	500 MG	IV	J9200
FLUCICLOVINE F-18, DIAGNOSTIC	1 MCI	IV	A9588
FLUCONAZOLE	200 MG	IV	J1450
FLUDARA	50 MG	IV	J9185
FLUDARABINE PHOSPHATE	10 MG	ORAL	J8562
FLUDARABINE PHOSPHATE	50 MG	IV	J9185
FLUDEOXYGLUCOSE F18	STUDY DOSE UP TO 45 MCI	IV	A9552
FLUID FLOW, FLUID GF	1 CC	OTH	Q4206
FLULAVAL	EA	IM	Q2036
FLUMADINE (DEMONSTATION PROJECT)	100 MG	ORAL	G9036
FLUNISOLIDE, COMPOUNDED, UNIT DOSE	1 MG	INH	J7641
FLUOCINOLONE ACETONIDE INTRAVITREAL IMPLANT	IMPLANT	OTH	J7311
FLUOCINOLONE ACETONIDE, INTRAVITREAL IMPLANT	0.01 MG	OTH	J7313
FLUOCINOLONE ACETONIDE, INTRAVITREAL IMPLANT	0.01 MG	OTH	J7314
FLUORODEOXYGLUCOSE F-18 FDG, DIAGNOSTIC	STUDY DOSE UP TO 45 MCI	IV	A9552
FLUOROESTRADIOL F 18, DIAGNOSTIC	1 MCI	IV	A9591
FLUOROURACIL	500 MG	IV	J9190
FLUPHENAZINE DECANOATE	25 MG	SC, IM	J2680
FLUTAMIDE	125 MG	ORAL	S0175

Drug Name	Unit Per	Route	Code
FLUTEMETAMOL F18, DIAGNOSTIC	STUDY DOSE UP TO 5 MCI	IV	Q9982
FLUVIRIN	EA	IM	Q2037
FLUZONE	EA	IM	Q2038
FOLEX	5 MG	IV, IM, IT, IA	J9250
FOLEX	50 MG	IV, IM, IT, IA	J9260
FOLEX PFS	5 MG	IV, IM, IT, IA	J9250
FOLEX PFS	50 MG	IV, IM, IT, IA	J9260
FOLLISTIM	75 IU	SC, IM	S0128
FOLLITROPIN ALFA	75 IU	SC	S0126
FOLLITROPIN BETA	75 IU	SC, IM	S0128
FOLOTYN	1 MG	IV	J9307
FOMEPIZOLE	15 MG	IV	J1451
FOMIVIRSEN SODIUM	1.65 MG	OTH	J1452
FONDAPARINUX SODIUM	0.5 MG	SC	J1652
FORMOTEROL FUMERATE NONCOMPOUNDED UNIT DOSE FORM	20 MCG	INH	J7606
FORMOTEROL, COMPOUNDED, UNIT DOSE	12 MCG	INH	J7640
FORTAZ	500 MG	IM, IV	J0713
FORTEO	10 MCG	SC	J3110
FORTOVASE	200 MG	ORAL	S0140
FOSAPREPITANT	1 MG	IV	J1453
FOSCARNET SODIUM	1,000 MG	IV	J1455
FOSCAVIR	1,000 MG	IV	J1455
FOSNETUPITANT AND PALONOSETRON	235 MG/0.25 MG	IV	J1454
FOSPHENYTOIN	50 MG	IM, IV	Q2009
FOSPHENYTOIN SODIUM	750 MG	IM, IV	S0078
FRAGMIN	2,500 IU	SC	J1645
FREMANEZUMAB-VFRM	1 MG	SC	J3031
FUDR	500 MG	IV	J9200
FULPHILA	0.5 MG	SC	Q5108
FULVESTRANT	25 MG	IM	J9395
FUNGIZONE	50 MG	IV	J0285
FUROSEMIDE	20 MG	IM, IV	J1940
FUZEON	1 MG	SC	J1324
GABLOFEN	10 MG	IT	J0475
GABLOFEN	50 MCG	IT	J0476
GADAVIST	0.1 ML	IV	A9585
GADOBENATE DIMEGLUMINE (MULTIHANCE MULTIPACK)	1 ML	IV	A9577
GADOBUTROL	0.1 ML	IV	A9585
GADOFOSVESET TRISODIUM	1 ML	IV	A9583
GADOTERATE MEGLUMINE	0.1 ML	IV	A9575
GADOTERIDOL (PROHANCE MULTIPACK)	1 ML	IV	A9576
GADOXETATE DISODIUM	1 ML	IV	A9581
GALLIUM GA-67	1 MCI	IV	A9556
GALLIUM GA-68 PSMA-11, DIAGNOSTIC, (UCLA)	1 MCI	IV	A9594
GALLIUM GA-68 PSMA-11, DIAGNOSTIC, (UCSF)	1 MCI	IV	A9593
GALLIUM GA-68, DOTATATE, DIAGNOSTIC	0.1 MCI	IV	A9587

Drug Name	Unit Per	Route	Code
GALLIUM GA-68, DOTATOC, DIAGNOSTIC	0.01 MCI	IV	C9067
GALLIUM NITRATE	1 MG	IV	J1457
GALSULFASE	1 MG	IV	J1458
GAMASTAN	1 CC	IM	J1460
GAMASTAN	OVER 10 CC	IM	J1560
GAMASTAN SD	1 CC	IM	J1460
GAMASTAN SD	OVER 10 CC	IM	J1560
GAMIFANT	1 MG	IV	J9210
GAMMA GLOBULIN	1 CC	IM	J1460
GAMMA GLOBULIN	OVER 10 CC	IM	J1560
GAMMAGARD	500 MG	IV	J1569
GAMMAGRAFT	SQ CM	OTH	Q4111
GAMMAKED	500 MG	IV, SC	J1561
GAMMAPLEX	500 MG	IV	J1557
GAMUNEX	500 MG	IV, SQ	J1561
GAMUNEX-C	500 MG	IV, SC	J1561
GANCICLOVIR	4.5 MG	OTH	J7310
GANCICLOVIR SODIUM	500 MG	IV	J1570
GANIRELIX ACETATE	250 MCG	SC	S0132
GANITE	1 MG	IV	J1457
GARAMYCIN	80 MG	IM, IV	J1580
GASTROCROM	10 MG	INH	J7631
GASTROMARK	1 ML	ORAL	Q9954
GATIFLOXACIN	10 MG	IV	J1590
GAZYVA	10 MG	IV	J9301
GEFITINIB	250 MG	ORAL	J8565
GEL-ONE	PER DOSE	INJ	J7326
GELSYN-3	0.1 MG	INJ	J7328
GEMCITABINE HYDROCHLORIDE	100 MG	IV	J9198
GEMTUZUMAB OZOGAMICIN	0.1 MG	INF	J9203
GENESIS AMNIOTIC MEMBRANE	SQ CM	OTH	Q4198
GENGRAF	25 MG	ORAL	J7515
GENGRAF	100 MG	ORAL	J7502
GENOTROPIN	1 MG	SC	J2941
GENOTROPIN MINIQUICK	1 MG	SC	J2941
GENOTROPIN NUTROPIN	1 MG	SC	J2941
GENTAMICIN	80 MG	IM, IV	J1580
GENTRAN	500 ML	IV	J7100
GENTRAN 75	500 ML	IV	J7110
GENVISC 850	1 MG	INJ	J7320
GEODON	10 MG	IM	J3486
GEREF	1MCG	SC	Q0515
GIVLAARI	0.5 MG	SC	J0223
GIVOSIRAN	0.5 MG	SC	J0223
GLASSIA	10 MG	IV	J0257
GLATIRAMER ACETATE	20 MG	SC	J1595
GLEEVEC	100 MG	ORAL	S0088
GLOFIL-125	STUDY DOSE UP TO 10 UCI	IV	A9554
GLUCAGEN	1 MG	SC, IM, IV	J1610
GLUCAGON	1 MG	SC, IM, IV	J1610
GLUCOTOPE	STUDY DOSE UP TO 45 MCI	IV	A9552

Drug Name	Unit Per	Route	Code
GLYCOPYRROLATE, COMPOUNDED CONCENTRATED	PER MG	INH	J7642
GLYCOPYRROLATE, COMPOUNDED, UNIT DOSE	1 MG	INH	J7643
GOLD SODIUM THIOMALATE	50 MG	IM	J1600
GOLIMUMAB	1 MG	IV	J1602
GOLODIRSEN	10 MG	IV	J1429
GONADORELIN HCL	100 MCG	SC, IV	J1620
GONAL-F	75 IU	SC	S0126
GOPRELTO	1 MG	OTH	C9046
GOSERELIN ACETATE	3.6 MG	SC	J9202
GRAFIX CORE	SQ CM	OTH	Q4132
GRAFIX PRIME	SQ CM	OTH	Q4133
GRAFIXPL CORE	SQ CM	OTH	Q4132
GRAFIXPL PRIME	SQ CM	OTH	Q4133
GRAFTJACKET	SQ CM	OTH	Q4107
GRAFTJACKET EXPRESS	1 CC	INJ	Q4113
GRANISETRON HCL	1 MG	ORAL	Q0166
GRANISETRON HCL	100 MCG	IV	J1626
GRANISETRON HCL	1 MG	IV	S0091
GRANISETRON, EXTENDED-RELEASE	0.1 MG	SC	J1627
GRANIX	1 MCG	IV	J1447
GUARDIAN	SQ CM	OTH	Q4151
GUSELKUMAB	1 MG	SC	J1628
GYNOGEN L.A. 10	10 MG	IM	J1380
GYNOGEN L.A. 20	10 MG	IM	J1380
GYNOGEN L.A. 40	10 MG	IM	J1380
H.P. ACTHAR GEL	UP TO 40 UNITS	OTH	J0800
HAEGARDA	10 UNITS	SC	J0599
HALAVEN	0.1 MG	IV	J9179
HALDOL	5 MG	IM, IV	J1630
HALDOL DECANOATE	50 MG	IM	J1631
HALOPERIDOL	5 MG	IM, IV	J1630
HECTOROL	1 MG	IV	J1270
HELICOLL	SQ CM	OTH	Q4164
HEMIN	1 MG	IV	J1640
HEMLIBRA	0.5 MG	SC	J7170
HEMOFIL-M	1 IU	IV	J7190
HEMOSPRAY	UNKNOWN	OTH	C1052
HEMOSTATIC AGENT, GASTROINTESTINAL	UNKNOWN	OTH	C1052
HEP LOCK	10 U	IV	J1642
HEP-PAK	10 UNITS	IV	J1642
HEPAGAM B	0.5 ML	IM	J1571
HEPAGAM B	0.5 ML	IV	J1573
HEPARIN SODIUM	10 U	IV	J1642
HEPARIN SODIUM	1,000 U	IV, SC	J1644
HEPATITIS B IMMUNE GLOBULIN	0.5 ML	IV	J1573
HEPATOLITE	STUDY DOSE UP TO 15 MCI	IV	A9510
HERCEPTIN HYLECTA	10 MG	SC	J9356
HERCEPTIN, EXCLUDES BIOSIMILAR	10 MG	IV	J9355
HERZUMA	10 MG	IV	Q5113

Drug Name	Unit Per	Route	Code
HEXADROL	0.25 MG	ORAL	J8540
HEXAMINOLEVULINATE HYDROCHLORIDE	STUDY DOSE	OTH	A9589
HIGH OSMOLAR CONTRAST MATERIAL, UP TO 149 MG/ML IODINE CONCENTRATION	1 ML	IV	Q9958
HIGH OSMOLAR CONTRAST MATERIAL, UP TO 150-199 MG/ML IODINE CONCENTRATION	1 ML	IV	Q9959
HIGH OSMOLAR CONTRAST MATERIAL, UP TO 200-249 MG/ML IODINE CONCENTRATION	1 ML	IV	Q9960
HIGH OSMOLAR CONTRAST MATERIAL, UP TO 250-299 MG/ML IODINE CONCENTRATION	1 ML	IV	Q9961
HIGH OSMOLAR CONTRAST MATERIAL, UP TO 300-349 MG/ML IODINE CONCENTRATION	1 ML	IV	Q9962
HIGH OSMOLAR CONTRAST MATERIAL, UP TO 350-399 MG/ML IODINE CONCENTRATION	1 ML	IV	Q9963
HIGH OSMOLAR CONTRAST MATERIAL, UP TO 400 OR GREATER MG/ML IODINE CONCENTRATION	1 ML	IV	Q9964
HISTERLIN IMPLANT (VANTAS)	50 MG	OTH	J9225
HISTRELIN ACETATE	10 MG	INJ	J1675
HISTRELIN IMPLANT (SUPPRELIN LA)	50 MG	OTH	J9226
HIZENTRA	100 MG	SC	J1559
HMATRIX	SQ CM	OTH	Q4134
HUMALOG	5 U	SC	J1815
HUMALOG	50 U	SC	J1817
HUMAN FIBRINOGEN CONCENTRATE	1 MG	IV	J7177
HUMATE-P	1 IU	IV	J7187
HUMATROPE	1 MG	SC	J2941
HUMIRA	20 MG	SC	J0135
HUMULIN	5 U	SC	J1815
HUMULIN	50 U	SC	J1817
HUMULIN R	5 U	SC	J1815
HUMULIN R U-500	5 U	SC	J1815
HYALGAN	PER DOSE	INJ	J7321
HYALOMATRIX	SQ CM	OTH	Q4117
HYALURONAN	0.1 MG	INJ	J7328
HYALURONAN	1 MG	INJ	J7322
HYALURONAN	PER DOSE	INJ	J7324
HYALURONAN	PER DOSE	INJ	J7321
HYALURONAN	1 MG	INJ	J7325
HYALURONAN	PER DOSE	INJ	J7327
HYALURONAN	PER DOSE	INJ	J7326
HYALURONAN	1 MG	INJ	J7320
HYALURONAN	PER DOSE	INJ	J7323
~~HYALURONAN~~	~~PER DOSE~~	~~INJ~~	~~J7333~~
HYALURONAN	1 MG	INJ	J7332
HYALURONAN	1 MG	INJ	J7331
HYALURONAN	1 MG	INJ	J7329
HYALURONAN	1 MG	INJ	J7318
HYALURONIDASE	150 UNITS	VAR	J3470

Appendix 1 — Table of Drugs and Biologicals

Drug Name	Unit Per	Route	Code
HYALURONIDASE RECOMBINANT	1 USP UNIT	SC	J3473
HYALURONIDASE, OVINE, PRESERVATIVE FREE	1000 USP	OTH	J3472
HYALURONIDASE, OVINE, PRESERVATIVE FREE	1 USP	OTH	J3471
HYCAMTIN	0.1 MG	IV	J9351
HYCAMTIN	0.25 MG	ORAL	J8705
HYDRALAZINE HCL	20 MG	IV, IM	J0360
HYDRATE	50 MG	IM, IV	J1240
HYDREA	500 MG	ORAL	S0176
HYDROCORTISONE ACETATE	25 MG	IV, IM, SC	J1700
HYDROCORTISONE SODIUM PHOSPHATE	50 MG	IV, IM, SC	J1710
HYDROCORTISONE SODIUM SUCCINATE	100 MG	IV, IM, SC	J1720
HYDROCORTONE PHOSPHATE	50 MG	SC, IM, IV	J1710
HYDROMORPHONE HCL	250 MG	OTH	S0092
HYDROMORPHONE HCL	4 MG	SC, IM, IV	J1170
HYDROXOCOBALAMIN	1,000 MCG	IM, SC	J3420
HYDROXYCOBAL	1,000 MCG	IM, SC	J3420
HYDROXYPROGESTERONE CAPROATE (MAKENA)	10 MG	IM	J1726
HYDROXYUREA	500 MG	ORAL	S0176
HYDROXYZINE HCL	25 MG	IM	J3410
HYDROXYZINE PAMOATE	25 MG	ORAL	Q0177
HYMOVIS	1 MG	INJ	J7322
HYOSCYAMINE SULFATE	0.25 MG	SC, IM, IV	J1980
HYPERRHO S/D	300 MCG	IV	J2790
HYPERTET SD	UP TO 250 MG	IM	J1670
HYPERTONIC SALINE SOLUTION	1 ML	VAR	J7131
HYQVIA	100 MG	IV	J1575
HYREXIN	50 MG	IV, IM	J1200
HYZINE	25 MG	IM	J3410
HYZINE-50	25 MG	IM	J3410
IBALIZUMAB-UIYK	10 MG	IV	J1746
IBANDRONATE SODIUM	1 MG	IV	J1740
IBRITUMOMAB TUXETAN	STUDY DOSE UP TO 5 MCI	IV	A9542
IBUPROFEN	100 MG	IV	J1741
IBUTILIDE FUMARATE	1 MG	IV	J1742
ICATIBANT	1 MG	SC	J1744
IDAMYCIN	5 MG	IV	J9211
IDAMYCIN PFS	5 MG	IV	J9211
IDARUBICIN HCL	5 MG	IV	J9211
~~IDECABTAGENE VICLEUCEL~~	~~UP TO 460 MILLION CELLS~~	~~IV~~	~~C9081~~
IDECABTAGENE VICLEUCEL	UP TO 460 MILLION CELLS	IV	Q2055
IDELVION	1 IU	IV	J7202
IDURSULFASE	1 MG	IV	J1743
IFEX	1 G	IV	J9208
IFOSFAMIDE	1 G	IV	J9208
IL-2	1 VIAL	IV	J9015
ILARIS	1 MG	SC	J0638
ILETIN	5 UNITS	SC	J1815
ILETIN II NPH PORK	50 U	SC	J1817

Drug Name	Unit Per	Route	Code
ILETIN II REGULAR PORK	5 U	SC	J1815
ILOPROST INHALATION SOLUTION	PER DOSE UP TO 20 MCG	INH	Q4074
ILUMYA	1 MG	SC	J3245
ILUVIEN	0.01 MG	OTH	J7313
IMAGENT	1 ML	IV	Q9955
IMATINIB	100 MG	ORAL	S0088
IMFINZI	10 MG	IV	J9173
IMIGLUCERASE	10 U	IV	J1786
IMIPENEM, CILASTATIN, AND RELEBACTAM	4 MG/4 MG/2 MG	IV	J0742
IMITREX	6 MG	SC	J3030
IMLYGIC	1 MILLION	INTRALESIONAL	J9325
~~IMMUNE GLOBULIN (ASCENIV)~~	~~500 MG~~	~~IV~~	~~C9072~~
IMMUNE GLOBULIN (ASCENIV)	500 MG	IV	J1554
IMMUNE GLOBULIN (BIVIGAM)	500 MG	IV	J1556
IMMUNE GLOBULIN (CIVITRU)	100 MG	SC	J1555
IMMUNE GLOBULIN (FLEBOGAMMA, FLEBOGAMMA DIF)	500 MG	IV	J1572
IMMUNE GLOBULIN (GAMMAGARD LIQUID)	500 MG	IV	J1569
IMMUNE GLOBULIN (GAMMAPLEX)	500 MG	IV	J1557
IMMUNE GLOBULIN (GAMUNEX)	500 MG	IV	J1561
IMMUNE GLOBULIN (HIZENTRA)	100 MG	SC	J1559
IMMUNE GLOBULIN (OCTAGAM)	500 MG	IV	J1568
IMMUNE GLOBULIN (PRIVIGEN) NONLYOPHILIZED	500 MG	IV	J1459
IMMUNE GLOBULIN (RHOPHYLAC)	100 IU	IM, IV	J2791
IMMUNE GLOBULIN (XEMBIFY)	100 MG	SC	J1558
IMMUNE GLOBULIN SUBCUTANEOUS	100 MG	SC	J1562
IMMUNE GLOBULIN/HYALURONIDASE	100 MG	IV	J1575
IMPLANON	IMPLANT	OTH	J7307
IMURAN	50 MG	ORAL	J7500
IN-111 SATUMOMAB PENDETIDE	STUDY DOSE UP TO MCI	IV	A4642
INAPSINE	5 MG	IM, IV	J1790
INCOBUTULINUMTOXINA	1 UNIT	IM	J0588
INDERAL	1 MG	IV	J1800
INDIUM IN-111 IBRITUMOMAB TIUXETAN, DIAGNOSTIC	STUDY DOSE UP TO 5 MCI	IV	A9542
INDIUM IN-111 LABELED AUTOLOGOUS PLATELETS	STUDY DOSAGE	IV	A9571
INDIUM IN-111 LABELED AUTOLOGOUS WHITE BLOOD CELLS	STUDY DOSE	IV	A9570
INDIUM IN-111 OXYQUINOLINE	0.5 MCI	IV	A9547
INDIUM IN-111 PENTETREOTIDE	STUDY DOSE UP TO 6 MCI	IV	A9572
INDURSALFASE	1 MG	IV	J1743
INEBILIZUMAB-CDON	1 MG	IV	J1823
INFED	50 MG	IM, IV	J1750
INFERGEN	1 MCG	SC	J9212

Drug Name	Unit Per	Route	Code
INFLECTRA	10 MG	IV	Q5103
INFLIXIMAB	10 MG	IV	J1745
INFLIXIMAB-ABDA, BIOSIMILAR	10 MG	IV	Q5104
INFLIXIMAB-AXXQ, BIOSIMILAR	10 MG	IV	Q5121
INFLIXIMAB-DYYB, BIOSIMILAR	10 MG	IV	Q5103
INFLIXIMAB-QBTX, BIOSIMILAR	10 MG	IV	Q5109
INFLUENZA VACCINE, AGRIFLU	UNKNOWN	IM	Q2034
INFLUENZA VIRUS VACCINE (AFLURIA)	EA	IM	Q2035
INFLUENZA VIRUS VACCINE (FLULAVAL)	EA	IM	Q2036
INFLUENZA VIRUS VACCINE (FLUVIRIN)	EA	IM	Q2037
INFLUENZA VIRUS VACCINE (FLUZONE)	EA	IM	Q2038
INFUGEM	100 MG	IV	J9198
INFUMORPH	10 MG	IM, IV, SC	J2270
INJECTAFER	1 MG	IV	J1439
INNOHEP	1,000 IU	SC	J1655
INNOVAMATRIX AC	SQ CM	OTH	A2001
INOTUZUMAB OZOGAMICIN	0.1 MG	IV	J9229
INSULIN	5 U	SC	J1815
INSULIN	50 U	SC	J1817
INSULIN LISPRO	5 U	SC	S5551
INSULIN LISPRO	5 U	SC	J1815
INSULIN PURIFIED REGULAR PORK	5 U	SC	J1815
INTAL	10 MG	INH	J7631
INTEGRA BILAYER MATRIX DRESSING	SQ CM	OTH	Q4104
INTEGRA DERMAL REGENERATION TEMPLATE	SQ CM	OTH	Q4105
INTEGRA FLOWABLE WOUND MATRIX	1 CC	INJ	Q4114
INTEGRA MATRIX	SQ CM	OTH	Q4108
INTEGRA MESHED BILAYER WOUND MATRIX	SQ CM	OTH	C9363
INTEGRA MOZAIK OSTEOCONDUCTIVE SCAFFOLD PUTTY	0.5 CC	OTH	C9359
INTEGRA MOZAIK OSTEOCONDUCTIVE SCAFFOLD STRIP	0.5 CC	OTH	C9362
INTEGRA OMNIGRAFT DERMAL REGENERATION MATRIX	SQ CM	OTH	Q4105
INTEGRA OS OSTEOCONDUCTIVE SCAFFOLD PUTTY	0.5 CC	OTH	C9359
INTEGRILIN	5 MG	IM, IV	J1327
INTERFERON ALFA-2A	3,000,000 U	SC, IM	J9213
INTERFERON ALFA-2B	1,000,000 U	SC, IM	J9214
INTERFERON ALFA-N3	250,000 IU	IM	J9215
INTERFERON ALFACON-1	1 MCG	SC	J9212
INTERFERON BETA-1A	1 MCG	IM	Q3027
INTERFERON BETA-1A	30 MCG	IM, SC	J1826
INTERFERON BETA-1A	1 MCG	SC	Q3028
INTERFERON BETA-1B	0.25 MG	SC	J1830
INTERFERON, ALFA-2A, RECOMBINANT	3,000,000 U	SC, IM	J9213

Drug Name	Unit Per	Route	Code
INTERFERON, ALFA-2B, RECOMBINANT	1,000,000 U	SC, IM	J9214
INTERFERON, ALFA-N3, (HUMAN LEUKOCYTE DERIVED)	250,000 IU	IM	J9215
INTERFERON, GAMMA 1-B	3,000,000 U	SC	J9216
INTERFYL	1 MG	OTH	Q4171
INTERLUEKIN	1 VIAL	IV	J9015
INTRON A	1,000,000 U	SC, IM	J9214
INVANZ	500 MG	IM, IV	J1335
INVEGA SUSTENNA	1 MG	IM	J2426
INVIRASE	200 MG	ORAL	S0140
IOBENGUANE SULFATE I-131	0.5 MCI	IV	A9508
IOBENGUANE, I-123, DIAGNOSTIC	PER STUDY DOSE UP TO 15 MCI	IV	A9582
IODINE I-123 IOBENGUANE, DIAGNOSTIC	15 MCI	IV	A9582
IODINE I-123 IOFLUPANE	STUDY DOSE UP TO 5 MCI	IV	A9584
IODINE I-123 SODIUM IODIDE CAPSULE(S), DIAGNOSTIC	100-9999 UCI	ORAL	A9516
IODINE I-123 SODIUM IODIDE, DIAGNOSTIC	1 MCI	IV	A9509
IODINE I-125 SERUM ALBUMIN, DIAGNOSTIC	5 UCI	IV	A9532
IODINE I-125 SODIUM IOTHALAMATE, DIAGNOSTIC	STUDY DOSE UP TO 10 UCI	IV	A9554
IODINE I-125, SODIUM IODIDE SOLUTION, THERAPEUTIC	1 MCI	ORAL	A9527
IODINE I-131 IOBENGUANE SULFATE, DIAGNOSTIC	0.5 MCI	IV	A9508
IODINE I-131 IODINATED SERUM ALBUMIN, DIAGNOSTIC	PER 5 UCI	IV	A9524
IODINE I-131 SODIUM IODIDE CAPSULE(S), DIAGNOSTIC	1 MCI	ORAL	A9528
IODINE I-131 SODIUM IODIDE CAPSULE(S), THERAPEUTIC	1 MCI	ORAL	A9517
IODINE I-131 SODIUM IODIDE SOLUTION, DIAGNOSTIC	1 MCI	ORAL	A9529
IODINE I-131 SODIUM IODIDE SOLUTION, THERAPEUTIC	1 MCI	ORAL	A9530
IODINE I-131 SODIUM IODIDE, DIAGNOSTIC	PER UCI UP TO 100 UCI	IV	A9531
IODINE I-131, IOBENGUANE	1 MCI	IV	A9590
IODOTOPE THERAPEUTIC CAPSULE(S)	1 MCI	ORAL	A9517
IODOTOPE THERAPEUTIC SOLUTION	1 MCI	ORAL	A9530
IOFLUPANE	STUDY DOSE UP TO 5 MCI	IV	A9584
ION-BASED MAGNETIC RESONANCE CONTRAST AGENT	1 ML	IV	Q9953
IOTHALAMATE SODIUM I-125	STUDY DOSE UP TO 10 UCI	IV	A9554
IPILIMUMAB	1 MG	IV	J9228
IPLEX	1 MG	SC	J2170
IPRATROPIUM BROMIDE, NONCOMPOUNDED, UNIT DOSE	1 MG	INH	J7644
IPTRATROPIUM BROMIDE COMPOUNDED, UNIT DOSE	1 MG	INH	J7645

Drug Name	Unit Per	Route	Code
IRESSA	250 MG	ORAL	J8565
IRINOTECAN	20 MG	IV	J9206
IRINOTECAN LIPOSOME	1 MG	IV	J9205
IRON DEXTRAN, 50 MG	50 MG	IM, IV	J1750
IRON SUCROSE	1 MG	IV	J1756
ISATUXIMAB-IRFC	10 MG	IV	J9227
ISAVUCONAZONIUM	1 MG	IV	J1833
ISOCAINE	10 ML	VAR	J0670
ISOETHARINE HCL COMPOUNDED, CONCENTRATED	1 MG	INH	J7647
ISOETHARINE HCL COMPOUNDED, UNIT DOSE	1 MG	INH	J7650
ISOETHARINE HCL, NONCOMPOUNDED CONCENTRATED	PER MG	INH	J7648
ISOETHARINE HCL, NONCOMPOUNDED, UNIT DOSE	1 MG	INH	J7649
ISOJEX	5 UCI	IV	A9532
ISOPROTERENOL HCL COMPOUNDED, CONCENTRATED	1 MG	INH	J7657
ISOPROTERENOL HCL COMPOUNDED, UNIT DOSE	1 MG	INH	J7660
ISOPROTERENOL HCL, NONCOMPOUNDED CONCENTRATED	1 MG	INH	J7658
ISOPROTERNOL HCL, NONCOMPOUNDED, UNIT DOSE	1MG	INH	J7659
ISOSULFAN BLUE	1 MG	SC	Q9968
~~ISTODAX~~	~~1 MG~~	~~IV~~	~~J9315~~
ISTODAX	0.1 MG	IV	J9319
ISUPREL	1 MG	INH	J7658
ISUPREL	1 MG	INH	J7659
ITRACONAZOLE	50 MG	IV	J1835
IXABEPILONE	1 MG	IV	J9207
IXEMPRA	1 MG	IV	J9207
IXIFI	10 MG	IV	Q5109
JELMYTO	1 MG	OTH	J9281
~~JEMPERLI~~	~~100 MG~~	~~IV~~	~~C9082~~
JEMPERLI	10 MG	IV	J9272
JETREA	0.125 MG	OTH	J7316
JEVTANA	1 MG	IV	J9043
JIVI	1 IU	IV	J7208
KADCYLA	1 MG	IV	J9354
KALBITOR	1 MG	SC	J1290
KANAMYCIN	500 MG	IM, IV	J1840
KANAMYCIN	75 MG	IM, IV	J1850
KANJINTI	10 MG	IV	Q5117
KANTREX	75 MG	IM, IV	J1850
KANTREX	500 MG	IM, IV	J1840
KANUMA	1 MG	IV	J2840
~~KCENTRA~~	~~PER I.U.~~	~~IV~~	~~C9132~~
KCENTRA	PER IU	IV	J7168
KEFZOL	500 MG	IM, IV	J0690
KEPIVANCE	50 MCG	IV	J2425
KEPPRA	10 MG	IV	J1953
KERAMATRIX OR KERASORB	SQ CM	OTH	Q4165
KERECIS OMEGA3	SQ CM	OTH	Q4158

Drug Name	Unit Per	Route	Code
KEROXX	1 CC	OTH	Q4202
KESTRONE	1 MG	IV, IM	J1435
KETOROLAC TROMETHAMINE	15 MG	IM, IV	J1885
KEYTRUDA	1 MG	IV	J9271
KHAPZORY	0.5 MG	IV	J0642
KIMYRSA	10 MG	IV	J2406
KINEVAC	5 MCG	IV	J2805
KOATE-DVI	1 IU	IV	J7190
KONAKION	1 MG	SC, IM, IV	J3430
KONYNE 80	1 IU	IV	J7194
KOVALTRY	1 I.U.	IV	J7211
KRYSTEXXA	1 MG	IV	J2507
KYBELLA	1 MG	SC	J0591
KYLEENA	19.5 MG	OTH	J7296
KYMRIAH	UP TO 600 MILLION CELLS	IV	Q2042
KYPROLIS	1 MG	IV	J9047
KYTRIL	1 MG	IV	S0091
KYTRIL	1 MG	ORAL	Q0166
KYTRIL	100 MCG	IV	J1626
L.A.E. 20	10 MG	IM	J1380
LACOSAMIDE	1 MG	IV	C9254
LAETRILE	VAR	INJ	J3570
LANADELUMAB-FLYO	1 MG	SC	J0593
LANOXIN	0.5 MG	IM, IV	J1160
LANREOTIDE	1 MG	SC	J1930
LANTUS	5 U	SC	J1815
LARONIDASE	0.1 MG	IV	J1931
LARTRUVO	10 MG	INF	J9285
LASIX	20 MG	IM, IV	J1940
LEFAMULIN	1 MG	IV	J0691
LEMTRADA	1 MG	IV	J0202
LENTE ILETIN I	5 U	SC	J1815
LEPIRUDIN	50 MG	IV	J1945
LEUCOVORIN CALCIUM	50 MG	IM, IV	J0640
LEUKERAN	2 MG	ORAL	S0172
LEUKINE	50 MCG	IV	J2820
LEUPROLIDE	1 MG	SC	J1952
LEUPROLIDE ACETATE	7.5 MG	SC	J9217
LEUPROLIDE ACETATE	1 MG	IM	J9218
LEUPROLIDE ACETATE (FOR DEPOT SUSPENSION)	3.75 MG	IM	J1950
LEUPROLIDE ACETATE DEPOT	7.5 MG	SC	J9217
LEUPROLIDE ACETATE FOR DEPOT SUSPENSION	0.25 MG	SC	J1951
LEUPROLIDE ACETATE IMPLANT	65 MG	OTH	J9219
LEUSTATIN	1 MG	IV	J9065
LEVABUTEROL COMPOUNDED, UNIT DOSE	1 MG	INH	J7615
LEVABUTEROL, COMPOUNDED, CONCENTRATED	0.5 MG	INH	J7607
LEVALBUTEROL NONCOMPOUNDED, CONCENTRATED FORM	0.5 MG	INH	J7612
LEVALBUTEROL, NONCOMPOUNDED, UNIT DOSE	0.5 MG	INH	J7614

Drug Name	Unit Per	Route	Code
LEVAMISOLE HCL	50 MG	ORAL	S0177
LEVAQUIN	250 MG	IV	J1956
LEVEMIR	5 U	SC	J1815
LEVETIRACETAM	10 MG	IV	J1953
LEVO-DROMORAN	UP TO 2 MG	IV, IM	J1960
LEVOCARNITINE	1 G	IV	J1955
LEVOFLOXACIN	250 MG	IV	J1956
LEVOLEUCOVORIN	0.5 MG	IV	J0642
LEVONORGESTREL IMPLANT	IMPLANT	OTH	J7306
LEVONORGESTREL-RELEASING INTRAUTERINE CONTRACEPTIVE (MIRENA)	52 MG	OTH	J7298
LEVONORGESTREL-RELEASING INTRAUTERINE CONTRACEPTIVE (LILETTA)	52 MG	OTH	J7297
LEVONORGESTREL-RELEASING INTRAUTERINE CONTRACEPTIVE SYSTEM (KYLEENA)	19.5 MG	OTH	J7296
LEVONORGESTREL-RELEASING INTRAUTERINE CONTRACEPTIVE SYSTEM (SKYLA)	13.5 MG	OTH	J7301
LEVORPHANOL TARTRATE	2 MG	SC, IV, IM	J1960
LEVSIN	0.25 MG	SC, IM, IV	J1980
LEVULAN KERASTICK	354 MG	OTH	J7308
LEXISCAN	0.1 MG	IV	J2785
LIBRIUM	100 MG	IM, IV	J1990
LIBTAYO	1 MG	IV	J9119
LIDOCAINE 70 MG/TETRACAINE 70 MG	PATCH	OTH	C9285
LIDOCAINE HCL	10 MG	IV	J2001
LILETTA	52 MG	OTH	J7297
LINCOCIN HCL	300 MG	IV	J2010
LINCOMYCIN HCL	300 MG	IM, IV	J2010
LINEZOLID	200 MG	IV	J2020
LIORESAL	10 MG	IT	J0475
LIORESAL INTRATHECAL REFILL	50 MCG	IT	J0476
LIPODOX	10 MG	IV	Q2049
LIPOSOMAL, DAUNORUBICIN AND CYTARABINE	1 MG/2.27 MG	IV	J9153
LIQUAEMIN SODIUM	1,000 UNITS	SC, IV	J1644
LISOCABTAGENE MARALEUCEL	UP TO 110 MILLION CELLS	IV	C9076
LISOCABTAGENE MARALEUCEL	UP TO 110 MILLION CELLS	IV	Q2054
LISPRO-PFC	50 U	SC	J1817
LOK-PAK	10 UNITS	IV	J1642
LOMUSTINE	10 MG	ORAL	S0178
LONCASTUXIMAB TESIRINE-LPYL	0.1 MG	IV	C9084
LORAZEPAM	2 MG	IM, IV	J2060
LOVENOX	10 MG	SC	J1650
LOW OSMOLAR CONTRAST MATERIAL, 100-199 MG/ML IODINE CONCENTRATIONS	1 ML	IV	Q9965
LOW OSMOLAR CONTRAST MATERIAL, 200-299 MG/ML IODINE CONCENTRATION	1 ML	IV	Q9966
LOW OSMOLAR CONTRAST MATERIAL, 300-399 MG/ML IODINE CONCENTRATION	1 ML	IV	Q9967

Drug Name	Unit Per	Route	Code
LOW OSMOLAR CONTRAST MATERIAL, 400 OR GREATER MG/ML IODINE CONCENTRATION	1 ML	IV	Q9951
LOXAPINE	1 MG	INH	J2062
LUCENTIS	0.1 MG	IV	J2778
LUMASIRAN	0.5 MG	SC	C9074
LUMASIRAN	0.5 MG	SC	J0224
LUMASON	1 ML	IV	Q9950
LUMIZYME	10 MG	IV	J0221
LUMOXITI	0.01 MG	IV	J9313
LUPRON	1 MG	SC	J9218
LUPRON DEPOT	PER 3.75 MG	IM	J1950
LUPRON DEPOT	7.5 MG	SC	J9217
LUPRON IMPLANT	65 MG	OTH	J9219
LURBINECTEDIN	0.1 MG	IV	J9223
LUSPATERCEPT-AAMT	0.25 MG	SC	J0896
LUTATHERA	1 MCI	IM	A9513
LUTETIUM LU 177, DOTATATE, THERAPEUTIC	1 MCI	IM	A9513
LUTREPULSE	100 MCG	SC, IV	J1620
LUXTURNA	1 BILLION VECTOR GENOMES	OTH	J3398
LYMPHAZURIN	1 MG	SC	Q9968
LYMPHOCYTE IMMUNE GLOBULIN, ANTITHYMOCYTE GLOBULIN, EQUINE	250 MG	OTH	J7504
LYMPHOCYTE IMMUNE GLOBULIN, ANTITHYMOCYTE GLOBULIN, RABBIT	25 MG	OTH	J7511
LYMPHOSEEK	0.5 MCI	SC, OTH	A9520
MACUGEN	0.3 MG	OTH	J2503
MAGNESIUM SULFATE	500 MG	IV	J3475
MAGNETIC RESONANCE CONTRAST AGENT	1 ML	ORAL	Q9954
MAGROTEC	STUDY DOSE UP TO 10 MCI	IV	A9540
MAKENA	10 MG	IM	J1726
MANNITOL	25% IN 50 ML	IV	J2150
MANNITOL	5 MG	INH	J7665
MARCAINE HCL	30 ML	VAR	S0020
MARGENZA	5 MG	IV	J9353
MARGETUXIMAB-CMKB	5 MG	IV	J9353
MARINOL	2.5 MG	ORAL	Q0167
MARMINE	50 MG	IM, IV	J1240
MARQIBO KIT	5 MG	IV	J9371
MATRION	SQ CM	OTH	Q4201
MATRISTEM MICROMATRIX	1 MG	OTH	Q4118
MATULANE	50 MG	ORAL	S0182
MAXIPIME	500 MG	IV	J0692
MDP-BRACCO	STUDY DOSE UP TO 30 MCI	IV	A9503
MECASERMIN	1 MG	SC	J2170
MECHLORETHAMINE HCL (NITROGEN MUSTARD)	10 MG	IV	J9230
MEDIDEX	1 MG	IM, IV, OTH	J1100
MEDISKIN	SQ CM	OTH	Q4135

Drug Name	Unit Per	Route	Code
MEDROL	4 MG	ORAL	J7509
MEDROXYPROGESTERONE ACETATE	1 MG	IM	J1050
MEFOXIN	1 G	IV	J0694
MEGACE	20 MG	ORAL	S0179
MEGESTROL ACETATE	20 MG	ORAL	S0179
MELOXICAM	1 MG	IV	J1738
MELPHALAN	1 MG	IV	J9246
MELPHALAN FLUFENAMIDE	1 MG	IV	J9247
~~MELPHALAN FLUFENAMIDE HCL~~	~~1 MG~~	~~IV~~	~~C9080~~
MELPHALAN HCL	2 MG	ORAL	J8600
MEMBRANE GRAFT OR MEMBRANE WRAP	SQ CM	OTH	Q4205
MEMODERM	SQ CM	OTH	Q4126
MENADIONE	1 MG	IM, SC, IV	J3430
MENOTROPINS	75 IU	SC, IM, IV	S0122
MEPERGAN	50 MG	IM, IV	J2180
MEPERIDINE AND PROMETHAZINE HCL	50 MG	IM, IV	J2180
MEPERIDINE HCL	100 MG	IM, IV, SC	J2175
MEPIVACAINE HCL	10 ML	VAR	J0670
MEPOLIZUMAB	1 MG	SQ	J2182
MEPSEVII	1 MG	IV	J3397
MERCAPTOPURINE	50 MG	ORAL	S0108
MERITATE	150 MG	IV	J3520
MEROPENEM	100 MG	IV	J2185
MEROPENEM, VABORBACTAM	10 MG/10 MG	IV	J2186
MERREM	100 MG	IV	J2185
MESNA	200 MG	IV	J9209
MESNEX	200 MG	IV	J9209
METAPROTERENOL SULFATE COMPOUNDED, UNIT DOSE	10 MG	INH	J7670
METAPROTERENOL SULFATE, NONCOMPOUNDED, CONCENTRATED	10 MG	INH	J7668
METAPROTERENOL SULFATE, NONCOMPOUNDED, UNIT DOSE	10 MG	INH	J7669
METARAMINOL BITARTRATE	10 MG	IV, IM, SC	J0380
METASTRON STRONTIUM 89 CHLORIDE	1 MCI	IV	A9600
METATRACE	STUDY DOSE UP TO 45 MCI	IV	A9552
METHACHOLINE CHLORIDE	1 MG	INH	J7674
METHADONE	5 MG	ORAL	S0109
METHADONE HCL	10 MG	IM, SC	J1230
METHAPREL, COMPOUNDED, UNIT DOSE	10 MG	INH	J7670
METHAPREL, NONCOMPOUNDED, CONCENTRATED	10 MG	INH	J7668
METHAPREL, NONCOMPOUNDED, UNIT DOSE	10 MG	INH	J7669
METHERGINE	0.2 MG	IM, IV	J2210
METHOTREXATE	2.5 MG	ORAL	J8610
METHOTREXATE	5 MG	IV, IM, IT, IA	J9250
METHOTREXATE	50 MG	IV, IM, IT, IA	J9260
METHOTREXATE LPF	5 MG	IV, IM, IT, IA	J9250
METHOTREXATE LPF	50 MG	IV, IM, IT, IA	J9260

Drug Name	Unit Per	Route	Code
METHYL AMINOLEVULINATE 16.8%	1 G	OTH	J7309
METHYLCOTOLONE	80 MG	IM	J1040
METHYLDOPA HCL	UP TO 250 MG	IV	J0210
METHYLDOPATE HCL	UP TO 250 MG	IV	J0210
METHYLENE BLUE	1 MG	SC	Q9968
METHYLERGONOVINE MALEATE	0.2 MG	IM, IV	J2210
METHYLNALTREXONE	0.1 MG	SC	J2212
METHYLPRED	4 MG	ORAL	J7509
METHYLPREDNISOLONE	4 MG	ORAL	J7509
METHYLPREDNISOLONE	125 MG	IM, IV	J2930
METHYLPREDNISOLONE	UP TO 40 MG	IM, IV	J2920
METHYLPREDNISOLONE ACETATE	20 MG	IM	J1020
METHYLPREDNISOLONE ACETATE	80 MG	IM	J1040
METHYLPREDNISOLONE ACETATE	40 MG	IM	J1030
METOCLOPRAMIDE	10 MG	IV	J2765
METRONIDAZOLE	500 MG	IV	S0030
METVIXIA 16.8%	1 G	OTH	J7309
MIACALCIN	400 U	SC, IM	J0630
MIBG	0.5 MCI	IV	A9508
MICAFUNGIN SODIUM	1 MG	IV	J2248
MICRHOGAM	50 MCG	IV	J2788
MICROLYTE MATRIX	SQ CM	OTH	A2005
MICROPOROUS COLLAGEN IMPLANTABLE SLIT TUBE	1 CM LENGTH	OTH	C9353
MICROPOROUS COLLAGEN IMPLANTABLE TUBE	1 CM LENGTH	OTH	C9352
MIDAZOLAM HCI	1 MG	IM, IV	J2250
MIFEPRISTONE	200 MG	ORAL	S0190
MILRINONE LACTATE	5 MG	IV	J2260
MINOCIN	1 MG	IV	J2265
MINOCYCLINE HCL	1 MG	IV	J2265
MINOXIDIL	10 MG	ORAL	S0139
MIRCERA	1 MCG	IV	J0887
MIRCERA	1 MCG	SC	J0888
MIRENA	52 MG	OTH	J7298
MIRODERM	SQ CM	OTH	Q4175
MIRRAGEN ADVANCED WOUND MATRIX	SQ CM	OTH	A2002
MISOPROSTOL	200 MG	ORAL	S0191
MITHRACIN	2.5 MG	IV	J9270
MITOMYCIN	5 MG	IV	J9280
MITOMYCIN	0.2 MG	OTH	J7315
MITOMYCIN PYELOCALYCEAL INSTILLATION	1 MG	OTH	J9281
MITOSOL	0.2 MG	OTH	J7315
MITOXANA	1 G	IV	J9208
MITOXANTRONE HCL	5 MG	IV	J9293
MOGAMULIZUMAB-KPKC	1 MG	IV	J9204
~~MOMETASONE FUROATE SINUS IMPLANT~~	~~10 MCG~~	~~OTH~~	~~C9122~~
MOMETASONE FUROATE SINUS IMPLANT	10 MCG	OTH	J7402
~~MOMETASONE FUROATE SINUS IMPLANT~~	~~10 MCG~~	~~OTH~~	~~J7401~~
MONARC-M	1 IU	IV	J7190

Drug Name	Unit Per	Route	Code
~~MONJUVI~~	~~2 MG~~	~~IV~~	~~C9070~~
MONJUVI	2 MG	IV	J9349
MONOCLATE-P	1 IU	IV	J7190
MONOFERRIC	10 MG	IV	J1437
MONONINE	1 IU	IV	J7193
MONOPUR	75 IU	SC, IM	S0122
MONOVISC	PER DOSE	INJ	J7327
MORPHINE SULFATE	10 MG	IM, IV, SC	J2270
MORPHINE SULFATE	500 MG	OTH	S0093
MORPHINE SULFATE, PRESERVATIVE-FREE FOR EPIDURAL OR INTRATHECAL USE	10 MG	OTH	J2274
MOXETUMOMAB PASUDOTOX-TDFK	0.01 MG	IV	J9313
MOXIFLOXACIN	100 MG	IV	J2280
MOZOBIL	1 MG	SC	J2562
MPI INDIUM DTPA	0.5 MCI	IV	A9548
MS CONTIN	500 MG	OTH	S0093
MUCOMYST	1 G	INH	J7608
MUCOSIL	1 G	INH	J7608
MULTIHANCE	1 ML	IV	A9577
MULTIHANCE MULTIPACK	1 ML	IV	A9578
MUROMONAB-CD3	5 MG	OTH	J7505
MUSE	EA	OTH	J0275
MUSTARGEN	10 MG	IV	J9230
MUTAMYCIN	5 MG	IV	J9280
MVASI	10 MG	IV	Q5107
MYCAMINE	1 MG	IV	J2248
MYCOPHENOLATE MOFETIL	250 MG	ORAL	J7517
MYCOPHENOLIC ACID	180 MG	ORAL	J7518
MYFORTIC DELAYED RELEASE	180 MG	ORAL	J7518
MYLERAN	2 MG	ORAL	J8510
MYLOCEL	500 MG	ORAL	S0176
MYLOTARG	0.1 MG	INF	J9203
MYOBLOC	100 U	IM	J0587
MYOCHRYSINE	50 MG	IM	J1600
MYOWN SKIN	SQ CM	OTH	Q4226
MYOZYME	10 MG	IV	J0220
NABILONE	1 MG	ORAL	J8650
NAFCILLIN SODIUM	2 GM	IM, IV	S0032
NAGLAZYME	1 MG	IV	J1458
NALBUPHINE HCL	10 MG	IM, IV, SC	J2300
NALLPEN	2 GM	IM, IV	S0032
NALOXONE HCL	1 MG	IM, IV, SC	J2310
NALTREXONE, DEPOT FORM	1 MG	IM	J2315
NANDROLONE DECANOATE	50 MG	IM	J2320
NARCAN	1 MG	IM, IV, SC	J2310
NAROPIN	1 MG	VAR	J2795
NASALCROM	10 MG	INH	J7631
NATALIZUMAB	1 MG	IV	J2323
NATRECOR	0.1 MG	IV	J2325
NATURAL ESTROGENIC SUBSTANCE	1 MG	IM, IV	J1410
NAVELBINE	10 MG	IV	J9390
NAXITAMAB-GQGK	1 MG	IV	J9348

Drug Name	Unit Per	Route	Code
ND-STAT	10 MG	IM, SC, IV	J0945
NEBCIN	80 MG	IM, IV	J3260
NEBUPENT	300 MG	IM, IV	S0080
NEBUPENT	300 MG	INH	J2545
NECITUMUMAB	1 MG	IV	J9295
NELARABINE	50 MG	IV	J9261
NEMBUTAL SODIUM	50 MG	IM, IV, OTH	J2515
NEOPATCH	SQ CM	OTH	Q4176
NEORAL	25 MG	ORAL	J7515
NEORAL	250 MG	ORAL	J7516
NEOSAR	100 MG	IV	J9070
NEOSCAN	1 MCI	IV	A9556
NEOSTIGMINE METHYLSULFATE	0.5 MG	IM, IV	J2710
NEOTECT	STUDY DOSE UP TO 35 MCI	IV	A9536
NEOX 100	SQ CM	OTH	Q4156
NEOX CORD 1K	SQ CM	OTH	Q4148
NEOX CORD RT	SQ EM	OTH	Q4148
NEOXFLO	1 MG	OTH	Q4155
NESACAINE	30 ML	VAR	J2400
NESACAINE-MPF	30 ML	VAR	J2400
NESIRITIDE	0.1 MG	IV	J2325
NETSPOT	0.1 MCI	IV	A9587
NETUPITANT AND PALONOSETRON	300 MG/0.5 MG	ORAL	J8655
~~NEULASTA~~	~~6 MG~~	~~SC, SQ~~	~~J2505~~
NEULASTA	0.5 MG	SC	J2506
NEUMEGA	5 MG	SC	J2355
NEUPOGEN	1 MCG	SC, IV	J1442
NEURAGEN NERVE GUIDE	1 CM LENGTH	OTH	C9352
NEUROLITE	STUDY DOSE UP TO 25 MCI	IV	A9557
NEUROMATRIX	0.5 CM LENGTH	OTH	C9355
NEUROMEND NERVE WRAP	0.5 CM	OTH	C9361
NEUROWRAP NERVE PROTECTOR	1 CM LENGTH	OTH	C9353
NEUTREXIN	25 MG	IV	J3305
NEUTROSPEC	STUDY DOSE UP TO 25 MCI	IV	A9566
NEXPLANON	IMPLANT	OTH	J7307
NEXVIAZYME	4 MG	IV	C9085
NIPENT	10 MG	IV	J9268
NITROGEN MUSTARD	10 MG	IV	J9230
NITROGEN N-13 AMMONIA, DIAGNOSTIC	STUDY DOSE UP TO 40 MCI	INJ	A9526
NIVESTYM	1 MCG	INJ	Q5110
NIVOLUMAB	1 MG	IV	J9299
NOLVADEX	10 MG	ORAL	S0187
NORDITROPIN	1 MG	SC	J2941
NORDYL	50 MG	IV, IM	J1200
NORFLEX	60 MG	IV, IM	J2360
NORMAL SALINE SOLUTION	1000 CC	IV	J7030
NORMAL SALINE SOLUTION	250 CC	IV	J7050
NORMAL SALINE SOLUTION	500 ML	IV	J7040
NOVACHOR	SQ CM	OTH	Q4194
NOVAFIX	SQ CM	OTH	Q4208

Appendix 1 — Table of Drugs and Biologicals

Drug Name	Unit Per	Route	Code
NOVAFIX DL	SQ CM	OTH	Q4254
NOVANTRONE	5 MG	IV	J9293
NOVAREL	1,000 USP U	IM	J0725
NOVOEIGHT	IU	IV	J7182
NOVOLIN	50 U	SC	J1817
NOVOLIN R	5 U	SC	J1815
NOVOLOG	50 U	SC	J1817
NOVOSEVEN	1 MCG	IV	J7189
NOVOSORB SYNPATH DERMAL MATRIX	SQ CM	OTH	A2006
NPH	5 UNITS	SC	J1815
NPLATE	10 MCG	SC	J2796
NUBAIN	10 MG	IM, IV, SC	J2300
NUCALA	1 MG	SQ	J2182
NUDYN	0.5 CC	OTH	Q4233
NULOJIX	1 MG	IV	J0485
NUMORPHAN	1 MG	IV, SC, IM	J2410
NUSHIELD	SQ CM	OTH	Q4160
NUSINERSEN	0.1 MG	INJ	J2326
NUTRI-TWELVE	1,000 MCG	IM, SC	J3420
NUTROPIN	1 MG	SC	J2941
NUTROPIN A.Q.	1 MG	SC	J2941
NUVARING VAGINAL RING	EACH	OTH	J7303
NUVARING VAGINAL RING	0.015 MG/0.12 MG	OTH	J7295
NUWIQ	1 IU	IV	J7209
NUZYRA	1 MG	IV	J0121
NYVEPRIA	0.5 MG	SC	Q5122
OASIS BURN MATRIX	SQ CM	OTH	Q4103
OASIS ULTRA TRI-LAYER WOUND MATRIX	SQ CM	OTH	Q4124
OASIS WOUND MATRIX	SQ CM	OTH	Q4102
OBINUTUZUMAB	10 MG	IV	J9301
OBIZUR	IU	IV	J7188
OCRELIZUMAB	1 MG	INJ	J2350
OCREVUS	1 MG	INJ	J2350
OCRIPLASMIN	0.125 MG	OTH	J7316
OCTAFLUOROPROPANE UCISPHERES	1 ML	IV	Q9956
OCTAGAM	500 MG	IV	J1568
OCTREOSCAN	STUDY DOSE UP TO 6 MCI	IV	A9572
OCTREOTIDE ACETATE DEPOT	1 MG	IM	J2353
OCTREOTIDE, NON-DEPOT FORM	25 MCG	SC, IV	J2354
OFATUMUMAB	10 MG	IV	J9302
OFIRMEV	10 MG	IV	J0131
OFLOXACIN	400 MG	IV	S0034
OFORTA	10 MG	ORAL	J8562
OGIVRI	10 MG	IV	Q5114
OLANZAPINE	2.5 MG	IM	S0166
OLANZAPINE LONG ACTING	1 MG	IM	J2358
OLARATUMAB	10 MG	INF	J9285
OMACETAXINE MEPESUCCINATE	0.01 MG	SC	J9262
OMADACYCLINE	1 MG	IV	J0121
OMALIZUMAB	5 MG	SC	J2357

Drug Name	Unit Per	Route	Code
OMEGAVEN	10 G	IV	B4187
OMIDRIA	1 ML	OTH	J1097
OMNIPAQUE 140	PER ML	IV	Q9965
OMNIPAQUE 180	PER ML	IV	Q9965
OMNIPAQUE 240	PER ML	IV	Q9966
OMNIPAQUE 300	PER ML	IV	Q9967
OMNIPAQUE 350	PER ML	IV	Q9967
OMONTYS (FOR ESRD ON DIALYSIS)	0.1 MG	SC, IV	J0890
ONABOTULINUMTOXINA	1 UNIT	IM, OTH	J0585
ONASEMNOGENE ABEPARVOVEC-XIOI	UP TO 5X10^{15} VECTOR GENOMES	IV	J3399
ONCASPAR	VIAL	IM, IV	J9266
ONCOSCINT	STUDY DOSE, UP TO 6 MCI	IV	A4642
ONDANSETRON	1 MG	ORAL	Q0162
ONDANSETRON	4 MG	ORAL	S0119
ONDANSETRON HYDROCHLORIDE	1 MG	IV	J2405
ONIVYDE	1 MG	IV	J9205
ONPATTRO	0.1 MG	IV	J0222
ONTAK	300 MCG	IV	J9160
ONTRUZANT	10 MG	IV	Q5112
OPDIVO	1 MG	IV	J9299
OPRELVEKIN	5 MG	SC	J2355
OPTIRAY	PER ML	IV	Q9967
OPTIRAY 160	PER ML	IV	Q9965
OPTIRAY 240	PER ML	IV	Q9966
OPTIRAY 300	PER ML	IV	Q9967
OPTIRAY 320	PER ML	IV	Q9967
OPTISON	1 ML	IV	Q9956
ORAL MAGNETIC RESONANCE CONTRAST AGENT, PER 100 ML	100 ML	ORAL	Q9954
ORBACTIV	10 MG	IV	J2407
ORENCIA	10 MG	IV	J0129
ORITAVANCIN	10 MG	IV	J2407
ORITAVANCIN	10 MG	IV	J2406
ORPHENADRINE CITRATE	60 MG	IV, IM	J2360
ORTHADAPT BIOIMPLANT	SQ CM	OTH	C1781
ORTHOCLONE OKT3	5 MG	OTH	J7505
ORTHOVISC	PER DOSE	INJ	J7324
OSELTAMIVIR PHOSPHATE (BRAND NAME) (DEMONSTRATION PROJECT)	75 MG	ORAL	G9035
OSELTAMIVIR PHOSPHATE (GENERIC) (DEMONSTRATION PROJECT)	75 MG	ORAL	G9019
OSMITROL	25% IN 50 ML	IV	J2150
OTIPRIO	6 MG	OTIC	J7342
OXACILLIN SODIUM	250 MG	IM, IV	J2700
OXALIPLATIN	0.5 MG	IV	J9263
OXILAN 300	PER ML	IV	Q9967
OXILAN 350	PER ML	IV	Q9967
OXLUMO	0.5 MG	SC	C9074
OXLUMO	0.5 MG	SC	J0224
OXYMORPHONE HCL	1 MG	IV, SC, IM	J2410

Drug Name	Unit Per	Route	Code	Drug Name	Unit Per	Route	Code
OXYTETRACYCLINE HCL	50 MG	IM	J2460	PENICILLIN G POTASSIUM	600,000 U	IM, IV	J2540
OXYTOCIN	10 U	IV, IM	J2590	PENICILLIN G PROCAINE	600,000 U	IM, IV	J2510
OZURDEX	0.1 MG	OTH	J7312	PENTACARINAT	300 MG	INH	S0080
PACIS BCG	1 MG	OTH	J9030	PENTAM	300 MG	IM, IV	J2545
PACLITAXEL	1 MG	IV	J9267	PENTAM 300	300 MG	IM, IV	S0080
PACLITAXEL PROTEIN-BOUND PARTICLES	1 MG	IV	J9264	PENTAMIDINE ISETHIONATE	300 MG	IM, IV	S0080
PADCEV	0.25 MG	IV	J9177	PENTAMIDINE ISETHIONATE COMPOUNDED	PER 300 MG	INH	J7676
PALIFERMIN	50 MCG	IV	J2425	PENTAMIDINE ISETHIONATE NONCOMPOUNDED	300 MG	INH	J2545
PALINGEN OR PALINGEN XPLU	SQ CM	OTH	Q4173	PENTASPAN	100 ML	IV	J2513
PALINGEN OR PROMATRX	0.36 MG/0.25 CC	OTH	Q4174	PENTASTARCH 10% SOLUTION	100 ML	IV	J2513
PALIPERIDONE PALMITATE EXTENDED RELEASED	1 MG	IM	J2426	PENTATE CALCIUM TRISODIUM	STUDY DOSE UP TO 75 MCI	INH	A9567
PALONOSETRON HCL	25 MCG	IV	J2469	PENTATE CALCIUM TRISODIUM	STUDY DOSE UP TO 25 MCI	IV	A9539
PAMIDRONATE DISODIUM	30 MG	IV	J2430	PENTATE ZINC TRISODIUM	STUDY DOSE UP TO 25 MCI	IV	A9539
PANHEMATIN	1 MG	IV	J1640				
PANITUMUMAB	10 MG	IV	J9303	PENTATE ZINC TRISODIUM	STUDY DOSE UP TO 75 MCI	INH	A9567
PANTOPRAZOLE SODIUM	VIAL	IV	C9113				
PANTOPRAZOLE SODIUM	40 MG	IV	S0164	PENTAZOCINE	30 MG	IM, SC, IV	J3070
PAPAVERINE HCL	60 MG	IV, IM	J2440	PENTOBARBITAL SODIUM	50 MG	IM, IV, OTH	J2515
PARAGARD T380A	EA	OTH	J7300	PENTOSTATIN	10 MG	IV	J9268
PARAPLANTIN	50 MG	IV	J9045	PEPAXTO	~~1 MG~~	~~IV~~	~~C9080~~
PARICALCITOL	1 MCG	IV, IM	J2501	PEPAXTO	1 MG	IV	J9247
PARSABIV	0.1 MG	IV	J0606	PEPCID	20 MG	IV	S0028
PASIREOTIDE LONG ACTING	1 MG	IV	J2502	PERAMIVIR	1 MG	IV	J2547
PATISIRAN	0.1 MG	IV	J0222	PERFLEXANE LIPID MICROSPHERE	1 ML	IV	Q9955
PEDIAPRED	5 MG	ORAL	J7510	PERFLUTREN LIPID MICROSPHERE	1 ML	IV	Q9957
PEG-INTRON	180 MCG	SC	S0145				
PEGADEMASE BOVINE	25 IU	IM	J2504	PERFOROMIST	20 MCG	INH	J7606
PEGAPTANIB SODIUM	0.3 MG	OTH	J2503	PERJETA	1 MG	IV	J9306
PEGASPARGASE	VIAL	IM, IV	J9266	PERMACOL	SQ CM	OTH	C9364
~~PEGFILGRASTIM~~	~~6 MG~~	~~SC~~	~~J2505~~	PERPHENAZINE	5 MG	IM, IV	J3310
PEGFILGRASTIM, EXCLUDES BIOSIMILAR	0.5 MG	SC	J2506	PERPHENAZINE	4 MG	ORAL	Q0175
PEGFILGRASTIM-APGF, BIOSIMILAR	0.5 MG	SC	Q5122	PERSANTINE	10 MG	IV	J1245
PEGFILGRASTIM-BMEZ, BIOSIMILAR	0.5 MG	SC	Q5120	PERSERIS	0.5 MG	SC	J2798
PEGFILGRASTIM-CBQV, BIOSIMILAR	0.5 MG	SC	Q5111	PERTUZUMAB	1 MG	IV	J9306
PEGFILGRASTIM-JMDB, BIOSIMILAR	0.5 MG	SC	Q5108	PERTUZUMAB, TRASTUZUMAB, AND HYALURONIDASE-ZZXF	10 MG	SC	J9316
PEGINESATIDE (FOR ESRD ON DIALYSIS)	0.1 MG	SC, IV	J0890	PFIZERPEN A.S.	600,000 U	IM, IV	J2510
PEGINTERFERON ALFA-2A	180 MCG	SC	S0145	PHENERGAN	50 MG	IM, IV	J2550
PEGLOTICASE	1 MG	IV	J2507	PHENERGAN	12.5 MG	ORAL	Q0169
PEGYLATED INTERFERON ALFA-2A	180 MCG	SC	S0145	PHENOBARBITAL SODIUM	120 MG	IM, IV	J2560
				PHENTOLAMINE MESYLATE	5 MG	IM, IV	J2760
PEGYLATED INTERFERON ALFA-2B	10 MCG	SC	S0148	PHENYLEPHRINE 10.16 MG/ML AND KETOROLAC 2.88 MG/ML OPHTHALMIC IRRIGATION SOLUTION	1 ML	OTH	J1097
PEMBROLIZUMAB	1 MG	IV	J9271				
PEMETREXED	10 MG	IV	J9304	PHENYLEPHRINE HCL	1 ML	SC, IM, IV	J2370
PEMFEXY	10 MG	IV	J9304	PHENYTOIN SODIUM	50 MG	IM, IV	J1165
PENICILLIN G BENZATHINE	100,000 U	IM	J0561	PHESGO	10 MG	SC	J9316
				PHOSPHOCOL	1 MCI	IV	A9563
PENICILLIN G BENZATHINE AND PENICILLIN G PROCAINE	100,000 UNITS	IM	J0558	PHOSPHOTEC	STUDY DOSE UP TO 25 MCI	IV	A9538
				PHOTOFRIN	75 MG	IV	J9600

Appendix 1 — Table of Drugs and Biologicals

Drug Name	Unit Per	Route	Code
PHOTREXA VISCOUS	UP TO 3 ML	OTH	J2787
PHYTONADIONE	1 MG	IM, SC, IV	J3430
PIFLUFOLASTAT F-18, DIAGNOSTIC	1 MCI	IV	A9595
PIPERACILLIN SODIUM	500 MG	IM, IV	S0081
PIPERACILLIN SODIUM/TAZOBACTAM SODIUM	1 G/1.125 GM	IV	J2543
PITOCIN	10 U	IV, IM	J2590
PLATINOL AQ	10 MG	IV	J9060
PLAZOMICIN	5 MG	IV	J0291
PLERIXAFOR	1 MG	SC	J2562
PLICAMYCIN	2.5 MG	IV	J9270
PNEUMOCOCCAL CONJUGATE	EA	IM	S0195
PNEUMOVAX II	EA	IM	S0195
POLATUZUMAB VEDOTIN-PIIQ	1 MG	IV	J9309
POLIVY	1 MG	IV	J9309
POLOCAINE	10 ML	VAR	J0670
POLYCYTE	0.5 CC	OTH	Q4241
PORCINE IMPLANT, PERMACOL	SQ CM	OTH	C9364
PORFIMER SODIUM	75 MG	IV	J9600
PORK INSULIN	5 U	SC	J1815
POROUS PURIFIED COLLAGEN MATRIX BONE VOID FILLER	0.5 CC	OTH	C9362
POROUS PURIFIED COLLAGEN MATRIX BONE VOID FILLER, PUTTY	0.5 CC	OTH	C9359
PORTRAZZA.	1 MG	IV	J9295
POTASSIUM CHLORIDE	2 MEQ	IV	J3480
POTELIGEO	1 MG	IV	J9204
PRALATREXATE	1 MG	IV	J9307
PRALIDOXIME CHLORIDE	1 MG	IV, IM, SC	J2730
PREDNISOLONE	5 MG	ORAL	J7510
PREDNISOLONE ACETATE	1 ML	IM	J2650
PREDNISONE, IMMEDIATE RELEASE OR DELAYED RELEASE	1 MG	ORAL	J7512
PREDNORAL	5 MG	ORAL	J7510
PREGNYL	1,000 USP U	IM	J0725
PRELONE	5 MG	ORAL	J7510
PREMARIN	25 MG	IV, IM	J1410
PRENATAL VITAMINS	30 TABS	ORAL	S0197
PRI-METHYLATE	80 MG	IM	J1040
PRIALT	1 MCG	OTH	J2278
PRIMACOR	5 MG	IV	J2260
PRIMATRIX	SQ CM	OTH	Q4110
PRIMAXIN	250 MG	IV, IM	J0743
PRIMESTRIN AQUEOUS	1 MG	IM, IV	J1410
PRIMETHASONE	1 MG	IM, IV, OTH	J1100
PRIVIGEN	500 MG	IV	J1459
PROBUPHINE IMPLANT	74.2 MG	OTH	J0570
PROCAINAMIDE HCL	1 G	IM, IV	J2690
PROCARBAZINE HCL	50 MG	ORAL	S0182
PROCENTA	200 MG	OTH	Q4244
PROCHLOPERAZINE MALEATE	5 MG	ORAL	S0183
PROCHLORPERAZINE	10 MG	IM, IV	J0780
PROCHLORPERAZINE MALEATE	5 MG	ORAL	Q0164
PROCRIT, NON-ESRD USE	1,000 U	SC, IV	J0885

Drug Name	Unit Per	Route	Code
PROFILNINE HEAT-TREATED	1 IU	IV	J7194
PROFILNINE SD	1 IU	IV	J7194
PROFONIX	VIAL	INJ	C9113
PROGENAMATRIX	SQ CM	OTH	Q4222
PROGESTERONE	50 MG	IM	J2675
PROGRAF	5 MG	OTH	J7525
PROGRAF	1 MG	ORAL	J7507
PROLEUKIN	1 VIAL	VAR	J9015
PROLIA	1 MG	SC	J0897
PROLIXIN DECANOATE	25 MG	SC, IM	J2680
PROMAZINE HCL	25 MG	IM	J2950
PROMETHAZINE HCL	12.5 MG	ORAL	Q0169
PROMETHAZINE HCL	50 MG	IM, IV	J2550
PRONESTYL	1 G	IM, IV	J2690
PROPECIA	5 MG	ORAL	S0138
PROPLEX SX-T	1 IU	IV	J7194
PROPLEX T	1 IU	IV	J7194
PROPOFOL	10 MG	IV	J2704
PROPRANOLOL HCL	1 MG	IV	J1800
PROREX	50 MG	IM, IV	J2550
PROSCAR	5 MG	ORAL	S0138
PROSTASCINT	STUDY DOSE UP TO 10 MCI	IV	A9507
PROSTIGMIN	0.5 MG	IM, IV	J2710
PROSTIN VR	1.25 MCG	INJ	J0270
PROTAMINE SULFATE	10 MG	IV	J2720
PROTEIN C CONCENTRATE	10 IU	IV	J2724
PROTEXT	1 CC	OTH	Q4246
PROTHROMBIN COMPLEX CONCENTRATE (HUMAN)	PER IU	IV	J7168
PROTIRELIN	250 MCG	IV	J2725
PROTONIX IV	40 MG	IV	S0164
PROTONIX IV	VIAL	IV	C9113
PROTOPAM CHLORIDE	1 G	SC, IM, IV	J2730
PROTROPIN	1 MG	SC, IM	J2940
PROVENGE	INFUSION	IV	Q2043
PROVENTIL NONCOMPOUNDED, CONCENTRATED	1 MG	INH	J7611
PROVENTIL NONCOMPOUNDED, UNIT DOSE	1 MG	INH	J7613
PROVOCHOLINE POWDER	1 MG	INH	J7674
PROZINE-50	25 MG	IM	J2950
PULMICORT	0.25 MG	INH	J7633
PULMICORT RESPULES	0.5 MG	INH	J7627
PULMICORT RESPULES NONCOMPOUNDED, CONCETRATED	0.25 MG	INH	J7626
PULMOZYME	1 MG	INH	J7639
PURAPLY	SQ CM	OTH	Q4195
PURAPLY AM	SQ CM	OTH	Q4196
PURAPLY XT	SQ CM	OTH	Q4197
PURINETHOL	50 MG	ORAL	S0108
PYLARIFY	1 MCI	IV	A9595
PYRIDOXINE HCL	100 MG	IM, IV	J3415
QUADRAMET	PER DOSE UP TO 150 MCI	IV	A9604

Drug Name	Unit Per	Route	Code
QUELICIN	20 MG	IM, IV	J0330
QUINUPRISTIN/DALFOPRISTIN	500 MG	IV	J2770
QUTENZA	1 SQ CM	OTH	J7336
QUZYTIIR	0.5 MG	IV	J1201
RADICAVA	1 MG	IV	J1301
RADIESSE	0.1 ML	OTH	Q2026
RADIUM (RA) 223 DICHLORIDE THERAPEUTIC	PER MICROCURIE	IV	A9606
RAMUCIRUMAB	5 MG	IV	J9308
RANIBIZUMAB	0.1 MG	OTH	J2778
RANITIDINE HCL	25 MG	INJ	J2780
RAPAMUNE	1 MG	ORAL	J7520
RAPIVAB	1 MG	IV	J2547
RASBURICASE	0.5 MG	IM	J2783
RAVULIZUMAB-CWVZ	10 MG	IV	J1303
REBETRON KIT	1,000,000 U	SC, IM	J9214
REBIF	30 MCG	SC	J1826
REBIF	1 MCG	SC	Q3028
REBINYN	1 IU	IV	J7203
REBLOZYL	0.25 MG	SC	J0896
RECARBRIO	4 MG/4 MG/2 MG	IV	J0742
RECLAST	1 MG	IV	J3489
REDISOL	1,000 MCG	SC. IM	J3420
REFLUDAN	50 MG	IM, IV	J1945
REGADENOSON	0.1 MG	IV	J2785
REGEN-COV	1200 MG	IV	Q0244
REGITINE	5 MG	IM, IV	J2760
REGLAN	10 MG	IV	J2765
REGRANEX GEL	0.5 G	OTH	S0157
REGUARD	SQ CM	OTH	Q4255
REGULAR INSULIN	5 UNITS	SC	J1815
RELAXIN	10 ML	IV, IM	J2800
RELENZA (DEMONSTRATION PROJECT)	10 MG	INH	G9034
RELION	5 U	SC	J1815
RELION NOVOLIN	50 U	SC	J1817
RELISTOR	0.1 MG	SC	J2212
REMICADE	10 MG	IV	J1745
REMODULIN	1 MG	SC	J3285
RENFLEXIS	10 MG	IV	Q5104
REODULIN	1 MG	SC	J3285
REOPRO	10 MG	IV	J0130
REPRIZA	SQ CM	OTH	Q4143
REPRONEX	75 IU	SC, IM, IV	S0122
RESLIZUMAB	1 MG	IV	J2786
RESPIROL NONCOMPOUNDED, CONCENTRATED	1 MG	INH	J7611
RESPIROL NONCOMPOUNDED, UNIT DOSE	1 MG	INH	J7613
RESTORIGIN	1 CC	INJ	Q4192
RESTORIGIN	SQ CM	OTH	Q4191
RESTRATA	SQ CM	OTH	A2007
RETACRIT	100 UNITS	INJ, IV	Q5105
RETACRIT	1000 UNITS	INJ, IV	Q5106

Drug Name	Unit Per	Route	Code
RETAVASE	18.1 MG	IV	J2993
RETEPLASE	18.1 MG	IV	J2993
RETISERT	IMPLANT	OTH	J7311
RETROVIR	10 MG	IV	J3485
RETROVIR	100 MG	ORAL	S0104
REVEFENACIN INHALATION	1 MCG	INH	J7677
REVITA	SQ CM	OTH	Q4180
REVITALON	SQ CM	OTH	Q4157
RHEOMACRODEX	500 ML	IV	J7100
RHEUMATREX	2.5 MG	ORAL	J8610
RHEUMATREX DOSE PACK	2.5 MG	ORAL	J8610
RHO D IMMUNE GLOBULIN	300 MCG	IV	J2790
RHO D IMMUNE GLOBULIN (RHOPHYLAC)	100 IU	IM, IV	J2791
RHO D IMMUNE GLOBULIN MINIDOSE	50 MCG	IM	J2788
RHO D IMMUNE GLOBULIN SOLVENT DETERGENT	100 IU	IV	J2792
RHOGAM	50 MCG	IM	J2788
RHOGAM	300 MCG	IM	J2790
RHOPHYLAC	100 IU	IM, IV	J2791
RIABNI	10 MG	IV	Q5123
RIBOFLAVIN 5'-PHOSPHATE, OPHTHALMIC SOLUTION	UP TO 3 ML	OTH	J2787
RILONACEPT	1 MG	SC	J2793
RIMANTADINE HCL (DEMONSTRATION PROJECT)	100 MG	ORAL	G9020
RIMANTADINE HCL (DEMONSTRATION PROJECT)	100 MG	ORAL	G9036
RIMSO 50	50 ML	IV	J1212
RINGERS LACTATE INFUSION	UP TO 1000 CC	IV	J7120
RISPERDAL CONSTA	0.5 MG	IM	J2794
RISPERIDONE	0.5 MG	SC	J2798
RISPERIDONE	0.5 MG	IM	J2794
RITUXAN	10 MG	IV	J9312
RITUXAN HYCELA	10 MG	SC	J9311
RITUXIMAB	10 MG	IV	J9312
RITUXIMAB 10 MG AND HYALURONIDASE	10 MG	SC	J9311
RITUXIMAB-ABBS, BIOSIMILAR	10 MG	IV	Q5115
RITUXIMAB-ARRX, BIOSIMILAR	10 MG	IV	Q5123
RITUXIMAB-PVVR, BIOSIMILAR	10 MG	IV	Q5119
RIXUBIS	IU	IV	J7200
ROBAXIN	10 ML	IV, IM	J2800
ROCEPHIN	250 MG	IV, IM	J0696
ROFERON-A	3,000,000 U	SC, IM	J9213
ROLAPITANT	1 MG	ORAL	J8670
ROLAPITANT	0.5 MG	ORAL, IV	J2797
ROMIDEPSIN	1 MG	IV	J9315
ROMIDEPSIN, LYOPHILIZED	0.1 MG	IV	J9319
ROMIDEPSIN, NON-LYPOHILIZED	1 MG	IV	C9065
ROMIDEPSIN, NONLYOPHILIZED	0.1 MG	IV	J9318
ROMIPLOSTIM	10 MCG	SC	J2796
ROMOSOZUMAB-AQQG	1 MG	SC	J3111
ROPIVACAINE HYDROCHLORIDE	1 MG	VAR	J2795
RUBEX	10 MG	IV	J9000

Drug Name	Unit Per	Route	Code
RUBIDIUM RB-82	STUDY DOSE UP TO 60 MCI	IV	A9555
RUBRAMIN PC	1,000 MCG	SC, IM	J3420
RUBRATOPE 57	STUDY DOSE UP TO 1 UCI	ORAL	A9559
RUCONEST	10 UNITS	IV	J0596
RUXIENCE	10 MG	IV	Q5119
RYBREVANT	10 MG	IV	C9083
RYBREVANT	2 MG	IV	J9061
RYLAZE	0.1 MG	IM	J9021
SACITUZUMAB GOVITECAN-HZIY	2.5 MG	IV	J9317
SAIZEN	1 MG	SC	J2941
SAIZEN SOMATROPIN RDNA ORIGIN	1 MG	SC	J2941
SALINE OR STERILE WATER, METERED DOSE DISPENSER	10 ML	INH	A4218
SALINE, STERILE WATER, AND/OR DEXTROSE DILUENT/FLUSH	10 ML	VAR	A4216
SALINE/STERILE WATER	500 ML	VAR	A4217
SAMARIUM LEXIDRONAM	PER DOSE UP TO 150 MCI	IV	A9604
SANDIMMUNE	100 MG	ORAL	J7502
SANDIMMUNE	250 MG	IV	J7516
SANDIMMUNE	25 MG	ORAL	J7515
SANDOSTATIN	25 MCG	SC, IV	J2354
SANDOSTATIN LAR	1 MG	IM	J2353
SANGCYA	100 MG	ORAL	J7502
SANO-DROL	40 MG	IM	J1030
SANO-DROL	80 MG	IM	J1040
SAPHNELO	1 MG	IV	C9086
SAQUINAVIR	200 MG	ORAL	S0140
SARCLISA	10 MG	IV	J9227
SARGRAMOSTIM (GM-CSF)	50 MCG	IV	J2820
SCANDONEST	PER 10 ML	IV	J0670
SCENESSE	1 MG	OTH	J7352
SCULPTRA	0.5 ML	OTH	Q2028
SEBELIPASE ALFA	1 MG	IV	J2840
SECREFLO	1 MCG	IV	J2850
SECRETIN, SYNTHETIC, HUMAN	1 MCG	IV	J2850
SEGESTERONE ACETATE AND ETHINYL ESTRADIOL VAGINAL RING	0.15 MG/0.013 MG	OTH	J7294
SENSIPAR	1 MG	ORAL	J0604
SENSORCAINE	30 ML	VAR	S0020
SEPTRA IV	10 ML	IV	S0039
SERMORELIN ACETATE	1 MCG	IV	Q0515
SEROSTIM	1 MG	SC	J2941
SEROSTIM RDNA ORIGIN	1 MG	SC	J2941
SEVENFACT	1 MCG	IV	J7212
SIGNIFOR LAR	1 MG	IV	J2502
SILDENAFIL CITRATE	25 MG	ORAL	S0090
SILTUXIMAB	10 MG	IV	J2860
SIMPONI	1 MG	IV	J1602
SIMULECT	20 MG	IV	J0480
SINCALIDE	5 MCG	IV	J2805
SINUVA	10 MCG	OTH	C9122

Drug Name	Unit Per	Route	Code
SINUVA	10 MCG	OTH	J7402
SINUVA	10 MCG	OTH	J7401
SIPULEUCEL-T	INFUSION	IV	Q2043
SIROLIMUS	1 MG	ORAL	J7520
SIVEXTRO	1 MG	IV	J3090
SKIN SUBSTITUTE, SYNTHETIC, RESORBABLE	SQ CM	OTH	C1849
SKINTE	SQ CM	OTH	Q4200
SKYLA	13.5 MG	OTH	J7301
SMZ-TMP	10 ML	IV	S0039
SODIUM FERRIC GLUCONATE COMPLEX IN SUCROSE	12.5 MG	IV	J2916
SODIUM FLUORIDE F-18, DIAGNOSTIC	STUDY DOSE UP TO 30 MCI	IV	A9580
SODIUM IODIDE I-131 CAPSULE DIAGNOSTIC	1 MCI	ORAL	A9528
SODIUM IODIDE I-131 CAPSULE THERAPEUTIC	1 MCI	ORAL	A9517
SODIUM IODIDE I-131 SOLUTION THERAPEUTIC	1 MCI	ORAL	A9530
SODIUM PHOSPHATE P32	1 MCI	IV	A9563
SOLGANAL	50 MG	IM	J2910
SOLIRIS	10 MG	IV	J1300
SOLTAMOX	10 MG	ORAL	S0187
SOLU-CORTEF	100 MG	IV, IM, SC	J1720
SOLU-MEDROL	40 MG	IM, IV	J2920
SOLU-MEDROL	125 MG	IM, IV	J2930
SOLUREX	1 MG	IM, IV, OTH	J1100
SOMATREM	1 MG	SC, IM	J2940
SOMATROPIN	1 MG	SC	J2941
SOMATULINE	1 MG	SC	J1930
SOTALOL HYDROCHLORIDE	1 MG	IV	C9482
SOTROVIMAB	500 MG	IV	Q0247
SPECTINOMYCIN DIHYDROCHLORIDE	2 G	IM	J3320
SPECTRO-DEX	1 MG	IM, IV, OTH	J1100
SPINRAZA	0.1 MG	INJ	J2326
SPORANOX	50 MG	IV	J1835
SPRAVATO	1 MG	OTH	S0013
STADOL	1 MG	IM, IV	J0595
STADOL NS	25 MG	OTH	S0012
STELARA	1 MG	SC	J3357
STELARA	1 MG	SC, IV	J3358
STERILE WATER OR SALINE, METERED DOSE DISPENSER	10 ML	INH	A4218
STERILE WATER, SALINE, AND/OR DEXTROSE DILUENT/FLUSH	10 ML	VAR	A4216
STERILE WATER/SALINE	500 ML	VAR	A4217
STRATTICE TM	SQ CM	OTH	Q4130
STRAVIX	SQ CM	OTH	Q4133
STRAVIXPL	SQ CM	OTH	Q4133
STREPTASE	250,000 IU	IV	J2995
STREPTOKINASE	250,000 IU	IV	J2995
STREPTOMYCIN	1 G	IM	J3000
STREPTOZOCIN	1 G	IV	J9320
STRONTIUM 89 CHLORIDE	1 MCI	IV	A9600

Drug Name	Unit Per	Route	Code
SUBLIMAZE	0.1 MG	IM, IV	J3010
SUBLOCADE	≤ 100 MG	SC	Q9991
SUBLOCADE	> 100 MG	SC	Q9992
SUBOXONE	4 MG	ORAL	J0573
SUBOXONE	2 MG	ORAL	J0572
SUBOXONE	12 MG	ORAL	J0575
SUBOXONE	8 MG	ORAL	J0574
SUBUTEX	1 MG	ORAL	J0571
SUCCINYLCHOLINE CHLORIDE	20 MG	IM, IV	J0330
SULFAMETHOXAZOLE AND TRIMETHOPRIM	10 ML	IV	S0039
SULFUR HEXAFLUORIDE LIPID MICROSPHERES	1 ML	IV	Q9950
SULFUTRIM	10 ML	IV	S0039
SUMATRIPTAN SUCCINATE	6 MG	SC	J3030
SUPARTZ	PER DOSE	INJ	J7321
SUPPRELIN LA	10 MCG	OTH	J1675
SUREDERM	SQ CM	OTH	Q4220
SURFACTOR	0.5 CC	OTH	Q4233
SURGICORD	SQ CM	OTH	Q4218
SURGIGRAFT	SQ CM	OTH	Q4183
SURGIGRAFT-DUAL	SQ CM	OTH	Q4219
SURGIMEND COLLAGEN MATRIX, FETAL	0.5 SQ CM	OTH	C9358
SURGIMEND COLLAGEN MATRIX, NEONATAL	0.5 SQ CM	OTH	C9360
SURGRAFT	SQ CM	OTH	Q4209
SUSTOL	0.1 MG	SC	J1627
SYLVANT	10 MG	IV	J2860
SYMMETREL (DEMONSTRATION PROJECT)	100 MG	ORAL	G9033
SYMPHONY	SQ CM	OTH	A2009
SYNERA	70 MG/70 MG	OTH	C9285
SYNERCID	500 MG	IV	J2770
SYNOJOYNT	1 MG	INJ	J7331
SYNRIBO	0.01 MG	SC	J9262
SYNTOCINON	10 UNITS	IV	J2590
SYNVISC/SYNVISC-ONE	1 MG	INJ	J7325
SYTOBEX	1,000 MCG	SC, IM	J3420
T-GEN	250 MG	ORAL	Q0173
TACRINE HCL	10 MG	ORAL	S0014
TACROLIMUS	1 MG	ORAL	J7507
TACROLIMUS	5 MG	OTH	J7525
TACROLIMUS, EXTENDED RELEASE	0.25 MG	ORAL	J7503
TACROLIMUS, EXTENDED RELEASE	0.1 MG	ORAL	J7508
~~TAFASITAMAB-CXIX~~	~~2 MG~~	~~IV~~	~~C9070~~
TAFASITAMAB-CXIX	2 MG	IV	J9349
TAGAMET HCL	300 MG	IM, IV	S0023
TAGRAXOFUSP-ERZS	10 MCG	IV	J9269
TAKHZYRO	1 MG	SC	J0593
TALIGLUCERASE ALFA	10 U	IV	J3060
TALIMOGENE LAHERPAREPVEC	1 MILLION	INTRALESIONAL	J9325
TALWIN	30 MG	IM, SC, IV	J3070

Drug Name	Unit Per	Route	Code
TALYMED	SQ CM	OTH	Q4127
TAMIFLU (DEMONSTRATION PROJECT)	75 MG	ORAL	G9019
TAMIFLU (DEMONSTRATION PROJECT)	75 MG	ORAL	G9035
TAMOXIFEN CITRATE	10 MG	ORAL	S0187
TAXOL	1 MG	IV	J9267
TAXOTERE	1 MG	IV	J9171
TAZICEF	500 MG	IM, IV	J0713
TBO-FILGRASTIM	1 MCG	IV	J1447
TC 99M TILOMANOCEPT	0.5 MCI	SC, OTH	A9520
TEBAMIDE	250 MG	ORAL	Q0173
TEBOROXIME TECHNETIUM TC 99M	STUDY DOSE	IV	A9501
TEBOROXIME, TECHNETIUM	STUDY DOSE	IV	A9501
~~TECARTUS~~	~~UP TO 200 MILLION CELLS~~	~~IV~~	~~C9073~~
TECARTUS	UP TO 200 MILLION CELLS	IV	Q2053
TECENTRIQ	10 MG	INF	J9022
TECHNEPLEX	STUDY DOSE UP TO 25 MCI	IV	A9539
TECHNESCAN	STUDY DOSE UP TO 30 MCI	IV	A9561
TECHNESCAN FANOLESOMAB	STUDY DOSE UP TO 25 MCI	IV	A9566
TECHNESCAN MAA	STUDY DOSE UP TO 10 MCI	IV	A9540
TECHNESCAN MAG3	STUDY DOSE UP TO 15 MCI	IV	A9562
TECHNESCAN PYP	STUDY DOSE UP TO 25 MCI	IV	A9538
TECHNESCAN PYP KIT	STUDY DOSE UP TO 25 MCI	IV	A9538
TECHNETIUM SESTAMBI	STUDY DOSE	IV	A9500
TECHNETIUM TC 99M APCITIDE	STUDY DOSE UP TO 20 MCI	IV	A9504
TECHNETIUM TC 99M ARCITUMOMAB, DIAGNOSTIC	STUDY DOSE UP TO 45 MCI	IV	A9568
TECHNETIUM TC 99M BICISATE	STUDY DOSE UP TO 25 MCI	IV	A9557
TECHNETIUM TC 99M DEPREOTIDE	STUDY DOSE UP TO 35 MCI	IV	A9536
TECHNETIUM TC 99M EXAMETAZIME	STUDY DOSE UP TO 25 MCI	IV	A9521
TECHNETIUM TC 99M FANOLESOMAB	STUDY DOSE UP TO 25 MCI	IV	A9566
TECHNETIUM TC 99M LABELED RED BLOOD CELLS	STUDY DOSE UP TO 30 MCI	IV	A9560
TECHNETIUM TC 99M MACROAGGREGATED ALBUMIN	STUDY DOSE UP TO 10 MCI	IV	A9540
TECHNETIUM TC 99M MDI-MDP	STUDY DOSE UP TO 30 MCI	IV	A9503
TECHNETIUM TC 99M MEBROFENIN	STUDY DOSE UP TO 15 MCI	IV	A9537
TECHNETIUM TC 99M MEDRONATE	STUDY DOSE UP TO 30 MCI	IV	A9503
TECHNETIUM TC 99M MERTIATIDE	STUDY DOSE UP TO 15 MCI	IV	A9562

Appendix 1 — Table of Drugs and Biologicals

Drug Name	Unit Per	Route	Code
TECHNETIUM TC 99M OXIDRONATE	STUDY DOSE UP TO 30 MCI	IV	A9561
TECHNETIUM TC 99M PENTETATE	STUDY DOSE UP TO 25 MCI	IV	A9539
TECHNETIUM TC 99M PYROPHOSPHATE	STUDY DOSE UP TO 25 MCI	IV	A9538
TECHNETIUM TC 99M SODIUM GLUCEPATATE	STUDY DOSE UP TO 25 MCI	IV	A9550
TECHNETIUM TC 99M SUCCIMER	STUDY DOSE UP TO 10 MCI	IV	A9551
TECHNETIUM TC 99M SULFUR COLLOID	STUDY DOSE UP TO 20 MCI	IV	A9541
TECHNETIUM TC 99M TETROFOSMIN, DIAGNOSTIC	STUDY DOSE	IV	A9502
TECHNETIUM TC-99M EXAMETAZIME LABELED AUTOLOGOUS WHITE BLOOD CELLS	STUDY DOSE	IV	A9569
TECHNETIUM TC-99M TEBOROXIME	STUDY DOSE	IV	A9501
TECHNILITE	1 MCI	IV	A9512
TEDIZOLID PHOSPHATE	1 MG	IV	J3090
TEFLARO	10 MG	IV	J0712
TELAVANCIN	10 MG	IV	J3095
TEMODAR	5 MG	ORAL	J8700
TEMODAR	1 MG	IV	J9328
TEMOZOLOMIDE	5 MG	ORAL	J8700
TEMOZOLOMIDE	1 MG	IV	J9328
TEMSIROLIMUS	1 MG	IV	J9330
TENDON, POROUS MATRIX	SQ CM	OTH	C9356
TENDON, POROUS MATRIX CROSS-LINKED AND GLYCOSAMINOGLYCAN MATRIX	SQ CM	OTH	C9356
TENECTEPLASE	1 MG	IV	J3101
TENIPOSIDE	50 MG	IV	Q2017
TENOGLIDE TENDON PROTECTOR	SQ CM	OTH	C9356
TENOGLIDE TENDON PROTECTOR SHEET	SQ CM	OTH	C9356
TENSIX	SQ CM	OTH	Q4146
TEPEZZA	10 MG	IV	J3241
TEPROTUMUMAB-TRBW	10 MG	IV	J3241
TEQUIN	10 MG	IV	J1590
TERBUTALINE SULFATE	1 MG	SC, IV	J3105
TERBUTALINE SULFATE, COMPOUNDED, CONCENTRATED	1 MG	INH	J7680
TERBUTALINE SULFATE, COMPOUNDED, UNIT DOSE	1 MG	INH	J7681
TERIPARATIDE	10 MCG	SC	J3110
TERRAMYCIN	50 MG	IM	J2460
TESTOSTERONE CYPIONATE	1 MG	IM	J1071
TESTOSTERONE ENANTHATE	1 MG	IM	J3121
TESTOSTERONE PELLET	75 MG	OTH	S0189
TESTOSTERONE UNDECANOATE	1 MG	IM	J3145
TETANUS IMMUNE GLOBULIN	250 U	IM	J1670
TETRACYCLINE HCL	250 MG	IV	J0120
THALLOUS CHLORIDE	1 MCI	IV	A9505
THALLOUS CHLORIDE TL-201	1 MCI	IV	A9505
THALLOUS CHLORIDE USP	1 MCI	IV	A9505

Drug Name	Unit Per	Route	Code
THEELIN AQUEOUS	1 MG	IM, IV	J1435
THEOPHYLLINE	40 MG	IV	J2810
THERACYS	1 MG	OTH	J9030
THERAGENESIS	SQ CM	OTH	A2008
THERASKIN	SQ CM	OTH	Q4121
THERION	SQ CM	OTH	Q4176
THIAMINE HCL	100 MG	INJ	J3411
THIETHYLPERAZINE MALEATE	10 MG	IM	J3280
THIETHYLPERAZINE MALEATE	10 MG	ORAL	Q0174
THIMAZIDE	250 MG	ORAL	Q0173
THIOTEPA	15 MG	IV	J9340
THORAZINE	50 MG	IM, IV	J3230
THROMBATE III	1 IU	IV	J7197
THYMOGLOBULIN	25 MG	OTH	J7511
THYROGEN	0.9 MG	IM, SC	J3240
THYROTROPIN ALPHA	0.9 MG	IM, SC	J3240
TICARCILLIN DISODIUM AND CLAVULANATE	3.1 G	IV	S0040
TICE BCG	1 MG	OTH	J9030
TICON	250 MG	IM	Q0173
TIGAN	200 MG	IM	J3250
TIGECYCLINE	1 MG	IV	J3243
TIJECT-20	200 MG	IM	J3250
TILDRAKIZUMAB	1 MG	SC	J3245
TIMENTIN	3.1 G	IV	S0040
TINZAPARIN	1,000 IU	SC	J1655
TIROFIBAN HCL	0.25 MG	IM, IV	J3246
TISAGENLECLEUCEL	UP TO 600 MILLION CELLS	IV	Q2042
TNKASE	1 MG	IV	J3101
TOBI	300 MG	INH	J7682
TOBRAMYCIN COMPOUNDED, UNIT DOSE	300 MG	INH	J7685
TOBRAMYCIN SULFATE	80 MG	IM, IV	J3260
TOBRAMYCIN, NONCOMPOUNDED, UNIT DOSE	300 MG	INH	J7682
TOCILIZUMAB	1 MG	IV	J3262
TOCILIZUMAB	1 MG	IV	Q0249
TOLAZOLINE HCL	25 MG	IV	J2670
TOPOSAR	10 MG	IV	J9181
TOPOTECAN	0.25 MG	ORAL	J8705
TOPOTECAN	0.1 MG	IV	J9351
TORADOL	15 MG	IV	J1885
TORISEL	1 MG	IV	J9330
TORNALATE	PER MG	INH	J7629
TORNALATE CONCENTRATE	PER MG	INH	J7628
TORSEMIDE	10 MG	IV	J3265
TOSITUMOMAB	450 MG	IV	G3001
TOTECT	PER 250 MG	IV	J1190
TRABECTEDIN	0.1 MG	IV	J9352
TRANSCYTE	SQ CM	OTH	Q4182
TRASTUZUMAB AND HYALURONIDASE-OYSK	10 MG	SC	J9356
TRASTUZUMAB, EXCLUDES BIOSIMILAR	10 MG	IV	J9355

Drug Name	Unit Per	Route	Code
TRASTUZUMAB-ANNS, BIOSIMILAR	10 MG	IV	Q5117
TRASTUZUMAB-DKST, BIOSIMILAR	10 MG	IV	Q5114
TRASTUZUMAB-DTTB, BIOSIMILAR	10 MG	IV	Q5112
TRASTUZUMAB-PKRB, BIOSIMILAR	10 MG	IV	Q5113
TRASTUZUMAB-QYYP, BIOSIMILAR	10 MG	IV	Q5116
TRASYLOL	10,000 KIU	IV	J0365
TRAZIMERA	10 MG	IV	Q5116
TREANDA	1 MG	IV	J9033
TRELSTAR DEPOT	3.75 MG	IM	J3315
TRELSTAR DEPOT PLUS DEBIOCLIP KIT	3.75 MG	IM	J3315
TRELSTAR LA	3.75 MG	IM	J3315
TREMFYA	1 MG	SC	J1628
TREPROSTINIL	1 MG	SC	J3285
TREPROSTINIL, INHALATION SOLUTION	1.74 MG	INH	J7686
TRETINOIN	5 G	OTH	S0117
TRETTEN	10 IU	IV	J7181
TRIAMCINOLONE ACETONIDE, PRESERVATIVE FREE	1 MG	INJ	J3300
TRIAMCINOLONE ACETONIDE, PRESERVATIVE-FREE, EXTENDED-RELEASE, MICROSPHERE FORMULATION	1 MG	OTH	J3304
TRIAMCINOLONE DIACETATE	5 MG	IM	J3302
TRIAMCINOLONE HEXACETONIDE	5 MG	VAR	J3303
TRIAMCINOLONE, COMPOUNDED, CONCENTRATED	1 MG	INH	J7683
TRIAMCINOLONE, COMPOUNDED, UNIT DOSE	1 MG	INH	J7684
TRIBAN	250 MG	ORAL	Q0173
TRIESENCE	1 MG	OTH	J3300
TRIFERIC AVNU	0.1 MG	IV	J1445
TRIFERIC POWDER	0.1 MG	IV	J1444
TRIFERIC SOLUTION	0.1 MG	IV	J1443
TRIFLUPROMAZINE HCL	UP TO 20 MG	INJ	J3400
~~TRILACICLIB~~	~~1 MG~~	~~IV~~	~~C9078~~
TRILACICLIB	1 MG	IV	J1448
TRILIFON	4 MG	ORAL	Q0175
TRILONE	5 MG	IM	J3302
TRILURON	1 MG	INJ	J7332
TRIMETHOBENZAMIDE HCL	200 MG	IM	J3250
TRIMETHOBENZAMIDE HCL	250 MG	ORAL	Q0173
TRIMETREXATE GLUCURONATE	25 MG	IV	J3305
TRIPTODUR	3.75 MG	IM	J3316
TRIPTORELIN PAMOATE	3.75 MG	IM	J3315
TRIPTORELIN, EXTENDED-RELEASE	3.75 MG	IM	J3316
TRISENOX	1 MG	IV	J9017
TRIVARIS	1 MG	VAR	J3300
TRIVISC	1 MG	INJ	J7329
TROBICIN	2 G	IM	J3320
TRODELVY	2.5 MG	IV	J9317

Drug Name	Unit Per	Route	Code
TROGARZO	10 MG	IV	J1746
TRUSKIN	SQ CM	OTH	Q4167
TRUXADRYL	50 MG	IV, IM	J1200
TRUXIMA	10 MG	IV	Q5115
TYGACIL	1 MG	IV	J3243
TYPE A BOTOX	1 UNIT	IM, OTH	J0585
TYSABRI	1 MG	IV	J2323
TYVASO	1.74 MG	INH	J7686
UDENYCA	0.5 MG	SC	Q5111
ULTOMIRIS	10 MG	IV	J1303
ULTRA-TECHNEKOW	1 MCI	IV	A9512
ULTRALENTE	5 U	SC	J1815
ULTRATAG	STUDY DOSE UP TO 30 MCI	IV	A9560
ULTRAVIST 150	1 ML	IV	Q9965
ULTRAVIST 240	1 ML	IV	Q9966
ULTRAVIST 300	1 ML	IV	Q9967
ULTRAVIST 370	1 ML	IV	Q9967
UNASYN	1.5 G	IM, IV	J0295
UPLIZNA	1 MG	IV	J1823
UREA	40 G	IV	J3350
URECHOLINE	UP TO 5 MG	SC	J0520
UROFOLLITROPIN	75 IU	SC, IM	J3355
UROKINASE	5,000 IU	IV	J3364
UROKINASE	250,000 IU	IV	J3365
USTEKINUMAB	1 MG	SC	J3357
USTEKINUMAB	1 MG	SC, IV	J3358
VABOMERE	10 MG/10 MG	IV	J2186
VALERGEN	10 MG	IM	J1380
VALIUM	5 MG	IV, IM	J3360
VALRUBICIN INTRAVESICAL	200 MG	OTH	J9357
VALSTAR	200 MG	OTH	J9357
VANCOCIN	500 MG	IM, IV	J3370
VANCOMYCIN HCL	500 MG	IV, IM	J3370
VANTAS	50 MG	OTH	J9225
VAPRISOL	1 MG	INJ	C9488
VARUBI	1 MG	ORAL	J8670
VARUBI	0.5 MG	ORAL, IV	J2797
VECTIBIX	10 MG	IV	J9303
VEDOLIZUMAB	1 MG	IV	J3380
VELAGLUCERASE ALFA	100 U	IV	J3385
VELBAN	I MG	IV	J9360
VELCADE	0.1 MG	IV, SC	J9041
VELETRI	0.5 MG	IV	J1325
VELOSULIN	5 U	SC	J1815
VELOSULIN BR	5 U	SC	J1815
VENDAJE	SQ CM	OTH	Q4252
VENOFER	1 MG	IV	J1756
VENTOLIN NONCOMPOUNDED, CONCENTRATED	1 MG	INH	J7611
VENTOLIN NONCOMPOUNDED, UNIT DOSE	1 MG	INH	J7613
VEPESID	50 MG	ORAL	J8560
VEPESID	10 MG	IV	J9181
VERITAS	SQ CM	OTH	C9354

Drug Name	Unit Per	Route	Code
VERSED	1 MG	IM, IV	J2250
VERTEPORFIN	0.1 MG	IV	J3396
VESTRONIDASE ALFA-VJBK	1 MG	IV	J3397
VFEND	200 MG	IV	J3465
VIAGRA	25 MG	ORAL	S0090
VIBATIV	10 MG	IV	J3095
VIDAZA	1 MG	SC	J9025
VIDEX	25 MG	ORAL	S0137
~~VILTEPSO~~	~~10 MG~~	~~IV~~	~~C9071~~
VILTEPSO	10 MG	IV	J1427
~~VILTOLARSEN~~	~~10 MG~~	~~IV~~	~~C9071~~
VILTOLARSEN	10 MG	IV	J1427
VIM	SQ CM	OTH	Q4251
VIMIZIM	1 MG	IV	J1322
VIMPAT	1 MG	IV, ORAL	C9254
VINBLASTINE SULFATE	1 MG	IV	J9360
VINCASCAR	1 MG	IV	J9370
VINCRISTINE SULFATE	1 MG	IV	J9370
VINCRISTINE SULFATE LIPOSOME	5 MG	IV	J9371
VINORELBINE TARTRATE	10 MG	IV	J9390
VIRILON	1 CC, 200 MG	IM	J1080
~~VISCO-3~~	~~PER DOSE~~	~~INJ~~	~~J7333~~
VISCO-3	PER DOSE	INJ	J7321
VISTAJECT-25	25 MG	IM	J3410
VISTARIL	25 MG	IM	J3410
VISTARIL	25 MG	ORAL	Q0177
VISTIDE	375 MG	IV	J0740
VISUDYNE	0.1 MG	IV	J3396
VITAMIN B-12 CYANOCOBALAMIN	1,000 MCG	IM, SC	J3420
VITAMIN B-17	VAR	INJ	J3570
VITRASE	1 USP	OTH	J3471
VITRASE	1,000 USP	OTH	J3472
VITRASERT	4.5 MG	OTH	J7310
VITRAVENE	1.65 MG	OTH	J1452
VIVITROL	1 MG	IM	J2315
VON WILLEBRAND FACTOR (RECOMBINANT)	1 IU	IV	J7179
VON WILLEBRAND FACTOR COMPLEX (HUMAN) (WILATE)	1 IU	IV	J7183
VON WILLEBRAND FACTOR COMPLEX, HUMATE-P	1 IU	IV	J7187
VON WILLEBRAND FACTOR VIII COMPLEX, HUMAN	PER FACTOR VIII IU	IV	J7186
VONVENDI	1 IU	IV	J7179
VORAXAZE	10 UNITS	IV	C9293
VORETIGENE NEPARVOVEC-RZYL	1 BILLION VECTOR GENOMES	OTH	J3398
VORICONAZOLE	200 MG	IV	J3465
VPRIV	100 U	IV	J3385
VUMON	50 MG	IV	Q2017
VYEPTI	1 MG	IV	J3032
VYONDYS 53	10 MG	IV	J1429
VYXEOS	1 MG/2.27 MG	IV	J9153
WEHAMINE	50 MG	IM, IV	J1240

Drug Name	Unit Per	Route	Code
WEHDRYL	50 MG	IM, IV	J1200
WELBUTRIN SR	150 MG	ORAL	S0106
WILATE	1 IU	IV	J7183
WINRHO SDF	100 IU	IV	J2792
WOUNDEX	SQ CM	OTH	Q4163
WOUNDEX FLOW	0.5 CC	OTH	Q4162
WOUNDFIX, WOUNDFIX PLUS, WOUNDFIX XPLUS	SQ CM	OTH	Q4217
WYCILLIN	600,000 U	IM, IV	J2510
XARACOLL	1 MG	OTH	C9089
XCELLERATE	SQ CM	OTH	Q4234
XCELLISTEM	SQ CM	OTH	A2004
XCM BIOLOGIC TISSUE MATRIX	SQ CM	OTH	Q4142
XELODA	150 MG	ORAL	J8520
XELODA	500 MG	ORAL	J8521
XEMBIFY	100 MG	SC	J1558
XENLETA	1 MG	IV	J0691
XENON XE-133	10 MCI	INH	A9558
XEOMIN	1 UNIT	IM	J0588
XERAVA	1 MG	IV	J0122
XGEVA	1 MG	SC	J0897
XIAFLEX	0.01 MG	OTH	J0775
XOFIGO	PER MICROCURIE	IV	A9606
XOLAIR	5 MG	SC	J2357
XWRAP	SQ CM	OTH	Q4204
XYLOCAINE	10 MG	IV	J2001
XYNTHA	1 IU	IV	J7185
YERVOY	1 MG	IV	J9228
YESCARTA	UP TO 200 MILLION CELLS	IV	Q2041
YONDELIS	0.1 MG	IV	J9352
YTTRIUM 90 IBRITUMOMAB TIUXETAN	TX DOSE UP TO 40 MCI	IV	A9543
YUPELRI	1 MCG	INH	J7677
YUTIQ	0.01 MG	OTH	J7314
ZALTRAP	1 MG	IV	J9400
ZANAMIVIR (BRAND) (DEMONSTRATION PROJECT)	10 MG	INH	G9034
ZANAMIVIR (GENERIC) (DEMONSTRATION PROJECT)	10 MG	INH	G9018
ZANOSAR	1 GM	IV	J9320
ZANTAC	25 MG	INJ	J2780
ZARXIO	1 MCG	IV, SC	Q5101
ZEMDRI	5 MG	IV	J0291
ZEMPLAR	1 MCG	IV, IM	J2501
ZENAPAX	25 MG	OTH	J7513
ZENITH AMNIOTIC MEMBRANE	SQ CM	OTH	Q4253
ZEPZELCA	0.1 MG	IV	J9223
ZERBAXA	50 MG/25 MG	IV	J0695
ZEVALIN	STUDY DOSE UP TO 5 MCI	IV	A9542
ZEVALIN DIAGNOSTIC	STUDY DOSE UP TO 5 MCI	IV	A9542
ZEVALIN THERAPEUTIC	TX DOSE UP TO 40 MCI	IV	A9543

Drug Name	Unit Per	Route	Code
ZICONOTIDE	1 MCG	IT	J2278
ZIDOVUDINE	100 MG	ORAL	S0104
ZIDOVUDINE	10 MG	IV	J3485
ZIEXTENZO	0.5 MG	SC	Q5120
ZILRETTA	1 MG	OTH	J3304
ZINACEFT	PER 750 MG	IM, IV	J0697
ZINECARD	250 MG	IV	J1190
ZINPLAVA	10 MG	INF	J0565
ZIPRASIDONE MESYLATE	10 MG	IM	J3486
ZIRABEV	10 MG	IV	Q5118
ZITHROMAX	500 MG	IV	J0456
ZITHROMAX	1 G	ORAL	Q0144
ZIV-AFLIBERCEPT	1 MG	IV	J9400
ZOFRAN	1 MG	IV	J2405
ZOFRAN	4 MG	ORAL	S0119
ZOFRAN	1 MG	ORAL	Q0162
ZOLADEX	3.6 MG	SC	J9202
ZOLEDRONIC ACID	1 MG	IV	J3489
ZOLGENSMA	UP TO 5X10^{15} VECTOR GENOMES	IV	J3399
ZOMETA	1 MG	IV	J3489
ZORBTIVE	1 MG	SC	J2941
ZORTRESS	0.25 MG	ORAL	J7527
ZOSYN	1 G/1.125 GM	IV	J2543
ZOVIRAX	5 MG	IV	J0133
ZUBSOLV	1.4 MG	ORAL	J0572
ZUBSOLV	5.7 MG	ORAL	J0573
ZULRESSO	1 MG	IV	J1632
ZUPLENZ	4 MG	ORAL	S0119
ZUPLENZ	1 MG	ORAL	Q0162
ZYNLONTA	0.1 MG	IV	C9084
ZYNRELEF	1 MG/0.03 MG	OTH	C9088
ZYPREXA	2.5 MG	IM	S0166
ZYPREXA RELPREVV	1 MG	IM	J2358
ZYVOX	200 MG	IV	J2020

NOT OTHERWISE CLASSIFIED DRUGS

Drug Name	Unit Per	Route	Code
ALFENTANIL	500 MCG	IV	J3490
ALGLUCOSIDASE ALFA NOS	10 MG	IV	J0220
ALIMTA	10 MG	IV	J9305
ALKERAN	50 MG	IV	J9245
ALLOPURINOL SODIUM	500 MG	IV	J3490
ALPHA 1 - PROTEINASE INHIBITOR (HUMAN) NOS	10 MG	IV	J0256
AMINOCAPROIC ACID	250 MG	IV	J3490
ANTIEMETIC NOC	VAR	ORAL	Q0181
ANTIEMETIC DRUG NOC	VAR	OTH	J8498
ANTIEMETIC DRUG, ORAL, NOS	VAR	ORAL	J8597
ANTIEMETIC DRUG, RECTAL/SUPPOSITORY, NOS	1 EA	OTH	J8498
ANTIHEMOPHILIC FACTOR HUMAN METHOD M MONOCLONAL PURIFIED	1 IU	IV	J7192

Drug Name	Unit Per	Route	Code
ANTITHROMBIN III	1 IU	IV	J7195
ASPARAGINASE	10,000 U	IM, IV, SC	J9020
AZTREONAM	500 MG	IM, IV	J3490
BENEFIX	1 IU	IV	J7195
BIOCLATE	1 IU	IV	J7192
BORTEZOMIB, NOT OTHERWISE SPECIFIED	0.1 MG	IV, SC	J9044
BUMETANIDE	0.25 MG	IM, IV	J3490
BUPIVACAINE, 0.25%	1 ML	OTH	J3490
BUPIVACAINE, 0.50%	1 ML	OTH	J3490
BUPIVACAINE, 0.75%	1 ML	OTH	J3490
CALCIUM CHLORIDE	100 MG	IV	J3490
CARIMUNE	500 MG	IV	J1566
CENACORT A-40	10 MG	IM	J3301
CLAVULANTE POTASSIUM/ TICARCILLIN DISODIUM	0.1-3 GM	IV	J3490
CLEVIDIPINE BUTYRATE	1 MG	IV	J3490
CLINDAMYCIN PHOSPHATE	150 MG	IV	J3490
COMPOUNDED DRUG, NOT OTHERWISE CLASSIFIED	VAR	VAR	J7999
COPPER SULFATE	0.4 MG	INJ	J3490
DILTIAZEM HCL	5 MG	IV	J3490
DOXAPRAM HCL	20 MG	IV	J3490
DOXORUBICIN HYDROCHLORIDE, LIPOSOMAL, NOT OTHERWISE SPECIFIED, 10 MG	10 MG	IV	Q2050
DOXYCYCLINE HYCLATE	100 MG	INJ	J3490
DRUG OR BIOLOGICAL, PART B DRUG COMPETITIVE ACQUISITION PROGRAM (CAP)	VAR	VAR	Q4082
ELSPAR	10,000 U	IM, IV, SC	J9020
ENALAPRILAT	1.25 MG	IV	J3490
ESMOLOL HYDROCHLORIDE	10 MG	IV	J3490
ESOMEPRAZOLE SODIUM	20 MG	IV	J3490
ETOMIDATE	2 MG	IV	J3490
FACTOR IX RECOMBINANT	1 IU	IV	J7195
FACTOR VIII RECOMBINANT	1 IU	IV	J7192
FAMOTIDINE	10 MG	IV	J3490
FLUMAZENIL	0.1 MG	IV	J3490
FOLIC ACID	5 MG	SC, IM, IV	J3490
FOSPROPOFOL DISODIUM	35 MG	IV	J3490
GADOLINIUM -BASED CONTRAST NOS	1 ML	IV	A9579
GAMMAGARD S/D	500 MG	IV	J1566
GEMCITABINE HCL	200 MG	IV	J9201
GEMZAR	200 MG	IV	J9201
GLUCARPIDASE	10 U	IV	J3490
GLYCOPYRROLATE	0.2 MG	IM, IV	J3490
HEMOFIL-M	1 IU	IV	J7192
HEMOPHILIA CLOTTING FACTOR, NOC	VAR	INJ	J7199
HEXAMINOLEVULINATE HCL	100 MG PER STUDY DOSE	IV	J3490
HUMAN FIBRINOGEN CONCENTRATE, NOT OTHERWISE SPECIFIED	1 MG	IV	J7178

Drug Name	Unit Per	Route	Code
HYDROXYPROGESTERONE CAPROATE, NOT OTHERWISE SPECIFIED	10 MG	IM	J1729
IMMUNE GLOBULIN LYOPHILIZED	500 MG	IV	J1566
IMMUNE GLOBULIN, NONLYOPHILIZED (NOS)	500 MG	IV	J1599
IMMUNOSUPPRESSIVE DRUG, NOC	VAR	VAR	J7599
INFLUENZA VIRUS VACCINE, NOT OTHERWISE SPECIFIED	EA	IM	Q2039
IVEEGAM	500 MG	IV	J1566
KENAJECT-40	10 MG	IM	J3301
KENALOG-10	10 MG	IM	J3301
KENALOG-40	10 MG	IM	J3301
KOGENATE FS	1 IU	IV	J7192
L-PHENYLALANINE MUSTARD	50 MG	IV	J9245
LABETALOL HCL	5 MG	INJ	J3490
LEVOLEUCOVORIN, NOS	0.5 MG	IV	J0641
MAGNEVIST	1 ML	IV	A9579
MELPHALAN HCL, NOS	50 MG	IV	J9245
METOPROLOL TARTRATE	1 MG	IV	J3490
METRONIDAZOLE INJ	500 MG	IV	J3490
MORRHUATE SODIUM	50 MG	OTH	J3490
MULTIPLE VITAMINS, WITH OR WITHOUT MINERALS AND TRACE ELEMENTS	VAR	ORAL	A9153
NITROGLYCERIN	5 MG	IV	J3490
NOC DRUGS, INHALATION SOLUTION ADMINISTERED THROUGH DME	1 EA	OTH	J7699
NOC DRUGS, OTHER THAN INHALATION DRUGS, ADMINISTERED THROUGH DME	1 EA	OTH	J7799
NONRADIOACTIVE CONTRACT IMAGING MATERIAL	STUDY DOSE	IV	A9698
NOT OTHERWISE CLASSIFIED, ANTINEOPLASTIC DRUGS	VAR	VAR	J9999
OLANZAPINE SHORT ACTING INTRAMUSCULAR INJECTION	0.5 MG	IM	J3490
OMNISCAN	1 ML	IV	A9579
PEMETREXED NOS	10 MG	IV	J9305
PHENYLEPHRINE KETOROLAC	4 ML	IRR	J3490
POLYGAM	500 MG	IV	J1566
POLYGAM S/D	500 MG	IV	J1566
POSITRON EMISSION TOMOGRAPHY RADIOPHARMACEUTICAL, DIAGNOSTIC, FOR NON-TUMOR IDENTIFICATION	STUDY DOSE	IV	A9598
POSITRON EMISSION TOMOGRAPHY RADIOPHARMACEUTICAL, DIAGNOSTIC, FOR TUMOR IDENTIFICATION	STUDY DOSE	IV	A9597
PRESCRIPTION DRUG, ORAL, CHEMOTHERAPEUTIC, NOS	VAR	ORAL	J8999
PRESCRIPTION DRUG, ORAL, NONCHEMOTHERAPEUTIC, NOS	VAR	ORAL	J8499
PROLASTIN	10 MG	IV	J0256
PROTEINASE INHIBITOR (HUMAN)	10 MG	IV	J0256
RADIOPHARMACEUTICAL, DIAGNOSTIC, NOC	VAR	VAR	A4641
RADIOPHARMACEUTICAL, THERAPEUTIC	STUDY DOSE	IV	A9699
RECOMBINATE	1 IU	IV	J7192
REFACTO	1 IU	IV	J7192
RIFAMPIN	600 MG	IV	J3490
SINGLE VITAMIN/MINERAL/TRACE ELEMENT	VAR	ORAL	A9152
SKIN SUBSTITUTE, NOS	VAR	OTH	Q4100
SODIUM ACETATE	2 MEQ	IV	J3490
SODIUM CHLORIDE, HYPERTONIC (3%-5% INFUSION)	250 CC	IV	J3490
SULFAMETHOXAZOLE-TRIMETHOPRIM	80 MG/16 MG	IV	J3490
SURGIMEND	0.5 SQ CM	OTH	J3490
THROMBATE III	1 IU	IV	J7195
TRI-KORT	10 MG	IM	J3301
TRIAM-A	10 MG	IM	J3301
TRIAMCINOLONE ACETONIDE	10 MG	IM	J3301
TRILOG	10 MG	IM	J3301
UNCLASSIFIED BIOLOGICS	VAR	VAR	J3590
UNCLASSIFIED DRUG OR BIOLOGICAL USED FOR ESRD ON DIALYSIS	VAR	VAR	J3591
UNCLASSIFIED DRUGS OR BIOLOGICALS	VAR	VAR	C9399
VASOPRESSIN	20 UNITS	SC, IM	J3490
VECURONIUM BROMIDE	1 MG	IV	J3490
WOUND FILLER, DRY FORM, PER G, NOS	1 G	OTH	A6262
WOUND FILLER, GEL/PASTE, PER FL OZ, NOS	1 OZ	OTH	A6261
ZEMAIRA	10 MG	IV	J0256

Appendix 2 — Modifiers

A modifier is a two-position code that is added to the end of a code to clarify the services being billed. Modifiers provide a means by which a service can be altered without changing the procedure code. They add more information, such as the anatomical site, to the code. In addition, they help to eliminate the appearance of duplicate billing and unbundling. Modifiers are used to increase accuracy in reimbursement, coding consistency, editing, and to capture payment data.

A1	Dressing for one wound
A2	Dressing for two wounds
A3	Dressing for three wounds
A4	Dressing for four wounds
A5	Dressing for five wounds
A6	Dressing for six wounds
A7	Dressing for seven wounds
A8	Dressing for eight wounds
A9	Dressing for nine or more wounds
AA	Anesthesia services performed personally by anesthesiologist
AD	Medical supervision by a physician: more than four concurrent anesthesia procedures
AE	Registered dietician
AF	Specialty physician
AG	Primary physician
AH	Clinical psychologist
AI	Principal physician of record
AJ	Clinical social worker
AK	Nonparticipating physician
AM	Physician, team member service
AO	Alternate payment method declined by provider of service
AP	Determination of refractive state was not performed in the course of diagnostic ophthalmological examination
AQ	Physician providing a service in an unlisted health professional shortage area (HPSA)
AR	Physician provider services in a physician scarcity area
AS	Physician assistant, nurse practitioner, or clinical nurse specialist services for assistant at surgery
AT	Acute treatment (this modifier should be used when reporting service 98940, 98941, 98942)
AU	Item furnished in conjunction with a urological, ostomy, or tracheostomy supply
AV	Item furnished in conjunction with a prosthetic device, prosthetic or orthotic
AW	Item furnished in conjunction with a surgical dressing
AX	Item furnished in conjunction with dialysis services
AY	Item or service furnished to an ESRD patient that is not for the treatment of ESRD
AZ	Physician providing a service in a dental health professional shortage area for the purpose of an electronic health record incentive payment
BA	Item furnished in conjunction with parenteral enteral nutrition (PEN) services
BL	Special acquisition of blood and blood products
BO	Orally administered nutrition, not by feeding tube
BP	The beneficiary has been informed of the purchase and rental options and has elected to purchase the item
BR	The beneficiary has been informed of the purchase and rental options and has elected to rent the item
BU	The beneficiary has been informed of the purchase and rental options and after 30 days has not informed the supplier of his/her decision
CA	Procedure payable only in the inpatient setting when performed emergently on an outpatient who expires prior to admission
CB	Service ordered by a renal dialysis facility (RDF) physician as part of the ESRD beneficiary's dialysis benefit, is not part of the composite rate, and is separately reimbursable
CC	Procedure code change (use CC when the procedure code submitted was changed either for administrative reasons or because an incorrect code was filed)
CD	AMCC test has been ordered by an ESRD facility or MCP physician that is part of the composite rate and is not separately billable
CE	AMCC test has been ordered by an ESRD facility or MCP physician that is a composite rate test but is beyond the normal frequency covered under the rate and is separately reimbursable based on medical necessity
CF	AMCC test has been ordered by an ESRD facility or MCP physician that is not part of the composite rate and is separately billable
CG	Policy criteria applied
CH	Zero percent impaired, limited or restricted
CI	At least 1 percent but less than 20 percent impaired, limited or restricted
CJ	At least 20 percent but less than 40 percent impaired, limited or restricted
CK	At least 40 percent but less than 60 percent impaired, limited or restricted
CL	At least 60 percent but less than 80 percent impaired, limited or restricted
CM	At least 80 percent but less than 100 percent impaired, limited or restricted
CN	100 percent impaired, limited or restricted
CO	Outpatient occupational therapy services furnished in whole or in part by an occupational therapy assistant
CQ	Outpatient physical therapy services furnished in whole or in part by a physical therapist assistant
CR	Catastrophe/disaster related
CS	Cost-sharing waived for specified COVID-19 testing-related services that result in an order for or administration of a COVID-19 test and/or used for cost-sharing waived preventive services furnished via telehealth in rural health clinics and federally qualified health centers during the COVID-19 public health emergency
CT	Computed tomography services furnished using equipment that does not meet each of the attributes of the national electrical manufacturers association (NEMA) XR-29-2013 standard
DA	Oral health assessment by a licensed health professional other than a dentist
E1	Upper left, eyelid
E2	Lower left, eyelid
E3	Upper right, eyelid

E4	Lower right, eyelid		G3	Most recent URR reading of 65 to 69.9

E4 Lower right, eyelid

EA Erythropoetic stimulating agent (ESA) administered to treat anemia due to anticancer chemotherapy

EB Erythropoetic stimulating agent (ESA) administered to treat anemia due to anticancer radiotherapy

EC Erythropoetic stimulating agent (ESA) administered to treat anemia not due to anticancer radiotherapy or anticancer chemotherapy

ED Hematocrit level has exceeded 39 percent (or hemoglobin level has exceeded 13.0 G/dl) for three or more consecutive billing cycles immediately prior to and including the current cycle

EE Hematocrit level has not exceeded 39 percent (or hemoglobin level has not exceeded 13.0 G/dl) for three or more consecutive billing cycles immediately prior to and including the current cycle

EJ Subsequent claims for a defined course of therapy, e.g., EPO, sodium hyaluronate, infliximab

EM Emergency reserve supply (for ESRD benefit only)

EP Service provided as part of Medicaid early periodic screening diagnosis and treatment (EPSDT) program

ER Items and services furnished by a provider-based, off-campus emergency department

ET Emergency services

EX Expatriate beneficiary

EY No physician or other licensed health care provider order for this item or service

F1 Left hand, second digit

F2 Left hand, third digit

F3 Left hand, fourth digit

F4 Left hand, fifth digit

F5 Right hand, thumb

F6 Right hand, second digit

F7 Right hand, third digit

F8 Right hand, fourth digit

F9 Right hand, fifth digit

FA Left hand, thumb

FB Item provided without cost to provider, supplier or practitioner, or full credit received for replaced device (examples, but not limited to, covered under warranty, replaced due to defect, free samples)

FC Partial credit received for replaced device

FP Service provided as part of family planning program

● FQ The service was furnished using audio-only communication technology

● FR The supervising practitioner was present through two-way, audio/video communication technology

● FS Split (or shared) evaluation and management visit

● FT Unrelated evaluation and management (E/M) visit during a postoperative period, or on the same day as a procedure or another E/M visit. (Report when an E/M visit is furnished within the global period but is unrelated, or when one or more additional E/M visits furnished on the same day are unrelated)

FX X-ray taken using film

FY X-ray taken using computed radiography technology/cassette-based imaging

G0 Telehealth services for diagnosis, evaluation, or treatment, of symptoms of an acute stroke

G1 Most recent URR reading of less than 60

G2 Most recent URR reading of 60 to 64.9

G3 Most recent URR reading of 65 to 69.9

G4 Most recent URR reading of 70 to 74.9

G5 Most recent URR reading of 75 or greater

G6 ESRD patient for whom less than six dialysis sessions have been provided in a month

G7 Pregnancy resulted from rape or incest or pregnancy certified by physician as life threatening

G8 Monitored anesthesia care (MAC) for deep complex, complicated, or markedly invasive surgical procedure

G9 Monitored anesthesia care for patient who has history of severe cardiopulmonary condition

GA Waiver of liability statement issued as required by payer policy, individual case

GB Claim being resubmitted for payment because it is no longer covered under a global payment demonstration

GC This service has been performed in part by a resident under the direction of a teaching physician

GE This service has been performed by a resident without the presence of a teaching physician under the primary care exception

GF Nonphysician (e.g., nurse practitioner (NP), certified registered nurse anesthetist (CRNA), certified registered nurse (CRN), clinical nurse specialist (CNS), physician assistant (PA)) services in a critical access hospital

GG Performance and payment of a screening mammogram and diagnostic mammogram on the same patient, same day

GH Diagnostic mammogram converted from screening mammogram on same day

GJ "Opt out" physician or practitioner emergency or urgent service

GK Reasonable and necessary item/service associated with a GA or GZ modifier

GL Medically unnecessary upgrade provided instead of nonupgraded item, no charge, no advance beneficiary notice (ABN)

GM Multiple patients on one ambulance trip

GN Services delivered under an outpatient speech language pathology plan of care

GO Services delivered under an outpatient occupational therapy plan of care

GP Services delivered under an outpatient physical therapy plan of care

GQ Via asynchronous telecommunications system

GR This service was performed in whole or in part by a resident in a Department of Veterans Affairs medical center or clinic, supervised in accordance with VA policy

GS Dosage of erythropoietin stimulating agent has been reduced and maintained in response to hematocrit or hemoglobin level

GT Via interactive audio and video telecommunication systems

GU Waiver of liability statement issued as required by payer policy, routine notice

GV Attending physician not employed or paid under arrangement by the patient's hospice provider

GW Service not related to the hospice patient's terminal condition

GX Notice of liability issued, voluntary under payer policy

GY Item or service statutorily excluded, does not meet the definition of any Medicare benefit or, for non-Medicare insurers, is not a contract benefit

GZ Item or service expected to be denied as not reasonable and necessary

H9 Court-ordered

HA	Child/adolescent program
HB	Adult program, nongeriatric
HC	Adult program, geriatric
HD	Pregnant/parenting women's program
HE	Mental health program
HF	Substance abuse program
HG	Opioid addiction treatment program
HH	Integrated mental health/substance abuse program
HI	Integrated mental health and intellectual disability/developmental disabilities program
HJ	Employee assistance program
HK	Specialized mental health programs for high-risk populations
HL	Intern
HM	Less than bachelor degree level
HN	Bachelors degree level
HO	Masters degree level
HP	Doctoral level
HQ	Group setting
HR	Family/couple with client present
HS	Family/couple without client present
HT	Multidisciplinary team
HU	Funded by child welfare agency
HV	Funded state addictions agency
HW	Funded by state mental health agency
HX	Funded by county/local agency
HY	Funded by juvenile justice agency
HZ	Funded by criminal justice agency
J1	Competitive acquisition program no-pay submission for a prescription number
J2	Competitive acquisition program, restocking of emergency drugs after emergency administration
J3	Competitive acquisition program (CAP), drug not available through CAP as written, reimbursed under average sales price methodology
J4	DMEPOS item subject to DMEPOS competitive bidding program that is furnished by a hospital upon discharge
J5	Off-the-shelf orthotic subject to DMEPOS competitive bidding program that is furnished as part of a physical therapist or occupational therapist professional service
JA	Administered intravenously
JB	Administered subcutaneously
JC	Skin substitute used as a graft
JD	Skin substitute not used as a graft
JE	Administered via dialysate
JF	Compounded drug
JG	Drug or biological acquired with 340B drug pricing program discount
JW	Drug amount discarded/not administered to any patient
K0	Lower extremity prosthesis functional level 0 - does not have the ability or potential to ambulate or transfer safely with or without assistance and a prosthesis does not enhance their quality of life or mobility.
K1	Lower extremity prosthesis functional level 1 - has the ability or potential to use a prosthesis for transfers or ambulation on level surfaces at fixed cadence, typical of the limited and unlimited household ambulator
K2	Lower extremity prosthesis functional level 2 - has the ability or potential for ambulation with the ability to traverse low level environmental barriers such as curbs, stairs or uneven surfaces, typical of the limited community ambulator
K3	Lower extremity prosthesis functional level 3 - has the ability or potential for ambulation with variable cadence, typical of the community ambulator who has the ability to transverse most environmental barriers and may have vocational, therapeutic, or exercise activity that demands prosthetic utilization beyond simple locomotion
K4	Lower extremity prosthesis functional level 4 - has the ability or potential for prosthetic ambulation that exceeds the basic ambulation skills, exhibiting high impact, stress, or energy levels, typical of the prosthetic demands of the child, active adult, or athlete
KA	Add on option/accessory for wheelchair
KB	Beneficiary requested upgrade for ABN, more than four modifiers identified on claim
KC	Replacement of special power wheelchair interface
KD	Drug or biological infused through DME
KE	Bid under round one of the DMEPOS competitive bidding program for use with noncompetitive bid base equipment
KF	Item designated by FDA as Class III device
KG	DMEPOS item subject to DMEPOS competitive bidding program number 1
KH	DMEPOS item, initial claim, purchase or first month rental
KI	DMEPOS item, second or third month rental
KJ	DMEPOS item, parenteral enteral nutrition (PEN) pump or capped rental, months four to fifteen
KK	DMEPOS item subject to DMEPOS competitive bidding program number 2
KL	DMEPOS item delivered via mail
KM	Replacement of facial prosthesis including new impression/moulage
KN	Replacement of facial prosthesis using previous master model
KO	Single drug unit dose formulation
KP	First drug of a multiple drug unit dose formulation
KQ	Second or subsequent drug of a multiple drug unit dose formulation
KR	Rental item, billing for partial month
KS	Glucose monitor supply for diabetic beneficiary not treated with insulin
KT	Beneficiary resides in a competitive bidding area and travels outside that competitive bidding area and receives a competitive bid item
KU	DMEPOS item subject to DMEPOS competitive bidding program number 3
KV	DMEPOS item subject to DMEPOS competitive bidding program that is furnished as part of a professional service
KW	DMEPOS item subject to DMEPOS competitive bidding program number 4
KX	Requirements specified in the medical policy have been met
KY	DMEPOS item subject to DMEPOS competitive bidding program number 5
KZ	New coverage not implemented by managed care
LC	Left circumflex coronary artery
LD	Left anterior descending coronary artery
LL	Lease/rental (use the LL modifier when DME equipment rental is to be applied against the purchase price)
LM	Left main coronary artery
LR	Laboratory round trip

LS FDA-monitored intraocular lens implant

LT Left side (used to identify procedures performed on the left side of the body)

M2 Medicare secondary payer (MSP)

MA Ordering professional is not required to consult a Clinical Decision Support Mechanism due to service being rendered to a patient with a suspected or confirmed emergency medical condition

MB Ordering professional is not required to consult a Clinical Decision Support Mechanism due to the significant hardship exception of insufficient internet access

MC Ordering professional is not required to consult a Clinical Decision Support Mechanism due to the significant hardship exception of electronic health record or Clinical Decision Support Mechanism vendor issues

MD Ordering professional is not required to consult a Clinical Decision Support Mechanism due to the significant hardship exception of extreme and uncontrollable circumstances

ME The order for this service adheres to Appropriate Use Criteria in the Clinical Decision Support Mechanism consulted by the ordering professional

MF The order for this service does not adhere to the Appropriate Use Criteria in the Clinical Decision Support Mechanism consulted by the ordering professional

MG The order for this service does not have applicable Appropriate Use Criteria in the qualified Clinical Decision Support Mechanism consulted by the ordering professional

MH Unknown if ordering professional consulted a Clinical Decision Support Mechanism for this service, related information was not provided to the furnishing professional or provider

MS Six month maintenance and servicing fee for reasonable and necessary parts and labor which are not covered under any manufacturer or supplier warranty

NB Nebulizer system, any type, FDA-cleared for use with specific drug

NR New when rented (use the NR modifier when DME which was new at the time of rental is subsequently purchased)

NU New equipment

P1 A normal healthy patient

P2 A patient with mild systemic disease

P3 A patient with severe systemic disease

P4 A patient with severe systemic disease that is a constant threat to life

P5 A moribund patient who is not expected to survive without the operation

P6 A declared brain-dead patient whose organs are being removed for donor purposes

PA Surgical or other invasive procedure on wrong body part

PB Surgical or other invasive procedure on wrong patient

PC Wrong surgery or other invasive procedure on patient

PD Diagnostic or related nondiagnostic item or service provided in a wholly owned or operated entity to a patient who is admitted as an inpatient within three days

PI Positron emission tomography (PET) or pet/computed tomography (CT) to inform the initial treatment strategy of tumors that are biopsy proven or strongly suspected of being cancerous based on other diagnostic testing

PL Progressive addition lenses

PM Post mortem

PN Nonexcepted service provided at an off-campus, outpatient, provider-based department of a hospital

PO Excepted service provided at an off-campus, outpatient, provider-based department of a hospital

PS Positron emission tomography (PET) or pet/computed tomography (CT) to inform the subsequent treatment strategy of cancerous tumors when the beneficiary's treating physician determines that the PET study is needed to inform subsequent antitumor strategy

PT Colorectal cancer screening test; converted to diagnostic test or other procedure

Q0 Investigational clinical service provided in a clinical research study that is in an approved clinical research study

Q1 Routine clinical service provided in a clinical research study that is in an approved clinical research study

Q2 Demonstration procedure/service

Q3 Live kidney donor surgery and related services

Q4 Service for ordering/referring physician qualifies as a service exemption

Q5 Service furnished under a reciprocal billing arrangement by a substitute physician or by a substitute physical therapist furnishing outpatient physical therapy services in a health professional shortage area, a medically underserved area, or a rural area

Q6 Service furnished under a fee-for-time compensation arrangement by a substitute physician or by a substitute physical therapist furnishing outpatient physical therapy services in a health professional shortage area, a medically underserved area, or a rural area

Q7 One Class A finding

Q8 Two Class B findings

Q9 One Class B and two Class C findings

QA Prescribed amounts of stationary oxygen for daytime use while at rest and nighttime use differ and the average of the two amounts is less than 1 liter per minute (LPM)

QB Prescribed amounts of stationary oxygen for daytime use while at rest and nighttime use differ and the average of the two amounts exceeds 4 liters per minute (LPM) and portable oxygen is prescribed

QC Single channel monitoring

QD Recording and storage in solid state memory by a digital recorder

QE Prescribed amount of stationary oxygen while at rest is less than 1 liter per minute (LPM)

QF Prescribed amount of stationary oxygen while at rest exceeds 4 liters per minute (LPM) and portable oxygen is prescribed

QG Prescribed amount of stationary oxygen while at rest is greater than 4 liters per minute (LPM)

QH Oxygen conserving device is being used with an oxygen delivery system

QJ Services/items provided to a prisoner or patient in state or local custody; however, the state or local government, as applicable, meets the requirements in 42 CFR 411.4 (B)

QK Medical direction of two, three, or four concurrent anesthesia procedures involving qualified individuals

QL Patient pronounced dead after ambulance called

QM Ambulance service provided under arrangement by a provider of services

QN Ambulance service furnished directly by a provider of services

QP Documentation is on file showing that the laboratory test(s) was ordered individually or ordered as a CPT-recognized panel other than automated profile codes 80002-80019, G0058, G0059, and G0060.

QQ Ordering professional consulted a qualified clinical decision support mechanism for this service and the related data was provided to the furnishing professional

QR Prescribed amounts of stationary oxygen for daytime use while at rest and nighttime use differ and the average of the two amounts is greater than 4 liters per minute (LPM)

QS	Monitored anesthesiology care service
QT	Recording and storage on tape by an analog tape recorder
QW	CLIA waived test
QX	CRNA service: with medical direction by a physician
QY	Medical direction of one certified registered nurse anesthetist (CRNA) by an anesthesiologist
QZ	CRNA service: without medical direction by a physician
RA	Replacement of a DME, orthotic or prosthetic item
RB	Replacement of a part of a DME, orthotic or prosthetic item furnished as part of a repair
RC	Right coronary artery
RD	Drug provided to beneficiary, but not administered "incident-to"
RE	Furnished in full compliance with FDA-mandated risk evaluation and mitigation strategy (REMS)
RI	Ramus intermedius coronary artery
RR	Rental (use the RR modifier when DME is to be rented)
RT	Right side (used to identify procedures performed on the right side of the body)
SA	Nurse practitioner rendering service in collaboration with a physician
SB	Nurse midwife
SC	Medically necessary service or supply
SD	Services provided by registered nurse with specialized, highly technical home infusion training
SE	State and/or federally-funded programs/services
SF	Second opinion ordered by a professional review organization (PRO) per section 9401, p.l. 99-272 (100 percent reimbursement - no Medicare deductible or coinsurance)
SG	Ambulatory surgical center (ASC) facility service
SH	Second concurrently administered infusion therapy
SJ	Third or more concurrently administered infusion therapy
SK	Member of high risk population (use only with codes for immunization)
SL	State supplied vaccine
SM	Second surgical opinion
SN	Third surgical opinion
SQ	Item ordered by home health
SS	Home infusion services provided in the infusion suite of the IV therapy provider
ST	Related to trauma or injury
SU	Procedure performed in physician's office (to denote use of facility and equipment)
SV	Pharmaceuticals delivered to patient's home but not utilized
SW	Services provided by a certified diabetic educator
SY	Persons who are in close contact with member of high-risk population (use only with codes for immunization)
SZ	Habilitative services
T1	Left foot, second digit
T2	Left foot, third digit
T3	Left foot, fourth digit
T4	Left foot, fifth digit
T5	Right foot, great toe
T6	Right foot, second digit
T7	Right foot, third digit
T8	Right foot, fourth digit
T9	Right foot, fifth digit
TA	Left foot, great toe
TB	Drug or biological acquired with 340B drug pricing program discount, reported for informational purposes
TC	Technical component; under certain circumstances, a charge may be made for the technical component alone; under those circumstances the technical component charge is identified by adding modifier TC to the usual procedure number; technical component charges are institutional charges and not billed separately by physicians; however, portable x-ray suppliers only bill for technical component and should utilize modifier TC; the charge data from portable x-ray suppliers will then be used to build customary and prevailing profiles
TD	RN
TE	LPN/LVN
TF	Intermediate level of care
TG	Complex/high tech level of care
TH	Obstetrical treatment/services, prenatal or postpartum
TJ	Program group, child and/or adolescent
TK	Extra patient or passenger, nonambulance
TL	Early intervention/individualized family service plan (IFSP)
TM	Individualized education program (IEP)
TN	Rural/outside providers' customary service area
TP	Medical transport, unloaded vehicle
TQ	Basic life support transport by a volunteer ambulance provider
TR	School-based individualized education program (IEP) services provided outside the public school district responsible for the student
TS	Follow-up service
TT	Individualized service provided to more than one patient in same setting
TU	Special payment rate, overtime
TV	Special payment rates, holidays/weekends
TW	Back-up equipment
U1	Medicaid level of care 1, as defined by each state
U2	Medicaid level of care 2, as defined by each state
U3	Medicaid level of care 3, as defined by each state
U4	Medicaid level of care 4, as defined by each state
U5	Medicaid level of care 5, as defined by each state
U6	Medicaid level of care 6, as defined by each state
U7	Medicaid level of care 7, as defined by each state
U8	Medicaid level of care 8, as defined by each state
U9	Medicaid level of care 9, as defined by each state
UA	Medicaid level of care 10, as defined by each state
UB	Medicaid level of care 11, as defined by each state
UC	Medicaid level of care 12, as defined by each state
UD	Medicaid level of care 13, as defined by each state
UE	Used durable medical equipment
UF	Services provided in the morning
UG	Services provided in the afternoon
UH	Services provided in the evening
UJ	Services provided at night
UK	Services provided on behalf of the client to someone other than the client (collateral relationship)
UN	Two patients served

UP	Three patients served
UQ	Four patients served
UR	Five patients served
US	Six or more patients served
V1	Demonstration modifier 1
V2	Demonstration modifier 2
V3	Demonstration modifier 3
V4	Demonstration modifier 4
V5	Vascular catheter (alone or with any other vascular access)
V6	Arteriovenous graft (or other vascular access not including a vascular catheter)
V7	Arteriovenous fistula only (in use with two needles)
V8	Infection present
V9	No infection present
VM	Medicare Diabetes Prevention Program (MDPP) virtual make-up session
VP	Aphakic patient
X1	Continuous/broad services: for reporting services by clinicians, who provide the principal care for a patient, with no planned endpoint of the relationship; services in this category represent comprehensive care, dealing with the entire scope of patient problems, either directly or in a care coordination role; reporting clinician service examples include, but are not limited to, primary care, and clinicians providing comprehensive care to patients in addition to specialty care
X2	Continuous/focused services: for reporting services by clinicians whose expertise is needed for the ongoing management of a chronic disease or a condition that needs to be managed and followed with no planned endpoint to the relationship; reporting clinician service examples include, but are not limited to, a rheumatologist taking care of the patient's rheumatoid arthritis longitudinally but not providing general primary care services
X3	Episodic/broad servies: for reporting services by clinicians who have broad responsibility for the comprehensive needs of the patient that is limited to a defined period and circumstance such as a hospitalization; reporting clinician service examples include, but are not limited to, the hospitalist's services rendered providing comprehensive and general care to a patient while admitted to the hospital
X4	Episodic/focused services: for reporting services by clinicians who provide focused care on particular types of treatment limited to a defined period and circumstance; the patient has a problem, acute or chronic, that will be treated with surgery, radiation, or some other type of generally time-limited intervention; reporting clinician service examples include, but are not limited to, the orthopedic surgeon performing a knee replacement and seeing the patient through the postoperative period
X5	Diagnostic services requested by another clinician: for reporting services by a clinician who furnishes care to the patient only as requested by another clinician or subsequent and related services requested by another clinician; this modifier is reported for patient relationships that may not be adequately captured by the above alternative categories; reporting clinician service examples include, but are not limited to, the radiologist's interpretation of an imaging study requested by another clinician
XE	Separate encounter, a service that is distinct because it occurred during a separate encounter
XP	Separate practitioner, a service that is distinct because it was performed by a different practitioner
XS	Separate structure, a service that is distinct because it was performed on a separate organ/structure
XU	Unusual nonoverlapping service, the use of a service that is distinct because it does not overlap usual components of the main service

Appendix 3 — Abbreviations and Acronyms

HCPCS Abbreviations and Acronyms

The following abbreviations and acronyms are used in the HCPCS descriptions:

/	or
<	less than
<=	less than equal to
>	greater than
>=	greater than equal to
AC	alternating current
AFO	ankle-foot orthosis
AICC	anti-inhibitor coagulant complex
AK	above the knee
AKA	above knee amputation
ALS	advanced life support
AMP	ampule
ART	artery
ART	arterial
ASC	ambulatory surgery center
ATT	attached
A-V	arteriovenous
AVF	arteriovenous fistula
BICROS	bilateral routing of signals
BK	below the knee
BLS	basic life support
BMI	body mass index
BP	blood pressure
BTE	behind the ear (hearing aid)
CAPD	continuous ambulatory peritoneal dialysis
Carb	carbohydrate
CBC	complete blood count
cc	cubic centimeter
CCPD	continuous cycling peritoneal analysis
CHF	congestive heart failure
CIC	completely in the canal (hearing aid)
CIM	Coverage Issue Manual
Clsd	closed
cm	centimeter
CMN	certificate of medical necessity
CMS	Centers for Medicare and Medicaid Services
CMV	cytomegalovirus
Conc	concentrate
Conc	concentrated
Cont	continuous
CP	clinical psychologist
CPAP	continuous positive airway pressure
CPT	Current Procedural Terminology
CRF	chronic renal failure
CRNA	certified registered nurse anesthetist
CROS	contralateral routing of signals
CSW	clinical social worker
CT	computed tomography
CTLSO	cervical-thoracic-lumbar-sacral orthosis
cu	cubic
DC	direct current
DI	diurnal rhythm
Dx	diagnosis
DLI	donor leukocyte infusion
DME	durable medical equipment
DME MAC	durable medical equipment Medicare administrative contractor
DMEPOS	durable medical equipment, prosthestics, orthotics and other supplies
DMERC	durable medical equipment regional carrier
DR	diagnostic radiology
DX	diagnostic
e.g.	for example
Ea	each
ECF	extended care facility
EEG	electroencephalogram
EKG	electrocardiogram
EMG	electromyography
EO	elbow orthosis
EP	electrophysiologic
EPO	epoetin alfa
EPSDT	early periodic screening, diagnosis and treatment
ESRD	end-stage renal disease
EWHO	elbow-wrist-hand orthotic
Ex	extended
Exper	experimental
Ext	external
F	french
FDA	Food and Drug Administration
FDG-PET	positron emission with tomography with 18 fluorodeoxyglucose
Fem	female
FO	finger orthosis
FPD	fixed partial denture
Fr	french
ft	foot
G-CSF	filgrastim (granulocyte colony-stimulating factor)
gm	gram (g)
H2O	water
HCl	hydrochloric acid, hydrochloride
HCPCS	Healthcare Common Procedural Coding System
HCT	hematocrit
HFO	hand-finger orthosis
HHA	home health agency
HI	high
HI-LO	high-low
HIT	home infusion therapy
HKAFO	hip-knee-ankle foot orthosis
HLA	human leukocyte antigen
HMES	heat and moisture exchange system
HNPCC	hereditary non-polyposis colorectal cancer
HO	hip orthosis
HPSA	health professional shortage area
HST	home sleep test
IA	intra-arterial administration
ip	interphalangeal
I-131	Iodine 131
ICF	intermediate care facility
ICU	intensive care unit

IM	intramuscular
in	inch
INF	infusion
INH	inhalation solution
INJ	injection
IOL	intraocular lens
IPD	intermittent peritoneal dialysis
IPPB	intermittent positive pressure breathing
IT	intrathecal administration
ITC	in the canal (hearing aid)
ITE	in the ear (hearing aid)
IU	international units
IV	intravenous
IVF	in vitro fertilization
KAFO	knee-ankle-foot orthosis
KO	knee orthosis
KOH	potassium hydroxide
L	left
LASIK	laser in situ keratomileusis
LAUP	laser assisted uvulopalatoplasty
lbs	pounds
LDL	low density lipoprotein
LDS	lipodystrophy syndrome
Lo	low
LPM	liters per minute
LPN/LVN	Licensed Practical Nurse/Licensed Vocational Nurse
LSO	lumbar-sacral orthosis
MAC	Medicare administrative contractor
mp	metacarpophalangeal
mcg	microgram
mCi	millicurie
MCM	Medicare Carriers Manual
MCP	metacarparpophalangeal joint
MCP	monthly capitation payment
mEq	milliequivalent
MESA	microsurgical epididymal sperm aspiration
mg	milligram
mgs	milligrams
MHT	megahertz
ml	milliliter
mm	millimeter
mmHg	millimeters of Mercury
MRA	magnetic resonance angiography
MRI	magnetic resonance imaging
NA	sodium
NCI	National Cancer Institute
NEC	not elsewhere classified
NG	nasogastric
NH	nursing home
NMES	neuromuscular electrical stimulation
NOC	not otherwise classified
NOS	not otherwise specified
O2	oxygen
OBRA	Omnibus Budget Reconciliation Act
OMT	osteopathic manipulation therapy
OPPS	outpatient prospective payment system
ORAL	oral administration
OSA	obstructive sleep apnea
Ost	ostomy
OTH	other routes of administration
oz	ounce
PA	physician's assistant
PAR	parenteral
PCA	patient controlled analgesia

PCH	pouch
PEN	parenteral and enteral nutrition
PENS	percutaneous electrical nerve stimulation
PET	positron emission tomography
PHP	pre-paid health plan
PHP	physician hospital plan
PI	paramedic intercept
PICC	peripherally inserted central venous catheter
PKR	photorefractive keratotomy
Pow	powder
PRK	photoreactive keratectomy
PRO	peer review organization
PSA	prostate specific antigen
PTB	patellar tendon bearing
PTK	phototherapeutic keratectomy
PVC	polyvinyl chloride
QPP	Quality Payment Program
R	right
Repl	replace
RN	registered nurse
RP	retrograde pyelogram
Rx	prescription
SACH	solid ankle, cushion heel
SC	subcutaneous
SCT	specialty care transport
SEO	shoulder-elbow orthosis
SEWHO	shoulder-elbow-wrist-hand orthosis
SEXA	single energy x-ray absorptiometry
SGD	speech generating device
SGD	sinus rhythm
SM	samarium
SNCT	sensory nerve conduction test
SNF	skilled nursing facility
SO	sacroilliac othrosis
SO	shoulder orthosis
Sol	solution
SQ	square
SR	screen
ST	standard
ST	sustained release
Syr	syrup
TABS	tablets
Tc	technetium
Tc 99m	technetium isotope
TENS	transcutaneous electrical nerve stimulator
THKAO	thoracic-hip-knee-ankle orthosis
TLSO	thoracic-lumbar-sacral-orthosis
TM	temporomandibular
TMJ	temporomandibular joint
TPN	total parenteral nutrition
U	unit
uCi	microcurie
VAR	various routes of administration
w	with
w/	with
w/o	without
WAK	wearable artificial kidney
wc	wheelchair
WHFO	wrist-hand-finger orthotic
WHO	wrist-hand orthotic
Wk	week
w/o	without
Xe	xenon (isotope mass of xenon 133)

Appendix 4 — Medicare Internet-only Manuals (IOMs)

The Centers for Medicare and Medicaid Services (CMS) restructured its paper-based manual system as a web-based system on October 1, 2003. Called the online CMS manual system, it combines all of the various program instructions into Internet-only Manuals (IOMs), which are used by all CMS programs and contractors. In many instances, the references from the online manuals in appendix 4 contain a mention of the old paper manuals from which the current information was obtained when the manuals were converted. This information is shown in the header of the text, in the following format, when applicable, as A3-3101, HO-210, and B3-2049.

Effective with implementation of the IOMs, the former method of publishing program memoranda (PMs) to communicate program instructions was replaced by the following four templates:

- One-time notification
- Manual revisions
- Business requirements
- Confidential requirements

The web-based system has been organized by functional area (e.g., eligibility, entitlement, claims processing, benefit policy, program integrity) in an effort to eliminate redundancy within the manuals, simplify updating, and make CMS program instructions available more quickly. The web-based system contains the functional areas included below:

Pub. 100	Introduction
Pub. 100-01	Medicare General Information, Eligibility, and Entitlement Manual
Pub. 100-02	Medicare Benefit Policy Manual
Pub. 100-03	Medicare National Coverage Determinations (NCD) Manual
Pub. 100-04	Medicare Claims Processing Manual
Pub. 100-05	Medicare Secondary Payer Manual
Pub. 100-06	Medicare Financial Management Manual
Pub. 100-07	State Operations Manual
Pub. 100-08	Medicare Program Integrity Manual
Pub. 100-09	Medicare Contractor Beneficiary and Provider Communications Manual
Pub. 100-10	Quality Improvement Organization Manual
Pub. 100-11	Programs of All-Inclusive Care for the Elderly (PACE) Manual
Pub. 100-12	State Medicaid Manual (under development)
Pub. 100-13	Medicaid State Children's Health Insurance Program (under development)
Pub. 100-14	Medicare ESRD Network Organizations Manual
Pub. 100-15	Medicaid Integrity Program (MIP)
Pub. 100-16	Medicare Managed Care Manual
Pub. 100-17	CMS/Business Partners Systems Security Manual
Pub. 100-18	Medicare Prescription Drug Benefit Manual
Pub. 100-19	Demonstrations
Pub. 100-20	One-Time Notification
Pub. 100-21	Reserved
Pub. 100-22	Medicare Quality Reporting Incentive Programs Manual
Pub. 100-24	State Buy-In Manual
Pub. 100-25	Information Security Acceptable Risk Safeguards Manual

A brief description of the Medicare manuals primarily used for *HCPCS Level II* follows:

The ***National Coverage Determinations Manual*** (NCD), is organized according to categories such as diagnostic services, supplies, and medical procedures. The table of contents lists each category and subject within that category. Revision transmittals identify any new or background material, recap the changes, and provide an effective date for the change. The manual contains four sections and is organized in accordance with CPT category sequence and contains a list of HCPCS codes related to coverage determinations, where appropriate.

The ***Medicare Benefit Policy Manual*** contains Medicare general coverage instructions that are not national coverage determinations. As a general rule, in the past these instructions have been found in chapter II of the ***Medicare Carriers Manual***, the ***Medicare Intermediary Manual***, other provider manuals, and program memoranda.

The ***Medicare Claims Processing Manual*** contains instructions for processing claims for contractors and providers.

The ***Medicare Program Integrity Manual*** communicates the priorities and standards for the Medicare integrity programs.

Medicare IOM References

A printed version of the Medicare IOM references will no longer be published in Optum360's *HCPCS Level II* product. Complete versions of all the manuals can be found online at https://www.cms.gov/ Regulations-and-Guidance/Guidance /Manuals/Internet-Only-Manuals-IOMs.

Appendix 5 — New, Revised, and Deleted Codes for 2022

NEW CODES

A2001	InnovaMatrix AC, per sq cm
A2002	Mirragen Advanced Wound Matrix, per sq cm
A2003	bio-ConneKt Wound Matrix, per sq cm
A2004	XCelliStem, per sq cm
A2005	Microlyte Matrix, per sq cm
A2006	NovoSorb SynPath dermal matrix, per sq cm
A2007	Restrata, per sq cm
A2008	TheraGenesis, per sq cm
A2009	Symphony, per sq cm
A2010	Apis, per sq cm
A4436	Irrigation supply; sleeve, reusable, per month
A4437	Irrigation supply; sleeve, disposable, per month
A4453	Rectal catheter for use with the manual pump-operated enema system, replacement only
A9592	Copper Cu-64, dotatate, diagnostic, 1 mCi
A9593	Gallium Ga-68 PSMA-11, diagnostic, (UCSF), 1 mCi
A9594	Gallium Ga-68 PSMA-11, diagnostic, (UCLA), 1 mCi
A9595	Piflufolastat f-18, diagnostic, 1 mCi
C1761	Catheter, transluminal intravascular lithotripsy, coronary
C1831	Personalized, anterior and lateral interbody cage (implantable)
C1832	Autograft suspension, including cell processing and application, and all system components
C1833	Monitor, cardiac, including intracardiac lead and all system components (implantable)
C9084	Injection, loncastuximab tesirine-lpyl, 0.1 mg
C9085	Injection, avalglucosidase alfa-ngpt, 4 mg
C9086	Injection, anifrolumab-fnia, 1 mg
C9087	Injection, cyclophosphamide, (AuroMedics), 10 mg
C9088	Instillation, bupivacaine and meloxicam, 1 mg/0.03 mg
C9089	Bupivacaine, collagen-matrix implant, 1 mg
C9776	Intraoperative near-infrared fluorescence imaging of major extra-hepatic bile duct(s) (e.g., cystic duct, common bile duct and common hepatic duct) with intravenous administration of indocyanine green (ICG) (list separately in addition to code for primary procedure)
C9778	Colpopexy, vaginal; minimally invasive extraperitoneal approach (sacrospinous)
C9779	Endoscopic submucosal dissection (ESD), including endoscopy or colonoscopy, mucosal closure, when performed
C9780	Insertion of central venous catheter through central venous occlusion via inferior and superior approaches (e.g., inside-out technique), including imaging guidance
E1629	Tablo hemodialysis system for the billable dialysis service
G0028	Documentation of medical reason(s) for not screening for tobacco use (e.g., limited life expectancy, other medical reason)
G0029	Tobacco screening not performed or tobacco cessation intervention not provided on the date of the encounter or within the previous 12 months, reason not otherwise specified
G0030	Patient screened for tobacco use and received tobacco cessation intervention on the date of the encounter or within the previous 12 months (counseling, pharmacotherapy, or both), if identified as a tobacco user
G0031	Palliative care services given to patient any time during the measurement period
G0032	Two or more antipsychotic prescriptions ordered for patients who had a diagnosis of schizophrenia, schizoaffective disorder, or bipolar disorder on or between January 1 of the year prior to the measurement period and the index prescription start date (IPSD) for antipsychotics
G0033	Two or more benzodiazepine prescriptions ordered for patients who had a diagnosis of seizure disorders, rapid eye movement sleep behavior disorder, benzodiazepine withdrawal, ethanol withdrawal, or severe generalized anxiety disorder on or between January 1 of the year prior to the measurement period and the IPSD for benzodiazepines
G0034	Patients receiving palliative care during the measurement period
G0035	Patient has any emergency department encounter during the performance period with place of service indicator 23
G0036	Patient or care partner decline assessment
G0037	On date of encounter, patient is not able to participate in assessment or screening, including nonverbal patients, delirious, severely aphasic, severely developmentally delayed, severe visual or hearing impairment and for those patients, no knowledgeable informant available
G0038	Clinician determines patient does not require referral
G0039	Patient not referred, reason not otherwise specified
G0040	Patient already receiving physical/occupational/speech/recreational therapy during the measurement period
G0041	Patient and/or care partner decline referral
G0042	Referral to physical, occupational, speech, or recreational therapy
G0043	Patients with mechanical prosthetic heart valve
G0044	Patients with moderate or severe mitral stenosis
G0045	Clinical follow-up and MRS score assessed at 90 days following endovascular stroke intervention
G0046	Clinical follow-up and MRS score not assessed at 90 days following endovascular stroke intervention
G0047	Pediatric patient with minor blunt head trauma and PECARN prediction criteria are not assessed
G0048	Patients who receive palliative care services any time during the intake period through the end of the measurement year
G0049	With maintenance hemodialysis (in-center and home HD) for the complete reporting month
G0050	Patients with a catheter that have limited life expectancy
G0051	Patients under hospice care in the current reporting month
G0052	Patients on peritoneal dialysis for any portion of the reporting month
G0053	Advancing rheumatology patient care MIPS value pathways
G0054	Coordinating stroke care to promote prevention and cultivate positive outcomes MIPS value pathways
G0055	Advancing care for heart disease MIPS value pathways
G0056	Optimizing chronic disease management MIPS value pathways

NEW CODES (continued)

G0057	Proposed adopting best practices and promoting patient safety within emergency medicine MIPS value pathways
G0058	Improving care for lower extremity joint repair MIPS value pathways
G0059	Patient safety and support of positive experiences with anesthesia MIPS value pathways
G0060	Allergy/Immunology MIPS specialty set
G0061	Anesthesiology MIPS specialty set
G0062	Audiology MIPS specialty set
G0063	Cardiology MIPS specialty set
G0064	Certified Nurse Midwife MIPS specialty set
G0065	Chiropractic Medicine MIPS specialty set
G0066	Clinical Social Work MIPS specialty set
G0067	Dentistry MIPS specialty set
G0327	Colorectal cancer screening; blood-based biomarker
G0465	Autologous platelet rich plasma (PRP) for diabetic chronic wounds/ulcers, using an FDA-cleared device (includes administration, dressings, phlebotomy, centrifugation, and all other preparatory procedures, per treatment)
G1024	Clinical decision support mechanism Radrite, as defined by the Medicare Appropriate Use Criteria Program
G1025	Patient-months where there are more than one Medicare capitated payment (MCP) provider listed for the month
G1026	The number of adult patient-months in the denominator who were on maintenance hemodialysis using a catheter continuously for 3 months or longer under the care of the same practitioner or group partner as of the last hemodialysis session of the reporting month
G1027	The number of adult patient-months in the denominator who were on maintenance hemodialysis under the care of the same practitioner or group partner as of the last hemodialysis session of the reporting month using a catheter continuously for less than 3 months
G1028	Take-home supply of nasal naloxone; 2-pack of 8 mg per 0.1 ml nasal spray (provision of the services by a Medicare-enrolled Opioid Treatment Program); list separately in addition to code for primary procedure
G2020	Services for high intensity clinical services associated with the initial engagement and outreach of beneficiaries assigned to the SIP component of the PCF model (do not bill with chronic care management codes)
G2172	All inclusive payment for services related to highly coordinated and integrated opioid use disorder (OUD) treatment services furnished for the demonstration project
G4000	Dermatology MIPS specialty set
G4001	Diagnostic Radiology MIPS specialty set
G4002	Electrophysiology Cardiac Specialist MIPS specialty set
G4003	Emergency Medicine MIPS specialty set
G4004	Endocrinology MIPS specialty set
G4005	Family Medicine MIPS specialty set
G4006	Gastroenterology MIPS specialty set
G4007	General Surgery MIPSspecialty set
G4008	Geriatrics MIPS specialty set
G4009	Hospitalists MIPS specialty set
G4010	Infectious Disease MIPS specialty set
G4011	Internal Medicine MIPS specialty set
G4012	Interventional Radiology MIPS specialty set
G4013	Mental/Behavioral Health MIPS specialty set
G4014	Nephrology MIPS specialty set
G4015	Neurology MIPS specialty set

G4016	Neurosurgical MIPS specialty set
G4017	Nutrition/Dietician MIPS specialty set
G4018	Obstetrics/Gynecology MIPS specialty set
G4019	Oncology/Hematology MIPS specialty set
G4020	Ophthalmology MIPS specialty set
G4021	Orthopedic surgery MIPS specialty set
G4022	Otolaryngology MIPS specialty set
G4023	Pathology MIPS specialty set
G4024	Pediatrics MIPS specialty set
G4025	Physical Medicine MIPS specialty set
G4026	Physical Therapy/Occupational Therapy MIPS specialty set
G4027	Plastic Surgery MIPS specialty set
G4028	Podiatry MIPS specialty set
G4029	Preventive Medicine MIPS specialty set
G4030	Pulmonology MIPS specialty set
G4031	Radiation Oncology MIPS specialty set
G4032	Rheumatology MIPS specialty set
G4033	Skilled Nursing Facility MIPS specialty set
G4034	Speech Language Pathology MIPS specialty set
G4035	Thoracic Surgery MIPS specialty set
G4036	Urgent Care MIPS specialty set
G4037	Urology MIPS specialty set
G4038	Vascular Surgery MIPS specialty set
G9988	Palliative care services provided to patient any time during the measurement period
G9989	Documentation of medical reason(s) for not administering pneumococcal vaccine (e.g., adverse reaction to vaccine)
G9990	Pneumococcal vaccine was not administered on or after patient's 60th birthday and before the end of the measurement period, reason not otherwise specified
G9991	Pneumococcal vaccine administered on or after patient's 60th birthday and before the end of the measurement period
G9992	Palliative care services used by patient any time during the measurement period
G9993	Patient was provided pallative care services any time during the measurement period
G9994	Patient is using palliative care services any time during the measurement period
G9995	Patients who use palliative care services any time during the measurement period
G9996	Documentation stating the patient has received or is currently receiving palliative or hospice care
G9997	Documentation of patient pregnancy anytime during the measurement period prior to and including the current encounter
G9998	Documentation of medical reason(s) for an interval of less than 3 years since the last colonoscopy (e.g., last colonoscopy incomplete, last colonoscopy had inadequate prep, piecemeal removal of adenomas, last colonoscopy found greater than 10 adenomas, or patient at high risk for colon cancer [Crohn's disease, ulcerative colitis, lower gastrointestinal bleeding, personal or family history of colon cancer, hereditary colorectal cancer syndromes])
G9999	Documentation of system reason(s) for an interval of less than 3 years since the last colonoscopy (e.g., unable to locate previous colonoscopy report, previous colonoscopy report was incomplete)
J0172	Injection, aducanumab-avwa, 2 mg
J0224	Injection, lumasiran, 0.5 mg
J0699	Injection, cefiderocol, 10 mg

NEW CODES (continued)

J0741	Injection, cabotegravir and rilpivirine, 2 mg/3 mg
J1305	Injection, evinacumab-dgnb, 5 mg
J1426	Injection, casimersen, 10 mg
J1427	Injection, viltolarsen, 10 mg
J1445	Injection, ferric pyrophosphate citrate solution (Triferic AVNU), 0.1 mg of iron
J1448	Injection, trilaciclib, 1 mg
J1554	Injection, immune globulin (Asceniv), 500 mg
J1951	Injection, leuprolide acetate for depot suspension (Fensolvi), 0.25 mg
J1952	Leuprolide injectable, camcevi, 1 mg
J2406	Injection, oritavancin (Kimyrsa), 10 mg
J2506	Injection, pegfilgrastim, excludes biosimilar, 0.5 mg
J7168	Prothrombin complex concentrate (human), Kcentra, per IU of Factor IX activity
J7294	Segesterone acetate and ethinyl estradiol 0.15 mg, 0.013 mg per 24 hours; yearly vaginal system, each
J7295	Ethinyl estradiol and etonogestrel 0.015 mg, 0.12 mg per 24 hours; monthly vaginal ring, each
J7402	Mometasone furoate sinus implant, (Sinuva), 10 mcg
J9021	Injection, asparaginase, recombinant, (Rylaze), 0.1 mg
J9037	Injection, belantamab mafodontin-blmf, 0.5 mg
J9061	Injection, amivantamab-vmjw, 2 mg
J9247	Injection, melphalan flufenamide, 1 mg
J9272	Injection, dostarlimab-gxly, 10 mg
J9318	Injection, romidepsin, nonlyophilized, 0.1 mg
J9319	Injection, romidepsin, lyophilized, 0.1 mg
J9348	Injection, naxitamab-gqgk, 1 mg
J9349	Injection, tafasitamab-cxix, 2 mg
J9353	Injection, margetuximab-cmkb, 5 mg
K1014	Addition, endoskeletal knee-shin system, 4 bar linkage or multiaxial, fluid swing and stance phase control
K1015	Foot, adductus positioning device, adjustable
K1016	Transcutaneous electrical nerve stimulator for electrical stimulation of the trigeminal nerve
K1017	Monthly supplies for use of device coded at K1016
K1018	External upper limb tremor stimulator of the peripheral nerves of the wrist
K1019	Monthly supplies for use of device coded at K1018
K1020	Noninvasive vagus nerve stimulator
K1021	Exsufflation belt, includes all supplies and accessories
K1022	Addition to lower extremity prosthesis, endoskeletal, knee disarticulation, above knee, hip disarticulation, positional rotation unit, any type
K1023	Distal transcutaneous electrical nerve stimulator, stimulates peripheral nerves of the upper arm
K1024	Nonpneumatic compression controller with sequential calibrated gradient pressure
K1025	Nonpneumatic sequential compression garment, full arm
K1026	Mechanical allergen particle barrier/inhalation filter, cream, nasal, topical
K1027	Oral device/appliance used to reduce upper airway collapsibility, without fixed mechanical hinge, custom fabricated, includes fitting and adjustment

M0201	COVID-19 vaccine administration inside a patient's home; reported only once per individual home, per date of service, when only COVID-19 vaccine administration is performed at the patient's home
M0240	Intravenous infusion or subcutaneous injection, casirivimab and imdevimab includes infusion or injection, and post administration monitoring, subsequent repeat doses
M0241	Intravenous infusion or subcutaneous injection, casirivimab and imdevimab includes infusion or injection, and post administration monitoring in the home or residence, this includes a beneficiary's home that has been made provider-based to the hospital during the covid-19 public health emergency, subsequent repeat doses
M0245	Intravenous infusion, bamlanivimab and etesevimab, includes infusion and post administration monitoring
M0246	Intravenous infusion, bamlanivimab and etesevimab, includes infusion and post administration monitoring in the home or residence; this includes a beneficiary's home that has been made provider-based to the hospital during the COVID-19 public health emergency
M0247	Intravenous infusion, sotrovimab, includes infusion and post administration monitoring
M0248	Intravenous infusion, sotrovimab, includes infusion and post administration monitoring in the home or residence; this includes a beneficiary's home that has been made provider-based to the hospital during the COVID-19 public health emergency
M0249	Intravenous infusion, tocilizumab, for hospitalized adults and pediatric patients (2 years of age and older) with COVID-19 who are receiving systemic corticosteroids and require supplemental oxygen, non-invasive or invasive mechanical ventilation, or extracorporeal membrane oxygenation (ECMO) only, includes infusion and post administration monitoring, first dose
M0250	Intravenous infusion, tocilizumab, for hospitalized adults and pediatric patients (2 years of age and older) with COVID-19 who are receiving systemic corticosteroids and require supplemental oxygen, non-invasive or invasive mechanical ventilation, or extracorporeal membrane oxygenation (ECMO) only, includes infusion and post administration monitoring, second dose
M1072	Radiation therapy for anal cancer under the Radiation Oncology model, 90-day episode, professional component
M1073	Radiation therapy for anal cancer under the Radiation Oncology model, 90-day episode, technical component
M1074	Radiation therapy for bladder cancer under the Radiation Oncology model, 90-day episode, professional component
M1075	Radiation therapy for bladder cancer under the Radiation Oncology model, 90-day episode, technical component
M1076	Radiation therapy for bone metastases under the Radiation Oncology model, 90-day episode, professional component
M1077	Radiation therapy for bone metastases under the Radiation Oncology model, 90-day episode, technical component
M1078	Radiation therapy for brain metastases under the Radiation Oncology model, 90 day episode, professional component
M1079	Radiation therapy for brain metastases under the Radiation Oncology model, 90-day episode, technical component
M1080	Radiation therapy for breast cancer under the Radiation Oncology model, 90 day-episode, professional component
M1081	Radiation therapy for breast cancer under the Radiation Oncology model, 90-day episode, technical component
M1082	Radiation therapy for cervical cancer under the Radiation Oncology model, 90-day episode, professional component
M1083	Radiation therapy for cervical cancer under the Radiation Oncology model, 90-day episode, technical component
M1084	Radiation therapy for cns tumors under the Radiation Oncology model, 90-day episode, professional component
M1085	Radiation therapy for cns tumors under the Radiation Oncology model, 90-day episode, technical component

NEW CODES (continued)

M1086   Radiation therapy for colorectal cancer under the Radiation Oncology model, 90-day episode, professional component

M1087   Radiation therapy for colorectal cancer under the Radiation Oncology model, 90-day episode, technical component

M1088   Radiation therapy for head and neck cancer under the Radiation Oncology model, 90-day episode, professional component

M1089   Radiation therapy for head and neck cancer under the Radiation Oncology model, 90-day episode, technical component

M1094   Radiation therapy for lung cancer under the Radiation Oncology model, 90-day episode, professional component

M1095   Radiation therapy for lung cancer under the Radiation Oncology model, 90-day episode, technical component

M1096   Radiation therapy for lymphoma under the Radiation Oncology model, 90-day episode, professional component

M1097   Radiation therapy for lymphoma under the Radiation Oncology model, 90-day episode, technical component

M1098   Radiation therapy for pancreatic cancer under the Radiation Oncology model, 90-day episode, professional component

M1099   Radiation therapy for pancreatic cancer under the Radiation Oncology model, 90-day episode, technical component

M1100   Radiation therapy for prostate cancer under the Radiation Oncology model, 90-day episode, professional component

M1101   Radiation therapy for prostate cancer under the Radiation Oncology model, 90-day episode, technical component

M1102   Radiation therapy for upper GI cancer under the Radiation Oncology model, 90-day episode, professional component

M1103   Radiation therapy for upper GI cancer under the Radiation Oncology model, 90-day episode, technical component

M1104   Radiation therapy for uterine cancer under the Radiation Oncology model, 90-day episode, professional component

M1105   Radiation therapy for uterine cancer under the Radiation Oncology model, 90-day episode, technical component

P9025   Plasma, cryoprecipitate reduced, pathogen reduced, each unit

P9026   Cryoprecipitated fibrinogen complex, pathogen reduced, each unit

Q0240   Injection, casirivimab and imdevimab, 600 mg

Q0244   Injection, casirivimab and imdevimab, 1200 mg

Q0245   Injection, bamlanivimab and etesevimab, 2100 mg

Q0247   Injection, sotrovimab, 500 mg

Q0249   Injection, tocilizumab, for hospitalized adults and pediatric patients (2 years of age and older) with COVID-19 who are receiving systemic corticosteroids and require supplemental oxygen, non-invasive or invasive mechanical ventilation, or extracorporeal membrane oxygenation (ECMO) only, 1 mg

Q2053   Brexucabtagene autoleucel, up to 200 million autologous anti-CD19 CAR positive viable T cells, including leukapheresis and dose preparation procedures, per therapeutic dose

Q2054   Lisocabtagene maraleucel, up to 110 million autologous anti-CD19 CAR-positive viable T cells, including leukapheresis and dose preparation procedures, per therapeutic dose

Q2055   Idecabtagene vicleucel, up to 460 million autologous B-cell maturation antigen (BCMA) directed CAR-positive T cells, including leukapheresis and dose preparation procedures, per therapeutic dose

Q4199   Cygnus matrix, per sq cm

Q4251   Vim, per sq cm

Q4252   Vendaje, per sq cm

Q4253   Zenith Amniotic Membrane, per sq cm

Q5123   Injection, rituximab-arrx, biosimilar, (Riabni), 10 mg

Q9004   Department of veterans affairs whole health partner services

S1091   Stent, noncoronary, temporary, with delivery system (Propel)

S9432   Medical foods for noninborn errors of metabolism

REVISED CODES

C9761   Cystourethroscopy, with ureteroscopy and/or pyeloscopy, with lithotripsy, and ureteral catheterization for steerable vacuum aspiration of the kidney, collecting system, ureter, bladder, and urethra if applicable

C9777   Esophageal mucosal integrity testing by electrical impedance, transoral, includes esophagoscopy or esophagogastroduodenoscopy

G0460   Autologous platelet rich plasma for nondiabetic chronic wounds/ulcers, including phlebotomy, centrifugation, and all other preparatory procedures, administration and dressings, per treatment

G1013   Clinical Decision Support Mechanism EvidenceCare ImagingCare, as defined by the Medicare Appropriate Use Criteria Program

G2081   Patients age 66 and older in institutional special needs plans (SNP) or residing in long-term care with a POS code 32, 33, 34, 54 or 56 for more than 90 consecutive days during the measurement period

G2097   Episodes where the patient had a competing diagnosis on or within 3 days after the episode date (e.g., intestinal infection, pertussis, bacterial infection, Lyme disease, otitis media, acute sinusitis, chronic sinusitis, infection of the adenoids, prostatitis, cellulitis, mastoiditis, or bone infections, acute lymphadenitis, impetigo, skin staph infections, pneumonia/gonococcal infections, venereal disease (syphilis, chlamydia, inflammatory diseases [female reproductive organs]), infections of the kidney, cystitis or UTI)

G2121   Depression, anxiety, apathy, and psychosis assessed

G2122   Depression, anxiety, apathy, and psychosis not assessed

G2140   Leg pain measured by the visual analog scale (VAS) at 3 months (6 to 20 weeks) postoperatively was less than or equal to 3.0 or leg pain measured by the visual analog scale (VAS) within 3 months preoperatively and at 3 months (6 to 20 weeks) postoperatively demonstrated an improvement of 5.0 points or greater

G2142   Functional status measured by the Oswestry Disability Index (ODI version 2.1a) at 1 year (9 to 15 months) postoperatively was less than or equal to 22 or functional status measured by the ODI version 2.1a within 3 months preoperatively and at 1 year (9 to 15 months) postoperatively demonstrated an improvement of 30 points or greater

G2143   Functional status measured by the Oswestry Disability Index (ODI version 2.1a) at 1 year (9 to 15 months) postoperatively was greater than 22 and functional status measured by the ODI version 2.1a within 3 months preoperatively and at 1 year (9 to 15 months) postoperatively demonstrated an improvement of less than 30 points

G2144   Functional status measured by the Oswestry Disability Index (ODI version 2.1a) at 3 months (6 to 20 weeks) postoperatively was less than or equal to 22 or functional status measured by the ODI version 2.1a within 3 months preoperatively and at 3 months (6 to 20 weeks) postoperatively demonstrated an improvement of 30 points or greater

G2145   Functional status measured by the Oswestry Disability Index (ODI version 2.1a) at 3 months (6 to 20 weeks) postoperatively was greater than 22 and functional status measured by the ODI version 2.1a within 3 months preoperatively and at 3 months (6 to 20 weeks) postoperatively demonstrated an improvement of less than 30 points

G2148   Multimodal pain management was used

G2150   Multimodal pain management was not used

G2173   URI episodes where the patient had a comorbid condition during the 12 months prior to or on the episode date (e.g., tuberculosis, neutropenia, cystic fibrosis, chronic bronchitis, pulmonary edema, respiratory failure, rheumatoid lung disease)

G2174   URI episodes when the patient had an active prescription of antibiotics (table 1) in the 30 days prior to the episode date

REVISED CODES (continued)

G2175 Episodes where the patient had a comorbid condition during the 12 months prior to or on the episode date (e.g., tuberculosis, neutropenia, cystic fibrosis, chronic bronchitis, pulmonary edema, respiratory failure, rheumatoid lung disease)

G2177 Acute bronchitis/bronchiolitis episodes when the patient had a new or refill prescription of antibiotics (table 1) in the 30 days prior to the episode date

G2215 Take home supply of nasal naloxone; 2-pack of 4 mg per 0.1 ml nasal spray (provision of the services by a Medicare-enrolled Opioid Treatment Program); list separately in addition to code for primary procedure

G8433 Screening for depression not completed, documented patient or medical reason

G8711 Prescribed or dispensed antibiotic on or within 3 days after the episode date

G8950 Elevated or hypertensive blood pressure reading documented, and the indicated follow-up is documented

G8952 Elevated or hypertensive blood pressure reading documented, indicated follow-up not documented, reason not given

G8967 FDA approved oral anticoagulant is prescribed

G8968 Documentation of medical reason(s) for not prescribing an FDA-approved anticoagulant to a patient with a CHA2DS-VASc score of 0 or 1 for men; or 0, 1, or 2 for women (e.g., present or planned atrial appendage occlusion or ligation)

G8969 Documentation of patient reason(s) for not prescribing an oral anticoagulant that is FDA-approved for the prevention of thromboembolism (e.g., patient preference for not receiving anticoagulation)

G9355 Elective delivery (without medical indication) by Cesarean birth or induction of labor not performed (<39 weeks of gestation)

G9356 Elective delivery (without medical indication) by Cesarean birth or induction of labor performed (<39 weeks of gestation)

G9359 Documentation of negative or managed positive TB screen with further evidence that TB is not active prior to treatment with a biologic immune response modifier

G9361 Medical indication for delivery by Cesarean birth or induction of labor (<39 weeks of gestation) [documentation of reason(s) for elective delivery (e.g., hemorrhage and placental complications, hypertension, preeclampsia and eclampsia, rupture of membranes (premature or prolonged), maternal conditions complicating pregnancy/delivery, fetal conditions complicating pregnancy/delivery, late pregnancy, prior uterine surgery, or participation in clinical trial)]

G9367 At least two orders for high risk medications from the same drug class

G9368 At least two orders for high risk medications from the same drug class not ordered

G9418 Primary nonsmall cell lung cancer biopsy and cytology specimen report documents classification into specific histologic type following IASLC guidance or classified as NSCLC-NOS with an explanation

G9419 Documentation of medical reason(s) for not including the histological type or NSCLC-NOS classification with an explanation (e.g. specimen insufficient or non-diagnostic, specimen does not contain cancer, or other documented medical reasons)

G9421 Primary nonsmall cell lung cancer lung biopsy and cytology specimen report does not document classification into specific histologic type or histologic type does not follow IASLC guidance or is classified as NSCLC-NOS but without an explanation

G9422 Primary lung carcinoma resection report documents PT category, PN category and for nonsmall cell lung cancer, histologic type (e.g., squamous cell carcinoma, adenocarcinoma and not NSCLC-NOS)

G9425 Primary lung carcinoma resection report does not document PT category, PN category and for nonsmall cell lung cancer, histologic type (e.g., squamous cell carcinoma, adenocarcinoma)

G9428 Pathology report includes the PT category, thickness, ulceration and mitotic rate, peripheral and deep margin status and presence or absence of microsatellitosis for invasive tumors

G9429 Documentation of medical reason(s) for not including PT category, thickness, ulceration and mitotic rate, peripheral and deep margin status and presence or absence of microsatellitosis for invasive tumors (e.g., negative skin biopsies, insufficient tissue, or other documented medical reasons)

G9431 Pathology report does not include the PT category, thickness, ulceration and mitotic rate, peripheral and deep margin status and presence or absence of microsatellitosis for invasive tumors

G9554 Final reports for CT, CTA, MRI or MRA of the chest or neck with follow-up imaging recommended

G9556 Final reports for CT, CTA, MRI or MRA of the chest or neck with follow-up imaging not recommended

G9557 Final reports for CT, CTA, MRI or MRA studies of the chest or neck without an incidentally found thyroid nodule < 1.0 cm noted or no nodule found

G9580 Door to puncture time of 90 minutes or less

G9582 Door to puncture time of greater than 90 minutes, no reason given

G9662 Previously diagnosed or have an active diagnosis of clinical ASCVD, including ASCVD procedure

G9663 Any LDL-C laboratory test result >= 190 mg/dl

G9703 Episodes where the patient is taking antibiotics (table 1) in the 30 days prior to the episode date, or had an active prescription on the episode date

G9716 BMI is documented as being outside of normal parameters, follow-up plan is not completed for documented medical reason

G9778 Patients who have a diagnosis of pregnancy at any time during the measurement period

G9779 Patients who are breastfeeding at any time during the measurement period

G9780 Patients who have a diagnosis of rhabdomyolysis at any time during the measurement period

G9781 Documentation of medical reason(s) for not currently being a statin therapy user or receiving an order (prescription) for statin therapy (e.g., patients with statin-associated muscle symptoms or an allergy to statin medication therapy, patients who are receiving palliative or hospice care, patients with active liver disease or hepatic disease or insufficiency, and patients with end stage renal disease [ESRD])

G9782 History of or active diagnosis of familial hypercholesterolemia

G9822 Patients who had an endometrial ablation procedure during the 12 months prior to the index date (exclusive of the index date)

G9823 Endometrial sampling or hysteroscopy with biopsy and results documented during the 12 months prior to the index date (exclusive of the index date) of the endometrial ablation

G9824 Endometrial sampling or hysteroscopy with biopsy and results not documented during the 12 months prior to the index date (exclusive of the index date) of the endometrial ablation

G9868 Receipt and analysis of remote, asynchronous images for dermatologic and/or ophthalmologic evaluation, for use only in a Medicare-approved CMMI model, less than 10 minutes

G9869 Receipt and analysis of remote, asynchronous images for dermatologic and/or ophthalmologic evaluation, for use only in a Medicare-approved CMMI model, 10 to 20 minutes

G9870 Receipt and analysis of remote, asynchronous images for dermatologic and/or ophthalmologic evaluation, for use only in a Medicare-approved CMMI model, more than 20 minutes

G9906 Patient identified as a tobacco user received tobacco cessation intervention on the date of the encounter or within the previous 12 months (counseling and/or pharmacotherapy)

G9907 Documentation of medical reason(s) for not providing tobacco cessation intervention on the date of the encounter or within the previous 12 months (e.g., limited life expectancy, other medical reason)

REVISED CODES (continued)

G9908 Patient identified as tobacco user did not receive tobacco cessation intervention on the date of the encounter or within the previous 12 months (counseling and/or pharmacotherapy), reason not given

G9909 Documentation of medical reason(s) for not providing tobacco cessation intervention on the date of the encounter or within the previous 12 months if identified as a tobacco user (e.g., limited life expectancy, other medical reason)

G9927 Documentation of system reason(s) for not prescribing an FDA-approved anticoagulation due to patient being currently enrolled in a clinical trial related to AF/atrial flutter treatment

G9928 FDA-approved anticoagulant not prescribed, reason not given

J7321 Hyaluronan or derivative, Hyalgan, Supartz or Visco-3, for intra-articular injection, per dose

K1013 Enema tube, with or without adapter, any type, replacement only, each

M0243 Intravenous infusion or subcutaneous injection, casirivimab and imdevimab includes infusion or injection, and post administration monitoring

M0244 Intravenous infusion or subcutaneous injection, casirivimab and imdevimab includes infusion or injection, and post administration monitoring in the home or residence; this includes a beneficiary's home that has been made provider-based to the hospital during the COVID-19 public health emergency

DELETED CODES

A4397	C9081	C9068	C9069	C9070	C9071	C9072
C9065	C9073	C9074	C9075	C9076	C9077	C9078
C9079	C9080	C9082	C9083	C9122	C9132	C9752
C9753	G0424	G2061	G2062	G2063	G2064	G2065
G8422	G8925	G8926	G8938	G9267	G9268	G9269
G9270	G9348	G9349	G9350	G9399	G9400	G9401
G9448	G9449	G9450	G9561	G9562	G9563	G9577
G9578	G9579	G9583	G9584	G9585	G9634	G9635
G9636	G9639	G9640	G9641	G9647	G9666	G9783
J0693	J2505	J7303	J7333	J7401	J9315	K1010
K1011	K1012	M0239	M1022	M1025	M1026	M1031
Q0239	Q4228	Q4236				

Appendix 6 — Place of Service and Type of Service

Place-of-Service Codes for Professional Claims

Listed below are place of service codes and descriptions. These codes should be used on professional claims to specify the entity where service(s) were rendered. Check with individual payers (e.g., Medicare, Medicaid, other private insurance) for reimbursement policies regarding these codes. To comment on a code(s) or description(s), please send your request to posinfo@cms.gov.

01	Pharmacy	A facility or location where drugs and other medically related items and services are sold, dispensed, or otherwise provided directly to patients.
02	Telehealth Provided Other than in Patient's Home	The location where health services and health related services are provided or received, through telecommunication technology. Patient is not located in their home when receiving health services or health related services through telecommunication technology.
03	School	A facility whose primary purpose is education.
04	Homeless Shelter	A facility or location whose primary purpose is to provide temporary housing to homeless individuals (e.g., emergency shelters, individual or family shelters).
05	Indian Health Service Free-Standing Facility	A facility or location, owned and operated by the Indian Health Service, which provides diagnostic, therapeutic (surgical and nonsurgical), and rehabilitation services to American Indians and Alaska Natives who do not require hospitalization.
06	Indian Health Service Provider-based Facility	A facility or location, owned and operated by the Indian Health Service, which provides diagnostic, therapeutic (surgical and nonsurgical), and rehabilitation services rendered by, or under the supervision of, physicians to American Indians and Alaska Natives admitted as inpatients or outpatients.
07	Tribal 638 Free-Standing Facility	A facility or location owned and operated by a federally recognized American Indian or Alaska Native tribe or tribal organization under a 638 agreement, which provides diagnostic, therapeutic (surgical and nonsurgical), and rehabilitation services to tribal members who do not require hospitalization.
08	Tribal 638 Provider-based Facility	A facility or location owned and operated by a federally recognized American Indian or Alaska Native tribe or tribal organization under a 638 agreement, which provides diagnostic, therapeutic (surgical and nonsurgical), and rehabilitation services to tribal members admitted as inpatients or outpatients.
09	Prison/Correctional Facility	A prison, jail, reformatory, work farm, detention center, or any other similar facility maintained by either Federal, State or local authorities for the purpose of confinement or rehabilitation of adult or juvenile criminal offenders.
10	Telehealth Provided in Patient's Home	The location where health services and health related services are provided or received, through telecommunication technology. Patient is located in their home (which is a location other than a hospital or other facility where the patient receives care in a private residence) when receiving health services or health related services through telecommunication technology.
11	Office	Location, other than a hospital, skilled nursing facility (SNF), military treatment facility, community health center, State or local public health clinic, or intermediate care facility (ICF), where the health professional routinely provides health examinations, diagnosis, and treatment of illness or injury on an ambulatory basis.
12	Home	Location, other than a hospital or other facility, where the patient receives care in a private residence.
13	Assisted Living Facility	Congregate residential facility with self-contained living units providing assessment of each resident's needs and on-site support 24 hours a day, 7 days a week, with the capacity to deliver or arrange for services including some health care and other services.
14	Group home	A residence, with shared living areas, where clients receive supervision and other services such as social and/or behavioral services, custodial service, and minimal services (e.g., medication administration).
15	Mobile Unit	A facility/unit that moves from place-to-place equipped to provide preventive, screening, diagnostic, and/or treatment services.
16	Temporary Lodging	A short-term accommodation such as a hotel, campground, hostel, cruise ship or resort where the patient receives care, and which is not identified by any other POS code.
17	Walk-in Retail Health Clinic	A walk-in health clinic, other than an office, urgent care facility, pharmacy, or independent clinic and not described by any other place of service code, that is located within a retail operation and provides, on an ambulatory basis, preventive and primary care services.
18	Place of Employment-Worksite	A location, not described by any other POS code, owned or operated by a public or private entity where the patient is employed, and where a health professional provides on-going or episodic occupational medical, therapeutic or rehabilitative services to the individual.

19	Off Campus-Outpatient Hospital	A portion of an off-campus hospital provider based department which provides diagnostic, therapeutic (both surgical and nonsurgical), and rehabilitation services to sick or injured persons who do not require hospitalization or institutionalization.
20	Urgent Care Facility	Location, distinct from a hospital emergency room, an office, or a clinic, whose purpose is to diagnose and treat illness or injury for unscheduled, ambulatory patients seeking immediate medical attention.
21	Inpatient Hospital	A facility, other than psychiatric, which primarily provides diagnostic, therapeutic (both surgical and nonsurgical), and rehabilitation services by, or under, the supervision of physicians to patients admitted for a variety of medical conditions.
22	On Campus-Outpatient Hospital	A portion of a hospital's main campus which provides diagnostic, therapeutic (both surgical and nonsurgical), and rehabilitation services to sick or injured persons who do not require hospitalization or institutionalization.
23	Emergency Room—Hospital	A portion of a hospital where emergency diagnosis and treatment of illness or injury is provided.
24	Ambulatory Surgical Center	A freestanding facility, other than a physician's office, where surgical and diagnostic services are provided on an ambulatory basis.
25	Birthing center	A facility, other than a hospital's maternity facilities or a physician's office, which provides a setting for labor, delivery, and immediate post-partum care as well as immediate care of new born infants.
26	Military Treatment Facility	A medical facility operated by one or more of the Uniformed services. Military Treatment Facility (MTF) also refers to certain former US Public Health Service (USPHS) facilities now designated as Uniformed Service Treatment Facilities (USTF).
27-30	Unassigned	N/A
31	Skilled Nursing Facility	A facility which primarily provides inpatient skilled nursing care and related services to patients who require medical, nursing, or rehabilitative services but does not provide the level of care or treatment available in a hospital.
32	Nursing Facility	A facility which primarily provides to residents skilled nursing care and related services for the rehabilitation of injured, disabled, or sick persons, or, on a regular basis, health-related care services above the level of custodial care to individuals other than those with intellectual disabilities.
33	Custodial Care Facility	A facility which provides room, board, and other personal assistance services, generally on a long-term basis, and which does not include a medical component.
34	Hospice	A facility, other than a patient's home, in which palliative and supportive care for terminally ill patients and their families are provided.
35-40	Unassigned	N/A
41	Ambulance—Land	A land vehicle specifically designed, equipped and staffed for lifesaving and transporting the sick or injured.
42	Ambulance—Air or Water	An air or water vehicle specifically designed, equipped and staffed for lifesaving and transporting the sick or injured.
43-48	Unassigned	N/A
49	Independent Clinic	A location, not part of a hospital and not described by any other Place-of-Service code, that is organized and operated to provide preventive, diagnostic, therapeutic, rehabilitative, or palliative services to outpatients only.
50	Federally Qualified Health Center	A facility located in a medically underserved area that provides Medicare beneficiaries preventive primary medical care under the general direction of a physician.
51	Inpatient Psychiatric Facility	A facility that provides inpatient psychiatric services for the diagnosis and treatment of mental illness on a 24-hour basis, by or under the supervision of a physician.
52	Psychiatric Facility-Partial Hospitalization	A facility for the diagnosis and treatment of mental illness that provides a planned therapeutic program for patients who do not require full time hospitalization, but who need broader programs than are possible from outpatient visits to a hospital-based or hospital-affiliated facility.
53	Community Mental Health Center	A facility that provides the following services: outpatient services, including specialized outpatient services for children, the elderly, individuals who are chronically ill, and residents of the CMHC's mental health services area who have been discharged from inpatient treatment at a mental health facility; 24 hour a day emergency care services; day treatment, other partial hospitalization services, or psychosocial rehabilitation services; screening for patients being considered for admission to State mental health facilities to determine the appropriateness of such admission; and consultation and education services.
54	Intermediate Care Facility/Individuals with Intellectual Disabilities	A facility which primarily provides health-related care and services above the level of custodial care to individuals but does not provide the level of care or treatment available in a hospital or SNF.
55	Residential Substance Abuse Treatment Facility	A facility which provides treatment for substance (alcohol and drug) abuse to live-in residents who do not require acute medical care. Services include individual and group therapy and counseling, family counseling, laboratory tests, drugs and supplies, psychological testing, and room and board.
56	Psychiatric Residential Treatment Center	A facility or distinct part of a facility for psychiatric care which provides a total 24-hour therapeutically planned and professionally staffed group living and learning environment.
57	Non-residential Substance Abuse Treatment Facility	A location which provides treatment for substance (alcohol and drug) abuse on an ambulatory basis. Services include individual and group therapy and counseling, family counseling, laboratory tests, drugs and supplies, and psychological testing.

58	Non-residential Opioid Treatment Facility	A location that provides treatment for opioid use disorder on an ambulatory basis. Services include methadone and other forms of Medication Assisted Treatment (MAT).
59	Unassigned	N/A
60	Mass Immunization Center	A location where providers administer pneumococcal pneumonia and influenza virus vaccinations and submit these services as electronic media claims, paper claims, or using the roster billing method. This generally takes place in a mass immunization setting, such as, a public health center, pharmacy, or mall but may include a physician office setting.
61	Comprehensive Inpatient Rehabilitation Facility	A facility that provides comprehensive rehabilitation services under the supervision of a physician to inpatients with physical disabilities. Services include physical therapy, occupational therapy, speech pathology, social or psychological services, and orthotics and prosthetics services.
62	Comprehensive Outpatient Rehabilitation Facility	A facility that provides comprehensive rehabilitation services under the supervision of a physician to outpatients with physical disabilities. Services include physical therapy, occupational therapy, and speech pathology services.
63-64	Unassigned	N/A
65	End-Stage Renal Disease Treatment Facility	A facility other than a hospital, which provides dialysis treatment, maintenance, and/or training to patients or caregivers on an ambulatory or home-care basis.
66-70	Unassigned	N/A
71	Public Health Clinic	A facility maintained by either State or local health departments that provides ambulatory primary medical care under the general direction of a physician.
72	Rural Health Clinic	A certified facility which is located in a rural medically underserved area that provides ambulatory primary medical care under the general direction of a physician.
73-80	Unassigned	N/A
81	Independent Laboratory	A laboratory certified to perform diagnostic and/or clinical tests independent of an institution or a physician's office.
82-98	Unassigned	N/A
99	Other Place of Service	Other place of service not identified above.

Type of Service

Common Working File Type of Service (TOS) Indicators

For submitting a claim to the Common Working File (CWF), use the following table to assign the proper TOS. Some procedures may have more than one applicable TOS. CWF will reject codes with incorrect TOS designations. CWF will produce alerts on codes with incorrect TOS designations.

The only exceptions to this annual update are:

- Surgical services billed for dates of service through December 31, 2007, containing the ASC facility service modifier SG must be reported as TOS F. Effective for services on or after January 1, 2008, the SG modifier is no longer applicable for Medicare services. ASC providers should discontinue applying the SG modifier on ASC facility claims. The indicator F does not appear in the TOS table because its use depends upon claims submitted with POS 24 (ASC facility) from

an ASC (specialty 49). This became effective for dates of service January 1, 2008, or after.

- Surgical services billed with an assistant-at-surgery modifier (80-82, AS,) must be reported with TOS 8. The 8 indicator does not appear on the TOS table because its use is dependent upon the use of the appropriate modifier. (See Pub. 100-04 *Medicare Claims Processing Manual*, chapter 12, "Physician/Practitioner Billing," for instructions on when assistant-at-surgery is allowable.)

- TOS H appears in the list of descriptors. However, it does not appear in the table. In CWF, "H" is used only as an indicator for hospice. The contractor should not submit TOS H to CWF at this time.

- For outpatient services, when a transfusion medicine code appears on a claim that also contains a blood product, the service is paid under reasonable charge at 80 percent; coinsurance and deductible apply. When transfusion medicine codes are paid under the clinical laboratory fee schedule they are paid at 100 percent; coinsurance and deductible do not apply.

Note: For injection codes with more than one possible TOS designation, use the following guidelines when assigning the TOS:

When the choice is L or 1:

- Use TOS L when the drug is used related to ESRD; or
- Use TOS 1 when the drug is not related to ESRD and is administered in the office.

When the choice is G or 1:

- Use TOS G when the drug is an immunosuppressive drug; or
- Use TOS 1 when the drug is used for other than immunosuppression.

When the choice is P or 1:

- Use TOS P if the drug is administered through durable medical equipment (DME); or
- Use TOS 1 if the drug is administered in the office.

The place of service or diagnosis may be considered when determining the appropriate TOS. The descriptors for each of the TOS codes listed in the annual HCPCS update are:

0	Whole blood
1	Medical care
2	Surgery
3	Consultation
4	Diagnostic radiology
5	Diagnostic laboratory
6	Therapeutic radiology
7	Anesthesia
8	Assistant at surgery
9	Other medical items or services
A	Used durable medical equipment (DME)
D	Ambulance
E	Enteral/parenteral nutrients/supplies
F	Ambulatory surgical center (facility usage for surgical services)
G	Immunosuppressive drugs
J	Diabetic shoes
K	Hearing items and services
L	ESRD supplies
M	Monthly capitation payment for dialysis
N	Kidney donor
P	Lump sum purchase of DME, prosthetics, orthotics
Q	Vision items or services
R	Rental of DME
S	Surgical dressings or other medical supplies
T	Outpatient mental health limitation
U	Occupational therapy
V	Pneumococcal/flu vaccine
W	Physical therapy

Appendix 7 — Deleted Code Crosswalk

Code	Cross Reference
C9081	To report, see ~Q2055
C9082	To report, see ~J9272
C9083	To report, see ~J9061
C9752	To report, see ~64628
C9753	To report, see ~64629

Appendix 8 — Glossary

accession. Process of identifying a specimen and entering a unique specimen identifier into laboratory records.

alveoplasty. Procedure in which the physician alters the contours of the alveolus by removing sharp areas or undercuts of alveolar bone.

angiography. Radiographic imaging of the arteries. Imaging may be performed to study the vasculature of any given organ, body system, or area of circulation such as the brain, heart, chest, kidneys, limbs, gastrointestinal tract, aorta, and pulmonary circulation to visualize the formation and the function of the blood vessels to detect problems such as a blockage or stricture. A catheter is inserted through an accessible blood vessel and the artery is injected with a radiopaque contrast material after which x-rays are taken.

apnea. Absence of breathing or breath.

apnea monitor. Device used to monitor breathing during sleep that sounds an alarm if breathing stops for more than the specified amount of time.

aqueous shunt. Silicone tube inserted into the anterior chamber of the eye and connected to a reservoir plate behind the pars plana to enhance drainage in the eye's anterior chamber and improve aqueous flow.

ballistocardiogram. Graphic recording of the movements of the body caused by cardiac contractions and blood flow, used to evaluate cardiac function.

BMI. Body mass index. Tool for calculating weight appropriateness in adults. The Centers for Disease Control and Prevention places adult BMIs in the following categories: below 18.5, underweight; 18.5 to 24.9, normal; 25.0 to 29.9 overweight; 30.0 and above, obese. BMI may be a factor in determining medical necessity for bariatric procedures.

brace. Orthotic device that supports, in correct position, any moveable body part, and allows for limited movement. Medicare has a strict definition of a brace that includes only rigid or semirigid devices.

brachytherapy. Form of radiation therapy in which radioactive pellets or seeds are implanted directly into the tissue being treated to deliver their dose of radiation in a more directed fashion. Brachytherapy provides radiation to the prescribed body area while minimizing exposure to normal tissue.

cardiointegram. Experimental, noninvasive analysis of electrical signals of the heart. Cardiointegram converts analog EKG signals to digital and performs a computer analysis that considers the time element.

cardiokymography. Noninvasive test that measures left anterior ventricle segmental wall motion.

cardioverter-defibrillator. Device that uses both low energy cardioversion or defibrillating shocks and antitachycardia pacing to treat ventricular tachycardia or ventricular fibrillation.

cast. *1)* Rigid encasement or dressing molded to the body from a substance that hardens upon drying to hold a body part immobile during the healing period; a model or reproduction made from an impression or mold. Generally, the supply of a cast is included in the codes describing the reduction. *2)* In dentistry and some other specialties, model or reproduction made from taking an impression or mold.

catheter. Flexible tube inserted into an area of the body for introducing or withdrawing fluid.

cervical cap. Contraceptive device similar in form and function to the diaphragm but that can be left in place for 48 hours.

chemotherapy. Treatment of disease, especially cancerous conditions, using chemical agents.

CMS. Centers for Medicare and Medicaid Services. Federal agency that administers the public health programs.

CMV. *1)* Controlled mechanical ventilation. *2)* Cytomegalovirus.

collagen. Protein based substance of strength and flexibility that is the major component of connective tissue, found in cartilage, bone, tendons, and skin.

colorectal cancer screening test. One of the following procedures performed for the purpose of detecting colorectal cancer: screening barium enema, screening fecal-occult blood test, screening flexible sigmoidoscopy, screening colonography, and screening colonoscopy.

compression sleeve. Fitted wrap that accelerates recovery in patients with vein disease, lymphedema, or diabetes. Compression sleeves increase circulation and decrease swelling and fluid buildup following surgery.

contrast material. Radiopaque substance placed into the body to enable a system or body structure to be visualized, such as nonionic and low osmolar contrast media (LOCM), ionic and high osmolar contrast media (HOCM), barium, and gadolinium.

covered osteoporosis drug. Injectable drug approved for treating post-menopausal osteoporosis provided to an individual that has suffered a bone fracture related to post-menopausal osteoporosis.

dermis. Skin layer found under the epidermis that contains a papillary upper layer and the deep reticular layer of collagen, vascular bed, and nerves.

dermis graft. Skin graft that has been separated from the epidermal tissue and the underlying subcutaneous fat, used primarily as a substitute for fascia grafts in plastic surgery.

dialysis. Artificial filtering of the blood to remove contaminating waste elements and restore normal balance.

disarticulation. Removal of a limb through a joint.

diskectomy. Surgical excision of an intervertebral disk.

DME MAC. Durable medical equipment Medicare administrative contractor. Entity where claims for specific DMEPOS must be submitted for processing and reimbursement.

DME PDAC. Durable Medical Equipment Pricing Data Analysis and Coding. Medicare contractor responsible for maintaining the durable medical equipment classification system (DMECS), including HCPCS coding determinations, and providing durable medical equipment, prosthetics, orthotics, and supplies (DMEPOS) allowables.

drug eluting stent. Specialized device placed inside blood vessels for intraluminal support that is coated with a controlled time-release drug that enters the surrounding tissue and helps prevent or slow the growth of plaque or stenotic tissue.

drug formulary. List of prescription medications preferred for use by a health plan and dispensed through participating pharmacies to covered persons.

drugs and biologicals. Drugs and biologicals included - or approved for inclusion - in the United States Pharmacopoeia, the National Formulary, the United States Homeopathic Pharmacopoeia, in New Drugs or Accepted Dental Remedies, or approved by the pharmacy and drug therapeutics committee of the medical staff of the hospital. Also included are medically accepted and FDA approved drugs used in an anticancer chemotherapeutic regimen. The carrier determines medical acceptance based on supportive clinical evidence.

dual-lead device. Implantable cardiac device (pacemaker or implantable cardioverter-defibrillator [ICD]) in which pacing and sensing components are placed in only two chambers of the heart.

durable medical equipment. Medical equipment that can withstand repeated use, is not disposable, is used to serve a medical purpose, is generally not useful to a person in the absence of a sickness or injury, and is appropriate for use in the home. Examples of durable medical equipment include hospital beds, wheelchairs, and oxygen equipment.

Dx. Diagnosis.

electrocardiogram. Recording of the electrical activity of the heart on a moving strip of paper that detects and records the electrical potential of the heart during contraction.

electroencephalography. Testing involving amplification, recording, and analysis of the electrical activity of the brain.

electromyography. Test that measures muscle response to nerve stimulation determining if muscle weakness is present and if it is related to the muscles themselves or a problem with the nerves that supply the muscles.

enteral. Pertaining to the intestines; enteral is often used in the context of nutrition management: formulas, jejunostomy tubes, nasogastric devices, etc.

epidermis. Outermost, nonvascular layer of skin that contains four to five differentiated layers depending on its body location: stratum corneum, lucidum, granulosum, spinosum, and basale.

EPO. *1)* Epoetin alpha. *2)* Exclusive provider organization. In health care contracting, an organization similar to an HMO, but the member must remain within the provider network to receive benefits. EPOs are regulated under insurance statutes rather than HMO legislation.

ESRD. End stage renal disease. Progression of chronic renal failure to lasting and irreparable kidney damage that requires dialysis or renal transplant for survival.

EVAR. Endovascular aortic repair. Deployment of a prosthetic stent via a catheter into the site of an abdominal aortic aneurysm (AAA). The stent provides a safe conduit for blood flow to relieve pressure on the aneurysm as the blood flows through the stent instead of continuing to bulge the sac formed by the aorta wall dilation.

event recorder. Portable, ambulatory heart monitor worn by the patient that makes electrocardiographic recordings of the length and frequency of aberrant cardiac rhythm to help diagnose heart conditions and to assess pacemaker functioning or programming.

Food and Drug Administration (FDA). Federal agency responsible for protecting public health by substantiating the safety, efficacy, and security of human and veterinary drugs, biological products, medical devices, national food supply, cosmetics, and items that give off radiation.

FOTO. Focus on therapeutic outcomes.

gait. Manner in which a person walks.

gene. Basic unit of heredity that contains nucleic acid. Genes are arranged in different and unique sequences or strings that determine the gene's function. Human genes usually include multiple protein coding regions such as exons separated by introns which are nonprotein coding sections.

genetic test. Test that is able to detect a gene mutation, either inherited or caused by the environment.

gingivoplasty. Repair or reconstruction of the gum tissue, altering the gingival contours by excising areas of gum tissue or making incisions through the gingiva to create a gingival flap.

glaucoma. Rise in intraocular pressure, restricting blood flow and decreasing vision.

habilitative services. Procedures or services provided to assist a patient in learning, keeping, and improving new skills needed to perform daily living activities. Habilitative services assist patients in acquiring a skill for the first time.

halo. Tool for stabilizing the head and spine.

health care provider. Entity that administers diagnostic and therapeutic services.

hemodialysis. Cleansing of wastes and contaminating elements from the blood by virtue of different diffusion rates through a semipermeable membrane, which separates blood from a filtration solution that diffuses other elements out of the blood.

home health services. Services furnished to patients in their homes under the care of physicians. These services include part-time or intermittent skilled nursing care, physical therapy, medical social services, medical supplies, and some rehabilitation equipment. Home health supplies and services must be prescribed by a physician, and the beneficiary must be confined at home in order for Medicare to pay the benefits in full.

hospice. Organization that furnishes inpatient, outpatient, and home health care for the terminally ill. Hospices emphasize support and counseling services for terminally ill people and their families, pain relief, and symptom management. When the Medicare beneficiary chooses hospice benefits, all other Medicare benefits are discontinued, except physician services and treatment of conditions not related to the terminal illness.

hypertrophic. Enlarged or overgrown from an increase in cell size of the affected tissue.

implant. Material or device inserted or placed within the body for therapeutic, reconstructive, or diagnostic purposes.

implantable cardioverter-defibrillator. Implantable electronic cardiac device used to control rhythm abnormalities such as tachycardia, fibrillation, or bradycardia by producing high- or low-energy stimulation and pacemaker functions. It may also have the capability to provide the functions of an implantable loop recorder or implantable cardiovascular monitor.

in situ. Located in the natural position or contained within the origin site, not spread into neighboring tissue.

incontinence. Inability to control urination or defecation.

infusion. Introduction of a therapeutic fluid, other than blood, into the bloodstream.

infusion pump. Device that delivers a measured amount of drug or intravenous solution through injection over a period of time.

intra-arterial. Within an artery or arteries.

intramuscular. Within a muscle.

intraocular lens. Artificial lens implanted into the eye to replace a damaged natural lens or cataract.

intravenous. Within a vein or veins.

introducer. Instrument, such as a catheter, needle, or tube, through which another instrument or device is introduced into the body.

keratoprosthesis. Surgical procedure in which the physician creates a new anterior chamber with a plastic optical implant to replace a severely damaged cornea that cannot be repaired.

LDS. Lipodystrophy syndrome. Syndrome which involves the partial or total absence of fat and/or the abnormal deposition and distribution of fat in the body due to a disturbance of the lipid metabolism.

magnetic resonance angiography. Diagnostic technique utilizing magnetic fields and radio waves rather than radiation to produce detailed, cross-sectional images of internal body structures.

multiple-lead device. Implantable cardiac device (pacemaker or implantable cardioverter-defibrillator [ICD]) in which pacing and sensing components are placed in at least three chambers of the heart.

mutation. Alteration in gene function that results in changes to a gene or chromosome. Can cause deficits or disease that can be inherited, can have beneficial effects, or result in no noticeable change.

nasogastric tube. Long, hollow, cylindrical catheter made of soft rubber or plastic that is inserted through the nose down into the stomach, and is used for feeding, instilling medication, or withdrawing gastric contents.

nebulizer. Latin for mist, a device that converts liquid into a fine spray and is commonly used to deliver medicine to the upper respiratory, bronchial, and lung areas.

negative pressure dressing. Adjunctive therapy used to speed wound healing in skin grafts or large wounds. It has been shown to increase blood flow, decrease bacterial count, and increase formation of granulation tissues. A foam pad is placed on the defect and covered with an occlusive drape. A small tube that is non-collapsible is placed into the foam and attached to a disposable pump that provides negative pressure up to -125 mmHg.

NMES. Neuromuscular electrical stimulation. Technology that uses percutaneous stimulation to deliver electrical impulses for muscle flexion to trigger action. NMES can, in some cases, create an ability to ambulate among paraplegic patients.

obturator. Prosthesis used to close an acquired or congenital opening in the palate that aids in speech and chewing.

occult blood test. Chemical or microscopic test to determine the presence of blood in a specimen.

occupational therapy. Training, education, and assistance intended to assist a person who is recovering from a serious illness or injury perform the activities of daily life.

ocular implant. Implant inside muscular cone.

omnicardiogram. Method of mathematically interpreting the usual linear form of the electrocardiogram in a different, roughly circular shape. This interpretation is then compared to a normal template and an analysis is performed on two randomly selected cycles from leads I, II, V4, V, and/or V6.

oral. Pertaining to the mouth.

ordering physician. Physician who orders nonphysician services (e.g., laboratory services, pharmaceutical services, imaging services, or durable medical equipment) for a patient.

orphan drugs. Drugs that treat diseases that affect fewer than 200,000 people in the United States, as designated by the FDA. Orphan drugs follow a varied process from other drugs regulated by the FDA.

orthosis. Derived from a Greek word meaning "to make straight," it is an artificial appliance that supports, aligns, or corrects an anatomical deformity or improves the use of a moveable body part. Unlike a prosthesis, an orthotic device is always functional in nature.

orthotic. Associated with the making and fitting of an orthosis(es).

osteo-. Having to do with bone.

osteogenesis stimulator. Device used to stimulate the growth of bone by electrical impulses or ultrasound.

ostomy. Artificial (surgical) opening in the body used for drainage or for delivery of medications or nutrients.

pacemaker. Implantable cardiac device that controls the heart's rhythm and maintains regular beats by artificial electric discharges. This device consists of the pulse generator with a battery and the electrodes, or leads, which are placed in single or dual chambers of the heart, usually transvenously.

parenteral. Other than the alimentary canal and is usually used in a method of delivery context: total parenteral nutrition (TPN) and parenteral nutrition therapy (PNT) formulas, kits, and devices.

parenteral nutrition. Nutrients provided subcutaneously, intravenously, intramuscularly, or intradermally for patients during the postoperative period and in other conditions, such as shock, coma, and renal failure.

partial hospitalization. Situation in which the patient only stays part of each day over a long period. Cardiac, rehabilitation, and chronic pain patients, for example, could use this service.

passive mobilization. Pressure, movement, or pulling of a limb or body part utilizing an apparatus or device.

periradicular. Surrounding part of the tooth's root.

peritoneal. Space between the lining of the abdominal wall, or parietal peritoneum, and the surface layer of the abdominal organs, or visceral peritoneum. It contains a thin, watery fluid that keeps the peritoneal surfaces moist.

peritoneal dialysis. Dialysis that filters waste from blood inside the body using the peritoneum, the natural lining of the abdomen, as the semipermeable membrane across which ultrafiltration is accomplished. A special catheter is inserted into the abdomen and a dialysis solution is drained into the abdomen. This solution extracts fluids and wastes, which are then discarded when the fluid is drained. Various forms of peritoneal dialysis include CAPD, CCPD, and NIDP.

peritoneal effusion. Persistent escape of fluid within the peritoneal cavity.

pessary. Device placed in the vagina to support and reposition a prolapsing or retropositioned uterus, rectum, or vagina.

photocoagulation. Application of an intense laser beam of light to disrupt tissue and condense protein material to a residual mass, used especially for treating ocular conditions.

physician. Legally authorized practitioners including a doctor of medicine or osteopathy, a doctor of dental surgery or of dental medicine, a doctor of podiatric medicine, a doctor of optometry, and a chiropractor only with respect to treatment by means of manual manipulation of the spine (to correct a subluxation).

PICC. Peripherally inserted central catheter. PICC is inserted into one of the large veins of the arm and threaded through the vein until the tip sits in a large vein just above the heart.

prehensile. Ability to grasp, seize, or hold.

prodrug. Inactive drug that goes through a metabolic process when given resulting in a chemical conversion that changes the drug into an active pharmacological agent.

prophylaxis. Intervention or protective therapy intended to prevent a disease.

prostate cancer screening tests. Test that consists of any (or all) of the procedures provided for the early detection of prostate cancer to a man 50 years of age or older who has not had a test during the preceding year. The procedures are as follows: A digital rectal examination; A prostate-specific antigen blood test. After 2002, the list of procedures may be expanded as appropriate for the early detection of prostate cancer, taking into account changes in technology and standards of medical practice, availability, effectiveness, costs, and other factors.

prosthetic. Device that replaces all or part of an internal body organ or body part, or that replaces part of the function of a permanently inoperable or malfunctioning internal body organ or body part.

pulse generator. Component of a pacemaker or an implantable cardioverter defibrillator that contains the battery and the electronics for producing the electrical discharge sent to the heart to control cardiac rhythm. Insertion or replacement of the pulse generator may be done alone, not in conjunction with insertion or replacement of the entire pacemaker system.

rehabilitation services. Therapy services provided primarily for assisting in a rehabilitation program of evaluation and service including cardiac rehabilitation, medical social services, occupational therapy, physical therapy, respiratory therapy, skilled nursing, speech therapy, psychiatric rehabilitation, and alcohol and substance abuse rehabilitation.

residual limb. Portion of an arm or leg that remains attached to the body after an amputation.

screening mammography. Radiologic images taken of the female breast for the early detection of breast cancer.

screening pap smear. Diagnostic laboratory test consisting of a routine exfoliative cytology test (Papanicolaou test) provided to a woman for the early detection of cervical or vaginal cancer. The exam includes a clinical breast examination and a physician's interpretation of the results.

sialodochoplasty. Surgical repair of a salivary gland duct.

single-lead device. Implantable cardiac device (pacemaker or implantable cardioverter-defibrillator [ICD]) in which pacing and sensing components are placed in only one chamber of the heart.

skin substitute. Non-autologous human or non-human skin that forms a base for skin growth, often considered a graft dressing.

speech prosthetic. Electronic speech aid device for patient who has had a laryngectomy. One operates by placing a vibrating head against the throat; the other amplifies sound waves through a tube which is inserted into the user's mouth.

splint. Brace or support. *1)* dynamic splint: brace that permits movement of an anatomical structure such as a hand, wrist, foot, or other part of the body after surgery or injury. *2)* static splint: brace that prevents movement and maintains support and position for an anatomical structure after surgery or injury.

stent. Tube to provide support in a body cavity or lumen.

stereotactic radiosurgery. Delivery of externally-generated ionizing radiation to specific targets for destruction or inactivation. Most often utilized in the treatment of brain or spinal tumors, high-resolution stereotactic imaging is used to identify the target and then deliver the treatment. Computer-assisted planning may also be employed. Simple and complex cranial lesions and spinal lesions are typically treated in a single planning and treatment session, although a maximum of five sessions may be required. No incision is made for stereotactic radiosurgery procedures.

subcutaneous. Below the skin.

TENS. Transcutaneous electrical nerve stimulator. TENS is applied by placing electrode pads over the area to be stimulated and connecting the electrodes to a transmitter box, which sends a current through the skin to sensory nerve fibers to help decrease pain in that nerve distribution.

terminal device. Addition to an upper limb prosthesis that replaces the function and/or appearance of a missing hand.

tracheostomy. Formation of a tracheal opening on the neck surface with tube insertion to allow for respiration in cases of obstruction or decreased patency. A tracheostomy may be planned or performed on an emergency basis for temporary or long-term use.

traction. Drawing out or holding tension on an area by applying a direct therapeutic pulling force.

transcutaneous electrical nerve stimulator. Device that delivers a controlled amount of electricity to an area of the body to stimulate healing and/or to mitigate post-surgical or post-traumatic pain.

transesophageal echocardiography. Guidance of a small probe into the esophagus under sedation to closely evaluate the heart and blood vessels within the chest.

type A emergency department. Emergency department licensed and advertised to be available to provide emergent care 24 hours a day, seven days a week. Type A emergency departments must meet both the CPT book definition of an emergency department and the EMTALA definition of a dedicated emergency department.

type B emergency department. Emergency department licensed and advertised to provide emergent care less than 24 hours a day, seven days a week. Type B emergency departments must meet the EMTALA definition of a dedicated emergency department.

vascular closure device. vascular closure devices seal femoral artery punctures caused by invasive or interventional procedures. The closure or seal is achieved by percutaneous delivery of the device's two primary structures, which are usually an anchor and a suture, clip or biologic substance (e.g., collagen, bioabsorbable polymer) or suture through the tissue tract.

Appendix 9 — Quality Payment Program

In 2015, Congress passed the Medicare Access and CHIP Reauthorization Act (MACRA), which included sweeping changes for practitioners who provide services reimbursed under the Medicare physician fee schedule (MPFS). The act focused on repealing the faulty Medicare sustainable growth rate, focusing on quality of patient outcomes, and controlling Medicare spending.

A MACRA final rule in October 2016 established the Quality Payment Program (QPP), which was effective January 1, 2017. This value-based payment model rewards eligible clinicians (ECs) who provide high-quality care and reduce the payments for those who fail to meet specific performance standards.

ECs can receive incentives under the QPP. Once the performance threshold is established, all ECs who score above that threshold are eligible to receive a positive payment adjustment. Keep in mind that the key requirement is that an EC **submit data** to avoid the negative payment adjustment and receive the incentives. The Centers for Medicare and Medicaid Services (CMS) has redesigned the scoring so that clinicians are able to know how well they are doing in the program, as benchmarks are known in advance of participating.

The QPP consists of two tracks that clinicians may choose from based on their practice size, location, specialty, or patient population:

- The merit-based incentive payment system (MIPS)

- Alternative payment models (APMs)

The 2017 QPP final rule established regulations for MIPS and APMs as well as related policies applicable to eligible clinicians who participate in the Shared Savings Program. These policies included requirements for Shared Savings Program accountable care organizations (ACOs) regarding reporting for the MIPS Quality performance category and a policy that gave ACOs full credit for the MIPS Improvement Activities performance category based on their participation in the Shared Savings Program. Since that time, revisions and modifications have been made to allow more focus on measurement efforts and to reduce barriers to entry into advanced APMs. Refinements will continue in order to reduce reporting burden and focus on patient outcomes.

MIPS provides specified performance categories under which payment adjustments may be earned for Part B covered professional services. Eligible clinicians can obtain a composite performance score (CPS) of up to 100 points from these weighted performance categories, which focus on patient care quality and cost, improvements in patient engagement and clinical care processes, and use of certified electronic health record technology (CEHRT). This performance score then defines the payment adjustments in the second calendar year after the year the score is obtained. For instance, the score obtained for the 2020 performance year is linked to payment for Medicare Part B services in 2022.

ECs currently have three available reporting frameworks, depending on individual needs and eligibility—traditional MIPS, MIPS Value Pathways (MVPs), and the alternative payment model (APM) performance pathway (APP). The majority of the proposed updates for CY 2022 focus on MIPS.

Traditional MIPS currently consists of the following performance categories:

- Quality

- Improvement Activities

- Promoting Interoperability (PI)

- Cost

MVPs, which were added as a result of complaints by some physicians of confusing quality measures, allow clinicians to report only on those measures that apply to their specialty. The CY 2022 proposed rule includes seven MVPs for the 2023 performance year related to the following clinical areas: anesthesia, chronic disease management, emergency medicine, heart disease, lower extremity joint repair, rheumatology, and stroke care and prevention. Additional MVPs will gradually be implemented for more specialties and subspecialties that participate in the program.

The APP is intended for MIPS-eligible ECs who also participate in MIPS APMs. Performance is measured across three areas (Quality, Improvement Activities, and Promoting Interoperability) in this reporting and scoring pathway, which aims to decrease reporting burden, encourage APM participation, and create new opportunities for scoring for existing MIPS APM participants. For performance year 2021, the APP Quality performance category accounted for 50 percent of the MIPS final score; the PI performance category weight was 30 percent; and the Improvement Activities performance category weight was 20 percent.

Proposed 2022/2023 Changes

As noted earlier, the majority of the proposed updates for CY 2022 focus on MIPS. In addition to the seven MVPs proposed for the 2023 performance year, other proposals in the CY 2022 proposed rule include:

- Additions to the MVP development criteria beginning with the 2022 performance year/2024 payment year related to relevant outcome measures, high-priority measures, outcomes-based administrative claims measures, and a qualified clinical data registry (QCDR) measure

- Timelines for transitioning to MVPs and for participant registration

- Establishment of subgroup reporting to provide more granular and comprehensive information that will be more clinically meaningful. Subgroup reporting is proposed to be limited to only those clinicians reporting through MVPs or APP

- MVP scoring policies by performance category and updating of the scoring hierarchy to include subgroups

- Revision of the definition of an MIPS-eligible clinician to include certified nurse midwives and clinical social workers

- Revision of the performance threshold

- Revisions and updates to the existing performance categories included in the traditional MIPS framework

- Proposals specific to the transition timeframe of accountable care organizations (ACOs) for reporting specific quality measures

Additionally, a request for public comments was made regarding an incremental timeline to transition to mandatory MVP reporting that will coincide with the sunset of traditional MIPS. The timeline currently being considered is the end of the CY 2027 performance period/2029 MIPS payment year, although this is not an official proposal at this time.

Detailed information regarding the Quality Payment Program may be found at https://qpp.cms.gov/. This website will also announce the final CMS determinations of advanced APMs and MIPS APMs for the 2022 performance period.